TRANSITION SERIES TOPICS FOR THE ADVANCED EMT

TRANSITION SERIES TOPICS FOR THE ADVANCED EMT

JOSEPH J. MISTOVICH, MED, NREMT-P
CHAIRPERSON, DEPARTMENT OF HEALTH PROFESSIONS
PROFESSOR OF HEALTH PROFESSIONS, YOUNGSTOWN STATE UNIVERSITY, YOUNGSTOWN, OHIO

DANIEL LIMMER, AS, EMT-P
EMS EDUCATOR, KENNEBUNKPORT, MAINE
PARAMEDIC, KENNEBUNKPORT EMS, KENNEBUNKPORT, MAINE

MEDICAL EDITOR

HOWARD A. WERMAN, MD, FACEP
PROFESSOR OF EMERGENCY MEDICINE, THE OHIO STATE UNIVERSITY COLLEGE OF MEDICINE, COLUMBUS, OHIO

Brady
is an imprint of

Pearson
Boston   Columbus   Indianapolis   New York   San Francisco   Upper Saddle River
Amsterdam   Cape Town   Dubai   London   Madrid   Milan Munich   Paris   Montreal   Toronto
Delhi   Mexico City   Sao Paulo   Sydney   Hong Kong   Seoul   Singapore   Taipei   Tokyo

Library of Congress Cataloging-in-Publication Data

Mistovich, Joseph J.
  Topics for the advanced EMT / Joseph J. Mistovich, Daniel Limmer ; medical editor, Howard A. Werman.
    p. ; cm. — (Transition series)
  Includes bibliographical references and index.
  ISBN-13: 978-0-13-708248-3
  ISBN-10: 0-13-708248-7
  I. Limmer, Daniel. II. Werman, Howard A. III. Title. IV. Series: Transitions series (Pearson Education, Inc.)
  [DNLM: 1. Emergency Treatment—methods—Problems and Exercises. 2. Emergency Medical Services—methods—Problems and Exercises. 3. Emergency Medical Technicians—Problems and Exercises. WB 18.2]

362.18—dc23   2011043724

Publisher: Julie Levin Alexander
Publisher's Assistant: Regina Bruno
Editor-in-Chief: Marlene McHugh Pratt
Acquisitions Editor: Sladjana Repic
Senior Managing Editor for Development:
  Lois Berlowitz
Project Manager: Deborah Wenger
Assistant Editor: Jonathan Cheung
Director of Marketing: David Gesell
Executive Marketing Manager: Derril Trakalo
Marketing Manager: Brian Hoehl
Marketing Specialist: Michael Sirinides
Marketing Assistant: Crystal Gonzalez

Managing Editor for Production: Patrick Walsh
Production Liaison: Patricia Gutierrez
Production Editor: Renata Butera
Manufacturing Manager: Alan Fischer
Editorial Media Manager: Amy Peltier
Media Project Manager: Lorena Cerisano
Art Director: Maria Guglielmo
Cover Design: Ilze Lemesis
Cover Image: Daniel Limmer
Interior Design: Ilze Lemesis
Composition: Aptara®, Inc.
Printer/Binder: R.R. Donnelley / Roanoke
Cover Printer: Lehigh-Phoenix Color

Photo Credits: Daniel Limmer, pp. 1, 7, 8, 9, 10, 72, 86, 91, 93, 98, 101, 102, 104, 141, 187; Vidacare Corporation, p. 386; Chad Johnson/Masterfile Corporation, p. 58; © Ken Kerr, pp. 80, 175; © Michal Heron, p. 115; Bryan E. Bledsoe, pp. 127, 250; © Edward T. Dickinson, MD, p. 134; © Charles Stewart, MD, Charles Stewart & Associates, p. 134; Dr. E. Walker / Photo Researchers, Inc., p. 166; Photo Researchers, Inc., p. 218; © Mark C. Ide, pp. 295, 348; © Ray Kemp/911 Imaging, p. 348; © Scott Metcalfe, pp. 360, 368; © Carl Leet, p. 380; Pearson Education, pp. 5, 10, 11, 14, 15, 29, 56, 60, 65, 77, 79, 80, 94, 95, 96, 97, 115, 121, 123, 128, 142, 144, 158, 160, 161, 172, 183, 185, 186, 187, 217, 229, 234, 235, 249, 250, 251, 265, 266, 270, 271, 295, 301, 323, 329, 330, 339, 344, 354, 367, 368; Richard Logan/Pearson Education/PH College, pp. 11, 19, 85, 187; Monkey Business Images/Shutterstock, p. 59; Pearson Education/PH College, p. 71; Pearson Education PH Chet, p. 71; Carl Leet/Pearson Education PH Chet, pp. 72, 276; Daniel Mihailescu / AFP/Daniel Limmer, p. 86; Carl Leet, YSU/Pearson Education, p. 72; Michal Heron/Pearson Education/PH College, pp. 59, 115; MorTan, Inc., p. 228; © Reprinted by permission of Nellcor Puritan Bennett LLC, Pleasanton, CA, p. 359; Floyd E. Jackson/Pearson Education/PH College, p. 366; Nathan Eldridge/Pearson Education/PH College, p. 367; Nathan Eldridge/Pearson Education, p. 195

Many of the designations by manufacturers and sellers to distinguish their products are claimed as trademarks. Where those designations appear in this book, and the publisher was aware of a trademark claim, the symbols® or ™ will appear at the first mention of the product.

Notice on Care Procedures: The author and the publisher of this book have taken care to make certain that the information given is correct and compatible with the standards generally accepted at the time of publication. Nevertheless, as new information becomes available, changes in treatment and in the use of equipment and procedures become necessary. The reader is advised to carefully consult the instruction and information material included with each piece of equipment or device before administration. Students are warned that the use of any techniques must be authorized by their medical adviser, where appropriate, in accord with local laws and regulations. The publisher disclaims any liability, loss, injury, or damage incurred as a consequence, directly or indirectly, of the use and application of any of the contents of this book.

Notice on Gender Usage: The English language has historically given preference to the male gender. Among many words, the pronouns "he" and "his" are commonly used to describe both genders. Society evolves faster than language, and the male pronouns still predominate in our speech. The authors have made great effort to treat the two genders equally, recognizing that a significant percentage of EMTs are female. However, in some instances, male pronouns may be used to describe both males and females solely for the purpose of brevity. This is not intended to offend any readers of the female gender.

Brady
is an imprint of

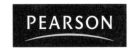

10 9 8 7 6 5 4 3 2 1

ISBN 13: 978-0-13-708248-3
ISBN 10:   0-13-708248-7

DEDICATION

To my best friend and beautiful wife, Andrea, for her unconditional love and inspiration to pursue my dreams. To my daughters Katie, Kristyn, Chelsea, Morgan, and Kara, who are my never-ending sources of love, laughter, and adventure and remind me why life is so precious. I love you all!

In memory of my father, Paul, who was a continuous source of encouragement and the epitome of perseverance. I have come to realize that he is my hero.

JJM

To Stephanie, Sarah, and Margo. A man is truly fortunate to be surrounded by such beauty, intelligence, and love. You are each amazing and wonderful—the foundation for all that I am.

DL

CONTENTS

Acknowledgments   xi

About the Authors   xiii

Transition to the National EMS Education Standards   xv

Instructor Resources   xxi

Preparatory   1

1   Research and EMS   1

2   Workforce Safety and Wellness   7

3   Therapeutic Communication   13

4   Legal Issues in EMS   18

Anatomy and Physiology   24

5   Anatomy and Physiology: Cellular Metabolism   24

Medical Terminology   29

6   Medical Terminology   29

Pathophysiology   35

7   Ambient Air, Airway, and Mechanics of Ventilation   35

8   Regulation of Ventilation, Ventilation/Perfusion Ratio, and Transport of Gases   41

9   Blood, Cardiac Function, and Vascular System   48

Life Span Development   56

10   Life Span Development   56

Public Health   62

11   Public Health and EMS   62

Principles of Pharmacology   67

12   EMS Pharmacology   67

Airway Management, Respiration, and Artificial Ventilation   75

13   Issues in Airway Management, Oxygenation, and Ventilation   75

Patient Assessment   83

14   Critical Thinking   83

15   Assessment of the Trauma Patient   90

16   Assessment of the Medical Patient   100

Medicine   106

17   Neurology: Altered Mental Status   106

18   Neurology: Stroke   111

19 Neurology: Seizures   119

20 Abdominal Emergencies and Gastrointestinal Bleeding   125

21 Immunology: Anaphylactic and Anaphylactoid Reactions   131

22 Infectious Disease   139

23 Endocrine Emergencies: Diabetes Mellitus and Hypoglycemia   147

24 Endocrine Emergencies: Hyperglycemic Disorders   152

25 Psychiatric Disorders   158

26 Cardiovascular Emergencies: Chest Pain and Acute Coronary Syndrome   164

27 Cardiovascular Emergencies: Congestive Heart Failure   171

28 Cardiovascular Emergencies: Hypertensive and Vascular Emergencies   177

29 Toxicology: Street Drugs   183

30 Respiratory Emergencies: Airway Resistance Disorders   190

31 Respiratory Emergencies: Lung and Gas Exchange Disorders   198

32 Respiratory Emergencies: Infectious Disorders   206

33 Hematology: Blood Disorders   212

34 Renal Disorders   217

35 Gynecologic Emergencies   221

36 Emergencies Involving the Eyes, Ears, Nose, and Throat   226

Shock and Resuscitation   231

37 Issues in Cardiac Arrest and Resuscitation   231

38 Shock   238

Trauma   248

39 Bleeding and Bleeding Control   248

40 Chest Trauma   253

41 Abdominal Trauma   262

42 Soft Tissue Injuries: Crush Injury and Compartment Syndrome   269

43 Head and Traumatic Brain Injury   273

44 Complete and Incomplete Spine and Spinal Cord Injuries   280

45 Trauma in Special Populations: Pediatrics   287

46 Trauma in Special Populations: Geriatrics   294

47 Trauma in Special Populations: Pregnancy   301

48 Diving Emergencies: Decompression Sickness and Arterial Embolism   305

Special Patient Populations   309

49 Obstetrics (Antepartum Complications)   309

50 Neonatology   315

51 Pediatrics   322

52 Geriatrics   328

53 Special Challenges   338

54 Bariatric Emergencies   346

EMS Operations   353

55   Multiple-Casualty Incidents and Incident Management   353

56   Advanced Skills for the AEMT   358

57   Additional Pharmacology for the AEMT   371

58   ECG Monitoring and Cardiac Dysrhythmias   378

Index   393

ACKNOWLEDGMENTS

Contributors

Thanks to the following people for their contributions to *Transition Series: Topics for the Advanced EMT.*

Dan Batsie, BA, NREMT
Regional Education Coordinator
North East Maine EMS
Bangor, ME

Nicole M. Beehler, BSAS, RN, CEN, EMT-P
Adjunct Faculty, Emergency Medical Technology Program
Department of Health Professions
Bitonte College of Health and Human Services
Youngstown State University
Youngstown, OH

Randall W. Benner, MEd, NREMT-P
Program Director, CFD
University of Cincinnati College of Medicine
Department of Emergency Medicine
Cincinnati, OH

Tom Brazelton, MD, MPH, FAAP
Associate Professor
Division of Critical Care Medicine
Department of Pediatrics
University of Wisconsin School of Medicine & Public Health
Madison, WI

Cornelia A. Bryan, MHHS, NREMT-P
Adjunct Faculty
Youngstown State University
Youngstown, OH

Keisha T. Robinson, DrPH, MPH
Assistant Professor/Director of Public Health Program/YSU MPH
    Program Coordinator
Department of Health Professions
Youngstown State University
Youngstown, OH

Reviewers

Thanks to the following reviewers for providing invaluable feedback, insight, and suggestions in the preparation of *Transition Series: Topics for the Advanced EMT.*

John L. Beckman, AA, BS, FF/EMT-P
EMS Instructor
Addison Fire Protection District
Fire Science Instructor, Technology
    Center of DuPage
Addison, IL

Richard Belle, BS, NREMT-P
Continuing Education Manager
Acadian Ambulance/National EMS
    Academy
Lafayette, LA

George Blankinship, FP I/C
Moraine Park Technical College
Fond du Lac, WI

Major Raymond W. Burton
Plymouth Regional Police/Corrections
    Academy
Plymouth, MA

Jerry Chaney, EMT-P/EMD
EMS Instructor
Onslow County Emergency Services
Jacksonville, NC

Helen T. Compton,
Associate Degree in Emergency Medical
    Services Paramedic
Mecklenburg County Rescue Squad
Clarksville, VA

Jesse N. Davis, NREMT-P, I/C
EMS Instructor/Chaves County Training
    Coordinator
Eastern New Mexico University—Roswell
Roswell, NM

Chuck Fedak, EMT-P, BS
EMT Program Director
Baldy View ROP–EMT Program
Ontario, CA

Robert Ferris
EMS Specialist, FF/EMT-P
Memorial Health System EMS
Colorado Springs, CO

Betty L. Holmes, BSE
Paramedic Instructor Rich Mountain
    Community College
Mena, AR

D. Randy Kuykendall, MLS, NREMT-P
Chief, Emergency Medical and Trauma
    Services Section
State of Colorado Department of Public
Health and Environment
Denver, CO

Peggy Lahren, BS, NREMT-P,
EMS Regional Coordinator
Arizona Department of Health,
    Bureau of EMS & Trauma
Phoenix, AZ

Alan Lambert, NREMT-P
Deputy Director
Louisiana Bureau of Emergency
    Medical Services
Baton Rouge, LA

James Massie, BS, NREMT-P
Assistant Professor of EMS Program
    College of Southern Idaho
Twin Falls, ID

Christopher Matthews, AGS, NREMT-P,
  EMS Instructor
Instructor
Truckee Meadows Community College
  EMS Programs
Reno, NV

Gregory S. Neiman, BA, NREMTP,
  CEMA (VA)
BLS Training Specialist
Virginia Office of EMS
Richmond, VA

Joel Perkins, EMT-P
Instructor
Westfield State University
Westfield, MA

Michael S. Vastano, AAS, NREMT-P
EMT Program Director
Captain James A. Lovell Federal Heath
  Care Center
North Chicago, IL

ABOUT THE AUTHORS

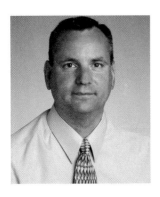

JOSEPH J. MISTOVICH

Joseph Mistovich is Chairperson of the Department of Health Professions and a Professor at Youngstown State University in Youngstown, Ohio. He has more than 25 years of experience as an educator in emergency medical services.

Mr. Mistovich received his Master of Education degree in Community Health Education from Kent State University in 1988. He completed a Bachelor of Science in Applied Science degree with a major in Allied Health in 1985, and an Associate in Applied Science degree in Emergency Medical Technology in 1982 from Youngstown State University.

Mr. Mistovich is an author or co-author of numerous EMS books and journal articles and is a frequent presenter at national and state EMS conferences.

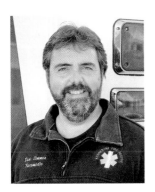

DANIEL LIMMER

Daniel Limmer has been involved in EMS for 31 years. He is active as a paramedic with Kennebunkport EMS in Kennebunkport, Maine. A passionate educator, he teaches basic, advanced, and continuing education EMS courses throughout Maine. He previously taught at George Washington University in Washington, D.C., where he coordinated international EMS education programs, and at the Hudson Valley Community College in Troy, New York. He is a charter member of the National Association of EMS Educators.

Mr. Limmer has also been involved in law enforcement, serving both as a dispatcher and police officer in Colonie, New York. He has received several awards and honors in law enforcement, including the distinguished service award (officer of the year), lifesaving award, and three command recognition awards. He also has served in the police department communications, patrol, juvenile, narcotics, and training units. Mr. Limmer retired from police work in New York but remains active as a police officer in Maine on a part-time basis.

In addition to authoring many EMS journal articles, Mr. Limmer has co-authored numerous EMS texts, including *Emergency Care*; *First Responder: A Skills Approach*; *EMT Complete: A Basic Worktext*; *Advanced Medical Life Support*; and *Active Learning Manual for EMTs*.

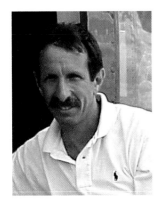

HOWARD A. WERMAN (MEDICAL EDITOR)

Howard Werman is Professor of Emergency Medicine at The Ohio State University. He is an active teacher of medical students in the College of Medicine and the residency training program in Emergency Medicine at The Ohio State University Medical Center. He has been a member of the faculty at Ohio State since 1984 and has been a contributing author to several prehospital and emergency medicine texts. He is past Chairman of the Board of the National Registry of Emergency Medical Technicians.

Dr. Werman has been active in medical direction of several emergency medical services and is currently Medical Director of MedFlight of Ohio, a critical care transport service that offers fixed-wing, helicopter, and mobile ICU services.

TRANSITION TO THE NATIONAL EMS EDUCATION STANDARDS

The National Highway Traffic Safety Administration (NHTSA) published the *National EMS Education Standards* in 2009 in response to the *EMS Education Agenda for the Future: A Systems Approach*. The National EMS Core Content and National EMS Scope of Practice Model served as the foundation for the development of the new Education Standards. The Education Standards replaced the 1985 Department of Transportation (DOT) Emergency Medical Technician–Intermediate Curriculum (I-85) and the 1999 EMT-Intermediate National Standard Curriculum (I-99). Unlike the old prescriptive DOT NSC, the Education Standards allow for much greater flexibility, adaptability, and creativity. Four levels of provider are given in the National EMS Education Standards: Emergency Medical Responder (EMR), Emergency Medical Technician (EMT—note "basic" has been deleted from the level), Advanced EMT (AEMT), and Paramedic. Two significant elements affect the AEMT: first, the EMT level has added significant content that the AEMT may or may not have originally received. Second, there are so many different definitions of "Intermediate" around the United States that an effort is under way to have a more defined and practical level of care for the AEMT that may be more consistent from state to state.

The Education Standards define the competencies, clinical behaviors, and judgments necessary for entry-level AEMTs to practice in the prehospital environment. For the Education Standards to be fully implemented, it is necessary for the education program and instructors or EMS service to work closely with the state EMS office to ensure that the National Scope of Practice Model has been adopted. Regardless of the adoption of the Education Standards, however, AEMT educators are obligated to present the most updated and current information to students. Likewise, practicing AEMTs have a responsibility to stay current with the latest medical information relevant to their respective level of prehospital practice through continuing education.

Transition Series: Topics for the Advanced EMT provides both an overview of new information contained within the Education Standards at the AEMT level and a source of continuing education for practicing AEMTs. If your initial EMT or AEMT training was under the old National Standard Curriculum, you will note new "topics" that were not contained in the prior curricula and previous "topics" that are presented at a much greater depth and breadth than what was contained previously. The EMT and AEMT educated and trained under the new Education Standards will be provided with a much greater foundation of knowledge for practicing prehospital care.

The National Registry of EMTs will no longer recognize two levels of EMT-Intermediate and will follow the certification levels outlines in the national EMS Education Standards. EMT-Intermediates who are currently registered at the I-85 level will need to complete a transition course and complete a skills examination to achieve registration at the AEMT level. I-99 Intermediates will be able to reregister at the AEMT level or complete a course to transition to the paramedic level. For more information on this contact your state EMS office or the NREMT (www.NREMT.org)

The National Association of State EMS Officials (NASEMSO) published a Gap Analysis Template in 2009 comparing the EMS knowledge and skills of the new National EMS Education Standards to the old Department of Transportation (DOT) National Standard Curricula (NSC). These changes, reflected as deletions, additions, and expansion from the previous NSC curriculum, identified by the Gap Analysis Template at the Advanced Emergency Medical Technician level, are as follows:

SKILLS NO LONGER TAUGHT TO ADVANCED EMTS

- Insertion of esophageal airways
- Administration of activated charcoal

SKILLS FOR THE EMT-INTERMEDIATE TRANSITIONING TO A 2009 ADVANCED EMT

- Administration of oxygen with the use of an oxygen humidifier
- Administration of oxygen via a partial rebreather mask
- Administration of oxygen via a simple face mask
- Administration of oxygen via a Venturi mask
- Use of Tracheostomy mask
- Tracheobronchial suctioning
- Supraglottic airways
- Intramuscular administration of epinephrine and glucagon
- Intranasal administration of naloxone
- IV administration of naloxone and 50 percent dextrose
- Use of an automatic transport ventilator
- Use of mechanical CPR devices (advanced training and protocol required)
- Revised patient restraint techniques (prone and hobbled restraint no longer appropriate and dangerous)
- Administration of beta-agonist medication via a small-volume nebulizer
- Self-administered nitrous oxide
- Administration of aspirin

NEW AEMT EDUCATION CONTENT

- Preparatory—EMS System
  - EMS systems provide more detailed discussion on patient safety, medical errors, and required affective characteristics.

- A research section was added addressing evidence-based decision making.
- Workforce safety and wellness section emphasizes the difference between Standard Precautions and personal protective equipment (PPE); bariatric issues and neonatal isolettes were added; and medical restraint techniques section was revised.
- Documentation includes HIPAA.
- A new section on therapeutic communications was added to improve patient communication.
- HIPAA was added to the medical/legal/ethics section in addition to living wills, surrogate decision makers, civil (tort) and criminal cases, and more information on ethics.

- Anatomy and Physiology includes more detailed information throughout the section.
- Medical Terminology section was added.
- Pathophysiology section was added with focus on understanding normal physiology and pathophysiology related primarily to airway, oxygenation, mechanics of ventilation, cardiovascular function, and perfusion.
- Life Span Development section was added.
- Public Health section was added as it pertains to EMS.
- Pharmacology changes include detailed information on medications carried by the AEMT plus classifications, naming, medication safety, legislation and pediatric/geriatric considerations:
  - Addition of "rights" of medical administration
- Airway Management, Respiration, and Oxygenation provides considerably more detail regarding anatomy and physiology, respiration and artificial ventilation.
- Patient Assessment changed to the following components with much more emphasis on critical thinking and clinical decision making:
  - Scene Size-Up
  - Primary Assessment (changed from Initial Assessment)
  - History Taking
  - Secondary Assessment (changed from Focused History and Physical Exam and Detailed Physical Exam)
    - Assessment of lung sounds
  - Monitoring Devices—pulse oximetry and blood glucose monitoring added to this section
  - Pediatric and geriatric considerations for assessment
- Medicine section includes the following areas and conditions:
  - Medical Overview incorporates assessment terminology relevant to the medical patient.
  - Neurology is drastically expanded to include stroke assessment and management, transient ischemic attack, altered mental status, seizure, status epilepticus, and headache.
  - Immunology section introduces significant and detailed information on the immune system.
  - Infectious Disease section includes updated information on infectious diseases such as MRSA and AIDS as well as disinfection and sterilization procedures.
  - Endocrine Disorders increased focus on pathophysiology and the relevance of diabetes in the community.
  - Psychiatric section includes material on excited delirium, patient restraint, and expanded information on psychiatric conditions, including acute psychosis and suicidal risk.
  - Cardiovascular section has an increased emphasis on anatomy, physiology, and pathophysiology and specific conditions such as acute coronary syndrome, thromboembolism, heart failure, and hypertensive emergencies.
  - Toxicology section expanded significantly and includes toxidromes.
  - Respiratory section includes more detailed assessment of the respiratory and expanded knowledge on conditions such as epiglottitis, spontaneous pneumothorax, pulmonary edema, asthma, COPD, toxic exposures, pertussis, cystic fibrosis, pulmonary embolism, pneumonia, and viral infections.
  - Hematology section includes a brief discussion of sickle cell disease and clotting disorders.
  - Genitourinary and Renal section includes more detailed discussion of the renal system and dialysis, catheter management, and kidney stones.
  - Gynecology section includes a brief discussion of sexually transmitted diseases and pelvic inflammatory disease.
  - Nontraumatic Musculoskeletal Disorder section provides information on nontraumatic fractures.
- Shock and Resuscitation section was added to emphasize shock as a multiple etiology syndrome with a much more comprehensive discussion. Cardiac arrest management now includes circulation assist devices.
- Trauma section includes the following areas and conditions:
  - Trauma Overview section includes CDC Field Triage Decision Scheme: The National Trauma Triage Protocol and assessment focused on trauma patients.
  - Bleeding section adds information on fluid resuscitation in bleeding and shock.
  - Chest Trauma section focuses on pathophysiology, assessment, and management of specific chest injuries.
  - Abdominal Trauma section focuses on pathophysiology, assessment, and management of specific abdominal injuries.
  - Head, Facial, Neck, and Spine Trauma section focuses on pathophysiology, assessment, and management of specific head, face, neck, and spine injuries.
  - Nervous System Trauma section focuses on pathophysiology, assessment, and management of specific brain and spinal cord injuries.
  - Special Considerations in Trauma section provides trauma assessment and management information specific to pediatric, elderly, cognitively impaired, and pregnant patients.
  - Multisystem Trauma includes discussion of kinematics of trauma and blast injuries.
- Special Patient Populations section includes the following areas and conditions:
  - Pregnant Patient section provides more detail on pregnancy, preeclampsia, eclampsia, and premature rupture of membranes.

- Pediatrics section provides more detail and conditions related to the pediatric patient.
- Geriatric section is separated into its own new section and focuses on the pathophysiology, assessment, and management of conditions related specifically to the geriatric patient.
- Patients with Special Challenges addresses elder abuse, homelessness, poverty, bariatric technology–dependent patients, hospice, sensory deficit, home care, and developmental disabilities.
- EMS Operations section includes the following areas:
  - Incident Management includes the federal requirements for compliance with incident management.
  - Multiple Casualty Incidents makes reference to the CDC Field Triage Scheme: The National Trauma Triage Protocol.
  - Air Medical section (same as Emergency Medical Technician).
  - Vehicle Extrication section (same as Emergency Medical Technician).
  - Hazardous Materials Awareness section (same as Emergency Medical Technician).
  - Mass Casualty Incidents Due to Terrorism or Disaster section (same as Emergency Medical Technician).

For the Advanced EMT trained under the 1985 Department of Transportation Emergency Medical Technician–Intermediate National Standard Curriculum, NASEMSO has identified *knowledge content* that is necessary to transition to an Advanced EMT under the new Education Standards. Depending on the individual state, this content may be delivered through continuing education or a structured and formal transition course. The information contained within *Transition Series: Topics for the Advanced EMT* can be used in either delivery format: a structured and formal transition course or various topics for continuing education. The topics presented in this book are contained within the Education Standards' competencies and provide a greater depth and breadth for the currently practicing EMT–Intermediate or the EMT–Intermediate who intends to transition to the new AEMT. The following table identifies the NASEMSO section and content necessary to transition to the "new" Advanced EMT and the related "Topic" numbers in this textbook.

Section (* = Education Standards Content Not Specifically Identified in the NASEMSO Essential Content: AEMT Gap Analysis)	Transition Topics: AEMT Topic Number	Transition Topics: AEMT Topic Title
Preparatory: EMS Systems	2 12	Workforce Safety and Wellness EMS Pharmacology
Preparatory: Research	1	NASEMSO recommends reviewing the importance of evidence-based decision-making process. Research was used in creating every topic in this text to ensure that it meets this standard.
Preparatory: Therapeutic Communication	3	Therapeutic Communication
Preparatory: Medical, Legal, Ethics	4	Legal Issues in EMS
Anatomy and Physiology; Pathophysiology	5 7 8 9	Anatomy and Physiology—Life Support Chain Pathophysiology: Part 1 (Ambient Air, Airway, and Mechanics of Ventilation) Pathophysiology: Part 2 (Minute and Alveolar Ventilation, Ventilation/Perfusion Ratio, Transport of Gases) Pathophysiology: Part 3 (Blood, Cardiac and Vascular System)
Medical Terminology*	6	Medical Terminology
Life Span Development*	10	Life Span Development
Public Health*	11	Public Health and EMS
Airway Management, Respiration and Oxygenation	13	Airway Management, Respiration, and Artificial Ventilation (Recognition of Respiratory Distress vs. Respiratory Failure; Intervention: Oxygenation, Positive Pressure Ventilation, CPAP)
Patient Assessment	14 15 16	Patient Assessment: Primary Assessment, Secondary Assessment, Taking a History, and Reassessment Trauma Assessment Medical Assessment
Patient Assessment: Monitoring Devices (Pulse Oximetry)	13	Airway Management, Respiration, and Artificial Ventilation (Recognition of Respiratory Distress vs. Respiratory Failure; Intervention: Oxygenation, Positive Pressure Ventilation, CPAP)

(Continued)

Section (* = Education Standards Content Not Specifically Identified in the NASEMSO Essential Content: AEMT Gap Analysis)	Transition Topics: AEMT Topic Number	Transition Topics: AEMT Topic Title
Medicine: Neurology	17	Neurology: Altered Mental Status*
	18	Neurology: Stroke
	19	Neurology: Seizures*
Medicine: Abdominal and Gastrointestinal Disorders	20	Acute Abdomen and Gastrointestinal Bleeding
Medicine: Infectious Disease	2, 22	NASEMSO recommends updated information on MRSA and HIV and cleaning and disinfecting ambulance and equipment.
Medicine: Immunology*	21	Immunology
Medicine: Endocrine Disorders	23	Endocrine Disorders: Hypoglycemia
	24	Endocrine Disorders: Hyperglycemic Emergencies (DKA and HHNS)
Medicine: Psychiatric	25	Psychiatric Disorders
Medicine: Cardiovascular	26	Cardiovascular Emergencies: Chest Pain and Acute Coronary Syndrome
	27	Cardiovascular Emergencies: Congestive Heart Failure
	28	Cardiovascular Emergencies: Hypertensive and Vascular Emergencies (Aortic Dissection, Aortic Aneurysm)
Medicine: Toxicology*	29	Toxicology: Street Drugs
Medicine: Respiratory	30	Respiratory Emergencies: Airway Resistance Disorders (Asthma, Bronchitis, Bronchiolitis)
	31	Respiratory Emergencies: Lung and Gas Exchange Disorders (Spontaneous Pneumothorax, Pulmonary Edema, Pulmonary Embolism, Cystic Fibrosis)
	32	Respiratory Emergencies: Infectious Disorders (Pneumonia, Pertussis, Viral Respiratory Infections)
Medicine: Hematology	33	Hematology: Blood Disorders
Medicine: Genitourinary/Renal	34	Renal Disorders
Medicine: Gynecologic Emergencies*	35	Gynecologic Emergencies
Medicine: Emergencies Involving the Eyes, Ears, Nose, and Throat*	36	Emergencies Involving the Eyes, Ears, Nose, and Throat
Shock and Resuscitation	37	Issues in Cardiac Arrest and Resuscitation
	38	Shock
Trauma: Overview	15	NASEMSO recommends familiarity with CDC Field Triage Decision Scheme: The National Trauma Triage Protocol
Trauma: Bleeding*	39	Bleeding and Bleeding Control
Trauma: Chest Trauma	40	Chest Trauma
Trauma: Abdominal and Genitourinary Trauma	41	Abdominal Trauma
Trauma: Soft-tissue Trauma*	42	Soft-Tissue Injuries: Crush Injury and Compartment Syndrome
Trauma: Head, Facial, Neck, and Spine Trauma	36	Emergencies Involving the Eyes, Ears, Nose, and Throat
	43	Head and Traumatic Brain Injury
Trauma: Nervous System Trauma	43	Head and Traumatic Brain Injuries
	44	Complete and Incomplete Spine and Spinal Cord Injuries

(Continued)

Section (* = Education Standards Content Not Specifically Identified in the NASEMSO Essential Content: AEMT Gap Analysis)	Transition Topics: AEMT Topic Number	Transition Topics: AEMT Topic Title
Trauma: Special Considerations in Trauma	45 46 47	Trauma in Special Populations: Pediatrics Trauma in Special Populations: Geriatrics Trauma in Special Populations: Pregnancy
Trauma: Environmental Emergencies*	48	Diving Emergencies: Decompression Sickness and Arterial Embolism
Special Patient Populations: Obstetrics	49	Special Populations: Obstetrics (Antepartum Complications)
Special Patient Populations: Newborn Care*	50	Special Populations: Neonatology
Special Patient Populations: Pediatrics*	51	Special Populations: Pediatrics
Special Patient Populations: Geriatrics*	52	Special Populations: Geriatrics
Special Patient Populations: Patients with Special Challenges*	53, 54	Special Populations: Patients with Special Challenges Special Populations—Bariatric Emergencies
EMS Operations: Incident Management	55	Multiple Casualty Incidents and Incident Management
EMS Operations: Hazardous Materials—Awareness	n/a	Note: NASEMSO recommends Hazardous Waste Operations and Emergency Response (HAZWOPER) First Responder Awareness Level training. Hazardous material awareness training is handled as stand-alone course/material.
EMS Operations: Mass Casualty Incidents Due to Terrorism and Disaster	55	Multiple-Casualty Incident and Incident Management
	56	Advanced Skills for the AEMT
	57	Additional Pharmacology for the AEMT
	58	ECG Monitoring and Cardiac Dysrhythmias

INSTRUCTOR RESOURCES

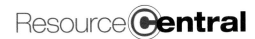

This *new* Web site contains all your instructor resources in one location! It provides all your teaching resources: PowerPoint program with instructor's notes and teaching tips, answer key to end-of-chapter questions, sample syllabi, and multiple-choice questions. To access Resource Central, go to **www.bradybooks.com** and select Resource Central.

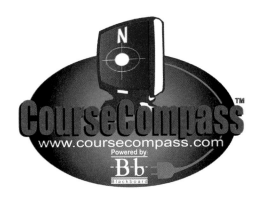

CourseCompass is a dynamic, interactive, online learning environment. You can easily create a course and customize it with your own materials. All instructor resources for this edition are already loaded to enable you to run your online course with ease.

Standard Preparatory

Competency Applies fundamental knowledge of the EMS system, safety/well-being of the AEMT, and medical/legal and ethical issues to the provision of emergency care.

TOPIC

1

RESEARCH AND EMS

INTRODUCTION

Every provider who steps into an ambulance would like to believe that what he is doing is really going to make a difference in the lives of his patients. We all hope that the therapies and interventions we deliver will be meaningful. Moreover, as budgets tighten and managers look for ways to control costs, it is more important than ever to ensure that what we do is both meaningful and cost effective.

In EMS, however, these are not simple questions. We spend nearly 3 billion dollars each year delivering care, but little of what we do has ever been truly evaluated. This presents some significant

TRANSITION *highlights*

- *Integration of research into EMS education and practice.*
- *Evidence-based decision making.*
- *The involvement of the AEMT in clinical and EMS systems research.*
- *Scientific theory.*
- *Types of research.*
- *Basics of analyzing and interpreting research.*

problems. How do we know we are being helpful? How do we know that the tools we use are effective? As the profession matures, the scientific experimentation to establish facts or measure outcomes—otherwise known as *research*—will offer us an opportunity to factually answer some of these questions and will help us guide our progress to better benefit our patients (▶ Figure 1-1).

This change is not simple. EMS is not an easy field in which to gather research, and serious challenges exist. As a provider, you should understand the value of research not only to your profession, but also to your everyday practice. You can take simple steps to improve your understanding and to help move EMS toward a more evidence-based approach. In this topic we discuss how EMS research is valuable and how you, as a provider, can improve the role of research in health care.

EMS RESEARCH AND YOU

Knowledge is power. Throughout health care, medicine is moving to a more *evidence-based* approach. This means that outcomes of therapies and interventions are carefully measured to ensure that they have the intended results. When changes are made, decisions are based on clear indications and outcomes that point to meaningful improvements in patient care.

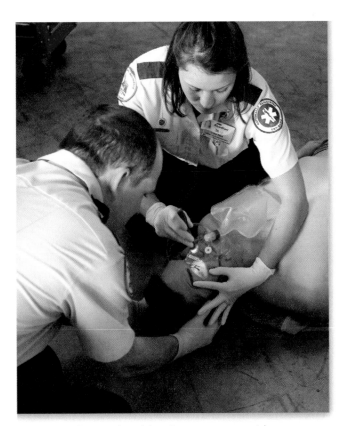

Figure 1-1 Research guides the care we provide.

As health care matures, more and more progress is achieved through an evidence-based approach. This means that the interventions we perform and the therapies we deliver must be meaningful and should be measurable. To assess the value of our care, we must turn to research. Quality studies and experimentation will separate important, relevant strategies from frivolous, wasteful endeavors. Consider the following situation:

> **To assess the value of our care, we must turn to research.**

You work as an advanced EMT for an ambulance service that has 20 ambulances. Staffing is tight—and the budget is tighter. Tomorrow a new device used to treat cardiac arrest will be released, at a cost of $1500 each. The company that created the device claims that it is the most important device the company has ever released and that it will significantly increase cardiac arrest survival rates.

As your company decides whether to buy the device, it must weigh the idea of improving survival rates against the high cost of the device. Of course, everyone would like to see patient care improve, but there is a significant cost to implementing this new device. If your company chooses to outfit its entire fleet, it will have to spend $30,000. If the device truly works, it makes a great deal of sense to purchase it; but if it doesn't work, $30,000 could pay for the addition of another AEMT.

How could your service make the correct decision? The answer is quality EMS research. If unbiased scientific experimentation existed showing that this device really did double survival rates of cardiac arrest, then this decision would be easy to make. Similarly, if a quality study demonstrated that the device did not improve cardiac arrest survival, then the service could invest its money in more meaningful areas.

If, as a profession, we were committed to an evidence-based approach, we could avoid spending time and money on ineffective therapies and focus our budgets on the elements of care that mean the most. This example is hypothetical, of course, but every day EMS agencies are faced with similar dilemmas. In addition to spending money, consider the dilemmas EMS leaders and providers are faced with in developing protocols, adopting new medications and devices, allotting staffing resources, and myriad other questions that desperately need thoughtful answers. In an age of slick marketing and ever-burgeoning technology, quality research and an evidence-based approach will help us answer questions and expend our resources wisely.

But what about the local level—how does EMS research affect the practice of a single AEMT? Consider your state, regional, or even service-level protocols. Decisions regarding scope of practice, equipment, and medications are made every day. Medical directors, state officials, and services consult relevant research to aid in choosing the paths and procedures that make the most sense.

Consider also the dynamic nature of health care. We know for sure that many of the treatments and therapies you are learning today may prove to be inappropriate on further examination in the future. The history of EMS is littered with ideas, medications, and other therapies that were considered state of the art until they were thoroughly examined and determined to be incorrect. Understanding how to interpret research will help you, as a provider, stay on the cutting edge of patient care. Decisions are made every day about how we conduct our business. Understanding research can help you contribute to these discussions.

The bottom line is that decision makers are consulting EMS research to make choices about your profession. EMS providers at every level are involved in making these decisions, but without a basic understanding of research, providers are routinely excluded from the conversation. Understanding research even at a very simple level allows you to speak the language of health care and can deliver to you a seat at the table. The best care possible results from an open dialogue among physicians, administrators, and providers and is best achieved by reviewing quality research.

THE BASICS OF EMS RESEARCH

Someone once said, "Not everything that is researched is true and not everything that is true has been researched." This statement certainly applies in the world of EMS. The dynamic nature of our treatment setting makes research difficult at best. We encounter many obstacles to research that simply are not there in other branches of the health care field. The environment in which we work can be unstable, our encounters are often brief, and our data collection is frequently disjointed and lacks centralization. Furthermore, we face many ethical dilemmas. Obtaining consent from a critical patient is often challenging at best. We do have many opportunities to create valid and important studies on prehospital care—but to do so, we must promote best practices of research so our outcomes can truly guide us to high-quality care.

Not all research is created equal. There are good studies, and there are bad studies. As we evolve in an evidence-based environment, we should strive to embrace the best practices of conducting and evaluating research. The finer points of medical research are by no means a simple topic, and a thorough examination of how to evaluate research is beyond the scope of this text. However, some broad concepts can be helpful to consider.

Remember that the process of research is the same whether you are an EMS researcher or a scientist in a laboratory. We each rely on the *scientific method*, developed by Galileo almost 400 years ago, as a process of experimentation for answering questions and acquiring new knowledge. In this method, general observations are stated as a *hypothesis* (or unproven theory). Predictions are then made, and these predictions, based on the hypothesis, are then tested to either prove or disprove the theory.

For example, you might notice that applying a bandage seems to control minor external bleeding. To use the scientific method, you might hypothesize that bandages do indeed control bleeding better than doing nothing at all. You could conduct a randomized control study to test your hypothesis by randomly assigning patients to the "bandage group" or to the "do-nothing group." You could then measure the amount of bleeding in each group and compare your results. Although there might be some ethical issues with your study, this experiment would help you either prove or disprove the value of bandaging. Furthermore, if your experiment was done properly, your results would hold up if the study was repeated, regardless of who conducted the experiment. That is the value of quality research. Unfortunately, not all research can live up to these quality markers.

In medicine, exacting and comprehensive studies are both difficult and time consuming. In most cases, we make decisions based on a broad variety of different sources. Unfortunately, much of what we do still relies on the "best guess strategy," but as we progress, we rely more and more on research and, in particular, research studies. When making decisions based on evidence (especially patient care decisions), it is clearly best to obtain an opinion based on many studies and not just a single work. The strength of your conclusion is increased significantly when a variety of studies point to the same conclusion.

The key is to obtain an objective opinion. When more than one study points to the same conclusion, it is more likely to be free from opinion and bias. Many individual studies are clouded by bias, which occurs when research is influenced by prior inclinations, beliefs, or prejudices. Bias influences a study when the outcomes are manipulated to fit an expected outcome instead of being measured objectively against the hypothesis. This can occur when researchers have a financial stake in a particular outcome, but more commonly it occurs simply as a result of poor methods used to conduct the research.

In the true scientific method, outcomes are not bent to conform to previously held notions, but rather are examined objectively and evaluated based solely on the facts. Valid research embraces this idea and uses methods designed to limit outside influences.

Different methods of research are considered more valid than others. This is typically judged by how well they avoid potential bias and exclude the possibility of error. Consider the following strategies:

PROSPECTIVE VERSUS RETROSPECTIVE
Retrospective reviews look at events that have occurred in the past. Health care frequently uses retrospective reviews to look back at the outcome of therapies previously performed. In contrast, prospective studies are designed to look forward. Methods are designed to test therapies and outcomes that will occur in the future. Prospective studies are generally easier to control, as rules and regulations can be put in place to control errors

and prevent bias. Retrospective studies cannot necessarily be controlled in such a way. Retrospective studies can certainly be considered valid, but a prospective method is generally considered more valid.

RANDOMIZATION
High-quality studies use randomization. In medicine, this type of study typically compares one therapy against another. Bias is controlled by randomly assigning a therapy to patients, as opposed to having predetermined groups. It also improves objectivity when analyzing outcomes. In high-quality studies, the researcher and the patients may not even know which therapy they are receiving. This process is called *blinding*. A research study can be either single-blinded (the researcher knows who gets what therapy) or double-blinded (neither the patient nor the researcher knows who gets what therapy). By blinding a study, it is very difficult to influence outcomes in any way, and the results are far more likely to be objective.

CONTROL GROUPS
The use of a control group helps to better evaluate outcomes fairly. In medicine, a control group is commonly a known or currently used therapy. In our previous bandaging study, we compared the bandaging group against a do-nothing group. In that case, the do-nothing group would be our control group. Including this group allows us not only to evaluate the outcome of bandaging, but also to compare those outcomes against a different strategy. This comparison adds weight and value to the analysis.

STUDY GROUP SIMILARITY
If a group of patients is being used to test a new treatment, it is important that subjects in that group have a certain degree of similarity. Let us say, for example, that we want to test a new airway device's impact on survival in trauma patients. We have designed and implemented a study to compare the use of the new device against a group of patients who received care without using the device. In our study, AEMTs were allowed to choose the patients on whom they wanted to use the new device.

When we look at our results, we find that the device group had a much higher mortality rate. At face, we could assume that this means the device did not work.

However, as we analyze the results, we find that the group assigned to the new device was much sicker than the group that did not receive the device. Here, the AEMTs just thought it would be better to use the new device only in the worse-off patients. Did more people die because of the device, or did more people die simply because they were hurt worse from the beginning? It is difficult to say—and therein lies the difficulty in comparing two vastly different groups. Consider also the challenges in comparing different age groups, different treatment protocols, or even different genders.

No study can be completely free from bias, but as you have seen, certain methods help to minimize the impact of subjectivity. Because of the dynamic and often sensitive nature of medicine, a large variety of research is used to make conclusions on therapies and treatment. Ideally, systematic reviews guide our most important decisions, but more commonly, a combination of research studies and research methods guides the decisions that are made. Consider the following types of medical research:

SYSTEMATIC REVIEW
In a systematic review, a series of studies pertaining to a single question are evaluated. Their results are reviewed, summarized, and used to draw evidence-based conclusions. It is important to remember that a systematic review is made up of not one, but many different research experiments.

RANDOMIZED CONTROLLED TRIALS (RCTs)
In an RCT, researchers randomly assign eligible subjects into groups to receive or not receive the intervention being tested. A control group is used to compare the tested theory against a known outcome. In 2000, for example, Marianne Gausche-Hill and her colleagues looked at pediatric intubation in Los Angeles County, California. In their study, children needing airway management were randomized, based on the day of the week, to either an intubation group or a bag-valve-mask (BVM) group. Outcomes of these patients were studied. Objectivity was improved because subjects were randomized and the results were more meaningful, as they could compare outcomes of the intubation group against the control BVM group.

In medicine, drugs are frequently tested in randomized studies using a placebo. To measure the outcome of a drug, patients are frequently randomized to receive either the real drug or a placebo, or "sugar pill," which has no effect. Frequently these studies use a double-blinding process so that even the providers carrying out the study, as well as the patients, do not know which path they are taking. In this type of study, the results of the new medication can be compared against the placebo control group to accurately assess the effect of the therapy.

COHORT/CONCURRENT CONTROL/ CASE-CONTROL STUDIES

In these types of studies, two groups or therapies or patients are compared, but subjects are not necessarily randomized. For example, you might compare the outcomes of one service that uses continuous positive airway pressure (CPAP) against the outcomes of another service that does not. A cohort study might follow patients who have a specific disease and compare them with a group of patients that does not have the disease. In both these studies, you are comparing two groups and have a control group, but the results are not truly randomized. Frequently, case-control studies are retrospective in nature, looking at two groups of events or outcomes that occurred in the past. All these studies can be valid and yield important information, but they also can be prone to bias in that it is difficult to control all aspects of similarity and methods among the different groups.

CASE SERIES/CASE REPORTS

Case studies and case reports review the treatment of a single patient or a series of patients. Frequently they report on unusual circumstances or outcomes. There is no control group, and these reports are always retrospective. They are certainly not as valid as randomized studies, but they often help us formulate larger questions to be investigated.

META-ANALYSIS

A meta-analysis is not truly a study itself, but rather a compilation of different studies looking at a single topic. A meta-analysis will summarize the work of others and frequently will comment on outcomes. In many cases, these are similar to a systematic review, but frequently are on a much smaller scale.

It is important to remember that every study should be reviewed independently.

The fact that it is a randomized controlled study does not ensure that its results are valid. That said, methodology does play a role in evaluating a study's importance. The American Heart Association qualifies the validity of research in a linear fashion using a "level of evidence" designation, which assigns varying levels of importance based on the way a study was conducted. This progression is useful in evaluating the importance of data and can be used as a framework for considering the utility of a particular study.

- **Level of Evidence 1:** In this sliding scale, the highest level (most valuable) set of data would result from RCTs or meta-analyses of RCTs.
- **Level of Evidence 2:** Studies using concurrent controls without true randomization. Because they are often retrospective and because the methods are more difficult to control without randomization, these types of studies are often less reliable.
- **Level of Evidence 3:** Studies using retrospective controls. There is little control of these experiments, as the testing is based on events that have already occurred. Because of this, it is difficult to ensure similar circumstances among research subjects. Although the data from retrospective studies may be useful, they can be prone to bias.
- **Level of Evidence 4:** Studies without a control group (e.g., case series). In these studies, only one group is looked at and is not compared to a second group. Here there is no control group against which to examine the results. Important information may be gained, but outcomes are difficult to truly understand without comparing to similar patients who received a different therapy.
- **Level of Evidence 5:** Studies not directly related to the specific patient/ population (e.g., a different patient/ population, animal models, mechanical models). These studies are common in EMS and are frequently used to evaluate prehospital treatments. Unfortunately, their data are prone to a wide range of interpretation, as we must make assumptions that what works in different populations or under different circumstances would work in the world of EMS.

Regardless of the type of study you are reading, you should always review research in a way that helps you identify bias or flaws

in the methodology. There is certainly a great deal more to learn about the evaluation of medical research, but there are some important questions to consider when reading a study. Consider the following questions:

- Was the study randomized, and was the randomization blinded?
- If more than one group was reviewed, were the groups similar at the start of the trial?
- Were all eligible patients analyzed, and if they were excluded, why were they excluded? Bias often occurs by removing data that lead in a different direction from your hypothesis. Often, the removal of patients from a study can identify potential problems.
- Were the outcomes really the result of the therapy? Consider the previously discussed example of the new airway device being used in only sicker patients. Occasionally, outcomes can be measured that would have happened randomly. For example, a company could invent a new device that it claims would make the sun rise tomorrow at 6:00 AM. Although the company could certainly produce a study that demonstrates the desired outcome, that outcome would have occurred whether the device was used or not. A powerful study is one that can be reproduced with the same results in relatively different circumstances.
- Is the outcome truly relevant? Many studies show differences among treatment but no real relevance. For example, a study might show that a new medication increases the return of spontaneous circulation in sudden cardiac arrest compared with a placebo control group. Getting a pulse back in more patients is important, but that result is not really relevant if exactly the same number of patients die at the conclusion of care as compared with the control group.

Many good resources on evaluating evidence-based medicine can be found, and there is a great deal more information to learn on evaluating research. Learning more about this topic as a provider will help you to understand the

> **Always review research in a way that helps you identify bias or flaws in the methodology.**

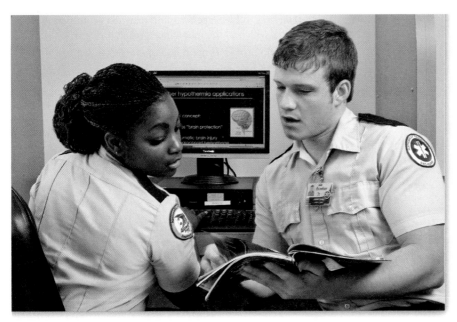

Figure 1-2 Read and evaluate research.

> **There is no better way to learn about research than to become involved in a research study.**

decisions and discussions that are ongoing both in EMS and in health care in general (▶ Figure 1-2). Classes, textbooks, and many other tutorials can improve your capability to read and evaluate research. However, there is no better way to learn about research than to become involved in a research study.

YOUR ROLE IN EMS RESEARCH

As previously stated, medicine in general is moving rapidly in a direction guided by evidence-based medicine. In EMS, we face a future in which payment will be based on validated outcomes. Therefore, your role as an advanced life support

(ALS) provider in research is especially important.

Aside from reading and discussing research, the ALS provider of the future will be on the front line of conducting research. We now know that the only way to truly prove our worth and prove the importance of our prehospital therapies is to evaluate them through clinical trials. As a provider, there are a variety of ways in which you may be involved in EMS research.

At the simplest level, your good documentation may help improve future studies. As EMS systems begin to collaborate and to centralize run-report data, this information may help guide any number of potential studies. EMS leaders will consider skills that are used, locations, times of day, and many other reported outcomes as they design the EMS system of the future. The time you take to document your call accurately and thoroughly

may be an essential component of evidence-based medicine and may have a significant impact on the decisions that are made regarding how you do business.

You may also take part in a research study. Your service, local hospital, or region may participate and enroll patients in a specifically designed experiment. In this case it is important to follow all the instructions you are given. Making exceptions or not following the instructions can insert bias or even eliminate your data from being considered. Participating in such a study is an important way to learn more about medical research. Not only might your service benefit from the information learned in the study, but often participation also gives you valuable insight into research methods and procedures.

As you progress as a provider, perhaps you will take part in designing a study. As an AEMT, you are on the forefront of prehospital medicine and can play an important role in shaping the future of our prehospital medicine. Many hospitals and EMS systems conduct research routinely. Your medical director or local state official may be able to offer opportunities if you would like to get involved.

CONCLUSIONS

EMS research is an important part of the future of our profession. Understanding the basic concepts of research offers you a role in shaping that direction. Remember that not all research is created equal. Take the time to learn more about reading and evaluating research literature, and you will improve your own importance to your chosen field. Remember that every EMS provider must play a role in conducting EMS research. Beyond just participating, becoming involved in research development offers a rewarding pathway for enlightened providers.

TRANSITIONING

REVIEW ITEMS

1. Evidence-based medicine means that _____.
   a. you must have evidence of the patient's condition to treat him
   b. our interventions must be measurable and researched
   c. you must present evidence to medical direction to perform interventions
   d. protocols must be pilot tested and researched before implementation

2. A hypothesis is _____.
   a. the endpoint of a research project
   b. an unproven theory
   c. the procedure used to guide a study
   d. a conclusion

3. A meta-analysis is _____.
   a. a randomized study
   b. a comparison of three or more hypotheses
   c. a compilation of studies looking at a topic
   d. a "blinded" study

4. According to the American Heart Association, a "Level of Evidence–5" means that the study _____.
   a. is not related directly to the patient population
   b. is of the highest value and credibility
   c. did not have a control group
   d. should be used to guide treatment protocols when possible

5. In reference to EMS agencies and providers conducting research, which of the following is true?
   a. EMS providers are not allowed to conduct research.
   b. EMS research is subject to the same rules as in-hospital research.
   c. Research conducted by EMS providers is considered less credible in evaluating prehospital care.
   d. EMS providers may conduct system research but not clinical research.

Standard Preparatory

Competency Applies fundamental knowledge of the EMS system, safety/well-being of the Advanced EMT, and medical/legal and ethical issues to the provision of emergency care.

TOPIC

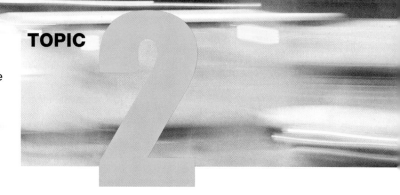

WORKFORCE SAFETY AND WELLNESS

INTRODUCTION

Anyone who was an Advanced EMT before the 1980s believed that the first priority at the scene was "airway, airway, airway." Although it is true that the airway is our first patient priority, EMS has matured and now realizes that the first priority at any scene is the safety of the EMS providers—for without this, there would be no patient care.

In times past, Standard Precautions were taken infrequently, and diseases such as HIV were not yet in the picture. The nature of EMS has changed dramatically since then. Workforce safety and wellness now have an appropriate and prominent place at the beginning of the EMS education standards. This topic covers infectious disease and Standard Precautions, scene safety, and a brief review of how to lift and move patients.

The topic "Workforce Safety and Wellness" is new to the education standards and combines what was traditionally in the "Well-Being of the EMS Provider" and the "Lifting and Moving Patients" lessons of prior curricula. This topic provides a brief and pertinent review of the older sections with attention to any changes in procedure and science that have occurred.

PROTECTION FROM DISEASE

Regardless of how long one has been certified as an AEMT, it is worth taking the time for a brief discussion of Standard Precautions. Previously called body substance isolation (BSI), the concept of Standard Precautions states that you will take precautions based on the likelihood of exposure (▶ Figure 2-1). This likelihood is based on the condition of the patient, the patient's illness or injuries, and the procedures you will likely perform.

As an AEMT, your use of modalities such as intravenous catheter insertion, medication administration, and advanced airways requires additional attention to Standard Precautions.

TRANSITION *highlights*

- *Importance of using Standard Precautions.*
- *The need to participate in exposure prevention strategies.*
- *Diseases of concern that the Advanced EMT is most likely to encounter in a prehospital setting.*
- *Discussion of certain EMS scenarios and how Advanced EMTs can best prevent themselves from becoming exposed, injured, or even killed.*
- *Techniques the Advanced EMT can employ when reacting to a dangerous situation.*

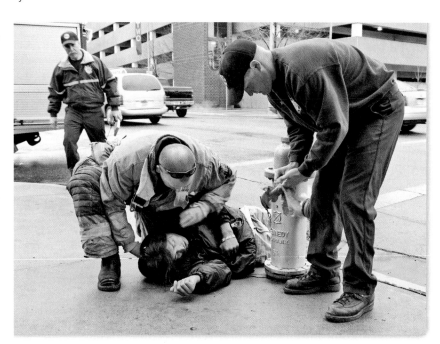

Figure 2-1 Standard Precautions will help prevent exposure to disease. They are taken after determining what risks of exposure are present.

Each of these modalities can cause a risk of exposure to disease if proper practices are not performed.

STANDARD PRECAUTIONS

One of the factors not involved in the Standard Precautions equation is the socioeconomic class or location of the patient (e.g., a patient in a "bad part of town"). These specifics should not matter because the precautions you take based on likelihood of exposure will protect you independent of other factors at the scene. Furthermore, those who live in higher socioeconomic classes and neighborhoods have exactly the same diseases as those who do not. You cannot tell if blood or body fluids are infectious by looking at the fluid or the person they come from. This is why we take Standard Precautions.

Taking Standard Precautions is a decision that an AEMT must make when sizing up a scene. It should not be made earlier or later. If you put on gloves before leaving the ambulance and before seeing the patient, you are making a decision before evaluating all the facts. In this case, you are also risking the integrity of the gloves you donned (▶ Figure 2-2) because carrying equipment to the scene and accessing the patient may cause tears in gloves that will cause body fluids to come into contact with your skin. If that skin is open, you will become exposed to the patient's blood or fluid.

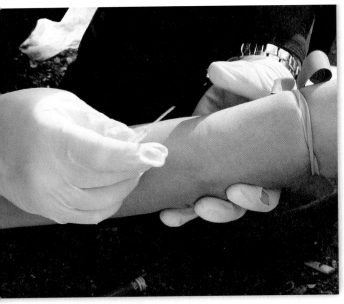

Figure 2-2 Taking Standard Precautions too early will render your efforts ineffective when you truly need them.

Face and respiratory protection often take a second position in the Standard Precautions hierarchy. This is partially because some providers don gloves before evaluating the scene and falsely believe they have taken precautions. When patients require suction or airway care or are unresponsive, vomiting, spitting, or otherwise likely to spray secretions toward your facial mucous membranes, you must protect your face. The use of advanced airways is an automatic indication for protection of the mucous membranes of the eyes, nose, and mouth with a mask and eye protection or, in some cases, a mask and face shield.

It is important to note that we contract many of the diseases we experience through this route. A friend or acquaintance sneezes into his hand. He then shakes your hand, or you touch an item he recently handled. You subsequently scratch your itchy eye and are then infected. Your eyes are designed with tear ducts to moisten the eye. That moisture drains through nasolacrimal ducts directly into your respiratory system.

Although the need for the use of gowns and other clothing protection is rare, at times (such as childbirth and multitrauma) this protection will be necessary.

The importance of hand washing must not be underestimated and is, in fact, the foremost protection from disease. Consider the following situations in which hand washing may be your only protection:

- You get into the passenger compartment of the ambulance and begin to enter run data on your mobile data terminal (MDT). The provider on the previous shift did not wash his hands before using the computer.
- You are removing the stretcher from your ambulance at the start of your shift to wash the floor. The stretcher had traces of blood on its rails from a prior call.
- You shake the hand of a colleague on her last day of work at your service. Her hand is contaminated with nasal secretions.

Thus, hand washing should be done after every call—and many times each day between calls—to prevent the transmission of disease. Although it is called hand washing, washing should continue up to the wrist and lower forearm (if exposed) and must include soap with vigorous scrubbing. Spend extra time on any visible soiled areas. While washing, your hands should always point down into the sink or basin to prevent contamination from reaching your arms or clothing. Rinse thoroughly and dry your hands. Use the paper towel to turn off the water to prevent recontamination by touching the faucet handles.

Alcohol-based hand cleaners also have a place in EMS. They are useful in the field when hand washing is not available. They are less effective than soap, however, and should not take the place of hand washing when hands are visibly soiled or contaminated with *Clostridium difficile* or other organisms.

EXPOSURE PREVENTION

Preventing exposure is part of a system that begins prior to a call and continues after a call.

Your EMS agency is required to provide training initially to employees, and yearly after that, in reference to protection from disease. The agency is also required to implement workplace practices and controls that are designed to prevent exposure to disease. The specifics are wide ranging but include everything from policies to equipment placement. It is important that you understand and follow these policies. Some of these controls include the following:

- Place equipment for Standard Precautions so it is readily available and accessible at the point of need. You may notice that gloves, glasses, and other equipment are available in both the cab and back of your ambulance. Personal protective equipment will also be available in kits should you need extras or if the equipment you are using suddenly fails.
- Provide training in dealing with needles used in patient care. Needles must be used and disposed of safely and appropriately.
- Provide equipment for decontamination. Most services use a commercially prepared disinfectant solution that is

used on the stretcher and surfaces in the back of the ambulance. Heavy-duty gloves should be used when cleaning surfaces that may tear standard disposable gloves.

- Use disposable equipment and supplies when they are likely to become contaminated.

DISEASES OF CONCERN

It is important for the AEMT to be aware of certain diseases. Understanding these diseases helps EMTs decide when certain Standard Precautions may be necessary. Although AEMTs recognize that we must not come in contact with any blood, knowledge of diseases such as tuberculosis and the H1N1 flu will help determine when respiratory precautions are necessary.

Table 2-1 reviews diseases with which an EMT may come in contact. Learn about these diseases to prepare and protect yourself appropriately. Remember that diseases are emerging all the time.

SCENE SAFETY

Most EMS personnel consider violence the biggest danger they will face. Television reports and the most dramatic news articles may involve violence, but experience shows that other dangers exist as well.

According to the National EMS Memorial Service Web page (www.nemsms.org), over the past several years more emergency medical personnel have been killed by air medical transportation crashes than by any other cause.

TABLE 2-1	Diseases of Concern	
Disease	**Mode of Transmission**	**Incubation Period**
AIDS (acquired immune deficiency syndrome)	Human immunodeficiency virus (HIV)-infected blood via intravenous drug use, unprotected sexual contact, blood transfusions, or (rarely) accidental needle sticks. Mothers also may pass HIV to their unborn children.	Several months or years
Chickenpox (varicella)	Airborne droplets. Can also be spread by contact with open sores	11 to 21 days
German measles (rubella)	Airborne droplets. Mothers may pass the disease to unborn children	10 to 12 days
H1N1 (flu)	Respiratory droplets	1 to 7 days
Hepatitis	Blood, stool, or other body fluids, or contaminated objects	Weeks to months, depending on type
Meningitis, bacterial	Oral and nasal secretions	2 to 10 days
Mumps	Droplets of saliva or objects contaminated by saliva	14 to 24 days
Pneumonia, bacterial and viral	Oral and nasal droplets and secretions	Several days
Staphylococcal skin infections	Direct contact with infected wounds or sores or with contaminated objects	Several days
Tuberculosis	Respiratory secretions, airborne or on contaminated objects	2 to 6 weeks
Whooping cough (pertussis)	Respiratory secretions or airborne droplets	6 to 20 days

The leading causes of death of on-duty EMS providers (excluding air medical transportation crashes) are motor vehicle crashes and cardiovascular disease. Motor vehicle crashes include those that occur in responding to and traveling from the scene as well as EMS providers being struck by vehicles while at accident scenes.

Highway Scenes

To protect yourself at highway scenes, always wear high-visibility American National Standards Institute (ANSI)-approved vests (▶ Figure 2-3) and stay out of the flow of traffic. Never depend on your vest or on the observation skills of motorists to stay safe. Remember that cars may spin out of control while trying to avoid the scene and thereby enter what was once considered a safe area.

When on any roadway, be sure the scene is blocked by vehicles with adequate lighting, size, or both. On highways, many agencies now require a heavy, high-visibility vehicle (fire apparatus or highway truck with warning lights) to physically block traffic lanes in which operations are being conducted.

Considerable attention is also being directed to AEMT safety in the patient compartment of the ambulance. Unsecured equipment will become a projectile in a crash. Any provider who is standing and/or unsecured in a crash may be injured or killed. New ambulance designs are creating workspaces in which EMS personnel can access vital supplies and equipment while seated and secured at the patient's side without moving around the passenger compartment.

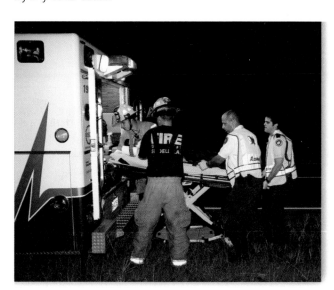

Figure 2-3 Wear high-visibility vests when working in and around a roadway.

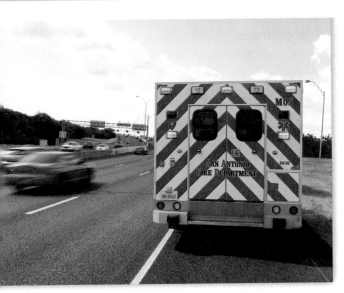

Figure 2-4 The chevron pattern is used to increase ambulance visibility.

A chevron design is being used on the back of many ambulances to promote visibility (▶ **Figure 2-4**). This design will be required in 2014.

Violence

Although not as statistically common as other causes of EMS provider death, violence remains a real concern to all levels of EMS providers. This section discusses the identification of and response to violence.

> **The best way to deal with violence is through observation and prevention.**

The best way to deal with violence is through observation and prevention. If this section dealt primarily with defensive tactics, you would be taught only how to fight and respond. The best defense, though, is actually prevention.

Your observation begins during the scene size-up—not when you pull up to the scene but, rather, for some time before. If you observe people fleeing the scene or acting violent or unruly, or if the call type might require police response, stage in a position out of sight of the scene.

If the outer perimeter appears secure, drive up to the scene. Here you will continue to observe. Look for continued indicators of violence. Does the scene appear "normal" (e.g., someone waving for you with a worried look) or suspicious (e.g., lights off, no activity)? If your observation of the scene does not reveal signs of

danger, you will exit your ambulance or response vehicle and approach. You will continue to be observant as you walk to the scene. You will observe for signs of danger, including loud voices, breaking glass, suspicious or furtive actions, and continued unusual silence.

The scene size-up does not stop once you safely reach the patient. The dynamics at the scene may change. Patients, family members, or bystanders may turn hostile or violent. Perpetrators may return to the scene. You must continue to be aware throughout the call.

One tactic used by police that often translates well to EMS providers is *contact and cover*. In police work, one officer is the primary contact officer, and the partner is the cover officer. The contact officer is the one who deals with and communicates with a suspect. The cover officer does not communicate with the suspect. He stands away (usually 90 degrees off to the side) from the contact officer and observes or "covers" the contact officer.

The 90-degree angle is multipurpose. It provides a separate and different view from that of the contact officer and prevents an attacker from attacking both officers at once.

Although there are obviously differences between suspects and patients, EMS and police operations are surprisingly similar. One AEMT often establishes a rapport with the patient and begins a history or physical exam. The other AEMT or AEMTs provide a support function, doing anything from recording vital signs to positioning the stretcher. This second AEMT will be in a much better position to observe the scene for subtle dangers that may be missed by the AEMT dealing with the patient.

Of course, both AEMTs (like both officers in the police example) have a role in safety. It is beneficial in the EMS setting for AEMTs to communicate with each other and with the dispatcher to warn of danger without alerting the aggressor. A simple predetermined code will accomplish this.

Reacting to Danger

There are four key ways to react to danger: calling for help, cover, concealment, and retreat. These four tactics can be performed together, but it is vitally important that they be done quickly and efficiently.

Calling for help is self-explanatory. Radio or phone your dispatcher as soon as it is safe for you to do so. Explain the nature of the danger and the help you will need. Be detailed. This will help the responding officers to remain safe and to quickly stabilize the scene. Calling for help also will prevent other units in a tiered response from encountering the same danger you did.

Cover (▶ **Figure 2-5**) is anything that hides your body and provides ballistic protection (protection from bullets). *Concealment* (▶ **Figure 2-6**) is anything that hides your body but does not offer ballistic protection. *Retreat* is rapidly fleeing danger.

You should use these four components as part of a plan for safe escape. For example, you may encounter a patient who becomes violent during your care or a perpetrator who returns to the scene to harm your patient again. Regardless of whether you know that the patient has a firearm, retreat from the scene immediately. While doing so, consider and take positions of cover (preferred) or concealment as you retreat. Do this until you are a considerable and totally safe distance from the danger. Remember that the

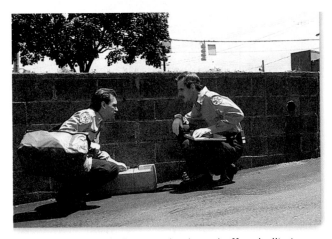

Figure 2-5 Cover hides your body and offers ballistic protection.

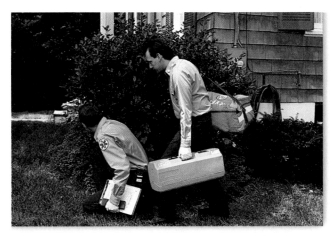

Figure 2-6 Concealment hides your body but offers no ballistic protection.

aggressor may chase you or move toward your position. Radio or call for help when it is safe to do so.

LIFTING AND MOVING

As an experienced AEMT, you have likely lifted and moved many patients. This topic is included here, though, because back injuries are a leading reason that AEMTs are forced to leave EMS. As such, a brief review of safe practices is warranted.

Remember that your brain is involved in the lift. Before moving any patient, be sure to develop a safe strategy for both of you. Consider the following:

- The location and obstacles present
- The weight of the patient
- The capabilities of personnel on scenes

- The device or devices needed
- The patient's condition
- The equipment that will be transported with the patient

Be sure to request extra assistance as soon as you know it will be needed. When you are prepared to lift, remember to follow these guidelines (▶ Figure 2-7):

- Lift with your legs, not your back.
- Place your feet shoulder-width apart and plant them firmly on the ground.
- Be sure you have a firm grip on the item being lifted. As much of your

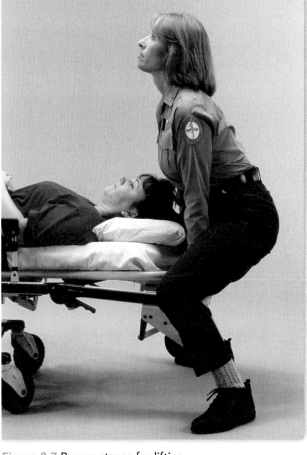

Figure 2-7 Proper stance for lifting.

hand as possible should be on the object.

- Keep the weight you are lifting close to your body.
- Do not reach or twist while lifting, pushing, or pulling.

TRANSITIONING • • • • • • • •

REVIEW ITEMS

1. The technique of "cover" _____.
   a. hides your body
   b. hides your body and offers ballistic protection
   c. offers ballistic protection but doesn't hide your body
   d. can be taken only when outdoors

2. Which of the following is *not* a method by which hepatitis C can be spread?
   a. blood   b. stool
   c. vaginal secretions   d. contaminated needle

3. The most important method to prevent the spread of disease is _____.
   a. hand washing
   b. always wearing protective gloves
   c. knowing the disease status of your patient
   d. wearing full protection on every call

4. Which of the following statements about care in the patient compartment is false?

   a. The patient should be securely strapped in the stretcher with a shoulder harness.

   b. It is the safest place to be in a crash.

   c. Unsecured items will become projectiles in a crash.

   d. The patient may fare better than the EMT in a crash.

5. When lifting a patient, the AEMT's feet should be _____.

   a. together

   b. shoulder-width apart

   c. as wide apart as possible to achieve ground stability

   d. one in front of the other to maintain center of gravity

CRITICAL THINKING

You are called to an 86-year-old patient with abdominal pain. You respond, and after examining the scene, you believe it is safe to enter. You find an alert, responsive patient who is experiencing abdominal pain. She does not appear to have any open wounds, appears to be in generally good health, is not vomiting, and is maintaining both bowel and bladder control.

1. What Standard Precautions are necessary for the following patient assessment and care tasks?

   a. Applying a nasal cannula

   b. Obtaining a radial pulse

   c. Obtaining a blood pressure

   d. Palpating the patient's abdomen

   e. Obtaining a history

The patient tells you she suddenly feels very ill. She becomes only verbally responsive. You hear some loud gurgling sounds coming from her abdomen and suspect she will vomit.

2. What Standard Precautions are necessary based on this new information?

The patient does vomit. Her level of responsiveness has continued to diminish. The patient requires suction.

3. What Standard Precautions are necessary based on this new information?

4. The patient codes and your protocols allow you to insert an advanced airway. What precautions would you take or continue for this procedure?

Standard Preparatory

Competency Applies fundamental knowledge of the EMS system, safety/well-being of the Advanced EMT, and medical/legal and ethical issues to the provision of emergency care.

TOPIC

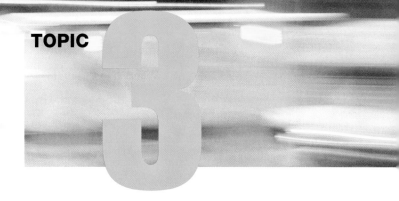

THERAPEUTIC COMMUNICATION

INTRODUCTION

As an Advanced EMT, you must be able to communicate effectively with all the people with whom you come in contact on a call. You must be able to adjust your communication strategies to meet the needs of those to whom you are speaking.

Communication is an active process that incorporates both verbal and nonverbal expressions into messages that are received by others. Many factors, such as age, gender, culture, and experiences, can influence how these messages are sent and interpreted. Effective communication can be used to establish a positive rapport with your patient so you can gain valuable information related to the call. To do this, you must be competent, confident, and compassionate.

TRANSITION *highlights*

● **Review of communication from a process perspective.**

● **Techniques to facilitate communication between individuals.**

● **Insight into communicating with patients from other cultural backgrounds.**

● **Strategies on how to communicate best with difficult patients.**

THE PROCESS OF COMMUNICATION

The process of communication begins when the sender creates and encodes a message based on the information he wants to convey to the receiver. For the receiver to understand the message, it must be decoded (▶ Figure 3-1). The process of decoding can be influenced by the receiver's beliefs, thoughts, perceptions, and values. It is important that the message be decoded accurately to ensure effective communication. The receiver should provide feedback by encoding a message back to the sender about the information that was received. In turn, the feedback should be decoded and interpreted. This exchange of messages and feedback is repeated continually during communication. If there is difficulty in interpreting the messages, communication will be impaired.

You should understand that both you and your patient will bring personal values, perceptions, and

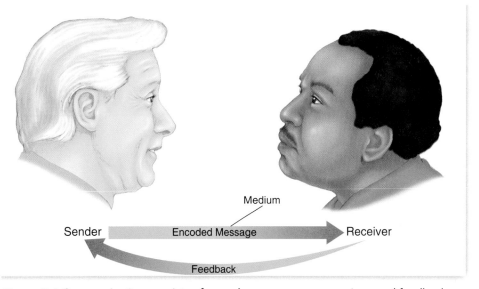

Sender   Encoded Message   Medium   Receiver

Feedback

Figure 3-1 Communication consists of a sender, a message, a receiver, and feedback.

TABLE 3-1	Techniques That May Facilitate Communication
Clarification	Ask more questions to clarify the patient's meaning.
Summary	Rephrase the response and ask whether this is what the patient meant.
Explanation	Present the information in a way the patient can understand.
Silence	Give the patient time to form an appropriate response.
Reflection	Redirect the patient's statements back to him empathetically.
Empathy	Try to understand how the patient feels and has been affected.
Confrontation	Avoid confrontation unless absolutely necessary. Always be respectful and act in the patient's best interest.
Facilitation	Help the patient express himself with the aid of communication devices.

experiences to your communication efforts. Some techniques that may help you facilitate communication with your patient are listed in Table 3-1.

GUIDELINES FOR INITIAL PATIENT CONTACT

As an AEMT, the first impression you give to a patient when you arrive on the scene provides a foundation for the rapport you will continue to develop with the patient. The rapport should be positive and help facilitate your understanding and care for the patient. Some guidelines involving the initial patient contact include the following:

- Dress and behave professionally.
- Introduce yourself and your team.
- Ask the patient how he would like to be addressed.
- Gain consent from the patient for everything you do.
- Be aware of defense mechanisms the patient may use.
- Speak clearly, calmly, and slowly, using a professional tone of voice.
- Respect the patient's privacy.
- Limit interruptions unless they are necessary for emergency care.
- Try to control the environment surrounding the patient.
- Be courteous, compassionate, respectful, and a good listener.

CONDUCTING THE PATIENT INTERVIEW

Conducting a patient interview is an important technique for an AEMT to have and use. When the patient interview is performed effectively, both the AEMT and the patient benefit from the process. The interview is used to gain valuable information about the patient's current problem and helps the AEMT determine an appropriate course of action. Although much of the interview is verbal, it is important for the AEMT to not overlook the nonverbal elements used throughout this process.

Nonverbal Communications

Nonverbal communications can convey valuable information between you and your patient. Nonverbal communication can include your posture, distance, gestures, use of eye contact, facial expressions, and touch. Suggested actions for using nonverbal communication appear in Table 3-2.

Each type of nonverbal communication technique conveys messages to your patient. It is important that you are aware of your patient's responses to nonverbal communications and that you react to them appropriately. Remember that what you *do not* say may be perceived by a patient as more important than what you *do* say.

Interviewing the Patient

When conducting the patient interview, you should use the following guidelines:

- Consider the patient's age and stage of development when asking a question. Use language the patient can understand.
- Ask one question at a time, and wait for a response before continuing.
- Initially, use open-ended questions to gain a detailed response from the patient. It is important to listen to what the patient has to say about the current problem.

TABLE 3-2	Nonverbal Communications
Type of Communication	Suggested Actions
Posture	Approach the patient with open arms, open hands, and relaxed shoulders. Remain at eye level with the patient.
Distance	Be aware of the distance between you and the patient. Ask for permission before entering your patient's personal space or intimate zone. (This rule may vary among cultures.)
Gestures	Be aware of any body movements or facial expressions you make. Watch your patient's facial expression for indications of how he feels.
Eye Contact	Maintain eye contact with the patient.
Haptics	Use touch to help calm the patient. It can convey compassion and empathy if you are sincere (▶ Figure 3-2).

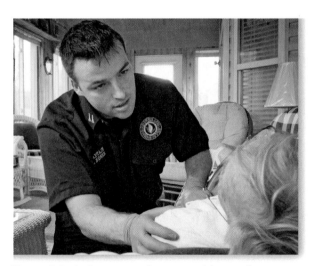

Figure 3-2 A sincere touch can provide comfort to a patient.

- Use closed questions (questions calling for a specific response) to clarify responses and obtain specific information. This type of questioning is also important to use if a patient is unable to respond in full sentences.
- Do not ask biased or leading questions. You may miss important information the patient has to offer, and you may inappropriately influence the patient's responses.
- Do not interrupt when the patient is speaking. Remember, what the patient has to say is important.
- Do not talk so much that you fail to actively listen to what the patient has to say.
- Do not provide false assurance to the patient. Be honest, but remain compassionate.
- Do not give inappropriate advice. Your patients view and value your input as a medical professional. Do not offer any form of diagnosis or discourage the patient from seeing a physician and receiving prompt medical treatment.
- Do not ask "why" questions that imply blame. Remain impartial and nonjudgmental.

TRANSCULTURAL CONSIDERATIONS

Culture is composed of the thoughts, communications, actions, and values of a racial, ethnic, social, or religious group. Both the AEMT and the patient bring their cultural experiences into the professional relationship. It is imperative to avoid ethnocentrism (a belief that one's own cultural group is of the most importance) and to respect the patient's culture. According to Bonita Stanton (2007), the following steps can be used to assist the AEMT in achieving cultural competence:

- Learn to value and understand other cultures, in part through self-awareness of your own cultural values.
- Learn basic fundamentals about other cultures, particularly those of the patients with whom you will interact.
- Develop the ability to apply cultural knowledge in patient encounters.
- Seek exposure to cross-cultural interactions.
- Be motivated to achieve all these steps.

The patient's culture affects how information is received, how illness is viewed, and what treatments are preferred. You should be aware of the sick role the patient may fill as part of his cultural beliefs and any types of folk medicines the patient may have used prior to your arrival. As an AEMT, you should understand that the acceptable use of distance and eye contact varies for different cultures, and you should use nonverbal cues to help guide your actions (▶ Figure 3-3).

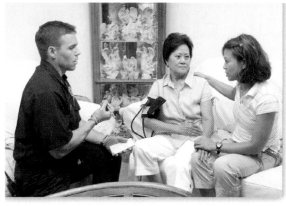

Figure 3-3 An AEMT should try to achieve cultural competence to facilitate communication.

CHALLENGES IN COMMUNICATION

Challenges in communication can come in different forms. As an AEMT, it is important for you to prepare for, rather than avoid, difficult situations that may cause challenges in communication.

Some specific situations that may cause communication challenges include the following:

- **Family preference issues.** Respect the family members' desire to help their loved one. Explain the patient's right to make his own decision if the patient is an adult and can provide informed consent. If it is necessary to use a different facility from the one the patient or family wants, explain kindly why using that particular facility is in the patient's best interest.
- **Motivating an unmotivated patient to talk to you.** Try to establish a good rapport. Make sure the patient understands your questions. Use closed questions if the patient has difficulty answering, or does not answer, your open-ended ones. Provide positive feedback.
- **Hostile patients.** Remember, your safety is paramount. Call for additional assistance if necessary. Advise the patient that you are there to help. Explain the benefits of cooperation. Establish guidelines for appropriate behavior. Conduct the interview as you would for other unmotivated patients.
- **Communicating with children.** Speak in a soft tone and use language that is age appropriate. Speak to children at their eye level. Remember that

children may take what you say literally, so be aware of your phrasing of words. Enlist the help of a parent or guardian when interviewing. Allow the child to have a comfort item if it does not impede care. Be honest about painful procedures.

- **Communicating with elderly patients.** Speak directly with your patient in a normal tone. Raise your voice only when a hearing problem exists. Make sure to give your patient time to respond to the questions you ask. Do not be condescending; show respect.

> It is important for you to prepare for, rather than avoid, difficult situations that may cause challenges in communication.

- **Communicating with patients who have disabilities.** If your patient is deaf, see whether he knows sign language. Use an interpreter if necessary. You can also write notes to obtain information from your patient. When patients have visual impairments, you must explain your actions before they are performed. Patients with cognitive impairments will require you to consider their developmental level in explaining procedures, involving caregivers, and the nature and complexity of the questions you ask.
- **Communicating with patients who do not speak English.** Language differences may be a barrier encountered by the AEMT when on a call. The use of an interpreter may be necessary. Some services and hospitals use a translation service that is available via telephone.

REVIEW ITEMS

1. This communication technique redirects the patient's own statements back to him:
   a. empathy
   b. clarification
   c. reflection
   d. silence

2. Which of the following is an acceptable action when interviewing a patient who does not speak English?
   a. Raise your voice so the patient can hear you.
   b. Address only bystanders for information.
   c. Leave the scene.
   d. Use an interpreter.

3. Cultural experiences and influences are brought to the patient relationship by _____.
   a. the patient only
   b. the AEMT only
   c. neither the patient nor the AEMT
   d. both the patient and the AEMT

4. Immediately following the encoding of a message, _____.
   a. the message should be sent to the receiver
   b. the sender should provide feedback to the receiver
   c. the receiver should give feedback to the sender
   d. the receiver should encode a message to the sender

5. Direct eye contact should be used _____.
   a. to intimidate your patient
   b. to show interest and respect for your patient
   c. regardless of the patient's cultural beliefs

APPLIED KNOWLEDGE

1. List steps an AEMT can take to become more culturally competent.

2. Explain how leading questions can impede effective communication.

3. Explain the process of communication.

4. What communication modifications may be necessary when interviewing a hostile patient?

5. When should an interpreter be used?

6. Why should open-ended questions be used before closed ones when interviewing a patient?

CLINICAL DECISION MAKING

You are called to the residence of a five-year-old male patient for an unknown injury. After determining that the scene is safe, you and your partner approach the residence in uniform with all your equipment. You are met at the door by the patient's mother. You introduce yourself and your partner and indicate that you are there to help.

1. Before entering the residence, what first impressions could you have already made on the mother?

The mother nods and leads you into the kitchen, where you see the child on the floor. There is one man in the room watching you. You ask the mother for her name and her son's name. She says her name is Olga and her son is Giovanni. You note a strong foreign accent when she speaks. As you ask the mother about the reason she called, she appears to have a bewildered look on her face. The woman states she speaks little English.

2. What could you do to help gain the information you need?

The woman turns to the man and says something in a language with which you are not familiar. The man then identifies himself as a neighbor and offers to help. You thank him. He says the mother called him after she called the ambulance. He said that her son cut himself on the hand with a kitchen knife. You look at the child, who is holding his hands together, and note a minimal amount of blood on the outside of his left hand.

3. How should you approach and communicate with this patient? What special considerations should you have when addressing a patient his age?

After completing your primary assessment, you advise the mother that her son should be seen by a physician. You anticipate that stitches will be needed, even though you were easily able to control the bleeding and bandage the wound. You found no other significant findings associated with the patient's current condition. You prepare the child for transport and proceed to the hospital; however, the interpreter cannot accompany you.

4. What techniques will you use to communicate with the patient while en route to the receiving facility? Why should you inform the receiving facility about the communication barrier before your arrival?

REFERENCE

Stanton, B. Cultural issues in pediatric care. In R. M. Kliegman, R. E. Behrman, H. B. Jenson, and B. F. Stanton (eds.), *Nelson Textbook of Pediatrics*, 18th ed. Philadelphia: Saunders Elsevier, 2007, pp. 24–26.

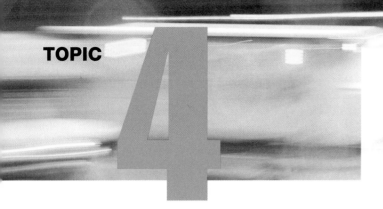

Standard Preparatory

Competency Applies fundamental knowledge of the EMS system, safety/well-being of the Advanced EMT, and medical/legal and ethical issues to the provision of emergency care.

LEGAL ISSUES IN EMS

TRANSITION highlights

- Legal terms commonly associated with pertinent EMS laws and regulations.
- Patient rights as applied to emergency and health care.
- The Advanced EMT's role in organ donation and other special reporting situations.

INTRODUCTION

Legal issues are integrated into every part of each call to which an Advanced EMT responds. They provide a basis for emergency care and serve to protect those who provide and receive the care. As an AEMT, you may be sued despite providing appropriate emergency care; however, if you behave ethically, act within your scope of practice, maintain the standard of care, and complete your documentation properly, your risk of being named in a lawsuit may be reduced. To do this, all EMS personnel must know and understand the laws, regulations, and policies that apply to them.

LEGAL TERMS

Scope of practice. The scope of practice refers to the actions and care that are legally allowed to be performed by the state in which the AEMT is providing emergency medical care. It defines the extent to which an AEMT may provide care and limits what the AEMT may do in response to an emergency. The scope of practice of the AEMT is greater than that of an EMT and contains advanced modalities that come with greater legal risks and ramifications.

Standard of care. The standard of care is the care that is expected to be provided by an AEMT with similar training

managing a patient in a similar situation. It is what a "reasonable person" with the same training in the same area would do for a similar patient. Unlike the scope of practice, which states *what* an AEMT can do, the standard of care focuses on *how* the AEMT does it.

Negligence. Negligence is a tort, or wrongful act, in which the AEMT had no intent to do any harm to the patient but in which a breach in the duty to act and harm have occurred. The plaintiff must prove the following four elements, or the suit will fail:

- The AEMT had a duty to act.
- The AEMT breached that duty to act.
- The patient suffered an injury or harm that is recognized by the law as a compensable injury. This means that by not providing the standard of care, the AEMT caused physical or psychological harm to the patient.
- The injuries were the direct (proximate) result of the breach of the duty. If a patient who files a negligence suit contributed in any manner to his own injury or illness, then the patient may be found guilty of contributory negligence.

Intentional torts. An intentional tort is an action knowingly committed by an individual that is considered to be civilly wrong according to the law. Common intentional torts in EMS include the following:

- *Abandonment* occurs when the treatment of a patient is stopped prior to transferring the care to another competent health care professional of an equal or higher level of training and certification or licensure.
- *Assault* is a willful threat to inflict harm on a patient.
- *Battery* is the act of physically touching a patient unlawfully without the patient's consent.
- *False imprisonment or kidnapping* is the intentional loading and transporting of a competent patient without the patient's consent.
- *Defamation* results when information damaging to a person's character or reputation is released to the public. The spoken form of defamation is slander; the written form is libel.

Duty to act. The concept known as duty to act refers to the AEMT's legal obligation to provide emergency care to a patient. An AEMT who is on duty and comes across an emergency is generally required to stop and provide care. An off-duty AEMT usually does not have the same legal duty to act. Always be sure you are familiar with the laws of your state. If an AEMT responds to an emergency scene and stops to provide emergency care, a duty to act will be created.

Good Samaritan laws. Good Samaritan laws have been developed in all states to provide immunity to individuals trying to help people in emergencies. Most of these laws will grant immunity from liability if the rescuer acts in good faith to provide care unless the actions taken constitute gross negligence. The laws governing private and public providers vary.

Sovereign immunity. Sovereign immunity, or governmental immunity, prevents patients who receive care from governmentally operated EMS services from suing the government for civil liability. Sovereign immunity does not apply to private EMS agencies, and it may not apply to EMS providers as individuals (only to the government agency itself).

Statute of limitations. Statute of limitations refers to the period of time during which an individual may file a negligence claim. The time begins when the injury or illness was caused or when it was first discovered that the problem existed.

Medical direction. Medical direction provides active physician interaction and oversight of the emergency care provided to patients within an EMS system. Because the AEMT acts as an extension of the physician in the field, it is necessary for the AEMT to communicate appropriately and follow the orders and protocols established by medical direction. Medical direction should be contacted whenever a question arises about the scope of practice or the direction of the emergency care.

Ethical behavior. Ethical behavior is expected from every AEMT. Ethics is a branch of philosophy specifically directed toward the study of morals or concepts such as what is right and wrong. All illegal actions are considered unethical. The National Association of Emergency Medical Technicians has issued a Code of Ethics for AEMTs. Some of the ethical responsibilities of all EMS personnel include the following:

- Providing competent and professional emergency care to every patient
- Respecting all persons and their rights
- Maintaining professional knowledge and skill mastery
- Participating in research and improving patient care outcomes
- Upholding all professional standards and conduct
- Reporting events thoroughly and honestly
- Working harmoniously with other health care professionals

PATIENTS' RIGHTS
Privacy and Confidentiality

As an AEMT, it is your responsibility to maintain the privacy and confidentiality of the patient's medical status, history, and records. The Health Insurance Portability and Accountability Act (HIPAA) of 1996 is a federal law that protects the privacy of patient health care information and gives the patient control over how the information is distributed and used. Releasing confidential information requires a written release form signed by the patient or a legal guardian. By law, you are allowed to release confidential patient information without the permission of the patient or the patient's guardian if:

- Another health care provider needs to know the information in order to continue medical care
- An official public health or other governmental agency requires mandatory reporting of information related to your contact with the patient
- You are requested by the police to provide the information as part of a potential criminal investigation

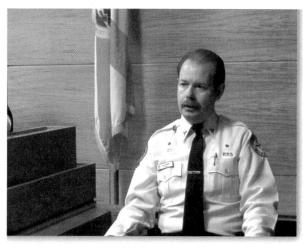

Figure 4-1 An AEMT may be required to testify in court in a variety of legal settings.

- A third-party billing form requires the information
- You are required by legal subpoena to provide the information in court (▶ **Figure 4-1**)

Access to Emergency Care

The Consolidated Omnibus Budget Reconciliation Act (COBRA) and the Emergency Medical Treatment and Active Labor Act (EMTALA) are federal regulations that ensure the public's access to emergency health care regardless of one's ability to pay. The regulations were intended to prevent "patient dumping," in which a patient requiring medical care is turned away or is transferred to a public hospital because of inability to pay for the services.

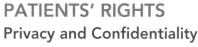

Medical direction should be contacted whenever a question arises about the scope of practice or the direction of the emergency care.

Consent

The conscious, competent, and rational patient has the right to accept or refuse emergency medical care. The patient must be informed of the care to be provided and the associated risks and consequences of receiving or refusing the care. This is referred to as *informed consent*. In addition, expressed consent from the patient must be obtained prior to initiating any care.

In a true emergency when a patient is unresponsive or is not competent, the law assumes that the patient would give consent for the treatment if able to do so. This is referred to as *implied consent*.

Some patients, such as those who are mentally incompetent or incarcerated, may not have the legal right to determine their own medical care. In these cases, it is necessary to gain consent for treatment from the legal authority that makes decisions on the patient's behalf. Minors, unless emancipated, are not considered legally competent to make their own medical decisions. Parental or legal guardian consent is needed before treating minors. If the parent or guardian is not present and cannot be reached, the concept of implied consent is used to initiate care.

With a greater skill set and assessment skills, the AEMT also has additional responsibility when it comes to patient consent and obtaining true informed consent. Although many would agree that the benefits of advanced modalities are significant, there are also greater risks. It is up to you to get the appropriate consent before beginning any care.

Refusing Care

Competent adult patients have the right to refuse emergency care and treatment, even if this may result in death. A patient who displays an altered mental status, is mentally ill (although a history of mental illness alone does not automatically preclude an individual from refusing), or is under the influence of drugs or alcohol may be considered incompetent or incapacitated. Before leaving the scene of a patient refusing care, you must do the following:

- Ensure that the patient is legally competent and is capable of making an informed decision.
- If you are unsure of the patient's competency, contact medical direction.
- If you are required to contact medical direction by protocol, do so.
- Inform the patient of the risks, including the possibility of death, associated with refusing emergency care and transport to a hospital.
- Ask the patient again to accept emergency care or transport.
- If the patient is competent and still refuses, ask him to sign a refusal form.

If possible, have a neutral third party witness the refusal.

- Encourage the patient to call back if he changes his mind or if other symptoms develop.
- Completely, accurately, and thoroughly document all aspects of the call.

Advance Directives

Patients are entitled to express their wishes about the events surrounding their end-of-life treatment and care. *Advance directives* are legal documents that state the patient's preferences about future medical and end-of-life care prior to serious injury or illness. Become familiar with the laws regarding living wills, do not resuscitate orders, and health care proxies for your region or state and the laws and rules governing their implementation.

- **Living wills** are written legal documents that indicate the patient's decision about the use of long-term life support and comfort measures, such as respirators and pain medications.
- **Medical power of attorney** (POA) is a legal document that designates a person, known as a *health care proxy*, to make medical decisions for a patient when the patient is unable to do so.
- **A do not resuscitate** (DNR) order is a written and signed request for health care providers to withhold resuscitative measures (▶ Figure 4-2). A DNR order may indicate a variety of detailed instructions for the AEMT to perform or omit, so it should be obtained and considered before beginning any resuscitative efforts. If the DNR order cannot be located immediately, it is best to err on the side of patient care and perform all resuscitative measures, and then contact medical direction.

You may also hear the term *surrogate decision maker*. This is another term for someone who is allowed to make health care decisions for another individual. This is often done through a *health care proxy* or durable power of attorney, which names someone to make decisions when the patient is incapacitated or incompetent.

Organ Donation

Patients may donate their organs if they sign a document giving permission to

have their organs harvested. If the patient is a potential organ donor, medical direction should be contacted. A patient who is an organ donor should not be treated differently from any other patient requiring emergency care.

Transport

In an emergency, it is important to transport the patient to the closest appropriate medical facility. As an AEMT, you should not bypass a medical facility that is able to treat the patient, unless you are instructed to do so by medical direction or the patient or predetermined protocol. If you bypass a facility, you should document the reason you did so. There are sometimes legitimate reasons to bypass a facility (e.g., if it is not a trauma hospital or stroke center) to provide the patient with appropriate care.

If you are transporting a patient from one facility to another, you should obtain informed consent, receive an accurate patient report, and receive proper documentation from the transferring facility before you place the patient on your cot. You should provide care only within your scope of practice and contact medical direction if any problems occur.

SPECIAL REPORTING SITUATIONS

AEMTs and other health care professionals are required to report certain types of incidents. Know the requirements in your state. Some special reporting situations include the following:

- **Suspected abuse or neglect.** Be careful to report and document the call objectively. Do not make accusations. Provide the proper emergency care to those involved, and follow local protocol. Safe haven laws allow a person who is unwilling or unable to care for a child to drop the child off at any police, fire, or EMS station. Some areas have also expanded this program to include elderly individuals.
- **Potential crime scenes.** The primary purpose for AEMTs at a crime scene is to assess and provide emergency care to the patient. They should attempt to not disturb evidence and should cooperate with other professionals on the scene.

PREHOSPITAL DO NOT RESUSCITATE ORDER

<u>ATTENDING PHYSICIAN</u>

In completing this prehospital DNR form, please check part A if no intervention by prehospital personnel is indicated. Please check Part A and options from Part B if specific interventions by prehospital personnel are indicated. To give a valid prehospital DNR order, this form must be completed by the patient's attending physician and must be provided to prehospital personnel.

A) _____ **Do Not Resuscitate (DNR):**
No Cardiopulmonary Resuscitation or Advanced Cardiac Life Support be performed by prehospital personnel

B) _____ **Modified Support**:
Prehospital personnel administer the following checked options:
_____ Oxygen administration
_____ Full airway support: intubation, airways, bag/valve/mask
_____ Venipuncture: IV crystalloids and/or blood draw
_____ External cardiac pacing
_____ Cardiopulmonary resuscitation
_____ Cardiac defibrillator
_____ Pneumatic anti-shock garment
_____ Ventilator
_____ ACLS meds
_____ Other interventions/medications (physician specify)
_____

Prehospital personnel are informed that (print patient name)_____
should receive no resuscitation (DNR) or should receive Modified Support as indicated. This directive is medically appropriate and is further documented by a physician's order and a progress note on the patient's permanent medical record. Informed consent from the capacitated patient or the incapacitated patient's legitimate surrogate is documented on the patient's permanent medical record. The DNR order is in full force and effect as of the date indicated below.

_____   _____
Attending Physician's Signature

_____   _____
Print Attending Physician's Name   Print Patient's Name and Location
                                             (Home Address or Health Care Facility)

_____
Attending Physician's Telephone

_____   _____
Date   Expiration Date (6 Mos from Signature)

Figure 4-2 Example of a do not resuscitate (DNR) order.

- **Suspected infectious disease exposure.** Certain diseases are tracked by health authorities. You will also be required to report exposures to your employer to receive workers' compensation benefits.

- **Treatment or transport of incapacitated patients or those who are patients against their will.** You will likely be transporting these patients in conjunction with law enforcement or mental health authorities.

- **Dog bites.** Because of the potential for rabies and required isolation periods, many states require reports of dog bites to the appropriate authorities.

REVIEW ITEMS

1. An alert and oriented adult patient initially refuses care and transport. He becomes unconscious before you leave. What type of consent will you have to obtain before emergency care may be provided in his current mental state?
   - a. expressed consent
   - b. implied consent
   - c. informed consent
   - d. false imprisonment

2. An alert and oriented adult patient is complaining of severe abdominal pain. What must be obtained prior to providing emergency care?
   - a. expressed and informed consent
   - b. expressed and implied consent
   - c. informed and implied consent
   - d. implied consent only

3. Which of the following must be proven for negligence?
   - a. There was not a requirement for the AEMT to provide care.
   - b. The AEMT caused the injury.
   - c. The AEMT followed his protocols.
   - d. There was not a breach of duty.

4. Your alert and oriented patient has stated he has a severe phobia of stethoscopes and has asked you and your partner not to use one during your assessment. Immediately following the conversation, your partner removes a stethoscope from the bag and states he is going to auscultate the patient's breath sounds. Which of the following charges could result from this action?
   - a. abandonment
   - b. negligence
   - c. assault
   - d. battery

5. Following the administration of nitroglycerin to an alert and oriented patient complaining of chest pain, you place the patient on the cot to transport her to the hospital. Prior to leaving, the patient states she has changed her mind and does not wish to go to the hospital. If you continue to take her to the hospital, it may result in which of the following charges?
   - a. abandonment
   - b. slander
   - c. kidnapping
   - d. defamation

6. You left your patient in the hallway of the hospital with the nursing assistant. You are guilty of _____.
   - a. assault
   - b. abandonment
   - c. battery
   - d. libel

APPLIED KNOWLEDGE

1. Name the four elements necessary to prove negligence.

2. Explain the difference between implied and expressed consent.

3. Explain why it is important for an AEMT to always behave ethically.

4. What determines an AEMT's standard of care?

5. What can an AEMT do to reduce the chance of being sued?

CLINICAL DECISION MAKING

Your supervisor calls you into her office as soon as you clock in for your morning shift at the station. She introduces you to the company's lawyer and informs you that you have been named in a lawsuit. She states that the plaintiff, Mrs. Smith, was a patient you treated more than three years ago and is now claiming that you were negligent.

1. Based on the scenario, what questions do you have?

2. On how many emergency calls have you been dispatched since that date?

3. Could you recall the specifics of that call based on this information?

4. What would you like to have to refresh your memory?

The lawyer hands you a copy of your run report of the call. As you read over your report, you are still unable to recall any specific details of the call. You look at the document and notice that you left a couple of blanks and misspelled several words on your report.

5. What concerns do you have now?

According to your prehospital care report, your patient was a 68-year-old woman whose daughter called 911 after her mother said she did not feel good. On your arrival, the patient was alert and oriented with no suspected injuries or impairments and refused any assessment or treatment.

6. At this point, what should you have done?

You and your partner attempted to persuade the patient to receive care, informed her of any risks associated with refusal, and contacted medical direction per your protocol. You advised the patient to call back if the symptoms progressed or if she changed her mind. You had her sign a refusal form.

7. What else should have been done?

8. What type of consent was rendered by the patient?

9. If you or your partner treated her at this time, of what would you be guilty?

As you were about to leave, the patient had a syncopal episode.

10. What should you have done next?

11. What type of consent was used? Why?

According to your protocol, you responded appropriately and performed emergency treatments that met the standard of care for your area. You loaded the patient into the ambulance and transported her to the closest hospital. You documented the call thoroughly.

12. Do you believe the plaintiff can prove negligence or kidnapping? Why?

13. Are you concerned about the lawsuit now? Why or why not?

TOPIC

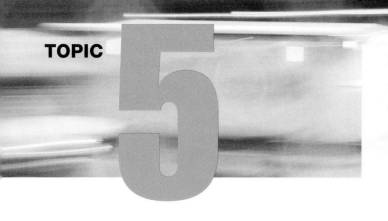

Standard Anatomy and Physiology

Competency Integrates complex knowledge of the anatomy and physiology of the airway, respiratory, and circulatory systems to the practice of EMS.

ANATOMY AND PHYSIOLOGY: CELLULAR METABOLISM

TRANSITION *highlights*

- *Understanding how cellular metabolism relates to the daily activities of the Advanced EMT during assessment and management of patients.*

- *Types of metabolic processes and how they influence the body's structure and function:*
    - *Anabolism.*
    - *Catabolism.*

- *Types of cellular respiration and how these activities can either maintain homeostasis or result in death of the patient:*
    - *Aerobic metabolism.*
    - *Anaerobic metabolism.*

- *Clinical illustration of how understanding metabolism and cellular respiration will better prepare the Advanced EMT to understand and interpret medical and traumatic emergencies in the patient.*

INTRODUCTION

EMS personnel, regardless of their level of certification, have always been taught that the most important aspect of any emergency care provided in the prehospital environment is to establish and maintain an airway, ventilation, oxygenation, and circulation. This fundamental care is aimed at keeping the patient alive until more definitive treatment can be administered through continuing advanced life support further into the call and at a medical facility.

To keep the patient alive, it is necessary to keep the cells alive. Most EMS providers do not think of prehospital care in this manner, but almost every aspect of emergency care provided is geared to keeping cells alive. Most think of the care in a much bigger patient picture such as keeping the patient conscious, relieving chest discomfort, reducing respiratory distress, and

increasing blood pressure. These are all potential indicators of continued or improved cellular function.

As cellular function deteriorates, subtle or obvious indicators in the form of signs and symptoms—such as a decreasing level of consciousness, decreasing blood pressure, motor and sensory deficits, and increasing heart rate—become evident. By understanding the most basic intention of emergency medical care—to keep the cells alive—establishing and maintaining the airway, ventilation, oxygenation, and circulation take on an even greater significance.

This topic is designed to provide the Advanced EMT with a basic understanding of normal cellular metabolism and a deviation from the normal state as it relates to assessment and emergency medical care.

METABOLISM

The cell is the basic functional unit of life. Every person who dies does so at a cellular level, regardless of the presenting injury or illness. A person with a massive traumatic brain injury resulting from a gunshot wound to the head, in which brain tissue is protruding from the skull, eventually dies from cellular dysfunction. The brain injury may have been the precursor to the organ system, organ, tissue, and cellular dysfunction, but it was the individual cell death that led to the patient's death. Thus, to keep a patient alive, the patient's cells must be kept alive.

For a cell to stay alive, it must maintain its metabolism, which requires a constant supply of fuel and oxygen and a normal cellular environment (milieu). The primary cellular fuel source is glucose. Once metabolized, the glucose provides energy for the cell to carry out its normal functions. A lack of glucose and oxygen will create a disturbance to cellular metabolism and may lead to dysfunction and eventual cell death.

Thousands of chemical reactions take place every second in the body and are essential to life. *Metabolism* is described as the sum total of the chemical reactions. Many of these reactions are linked—the product of one metabolic reaction is the impetus to start another set of reactions. Enzymes are special proteins that control these reactions.

Anabolism and Catabolism

The two types of metabolic processes are anabolism and catabolism. *Anabolism* is the process in which larger molecules are made from smaller ones, whereas *catabolism* is the process that breaks down large molecules into smaller ones. Anabolism uses energy and forms water in the process. The material provided is needed for continuous cellular growth and repair. An example of anabolism would be the formation of glycogen from glucose molecules; glycogen is then stored in the liver and other organs for return to the body for later use.

Catabolism requires specific enzymes to break down large molecules into smaller ones. The enzymes use water to split the molecules, and energy is released during the process. Thus, dehydration can have an impact on the effectiveness of catabolism.

The breakdown or energy-releasing reactions (catabolism) must occur at rates that meet the requirements of the reactions that build up or repair cells (anabolism) that are energy consuming. If a disturbance occurs in which the rate of catabolism does not meet the rate of anabolism, cell damage or death will result.

Cellular Respiration

Cellular respiration is the process in which energy is transferred from a glucose molecule and made available for use within the cell. *Oxidation* is the process of breaking down the glucose molecules in the cell. This reaction releases energy and

heat. The energy that is formed is carried as adenosine triphosphate (ATP) molecules that can be used by the cell. ATP is the primary energy-carrying molecule. Think of it as cellular energy that can be transferred to other molecules and allows the cell to work or change its function. An example of such work would be relaxation of bronchiole smooth muscle in response to sympathetic nervous system stimulation.

Without enough ATP, cells will quickly die. Thus, a constant source of energy in the form of ATP is necessary for normal cellular function. In addition, the breakdown of glucose (oxidation) is necessary to maintain body heat. Without an adequate rate of oxidation of glucose molecules in the cells, the body temperature will decrease, eventually leading to hypothermia.

Aerobic Cellular Metabolism

Three distinct but interrelated reactions occur during aerobic cellular metabolism: glycolysis, the citric acid cycle, and the electron transport chain. *Aerobic* refers to the fact that oxygen is available during the later part of the reaction (▶ Figure 5-1).

Lysis refers the splitting apart or disintegration of a substance. *Glyco-* is a prefix that refers to glucose. Thus, *glycolysis* is the breakdown of a glucose molecule. Glycolysis is the first process in cellular respiration, which takes a glucose molecule

that crosses the cell membrane and breaks it down into two pyruvic acid molecules. During this process two ATP (energy) molecules are released, along with high-energy electrons. This process is anaerobic—it does not require oxygen to be present.

The citric acid cycle, also known as the *Krebs cycle*, occurs in the mitochondria of the cell. The pyruvic acid that was produced during glycolysis enters the mitochondria, where carbon dioxide, more high-energy electrons, and more ATP are produced. The high-energy electrons are handed off to the electron transport chain, in which electrons are passed along the chain and energy is transferred to form more ATP.

The final electron carrier is oxygen. With oxygen available, the final by-product of aerobic cellular metabolism is water (H_2O), carbon dioxide (CO_2), a large amount of energy (32 to 34 molecules of ATP), and heat. The ATP, water, and heat are necessary for normal cell function; the carbon dioxide is passed to the blood and transported to the lungs, where it is eliminated during exhalation.

Anaerobic Cellular Metabolism

Anaerobic cellular metabolism refers to cellular respiration that occurs without the availability of oxygen (▶ Figure 5-2).

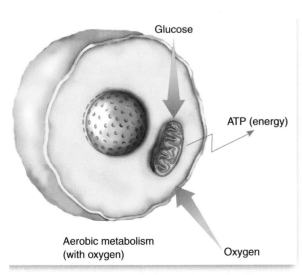

Figure 5-1 Aerobic metabolism. Glucose broken down in the presence of oxygen produces a large amount of energy (ATP).

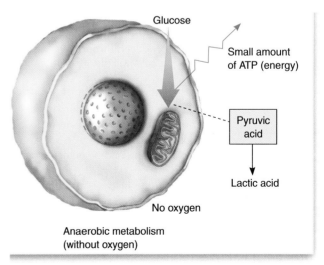

Figure 5-2 Anaerobic metabolism. Glucose broken down without the presence of oxygen produces pyruvic acid, which converts to lactic acid and only a small amount of energy (ATP). A lack of glucose and oxygen will create a disturbance to cellular metabolism and may lead to dysfunction and eventual cell death. Cell dysfunction and death lead to organ dysfunction. When a critical mass of cells dies within an organ, the organ itself then dies.

Sodium/Potassium Pump

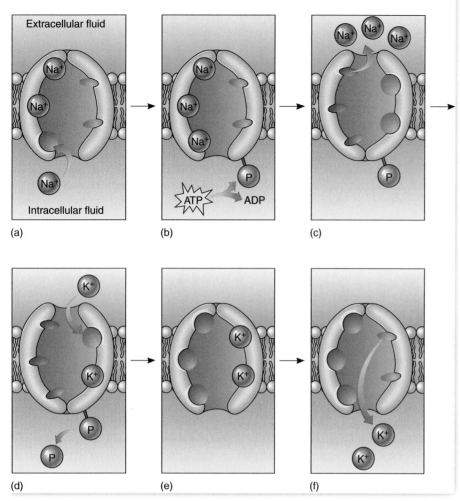

(a)   (b)   (c)

(d)   (e)   (f)

Figure 5-3 The sodium/potassium pump. Energy (ATP) is required to pump sodium (Na$^+$) molecules out of the cell against the concentration gradient. Potassium (K$^+$) then moves with the gradient to flow into the cell. Sodium and potassium are exchanged in a continuous cycle, which is necessary for proper cell function. The cycle continues as long as the cells produce energy through aerobic metabolism. When insufficient energy is produced through anaerobic metabolism, the sodium/potassium pump will fail, and cells will die.

Glycolysis does not require oxygen; thus, the process still occurs but produces only a very small amount of energy (two molecules of ATP), high-energy electrons, and two pyruvic acid molecules.

Without oxygen available in the mitochondria for the next reaction to occur, however, hydrogen molecules and the electrons are given back to the pyruvic acid, which then forms lactic acid. Lactic acid builds up within the cell, which inhibits glycolysis and leads to a further reduction in the already minimal production of ATP. The cell lacks the necessary ATP (energy) for normal function, and the environment becomes acidotic. The acid inactivates enzymes necessary to control the metabolic reactions and disrupts the cell membrane. If the integrity of the cell membrane is lost, the cell will die. The lactic acid will also diffuse out of the cell and enter the blood, making it acidotic as well.

Sodium/Potassium Pump

The primary intracellular (inside the cell) ion is potassium (K$^+$), and the primary extracellular (outside the cell) ion is sodium (Na$^+$). The cell membrane is less permeable to sodium ions than to potassium ions; thus, the sodium ions have a tendency to stay inside the cell. Sodium has an osmotic effect and draws water. If the sodium were allowed to stay inside the cell, the cell would eventually take on too much water, and the membrane would rupture (lyse), killing the cell.

The *sodium/potassium pump* exchanges three sodium molecules from inside the cell for two potassium molecules located outside the cell. This exchange maintains a normal balance of sodium and potassium and prevents the cell from swelling and rupturing (▶ Figure 5-3).

The Na$^+$/K$^+$ pump is an active process and requires energy to function. The energy is in the form of ATP. If ATP is not available, the pump does not function properly and allows Na$^+$ to collect inside the cell. Where sodium goes, water follows it. Therefore, the sodium draws water into the cell, where it causes it to swell, eventually rupturing the membrane and killing the cell.

CLINICAL APPLICATION OF CELLULAR METABOLISM

For cells to have normal function, an adequate amount of glucose and oxygen must be continuously delivered to them. With adequate delivery, high amounts of cellular energy (ATP), water, heat, and carbon dioxide are produced. The energy is used by the cell to carry out its function, such as muscular contraction or secretion of a hormone. The heat is used to maintain a normal body core temperature. The water is necessary for metabolic processes to occur. The carbon dioxide is transported by the blood and blown off during exhalation.

A lack of glucose and oxygen delivery results in inadequate energy production, a buildup of lactic acid, and a reduction in body heat. The cells may not have enough energy to carry out their normal function, such as forceful muscular contraction or the release of hormones from an endocrine gland. If ATP is not available to fuel the Na$^+$/K$^+$ pump, Na$^+$ stays inside the cell, draws water, causes the cell to swell, and eventually causes the membrane to rupture, leading to cell death.

Cell dysfunction and death lead to organ dysfunction. When a critical mass of cells dies within an organ, the organ itself first fails in its function, and then dies. This results ultimately from inadequate glucose and oxygen getting to cells.

Shock is defined as inadequate tissue perfusion. The inadequate perfusion refers directly to the lack of delivery of adequate amounts of oxygen and glucose to cells. If shock prevails, cells eventually die. A major sign of poor perfusion is altered mental status. The lack of oxygen and glucose delivery to the brain cells from poor perfusion—a direct result of the lack of ATP production and the buildup of lactic acid—leads to cerebral cell dysfunction. If the Na^+/K^+ pump fails because of inadequate ATP availability, brain cells begin to rupture and die.

Treatment of Shock

You arrive on the scene of an accident and find two traumatized patients. One is screaming, kicking, and pulling at you when you approach him. He is complaining of excruciating pain to his left humerus, which is fractured and protruding through the skin. His friend is lying quietly, is lethargic, and is not complaining. Which patient would you tend to first?

Most EMS providers would select the second patient. It takes a large amount of energy to kick, scream, and complain; thus, this patient likely has adequate amounts of oxygen and glucose being delivered to his cells. However, his friend has little energy to move or complain. It is likely that his lack of energy is a result of poor ATP energy production from anaerobic metabolism caused by inadequate perfusion of the cells (including the brain) with oxygen and glucose. He is much more likely to be in a shock state than the screaming patient is.

One of the basic principles of shock treatment is to keep the patient warm, even when the ambient temperature is considered hot. Why is hypothermia a problem for the shock patient? It takes energy to maintain normal body temperature and body function. This energy is not available when the patient is in shock. Shock results in the inadequate delivery of oxygen and glucose to cells, which leads to anaerobic metabolism. Aerobic metabolism produces a large amount of heat as a by-product, whereas anaerobic metabolism produces little heat, resulting in a decrease in the body core temperature. Hypothermia can ensue if the shock state is severe and of a longer duration.

Emergency care of a patient—including airway management, ventilation, oxygenation, bleeding control, administration of glucose and other medication, chest compressions, administration of fluids, and many other treatments—is geared to maintaining an adequate delivery of oxygen and glucose to cells. Lack of either substance may lead to cell, tissue, and organ dysfunction and, ultimately, death.

TRANSITIONING

REVIEW ITEMS

1. If glycolysis were the only component of cellular metabolism occurring, you would expect_____.
   a. excessive production of carbon dioxide
   b. the patient to exhibit little energy
   c. a minimal amount of lactic acid production
   d. the patient to have an increased body core temperature

2. A sudden increase in aerobic cellular metabolism would likely result in _____.
   a. pale, cool skin
   b. hypotension
   c. tachypnea
   d. bradycardia

3. A lack of the production of ATP would likely lead to _____.
   a. the movement of sodium ions out of the cell
   b. cell dehydration and shrinkage
   c. an increase in cellular activity
   d. cellular swelling and rupture of the membrane

4. The shock patient is at risk of becoming hypothermic because of _____.
   a. dysfunction of the sodium/potassium pump
   b. an increase in lactic acid production
   c. a decrease in glycolysis and aerobic metabolism
   d. an excessive amount of circulating carbon dioxide

5. What must be available in adequate amounts to reverse anaerobic metabolism and restore aerobic metabolism in the cell?
   a. carbon dioxide
   b. pyruvic acid
   c. potassium
   d. oxygen

APPLIED PATHOPHYSIOLOGY

1. Explain the difference between anabolism and catabolism.

2. Explain the difference between aerobic and anaerobic metabolism to include cellular by-products.

3. Describe the differences in how the patient with systemic anaerobic metabolism would present, as compared with the patient with aerobic metabolism.

4. List and explain the three distinct and interrelated reactions of aerobic metabolism.

5. Which of the reactions are common to both aerobic and anaerobic metabolism?

6. How much cellular energy production would occur in a patient who had glucose delivery to cells but no oxygen?

7. Explain why glucose is necessary to maintain normal movement of sodium and potassium in and out of the cell.

CLINICAL DECISION MAKING

You arrive on the scene and find a 26-year-old male patient who has been stabbed in the abdomen. A large pool of blood is on the ground near the patient. The patient is not alert and moans in response to a trapezius pinch. His airway is partially occluded with blood and vomit. His respirations are shallow and rapid. His skin is extremely pale, cool, and clammy.

1. After ensuring scene safety, what is your first immediate action on approaching this patient?

2. What are the life threats to this patient?

3. If his airway remains occluded, how would his metabolism be affected?

4. Why is this patient prone to hypothermia?

5. What does the pale, cool, and clammy skin indicate?

6. Why is the patient presenting with an altered mental status?

7. Based on the patient's presentation, what would you expect his cellular ATP production to be?

8. Why is this patient prone to acidosis?

Standard Medical Terminology

Competency Uses foundational anatomical and medical terms and abbreviations in written and oral communication with colleagues and other health care professionals.

TOPIC

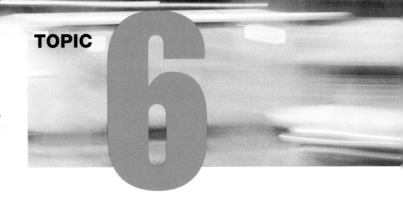

MEDICAL TERMINOLOGY

INTRODUCTION

Medical terminology is the language of health care. As an Advanced EMT, it is important that you establish a basic under-standing of medical terminology so you may communicate effectively with other professionals on the health care team. Although we adjust our communication styles for our patients, as health care professionals we should use proper medical terminology when addressing others on the health care team and when documenting patient care reports (▶ Figure 6-1).

> **Medical terminology is the language of health care.**

TRANSITION *highlights*

- *Review of what comprises a medical term:*
  - Prefix.
  - Suffix.
  - Combining form.
- *Comprehensive list of common medical terms with their definitions.*

MEDICAL TERM ORIGINS

At first glance, many medical terms may appear difficult to read, understand, or pronounce. One reason for this is because most medical terms are derived from Greek and Latin origins, with which we may not be very familiar. But if you know the common parts that compose the term, the words can become easier to understand and interpret.

To do this, it is necessary to memorize commonly encountered prefixes, suffixes, and combining forms. Many medical terms get their meaning from the anatomical structures, organs, and systems with which they are associated.

STRUCTURE OF MEDICAL TERMS

Most medical terms have three basic components: prefix, combining form, and suffix. The *combining form* is the subject or foundation of the word that gives the word its essential meaning.

Each combining form is composed of two parts: a root and a combining vowel. The *root* is the part of the term that pro-vides the foundation for the rest of the term. Combining vow-els are joined to the end of a root to connect the root to another root or to a suffix. Combining vowels make the word easier to pronounce. The most common combining vowel is *o*, followed by *i*. A combining vowel is not used if the suffix begins with a vowel.

Some medical terms may contain more than one combining form. For example, the term *cardiovascular* has two combining forms: cardi/o (heart) and vascul/o (vessel).

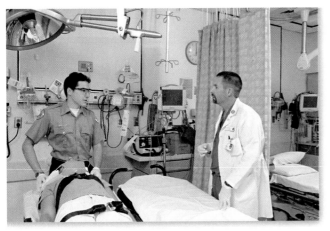

Figure 6-1 Use proper medical terminology to communicate with other health care professionals.

combining form + combining form + suffix

cardi/o + vascul/o + -ar

The *suffix* is the term located at the end of the word. It modifies the root and gives it an additional meaning. In this topic, suffixes appear with a hyphen in front of them, indicating that another term, usually a root, should precede them. For example, the suffix *-itis* means inflammation. The term *conjunctivitis* can be broken into the combining form *conjunctiv/o* followed by the suffix *-itis*. When the suffix is added to the root meaning conjunctiva, the term then refers to inflammation of the conjunctiva.

combining form + suffix

conjunctiv/o + -itis

(conjunctiva) + (inflammation)

A *prefix* is a term that begins the word. It is also used to modify the root. Some terms may not have a prefix, so it important to memorize which terms are roots and which are prefixes. Throughout this topic, prefixes appear with a hyphen after them, indicating that another term, usually a root word, should follow it. For example, the prefix *a-* means without. In the word *apnea*, the root *pne(a)* means breathing. By adding the prefix *a-* to the word, a specific modification has been made, and the meaning is changed to "without breathing."

prefix + combining form + suffix

a- + pne/o + -a

(without) + (breathing) + (condition)

HOW TO READ AND DEFINE MEDICAL TERMS

As in other words in English, medical terms are read from left to right. If a term has a prefix, it will be read first and will be followed by the combining form(s) and then the suffix (if one is present). For example, the term *hyperglycemia* contains the prefix *hyper-*, the combining form *glyc/o*, and the suffix *-emia*.

prefix + combining form + suffix

hyper- + glyc/o + -emia

(above or excessive) + (sugar) + (blood condition)

Many medical terms can be defined by determining the meaning of their parts. Unlike the method for reading the term, the definition is derived by determining the meaning of the suffix first, then the prefix, and finally the combining form(s). So in the preceding example of *hyperglycemia*, the meaning is derived from the suffix *-emia* (meaning blood condition), then the prefix *hyper-* (meaning above or excessive), followed by the combining form *glyc/o* (meaning glucose or sugar). So the meaning of the term *hyperglycemia* would be a blood condition that has an excessive amount of glucose (sugar) in it.

ACCEPTED MEDICAL TERMS AND ABBREVIATIONS

The meaning of every accepted medical term is not derived from the sum of its parts alone. Because of this, it is important for an AEMT to have access to a professional medical dictionary and use it appropriately. Throughout your medical career, you will continue to develop your vocabulary and use many medical terms in your documentation. Sometimes it will be more convenient to use an accepted medical abbreviation or symbol in your report instead of writing the entire term (▶ Figure 6-2).

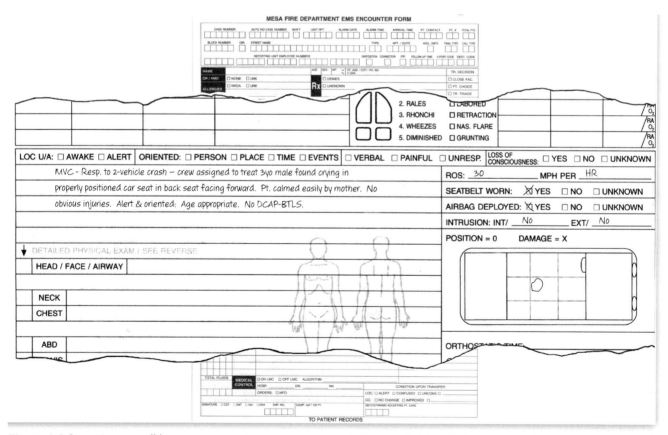

Figure 6-2 Sometimes it will be more convenient to use an accepted medical abbreviation or symbol in your report instead of writing the entire term.

It is important to understand that abbreviations can have more than one meaning and that you should use only those that are approved for use in your organization. The Joint Commission has published an official "do not use" list of abbreviations that should not be used in your documentation (www.jointcommission.org/patientsafety/donotuselist).

COMMON PREFIXES, SUFFIXES, AND COMBINING FORMS

Common prefixes, suffixes, and combining forms are depicted in Tables 6-1, 6-2, and 6-3, respectively. These tables are not all-inclusive, however.

TABLE 6-1 Common Prefixes in Medical Terms

Prefix	Meaning	Prefix	Meaning	Prefix	Meaning
a- , an-	without	en-, endo-	within	para-	alongside
ab-	away from	epi-	upon	peri-	around
ad-	to; toward, or near	eu-	good or normal	poly-	many
ante-	before	hemi-	half	post-	after or behind
anti-	against	hyper-	above or excessive	pre-, pro-	before
bi-	two or both	hypo-	below or deficient	quadr/i-	four
brady-	slow	infra-	below or deficient	sub-	below or deficient
circum-	around	inter-	between	super-, supra-	above or excessive
con-	together or with	intra-	within	tachy-	fast
contra-	against	macro-	large	uni-	one
de-	from, down, or not	micro-	small		
dys-	painful, difficult, or faulty	mono-	one		

TABLE 6-2 Common Suffixes in Medical Terms

Suffix	Meaning	Suffix	Meaning	Suffix	Meaning
-a,	condition of	-iatrics, -iatry	treatment	-otomy	cutting or separation
-ac, -al, -ar, -ary	pertaining to	-ic	pertaining to	-ous	pertaining to
-acusis	hearing	-ism	condition of	-plasty	surgical repair or reconstruction
-algia,	pain	-itis	inflammation	-plegia	paralysis
-arche	beginning	-ium	structure or tissue	-pnea	breathing
-ation	process	-lepsy	seizure	-rrhage, -rrhagia	to burst forth
-cele	pouching or hernia	-logist	one who specializes in the study of	-rrhea	discharge
-centesis	puncture for aspiration	-logy	study of	-scope	instrument for examination
-dynia	pain	-lysis	breakdown or dissolution	-scopy	process of examination
-eal	pertaining to	-malacia	softening	-spasm	involuntary contraction
-ectomy	excision	-megaly	enlargement	-stomy	creation of an opening
-emesis	vomiting	-meter	instrument for measuring	-tic	pertaining to
-emia	blood condition	-oma	tumor	-tomy	incision
-gram	record	-osis	condition or increase	-tripsy	crushing
-graphy	process of recording			-y	condition or process of
-ia	condition of				

TABLE 6-3   Common Combining Forms in Medical Terms

Related to the Cardiovascular System

Combining Form	Meaning
angi/o	vessel
aort/o	aorta
arteri/o	artery
ather/o	fatty paste
atri/o	atrium
cardi/o	heart
phleb/o	vein
sphygm/o	pulse
vas/o, vascul/o	vessel
ven/o	vein
ventricul/o	ventricle

Related to the Endocrine and Immune Systems

Combining Form	Meaning
aden/o	gland
adren/o, adrenal/o	adrenal gland
crin/o	to secrete
gluc/o, glyc/o	sugar
hormon/o	hormone
immune/o	safe
ket/o, keton/o	ketone bodies
pancreat/o	pancreas
thalm/o	thalamus
thym/o	thymus gland or mind
thyr/o, thyroid/o	thyroid gland

Related to the Eyes and Ears

Combining Form	Meaning
acous/o, audi/o	hearing
aque/o	water
aur/i	ear
blephar/o	eyelid
cerumen/o	wax
conjunctiv/o	conjunctiva
corne/o	cornea
kerat/o	cornea
myring/o	eardrum
ocul/o	eye
ot/o	ear
retin/o	retina
tympan/o	eardrum

Related to the Gastrointestinal System

Combining Form	Meaning
abdomin/o	abdomen
an/o	anus
appendic/o	appendix
bil/i	bile
bucc/o	cheek
celi/o	abdomen
chol/e	bile
col/o, colon/o	colon
duoden/o	duodenum
enter/o	small intestine
esophag/o	esophagus
gastr/o	stomach
hepat/o, hepatic/o	liver
herni/o	hernia
lapar/o	abdomen
or/o	mouth
peritone/o	peritoneum
phag/o	eat or swallow
proct/o	anus and rectum
rect/o	rectum
splen/o	spleen
stomat/o	mouth

Related to the Integumentary System

Combining Form	Meaning
adip/o	fat
cutane/o	skin
derm/o, dermat/o	skin
hist/o, histi/o	tissue
lip/o	fat
onych/o	nail
seb/o	oil
steat/o	fat
trich/o	hair

Related to the Musculoskeletal System

Combining Form	Meaning
ankyl/o	crooked or stiff
arthr/o, articulo	joint
brachi/o	arm
cephal/o	head
cervic/o	neck
chondr/o	cartilage
cost/o	rib
crani/o	skull
femor/o	femur
kyph/o	humped back
lord/o	bent
lumb/o	lower back
my/o, muscul/o, myos/o	muscle
oste/o	bone
patell/o	patella
pector/o	chest
pelv/i	pelvis
pod/o	foot
radi/o	radius or radiation
stern/o	sternum
steth/o	chest
ten/o, tend/o, tendin/o	tendon
thorac/o	chest
uln/o	ulna
vertebr/o	vertebra

Related to Neurology/Psychology

Combining Form	Meaning
cerebell/o	cerebellum
cerebr/o	cerebrum
encephal/o	entire brain
esthesi/o	sensation
mening/o, meningi/o	meninges
myel/o	bone marrow or spinal cord
neur/o	nerve
phas/o	speech
phob/o	exaggerated fear or sensitivity
phon/o	voice or sound
phren/o	diaphragm or mind
psych/o	mind
schiz/o	split or division

Related to the Reproductive System

Combining Form	Meaning
andr/o	man
balan/o	glans penis
colp/o	vagina
gynec/o	woman

Related to the Reproductive System

Combining Form	Meaning
hyster/o	uterus
mamm/o, mast/o	breast
metr/o	uterus
men/o	menstruation
oophor/o	ovary
orch/o, orchid/o	testis (testicle)
ovari/o	ovary
test/o	testis (testicle)
uter/o	uterus
vagin/o	vagina

Related to the Respiratory System

Combining Form	Meaning
aer/o	air or lung
alveol/o	alveolus (air sac)
bronch/o, bronchi/o	bronchus (airway)
bronchiol/o	bronchiole (little airway)
capn/o, carb/o	carbon dioxide
laryng/o	larynx
lob/o	lobe

nas/o	nose
pharyng/o	pharynx
pleur/o	pleura
pne(a)/o	breathing
pneum/o, pneumon/o	air or lung
pulmon/o	lung
rhin/o	nose
sinus/o	hollow
trache/o	trachea

Related to the Urinary System

Combining Form	Meaning
cyst/o	bladder or sac
glomerul/o	glomerulus (small ball)
lith/o	stone
nephr/o	kidney
ren/o	kidney
ur/o, urin/o	urine
ureter/o	ureter
urethr/o	urethra
vesic/o	bladder or sac

Other Common Combining Forms

Combining Form	Meaning
carcin/o	cancer
chrom/o, chromat/o	color
chyl/o	juice
cyan/o	blue
cyt/o	cell
diaphor/o	profuse sweating
dips/o	thirst
erythr/o	red
hem/o, hemat/o	blood
hydr/o	water
leuk/o	white
lingu/o	tongue
lymph/o	lymph
melan/o	black
necr/o	death
ox/o	oxygen
path/o	disease
purpur/o	purple
somat/o	body
thromb/o	clot
tox/o, toxic/o	toxic
xanth/o	yellow

TRANSITIONING

REVIEW ITEMS

1. A patient presents with hypotension. Based on the prefix in the term, you should suspect the patient's blood pressure to be _____.
   a. above normal
   b. below normal
   c. faster than usual
   d. slower than usual

2. You are called to the residence of a patient in respiratory distress. Dispatch advises the patient has recently had a tracheostomy. Based on this information, you expect to find a(n)_____.
   a. tube surgically placed in the stomach
   b. incision into the lungs
   c. artificial opening in the trachea
   d. excision of a lobe in the lungs

3. The term referring to the sac surrounding the heart is _____.
   a. myocardium
   b. pericardium
   c. epicardium
   d. endocardium

4. Which of the following terms refers to difficulty swallowing?
   a. parenteral
   b. esophagitis
   c. dysphagia
   d. dysphasia

5. A patient is vomiting blood. When documenting this finding, you should use the term _____.
   a. hematemesis
   b. rhinorrhea
   c. hematuria
   d. diarrhea

APPLIED KNOWLEDGE

1. If a patient has neuralgia, what body system is affected?

2. What does the term *subcutaneous* mean?

3. In what area does a gastroenterologist specialize?

4. If a patient has bradycardia, what does that mean?

5. Where are the suprarenal glands located?

CLINICAL DECISION MAKING

You are called to a nursing home for a 74-year-old male patient complaining of abdominopelvic pain. On arrival, the nurse informs you that the patient has had hematemesis, hematuria, and diarrhea that morning. According to the nurse, the patient has a colostomy and has recently had a suprapubic catheter inserted. The nurse states that the patient has a history of gastrointestinal reflux disease, colitis, acute renal failure, hypertension, diabetes, and a previous cerebral vascular attack with residual dysphasia.

1. Based on your knowledge of medical terminology, translate the medical terms and rewrite the preceding passage using common language.

You arrive at a residence of a 68-year-old female patient. As you approach your patient, she tells you she is "not feeling right." You begin to obtain a history and perform your assessment. You discover that she has low blood sugar, high blood pressure, a slow heart rate, difficulty breathing, chest pain, profuse sweating, and a bluish color around her lips. You also find that she had her left lung removed about two years ago. She has had regular checkups by her heart and lung doctor.

2. Based on your understanding of medical terminology, rewrite the passage using professional medical terminology.

Standard Pathophysiology

Competency Applies comprehensive knowledge of the pathophysiology of respiration and perfusion to patient assessment and management.

TOPIC

7

AMBIENT AIR, AIRWAY, AND MECHANICS OF VENTILATION

INTRODUCTION

Perfusion is the constant delivery of oxygen and glucose to cells and the adequate elimination of carbon dioxide and other waste products. To maintain adequate perfusion, the following components associated with the airway, ventilation, oxygenation, and circulation must work properly:

- Composition of ambient air
- Patency of the airway
- Mechanics of ventilation
- Regulation of ventilation
- Ventilation/perfusion ratio
- Transport of oxygen and carbon dioxide by the blood
- Blood volume
- Effectiveness of the pump function of the myocardium
- Systemic vascular resistance
- Microcirculation
- Blood pressure

A disturbance in any one of these components could lead to poor perfusion with a resultant inadequate delivery of oxygen and glucose to cells or an ineffective elimination of carbon dioxide and other waste products. For example, a heroin overdose patient has an occluded airway from excessive relaxation of the muscles controlling the tongue. This blocks the flow of air into the airway and subsequently into the alveoli, thereby limiting the amount of oxygen available for gas exchange. This reduces the amount of oxygen attached to hemoglobin in the blood, thereby reducing the amount of oxygen molecules available for offloading to cells.

Inadequate oxygen causes the cell to become hypoxic and switch to anaerobic metabolism. Anaerobic metabolism reduces ATP production, changes the effective function of the cell, and begins producing mass amounts of lactic acid, further reducing ATP production. If this continues, the cell will eventually dysfunction and die.

COMPOSITION OF AMBIENT AIR

The amount of oxygen in the ambient air will determine the concentration of oxygen breathed in by the patient, which in turn determines the amount reaching the alveoli for gas exchange.

TRANSITION highlights

- Gas composition in the ambient air, and how disturbances in this can have an ill effect on the metabolic processes of the body.

- Structure, function, and importance of the airway.

- Determinants of normal ventilation and alveolar ventilation.

- Ventilator components and how they pertain to cellular oxygenation:
  - Muscles used for breathing.
  - Airway resistance.
  - Airway compliance.
  - Pleural linings and cavity.

- Adequate and inadequate ventilation and the need to provide artificial ventilation.

A decrease in the concentration of oxygen in ambient air will directly reduce the amount of oxygen available for cell use.

Ambient air at sea level contains approximately 79 percent nitrogen, 21 percent oxygen, 0.9 percent argon, and 0.03 percent carbon dioxide. The partial pressures of the gases (see Table 7-1) play an important role in oxygenation and are discussed later.

Oxygen therapy is designed to increase the concentration of oxygen breathed in by the patient. By doing so, more oxygen is made available in the alveoli for gas exchange, and ultimately more oxygen is offloaded at the level of the cell. Therefore, cellular hypoxia (deficiency of oxygen reaching the tissues of the body) may be reversed or lessened by increasing the percentage of oxygen the patient breathes.

The concentration of oxygen breathed in by the patient is commonly referred to as the *fraction of inspired oxygen*, or the FiO_2. The FiO_2 is expressed as a fraction or decimal, not a percentage. Thus, at sea level the person would be inhaling

TABLE 7-1	Percentage and Partial Pressures of Gases in Ambient Air at Sea Level	
Gas	Percentage	Partial Pressure
Oxygen	21	159 mmHg
Nitrogen	79	597 mmHg
Argon	0.9	7 mmHg
Carbon dioxide	0.03	0.3 mmHg

21 percent oxygen, which would be expressed as an FiO_2 of 0.21.

A change in the composition of ambient air can lead to hypoxia. In some cases, it is severe enough to cause sudden death. A toxic gas can displace the oxygen and suffocate the patient. Other gases, such as carbon monoxide, may disrupt the ability of the blood to carry oxygen. Carbon monoxide will preferentially attach to hemoglobin over oxygen; thus, the red blood cells will become saturated with carbon monoxide and not oxygen.

Some toxic gases, such as cyanide, interfere with cells' ability to use the delivered oxygen. Other toxic gases may destroy lung tissue and impede gas exchange at the level of the alveoli. Regardless of the etiology or the gas, the cells become hypoxic and may eventually die.

> **If the epiglottis fails to function properly, the patient may aspirate substances into the trachea and lungs.**

PATENCY OF THE AIRWAY

One of the most basic and important steps in emergency care is to establish and maintain an open airway. Blood, vomitus, secretions, tissue, bone, teeth, food, and other substances may occlude the airway. However, one of the most common causes of an occluded airway is a result of the relaxation of the muscles controlling the mandible. This will allow the tongue to fall back into the pharynx and block the flow of air into the airway.

An airway obstruction can occur at several anatomic levels. An upper airway obstruction refers to occlusion in any structure above the trachea, whereas a lower airway obstruction is an occlusion to a structure below the larynx (▶ Figure 7-1).

Nasopharynx

Secretions, blood, vomitus, tissue swelling, bone fragments, and inserted foreign objects are causes of an occlusion of the nasopharynx. Blockage of this structure does not typically cause a major airway problem if the oropharynx remains clear. However, the substance, such as blood or vomitus, in the nasopharynx can drain down into the pharynx, causing the patient to aspirate or develop an occlusion in a distal airway structure. Thus, it is important to keep the nasopharynx clear.

Oropharynx and Pharynx

The oropharynx is the oral cavity that contains the tongue. The pharynx is distal to the oropharynx. The oropharynx and pharynx can become obstructed by foreign objects, the tongue, swelling of the tissue, hematomas, infection, food, blood, vomitus, and many other substances. Liquid substances may lead to aspiration, which may interfere with gas exchange at the level of the alveoli. Solid substances, such as the tongue, will block airflow mechanically, leading to a reduction of air entering the alveoli. In both cases, the decrease in oxygen exchange at the level of the alveoli will result in cellular hypoxia.

Epiglottis

The epiglottis is a flap of cartilaginous tissue that covers the opening of the larynx, known as the *glottic opening*, during swallowing. If the epiglottis fails to function properly, the patient may aspirate substances into the trachea and lungs. If injured or infected, the epiglottis may swell and occlude the glottic opening. Relaxation of the muscles controlling the mandible may also cause the flexible epiglottis to fall forward, occluding the glottic opening. The epiglottis can be lifted off the laryngeal opening by pulling the mandible forward when performing a chin lift or jaw thrust. Advanced airway adjuncts may be required to reverse obstruction of the epiglottis caused by swelling.

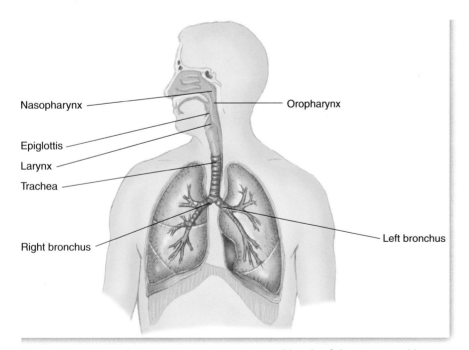

Nasopharynx
Oropharynx
Epiglottis
Larynx
Trachea
Right bronchus
Left bronchus

Figure 7-1 Airway obstruction can occur at several levels of the upper and lower airway, including the nasopharynx, oropharynx, posterior pharynx, epiglottis, larynx, trachea, and bronchi.

Larynx

The larynx is the structure in the upper airway that contains the vocal cords. The larynx can be obstructed by laryngeal spasm, also known as *laryngospasm*. This occurs when the vocal cords close together tightly, which prevents air from passing through the larynx and into the trachea. Injury, insertion of an airway, or some medications may cause laryngeal spasm. Laryngeal fracture or swelling may also cause obstruction of airflow into the trachea.

Trachea, Bronchi, and Bronchioles

Distal to the larynx is the trachea, which extends downward until it branches into the right and left main stem bronchi at the carina, which is located at the level of the second intercostal space anteriorly or the fourth thoracic vertebra posteriorly. The trachea is composed of C-shaped anterior cartilaginous rings and a posterior wall consisting of soft muscle.

The bronchi continue to branch into *bronchioles*. The terminal bronchioles end with alveolar sacs that contain alveoli. The alveolus is the site of gas exchange with blood.

Obstruction of the trachea, bronchi, and bronchioles can occur from food, objects, blood, vomitus, tissue swelling, bone, and other substances. The bronchioles can also be occluded from the constriction and spasm of the smooth muscle lining their walls. Blockage of the trachea, bronchi, or bronchioles reduces the flow of air into the alveoli and decreases gas exchange with the blood, which may lead to cellular hypoxia.

MECHANICS OF VENTILATION

A person breathes air into and out of the lungs based on changes in pressure within the chest cavity. The increase or decrease in pressure is a result of a change in the size of the thorax. According to the Boyle law, a volume of gas is inversely proportional to the pressure. It is summarized as follows:

- An *increase* in pressure (more positive) will *decrease* the volume of a gas.
- A *decrease* in pressure (more negative) will *increase* the volume of a gas.

When the diaphragm and external intercostal muscles contract, the size of the thorax increases. By increasing the size of a closed container, the intrathoracic pressure decreases (becomes more negative, thus creating a vacuum), based on the Boyle law. The difference in pressure between the outside air pressure and the decreased pressure within the thorax causes air to enter the lungs through the trachea.

At sea level, the atmospheric pressure is 760 mmHg. When the respiratory muscles contract during inhalation, the intrathoracic pressure drops to 758 mmHg. As noted previously, the drop in pressure allows air to be pulled into the lungs, causing inhalation.

On the other hand, when the diaphragm and external intercostal muscles relax, the ribs fall inward and the diaphragm moves upward, decreasing the size of the thorax. By decreasing the size of the thorax, the pressure inside becomes more positive. Based on the Boyle law, an increase in pressure decreases the volume of gas; thus, the air is forced out of the lungs.

When the respiratory muscles relax, the intrathoracic pressure increases to 761 mmHg. Because the intrathoracic pressure is greater than atmospheric pressure, it pushes the air out of the lungs, causing exhalation.

Accessory Muscles

Accessory muscles (see Table 7-2) are used to force greater airflow during inhalation or exhalation by contracting additional muscles. Forced inhalation requires the accessory muscles to increase the size of the thorax beyond normal. The increase in thoracic size will further

TABLE 7-2	Accessory Muscles of Ventilation

Accessory Muscles of Inhalation

- Sternocleidomastoid muscles lift the sternum upward.
- Scalene muscles elevate ribs 1 and 2.
- Pectoralis minor muscles elevate ribs 3 to 5.

Accessory Muscles of Exhalation

- Abdominal muscles force the diaphragm upward.
- Internal intercostal muscles pull the sternum and ribs inward.

decrease the intrathoracic size, making the pressure more negative and allowing more air to be drawn into the lungs.

During forced exhalation, the abdominal muscles contract and push the abdominal contents superiorly. This causes the diaphragm to be pushed upward. In addition, the internal intercostal muscles contract and pull the chest wall inward. Both these actions decrease the intrathoracic size beyond normal, make the intrathoracic pressure more positive, and create a higher pressure to force the air out.

Factors Affecting Ventilation

Two conditions that may require the use of accessory muscles to either generate a greater force to allow air to flow into the respiratory tract and lungs or force the air out are compliance and airway resistance.

COMPLIANCE   *Compliance* is a measure of the force that it takes for the lungs and chest wall to expand and distend. A condition, such as emphysema, that causes the chest wall and lungs to stiffen would lead to a decrease in compliance, making it more difficult for a patient to move air into and out of the lungs. You may experience poor compliance when it is more difficult than usual to deliver the ventilation when using a bag-valve-mask device.

AIRWAY RESISTANCE   Resistance to airflow through the respiratory tract is determined by the obstruction and internal diameter size of the lower airways. Mucus, swelling, and bronchiole constriction are the most common causes of obstructed airflow, resulting in a higher airway resistance (▶ Figure 7-2). A higher airway resistance requires the patient to work harder and expend more energy to move the air through the respiratory tract, which may lead to respiratory muscle fatigue and respiratory distress or failure.

Both poor compliance and higher airway resistance may lead to a decrease in the volume of air reaching the alveoli for gas exchange. This results in less oxygen attached to hemoglobin in the blood and, potentially, cellular hypoxia.

PLEURAL SPACE   The potential space between the visceral and parietal pleura maintains a negative pressure. Thus, if there is a break in the continuity of either or both pleura, air is drawn into the space between the pleura, creating an air-filled

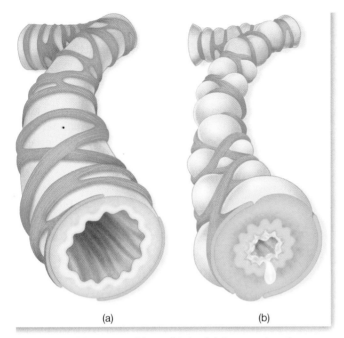

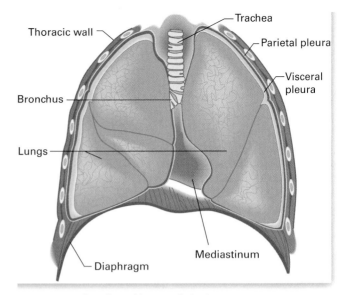

Figure 7-3 The pleural lining of the lung.

Figure 7-2 (a) A normal bronchiole. (b) A constricted bronchiole.

pleural space. Elastin, a component in the composition of the lung tissue, has an effect something like a rubber band: When elastin is stretched, its natural tendency is to recoil. Because of this property, the lungs are continuously pulling inward in an attempt to recoil, which allows them to collapse to about 5 percent of their normal size.

The parietal pleura is adhered to the thoracic cavity, whereas the visceral pleura is the outermost layer covering the lungs (▶ Figure 7-3). Between the two layers is serous fluid that primarily acts as a lubricant to reduce friction when the layers rub over each other during ventilation.

Because the lung tissue wants to recoil, the visceral pleura is continuously tugging inward against a relatively fixed parietal pleura. The serous fluid creates a "water glass" effect that is similar to what happens when a water glass is placed on a smooth surface (e.g., a drinking glass is placed in a puddle of water on a glass table) and pulled straight upward. The water creates a seal, and the pull on the glass creates a vacuum. A similar effect is created by the inward pull of the visceral, with the serous fluid acting like the water. Because of this effect, the intrapleural (inside the pleura) pressure remains negative and allows air to enter if either of the pleural layers is interrupted.

MINUTE VENTILATION *Minute ventilation*, also known as *minute volume*, is the amount of air moved in and out of the lungs in 1 minute. Minute ventilation is calculated by multiplying the tidal volume (V_T) by the frequency of ventilation (f), better known as the respiratory rate.

Minute ventilation = Tidal volume × Frequency of ventilation

Tidal volume is the amount of air breathed in and out with each individual breath. An average-size adult has a V_T of approximately 500 mL and a respiratory rate of 12 breaths per minute at rest. The minute ventilation will be calculated thus:

Minute ventilation = 500 mL × 12/minute

Minute ventilation = 6,000 mL/minute or 6 L/minute

Based on this calculation, an average-size adult moves approximately 6,000 mL of air into and out of the lungs every minute when breathing at a rate of 12 breaths per minute. Calculating the actual numbers is not necessary for EMS providers, but understanding what would cause the minute ventilation to decrease or increase is important. You must understand the following about minute ventilation:

- A *decrease* in tidal volume will *decrease* the minute ventilation.
- A *decrease* in frequency of ventilation (respiratory rate) will *decrease* the minute ventilation.

- A *decrease* in minute ventilation will *decrease* the amount of air available for gas exchange in the alveoli.
- A *decrease* in minute ventilation can lead to cellular hypoxia.

By increasing the respiratory rate, the patient can increase minute ventilation. For example, a patient with a low tidal volume (200 mL) increases his respiratory rate from 12 per minute to 28 per minute to compensate for the decrease in minute ventilation.

Low tidal volume with normal respiratory rate

Minute ventilation = 200 mL × 12/minute

Minute ventilation = 2,400 mL or 2.4 L

Low tidal volume with increased respiratory rate to compensate

Minute ventilation = 200 mL × 28 minute

Minute ventilation = 5,600 mL or 5.6 L

When the patient increases his respiratory rate to compensate for the low tidal volume, which would be present clinically as shallow breathing, his minute ventilation almost returns to normal. However, the patient would increase his work of breathing and expend the additional energy required to do so, as well as continuing to exhibit signs and symptoms of hypoxia, and he would continue to deteriorate. This extremely important concept is explained in the next section.

ALVEOLAR VENTILATION *Alveolar ventilation* is the amount of air that is moved into and out of the alveoli in 1 minute. The key word in this definition is *alveoli*. Minute ventilation accounts for only air moved into and out of the respiratory system and not specifically the alveoli, whereas alveolar ventilation specifically defines the amount of air reaching the alveoli for gas exchange.

Alveolar ventilation takes into account the concept of dead space. Dead space (V_D) consists of the areas in the respiratory tract during inhalation in which air collects but gas exchange does not occur. These areas include the nasopharynx, oropharynx, pharynx, larynx, trachea, bronchi, and bronchioles. Air will fill these areas first before reaching the alveoli; therefore, a decrease in the tidal volume would mean less air for the alveoli for gas exchange.

The average-size adult has 150 mL of dead air space. Because the tidal volume fills the dead space first, it must be removed from the total volume of air reaching the alveoli. It is calculated as follows:

Alveolar ventilation = (Tidal volume − Dead space) × Frequency of ventilation

In an average-size adult patient, the alveolar ventilation is calculated thus:

Alveolar ventilation = (500 mL − 150 mL) × 12/minute

Alveolar ventilation = 350 mL × 12/minute

Alveolar ventilation = 4,200 mL/minute or 4.2 L/minute

Recall that the minute ventilation in the average-size adult using the same tidal volume and respiratory rate was 6,000 mL/minute. Based on the alveolar minute ventilation calculation, of the 6 L of minute ventilation, only 4,200 mL, or 4.2 L, actually reaches the alveoli for gas exchange.

As with minute ventilation, the alveolar ventilation is affected by changes in the tidal volume and respiratory rate. However, a decrease in tidal volume affects alveolar ventilation much more profoundly than it affects minute ventilation. For example, recall the patient who increased his respiratory rate to 28 per minute to compensate for a decreased tidal volume (200 mL). By doing so, his minute ventilation almost returned to normal (5,600 mL); however, he was still displaying signs and symptoms of hypoxia and continued to deteriorate. Using the same patient data, the status of his alveolar ventilation is as follows:

Alveolar ventilation = (200 mL − 150 mL) × 28/minute

Alveolar ventilation = 50 mL × 28/minute

Alveolar ventilation = 1,400 mL/minute or 1.4 L/minute

Because the low tidal volume must still fill the dead air space, only 50 mL is reaching the alveoli for gas exchange. This explains the reason for the continued hypoxia, even though the patient's minute ventilation returned to close to normal.

The key points to remember with alveolar ventilation are the following:

- Although the patient may breathe faster to improve his minute ventilation, the amount of air available for gas exchange in the alveoli may be insufficient if the tidal volume is low.

- The dead space will fill first, regardless of the volume of air breathed in.

- To improve gas exchange in the patient with an inadequate tidal volume, you must provide positive pressure ventilation to increase tidal volume and move more air into the alveoli.

- By placing a patient with a low tidal volume on an oxygen mask, you will enrich the air in the dead air space with little getting to the alveoli. The patient needs ventilation.

- Assessing tidal volume is as important as assessing respiratory rate.

Inadequate ventilation is caused by either an inadequate respiratory rate or an insufficient tidal volume. If either one is inadequate, the patient requires positive pressure ventilation. For the patient to have adequate breathing, both the respiratory rate and tidal volume must be adequate.

TRANSITIONING

REVIEW ITEMS

1. The primary concern with obstruction of the nasopharynx by blood is _____.
   a. complete occlusion of the upper airway
   b. aspiration of the blood into the lungs
   c. continued blood loss, leading to hypovolemia
   d. swelling of the septum owing to irritation

2. You are administering oxygen to a patient via a nonrebreather mask at 15 lpm. You would report the FiO_2 to be _____.
   a. 0.50   b. 95%
   c. 79%   d. 0.95

3. Relaxation of the submandibular muscles controlling the mandible and tongue may cause _____.

   a. the epiglottis to fall closed over the glottic opening
   b. the tongue to be pulled forward, relieving an obstruction
   c. obstruction of airflow because of laryngeal spasm
   d. an obstruction at the inferior nasopharynx

4. You note exaggerated use of the muscles in the neck when the patient is breathing. You should suspect that the patient _____.
   a. is hyperventilating
   b. is having difficulty exhaling
   c. has a high airway resistance
   d. has a brain injury

5. A head-injured patient is responding to verbal stimuli with incomprehensible sounds. His respiratory rate is 32 per minute with little chest movement. You should suspect _____.

a. an adequate alveolar ventilation
b. an increased alveolar ventilation
c. an inadequate alveolar ventilation
d. a compensated alveolar ventilation

APPLIED PATHOPHYSIOLOGY

1. Explain how a change in the composition of ambient air can lead to cellular hypoxia.

2. Explain how an obstruction at the level of the oropharynx, nasopharynx, larynx, trachea, and bronchi can lead to cellular hypoxia.

3. Describe the types of obstruction that can occur at the level of the oropharynx, nasopharynx, larynx, trachea, and bronchi.

4. Explain the relationship between the tongue and epiglottis in airway obstruction.

5. Explain the Boyle law and its effect on the mechanics of ventilation.

6. Describe the changes in intrapulmonary pressures during inhalation and exhalation.

7. Explain how the accessory muscles assist in inhalation and exhalation.

8. Explain the difference between compliance and airway resistance and how each condition can lead to respiratory distress and failure.

9. Based on the "water glass" effect, explain what would result if a break in the continuity of the visceral or parietal pleura would occur.

10. Explain minute ventilation and how it applies to a patient's ventilatory status.

11. Explain alveolar ventilation and how it applies to a patient's ventilatory status.

CLINICAL DECISION MAKING

You are called for a patient having an asthma attack. You find a 26-year-old female patient sitting upright on a chair at the kitchen table. She appears to be in severe respiratory distress. As you approach her, you notice that she is pale and diaphoretic and has circumoral cyanosis. You also note use of her sternocleidomastoid muscles on inhalation.

During your primary assessment, you determine that the airway is open. Her respiratory rate is 34/minute with minimal chest wall movement. Her head is bobbing with each breath. Her radial pulse is 142/minute, and her skin is pale, cool, and clammy. Her SpO$_2$ is 74 percent on room air.

1. Are there any immediate life threats?

2. What emergency care should you provide based on the primary assessment findings?

3. Explain why the sternocleidomastoid muscles are being used.

4. Explain the cause for the pale, cool, and clammy skin.

5. If she was an average-size adult, what would you suspect her minute ventilation to be?

6. What would you suspect the alveolar ventilation status is? Why?

7. Explain the effect of the respiratory rate and tidal volume in this patient on minute ventilation and alveolar ventilation.

Standard Pathophysiology

Competency Applies comprehensive knowledge of the pathophysiology of respiration and perfusion to patient assessment and management.

TOPIC

8

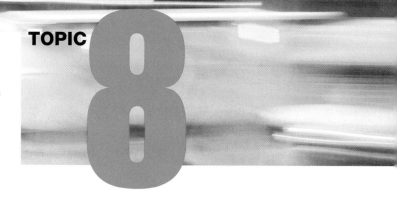

REGULATION OF VENTILATION, VENTILATION/PERFUSION RATIO, AND TRANSPORT OF GASES

INTRODUCTION

The pathophysiology included in this topic is among the most formative and challenging changes to the new education standards. Previously, Advanced EMTs had to know very little about the air moving in and out of the body—and, quite frankly, often in very simple terms and concepts. It was the belief, in creating the standards that include this information, that AEMTs would better understand the internal processes of perfusion and gas transport that would make assessment and care more intuitive and effective.

REGULATION OF VENTILATION

Although breathing can be altered voluntarily, it is primarily controlled involuntarily by the autonomic nervous system. A large part of the regulation is related to maintaining normal gas exchange and normal blood gas levels. Receptors within the body constantly measure the amount of oxygen (O_2), carbon dioxide (CO_2), and hydrogen ions (pH) and signal the brain to adjust the rate and depth of respiration (▶ Figure 8-1). Centers responsible for ventilatory control are the chemoreceptors, lung receptors, and specialized centers in the brain stem.

Chemoreceptors

Chemoreceptors are specialized receptors that monitor the number of hydrogen ions (pH) and the carbon dioxide and oxygen levels in the arterial blood. The two different types of chemoreceptors are central and peripheral.

CENTRAL CHEMORECEPTORS The central chemoreceptors are located near the respiratory center in the medulla. These receptors are most sensitive to changes in the amount of carbon dioxide in arterial blood and the pH of cerebrospinal fluid (CSF). The pH of CSF is directly related to the amount of carbon dioxide in the arterial blood. Carbon dioxide readily crosses the blood–brain barrier and moves into the CSF. In the CSF, the CO_2 combines with water (H_2O) to form carbonic acid (H_2CO_3). Thus

---

TRANSITION *highlights*

- The body's regulation of normal ventilation through blood chemistry values and the receptors that control them:
    - Central chemoreceptors.
    - Peripheral chemoreceptors.
    - Hypoxic and hypercarbic drive.

- How normal ventilation is affected by lung receptors and respiratory control centers in the brainstem.

- The ventilation/perfusion ratio and how it pertains to oxygenation of the bloodstream:
    - Illustration of how changes to the ventilation/perfusion ratio affect other bodily processes.

- The role blood, red blood cells, and hemoglobin play in cellular oxygenation and the removal of carbon dioxide from the cells.

- Alveolar and cellular gas exchange in the blood.

---

there is an association between CO_2 and the level of acid in the body as follows:

- An *increase* in the amount of CO_2 in the blood will *increase* the amount of acid in the blood.

- A *decrease* in the amount of CO_2 in the blood will *decrease* the amount of acid in the blood.

The central chemoreceptors are highly sensitive to the amount of hydrogen in the CSF. After the CO_2 and H_2O molecules combine to form H_2CO_3, the hydrogen ions (H^+) disassociate from the H_2CO_3, enter the CSF, and stimulate the central chemoreceptors. Small changes in the H^+ level in the CSF will stimulate a change in respirations. Because CO_2 is needed to produce H_2CO_3, the changes in the breathing rate and depth are geared toward increasing or decreasing the CO_2 level in the

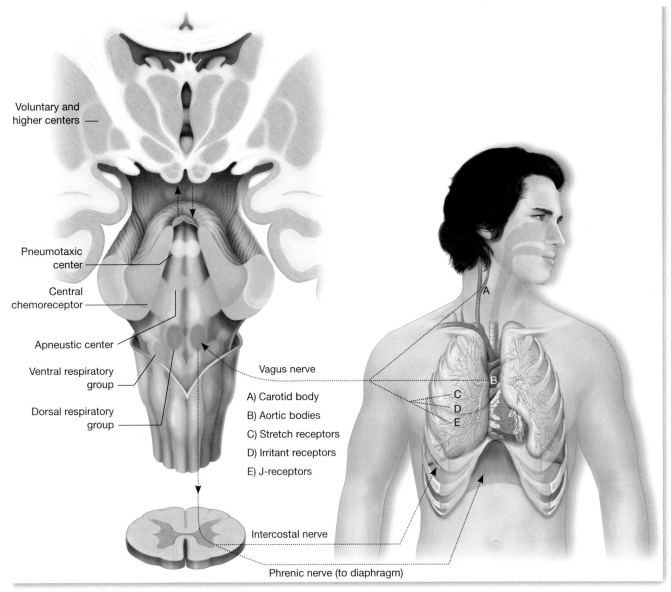

Voluntary and higher centers

Pneumotaxic center

Central chemoreceptor

Apneustic center

Ventral respiratory group

Dorsal respiratory group

Vagus nerve

A) Carotid body
B) Aortic bodies
C) Stretch receptors
D) Irritant receptors
E) J-receptors

Intercostal nerve

Phrenic nerve (to diaphragm)

Figure 8-1 Respiration is controlled by the autonomic nervous system. Receptors within the body measure oxygen, carbon dioxide, and hydrogen ions and send signals to the brain to adjust the rate and depth of respiration.

arterial blood. The response of ventilation can be summarized as follows:

- An *increase* in arterial CO_2 will *increase* the number of hydrogen ions in the CSF, stimulating an *increase* in the rate and depth of respiration to blow off more CO_2.

- A *decrease* in arterial CO_2 will *decrease* the number of hydrogen ions in the CSF, causing a *decrease* in the rate and depth of respiration to blow off less CO_2.

PERIPHERAL CHEMORECEPTORS The peripheral chemoreceptors are located in the aortic arch and carotid artery bodies in the neck. These chemoreceptors are also sensitive to CO_2 and pH; however, the arterial oxygen level is the strongest

stimulus. Thus, a change in the arterial oxygen level is what stimulates the brain to increase or decrease ventilation. It takes a significant decrease in the arterial oxygen content to trigger the peripheral chemoreceptors to stimulate the respiratory center to increase rate and depth of respiration. The activity of the peripheral chemoreceptors can be summarized as follows:

- A significant *decrease* in the arterial oxygen content will result in an *increase* in the rate and depth of ventilation aimed at *increasing* the arterial oxygen content.

Stimulation of both the central and peripheral chemoreceptors has a greater influence on changing the rate and depth of ventilation than either alone.

Hypoxic Drive

A person's ventilation is normally controlled by the strong stimulus provided by the amount of CO_2 in the arterial blood. This is referred to as a *hypercapnic drive* or *hypercarbic drive*. However, some patients with chronic obstructive pulmonary disease (COPD), such as emphysema or chronic bronchitis, have a tendency to retain carbon dioxide in their arterial blood from poor gas exchange. Because the CO_2 level is chronically elevated, the central chemoreceptors become desensitized to fluctuations that typically would stimulate a change in the rate or depth of ventilation. Because of the desensitization of the central chemoreceptors, the peripheral chemoreceptors become the primary stimulus to control ventilation.

Thus, hypoxia, rather than CO_2, becomes the stimulus for the person to breathe; this is referred to as a *hypoxic drive*.

Lung Receptors

Three different types of receptors are found within the lungs: irritant receptors, stretch receptors, and J-receptors. The irritant receptors are found in the airways and are sensitive to irritating gases, aerosols, and particles. Irritant receptors will cause a cough, bronchoconstriction, and an increase in the rate of ventilation.

The stretch receptors are located within the smooth muscle of the airways. These are responsible for measuring the size and volume of the lungs. To prevent overinflation when stimulated by high tidal volumes, these receptors decrease the rate and volume of ventilation when stretched.

J-receptors are located in the capillaries surrounding the alveoli and are sensitive to increases in pressure within the capillary. When activated, these receptors stimulate rapid, shallow respiration.

SPECIALIZED RESPIRATORY CENTERS IN THE BRAIN

The brainstem contains four respiratory control centers: the dorsal respiratory group, the ventral respiratory group, the apneustic center, and the pneumotaxic center. These centers stimulate the respiratory muscles to either contract or relax, depending on the impulse.

The dorsal respiratory group (DRG) is responsible for setting the basic rhythm of respiration. It consists of inspiratory neurons that send nerve impulses to the external intercostal muscles and diaphragm, stimulating them to contract, which results in inspiration. The DRG is active in every respiratory cycle, whether breathing is quiet or forced. In a typical respiratory cycle, the DRG stimulates the respiratory muscles to contract for 2 seconds, followed by 3 seconds with no stimulation, resulting in respiratory muscle relaxation.

The ventral respiratory group (VRG) has both inspiratory and expiratory neurons. However, the VRG is basically inactive during normal quiet breathing. The VRG becomes active when accessory muscles are needed to assist in inspiration

or expiration. The VRG_I, in which the *I* subscript indicates inspiratory VRG neurons, stimulates the pectoralis minor, scalene, and sternocleidomastoid muscles to force inspiration. The VRG_E, in which the *E* subscript indicates expiratory VRG neurons, stimulates the internal intercostal and abdominal muscles to force exhalation.

The apneustic center does not control the rhythm of respiration; however, it provides stimulation to the DRG and VRG_I to intensify the inhalation effort. The apneustic center may prolong inspiration, increasing the ventilatory volume.

The pneumotaxic center sends inhibitory impulses to the apneustic center to cease inhalation before the lungs become overinflated. It can promote passive exhalation both by shutting off the DRG and VRG_I and by activating the VRG_E.

VENTILATION/ PERFUSION RATIO

The ventilation/perfusion (V/Q) ratio describes the dynamic relationship between the amount of ventilation in the alveoli and the amount of perfusion through the alveolar capillaries. This relationship determines the quality of gas exchange across the alveolar–capillary membrane, which in turn determines the amount of oxygen entering the blood and CO_2 offloading from the blood. This relationship can be used to explain the etiology of hypoxemia.

In the ideal lung, each alveolus would receive an adequate amount of ventilation and a matching amount of blood flow through the surrounding capillary, resulting in a V/Q ratio of 1—that is, ventilation and perfusion are equal. This ideal condition never exists, though, because of the effects of gravity on blood flow, the structure of the lungs, and shunting of blood.

When a person is in a standing position, gravity pulls the lungs downward toward the diaphragm, compressing the lower lobes. As the lower lobes are compressed and blood is pulled down to the bases of the lungs, air travels upward to the apexes (tops) of the lungs and increases the residual volume. Interestingly, the alveoli in the apexes of the lungs have a greater residual volume of air, are larger, and have a higher surface tension, but they are fewer in number compared with other areas of the lungs. These larger alveoli in the apexes have a higher surface tension, which makes them less compliant

and harder to inflate during ventilation. Thus, the tidal volume is shifted to the lower lobes, where the lung is more compliant and there is less surface tension.

Because gravity pulls the blood downward, less pressure is required to perfuse the lower lobes of the lungs, as compared with the apexes, which are above the level of the heart. As a result, the bases of the lungs receive a greater amount of blood and are much better perfused than the apexes. This is a desirable condition, as the greatest amount of ventilation also exists in the base of the lungs.

The V/Q ratio is never at an ideal state in any zones of the lungs. In the apexes, the amount of available ventilation in the alveoli exceeds the amount of perfusion through the pulmonary capillaries; that is, more oxygen is available in the alveoli than the supply of blood is able to pick up and transport. This is considered to be wasted ventilation. In the bases, the amount of perfusion exceeds the amount of ventilation; this means more blood is moving through the pulmonary capillaries than there is alveolar oxygen available for it to pick up. This is considered to be wasted perfusion. Overall, under normal conditions, perfusion exceeds the amount of available ventilation.

Pressure Imbalances

The perfusion of blood through the pulmonary capillaries is affected by the amount of air and pressure inside the alveoli and the pressure of the blood flowing through the capillary bed (▶ Figure 8-2). If the pressure in an alveolus exceeds the hydrostatic pressure of blood in the capillary bed, blood flow through the capillary stops. This is most likely to occur in the apexes of the lungs, where the pressure inside the alveoli is highest and the blood

> In a typical respiratory cycle, the DRG stimulates the respiratory muscles to contract for 2 seconds, followed by 3 seconds with no stimulation.

> The bases of the lungs receive a greater amount of blood and are much better perfused than the apexes.

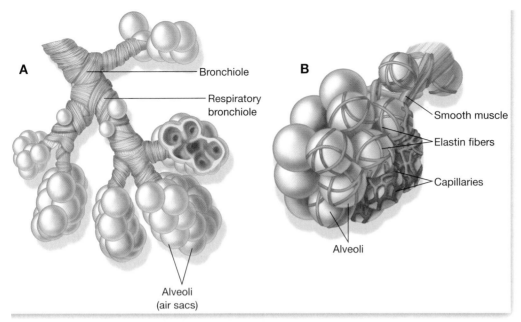

A

- Bronchiole
- Respiratory bronchiole
- Alveoli (air sacs)

B

- Smooth muscle
- Elastin fibers
- Capillaries
- Alveoli

Figure 8-2 Perfusion of the pulmonary capillaries is affected by pressure within the alveoli and pressure within the capillaries.

flow is lowest. However, it may also occur in the patient who is losing blood from an injury and has a decreasing blood pressure.

A decrease in the systemic blood pressure will also cause the pressure in the pulmonary capillaries to decrease. If the patient does not have a chest or lung injury, the lungs will continue to receive adequate volumes of air, creating adequate pressure in the alveoli. However, the reduction in blood pressure may allow the alveolar pressure to exceed the pulmonary capillary pressure and impede blood flow. This will result in poor alveolar perfusion, hypoxemia (reduced oxygen concentrations in the blood), and cellular hypoxia (oxygen deficiency in the cells).

Ventilatory Disturbances

A disturbance on the ventilation side of the V/Q ratio can lead to hypoxia. If a condition or injury causes less oxygenated air to be available in the alveoli for the amount of blood flowing through the pulmonary capillaries, the end result will be less oxygen saturating the blood and less oxygen delivered to the cells, creating hypoxemia and cellular hypoxia.

For example, if a patient is having an asthma attack and the bronchioles are

> **Hypoxia generally results from a ventilation or perfusion disturbance.**

inflamed and constricted, the restricted airways reduce airflow and provide less oxygenated air to the alveoli for gas exchange. The blood pressure is not affected; therefore, the amount of blood passing through the pulmonary capillaries remains normal. A ventilation disturbance has been created by making less oxygen available to the blood passing through the capillaries. In this condition, there is wasted perfusion, as the blood is available, but there is an inadequate amount of oxygen to be picked up. This disturbance in ventilation leads to hypoxemia and cellular hypoxia.

In the situation just described, in which an asthma attack has caused a ventilatory disturbance, the ventilation side of the V/Q ratio must be improved by relieving the bronchiole airway restriction and increasing the amount of oxygenated air entering the alveoli. An AEMT would achieve this by placing the patient on oxygen and administering a beta$_2$-agonist medication to dilate the bronchioles to improve airflow. Not only would this treatment increase the amount of air in the alveoli, but it would also increase the concentration of oxygen in the alveolar air, making more oxygen available for the blood moving through the pulmonary capillaries. This would reduce or eliminate the hypoxemia and cellular hypoxia.

Perfusion Disturbances

A perfusion disturbance may also lead to severe cellular hypoxia. Consider a patient

you encounter who has cut his radial artery on a saw and suffered severe blood loss. The patient has no chest or lung injury and has an increased rate and depth of ventilation. His minute ventilation and alveolar ventilation are increased; however, his cells are becoming hypoxic. Although he is moving more oxygenated air into the alveoli, his blood loss has significantly reduced the amount of blood flow through the pulmonary capillaries. This represents a perfusion disturbance because there is not enough blood to pick up the oxygen available in the alveoli. This would create a state of wasted ventilation, hypoxemia, and cellular hypoxia.

By placing the patient on oxygen, you might reduce some of the cellular hypoxia; however, it will not be eliminated until the perfusion disturbance is fixed. The bleeding must be stopped, and this patient needs to receive fluid and blood to increase the flow and pressure in the pulmonary capillaries so enough hemoglobin is available for oxygen in the alveoli to attach to and be transported to the cells.

Hypoxia generally results from a ventilation or perfusion disturbance. Myriad conditions can cause one of these disturbances to occur. The management of hypoxia resulting from a ventilatory disturbance should focus on improving ventilation and oxygenation. Managing a disturbance in perfusion must focus on increasing blood flow through the pulmonary capillaries, the availability of hemoglobin, and delivery of oxygen to the cells.

TRANSPORT OF OXYGEN AND CARBON DIOXIDE IN THE BLOOD

Oxygen must be continuously delivered by the blood to the cells for normal cellular metabolism to occur. Carbon dioxide, a by-product of aerobic metabolism, must be carried back to the lungs to be eliminated during exhalation. A disturbance in the transport system may lead to both cellular hypoxia (a lack of oxygen

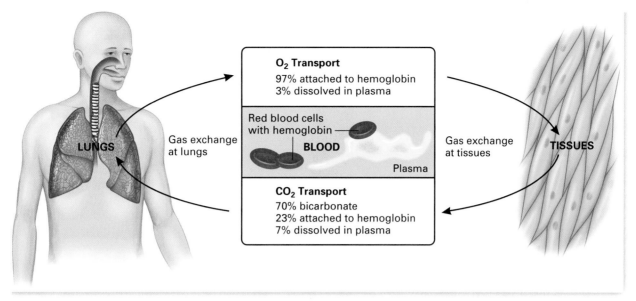

Figure 8-3 Oxygen is transported in the blood in two ways: attached to hemoglobin and dissolved in plasma. Carbon dioxide is transported in the blood in three ways: as bicarbonate, attached to hemoglobin, and dissolved in plasma.

available to the cells) and hypercarbia (a buildup of carbon dioxide in the blood). Both hypoxia and hypercarbia pose problems for normal cellular function and stability.

Both oxygen and carbon dioxide are transported by the blood but in different ways (▶ Figure 8-3). It is important to remember that oxygen and carbon dioxide move from areas of higher concentration to areas of lower concentration. This helps to explain the movement of gas molecules between alveoli and capillaries and between capillaries and cells.

A pulmonary embolus is another example of a common perfusion disturbance in which blood flow to a portion of the lung is physically blocked.

Oxygen Transport

Approximately 1000 mL of oxygen is delivered to the cells every minute. Oxygen is transported by the blood in two ways: dissolved in plasma and attached to hemoglobin. A small amount, only 1.5 percent to 3 percent, is dissolved in plasma. The majority of oxygen, approximately 97 percent to 98.5 percent, is attached to hemoglobin molecules.

Hemoglobin is a protein molecule that has four iron sites to which oxygen can bind. Thus, one hemoglobin molecule could carry up to four oxygen molecules. If one oxygen molecule is attached to the hemoglobin molecule, it is considered to have 25 percent saturation. Attachment of two oxygen molecules would be

considered 50 percent saturation, three molecules 75 percent saturation, and four molecules 100 percent saturation. The attachment of one oxygen molecule to a hemoglobin iron-binding site will increase the affinity for the other sites to also bind with oxygen.

Once an oxygen molecule binds with hemoglobin, the hemoglobin molecule is referred to as *oxyhemoglobin*. A hemoglobin molecule that has no oxygen attached is referred to as *deoxyhemoglobin*. Without hemoglobin, the negligible amount of oxygen that can be transported by plasma would not be enough to sustain normal cellular function or life. A loss of hemoglobin, which commonly occurs as a result of bleeding, can easily lead to severe cellular hypoxia, even though an adequate amount of oxygen is available in the alveoli.

Carbon Dioxide Transport

Carbon dioxide is transported in the blood in three ways: Approximately 7 percent is dissolved in plasma, 23 percent is attached to hemoglobin, and 70 percent is in the form of bicarbonate.

As CO_2 leaves the cells, it crosses over into the capillaries, where a small amount dissolves into the plasma. A larger amount of CO_2 attaches to hemoglobin. The largest amount of CO_2 diffuses into the red blood cells and combines with water to form H_2CO_3, which then dissociates into hydrogen and bicarbonate. The bicarbonate exits the cells and is transported in

the blood plasma. When the blood reaches the pulmonary circulation, the bicarbonate diffuses back into the red blood cells, where it combines with hydrogen and splits back into water and carbon dioxide. Regardless of the transport mechanism, the carbon dioxide diffuses into the alveoli, which are low in CO_2 concentration, and is eliminated during exhalation.

Alveolar/Capillary Gas Exchange

After inhalation, the alveoli are filled with oxygen-rich air that contains very little carbon dioxide. Conversely, the venous blood that flows through the capillaries surrounding the alveoli contains low levels of oxygen and higher amounts of carbon dioxide.

Because gas molecules naturally move from an area of high concentration to an area of low concentration, the high oxygen content in the alveoli moves across the membranes and into the capillaries, where the oxygen content is very low (▶ Figure 8-4). There, as described earlier, a small amount of oxygen dissolves in the plasma and a larger amount attaches to the hemoglobin. Simultaneously, CO_2 moves in the opposite direction, from the high levels contained in the capillaries into the alveoli, where the CO_2 content is low. It happens this way: The bicarbonate ions in the blood convert to water and CO_2, additional CO_2 diffuses out of the plasma and offloads from the

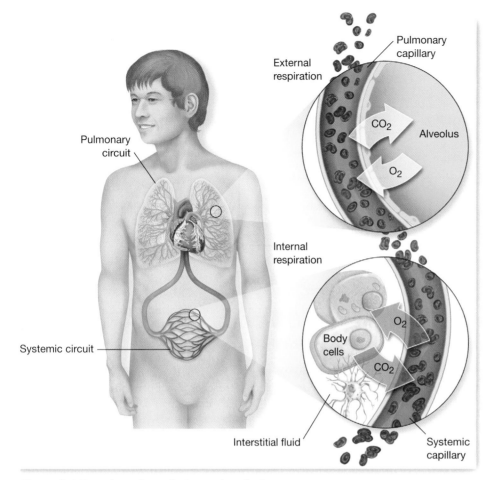

concentrations of oxygen and low concentrations of CO_2. This blood travels through an artery and then enters a smaller arteriole that leads to a capillary bed that is surrounded by cells. During cell metabolism, the cells have used oxygen and produced carbon dioxide as a byproduct. Thus, whereas the capillary beds contain blood that is high in oxygen and low in CO_2, the cells contain low levels of oxygen and high levels of CO_2.

As the blood enters the capillary, oxygen breaks free of the hemoglobin and diffuses out of the plasma, crosses the capillary membrane, and enters the cell. Simultaneously, CO_2 leaves the cell and crosses over into the capillary, where it dissolves in the plasma, attaches to hemoglobin, or enters the red blood cell to be converted to bicarbonate (Figure 8-4).

As the blood leaves the capillary, it enters a small venule, from which it is eventually dumped into a larger vein. The blood in the venules and veins contains low concentrations of oxygen and high concentrations of CO_2. This CO_2-carrying blood is transported to the right atrium of the heart, from which it enters the right ventricle and is pumped to the lungs. There, the blood enters the pulmonary capillaries to give off CO_2 and pick up oxygen in the alveolar/capillary gas exchange, as described earlier.

For the cells to receive an adequate amount of oxygen and eliminate CO_2, both the alveolar/capillary gas exchange and cell/capillary gas exchange must be functioning properly. A disturbance in either will result in either inadequate amounts of oxygen being delivered to the cells or the accumulation of CO_2.

Figure 8-4 Overview of ventilation and perfusion.

hemoglobin, and all this CO_2 crosses from the capillaries into the alveoli.

After these exchanges—from alveoli to capillaries and from capillaries to alveoli—the alveoli contain low levels of oxygen and high levels of CO_2, whereas the blood in the capillaries contains high levels of oxygen and low levels of CO_2. Basically, the gases have switched concentrations. The CO_2-rich air in the alveoli is exhaled from the lungs. The oxygen-rich blood in the capillaries is transported

from the pulmonary circulation to the left atrium and then to the left ventricle of the heart, from which it is ejected into the aorta and to the arteries throughout the body. This blood that is circulating throughout the body will be used in the cell/capillary gas exchange described next.

Cell/Capillary Gas Exchange

The blood that was ejected from the left ventricle into the arteries contains high

REVIEW ITEMS

1. An increase in the level of carbon dioxide in the arterial blood will result in _____.
   a. a decrease in the respiratory tidal volume
   b. a decrease in the number of hydrogen ions
   c. an increase in the respiratory rate
   d. an increase in bicarbonate

2. Increasing the oxygen content in the arterial blood in a patient breathing on a hypoxic drive will possibly lead to _____.
   a. stimulation of the central chemoreceptors
   b. a decrease in the rate and depth of respiration
   c. an increase in the amount of carbonic acid
   d. collection of hydrogen ions in the CSF

3. A patient presents with use of the sternocleidomastoid muscle and retractions during respiration. You would suspect that which of the following respiratory centers is providing respiratory muscle stimulation?
   a. DRG
   b. VRG_I
   c. VRG_E
   d. pneumotaxic center

4. Hypoxia associated with an acute asthma attack would likely result from _____.
   a. a ventilation disturbance
   b. an upper airway occlusion
   c. a perfusion disturbance
   d. chemoreceptor dysfunction

5. The primary method of transport of carbon dioxide in the blood is _____.
   a. dissolved in plasma
   b. attached to hemoglobin
   c. as carbonic acid
   d. in the form of bicarbonate

APPLIED PATHOPHYSIOLOGY

1. Explain how the central chemoreceptors regulate the rate and depth of respiration.

2. Explain how the peripheral chemoreceptors regulate the rate and depth of respiration.

3. Describe how administration of a high concentration of oxygen in a patient with a hypoxic drive may lead to respiratory depression and failure.

4. Explain a normal respiratory cycle based on activity of the DRG.

5. Explain the respiratory cycle in forced breathing based on activity of the VRG.

6. Explain hypoxia based on the ventilation/perfusion ratio.

7. Explain how a ventilation disturbance would lead to hypoxia.

8. Explain how a perfusion disturbance would lead to hypoxia.

9. Explain two ways oxygen is transported in the blood.

10. Explain three ways carbon dioxide is transported in the blood.

11. Explain gas exchange at the alveolar/capillary level.

12. Explain gas exchange at the tissue/capillary level.

CLINICAL DECISION MAKING

You arrive on the scene and find a 28-year-old male patient who was shot in the chest. The patient complains that he is struggling to breathe. His airway is open, and his respirations are rapid. His skin is pale, cool, and clammy, and he is exhibiting circumoral cyanosis. His SpO_2 reading is 76 percent on room air.

1. Following scene safety, what is your first immediate action after approaching this patient?

2. What are the life threats to this patient?

3. What do you suspect is causing the cyanosis and poor SpO_2 reading?

4. Would the hypoxia be related to a ventilation or perfusion disturbance?

5. Based on stimulation of the chemoreceptors, what is causing an increase in the respiratory rate?

TOPIC

9

Standard Pathophysiology

Competency Applies comprehensive knowledge of the pathophysiology of respiration and perfusion to patient assessment and management.

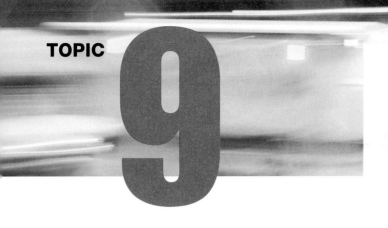

BLOOD, CARDIAC FUNCTION, AND VASCULAR SYSTEM

TRANSITION *highlights*

- *Blood volume (fluid and formed elements) and normal perfusion.*

- *Distribution of blood within the vascular compartment and the physiologic determinants that affect movement of fluid into and out of the vascular compartment:*
  – Hydrostatic pressure.
  – Plasma oncotic pressure.

- *Normal cardiac output, and how certain variables can alter it from normal:*
  – Changes in heart rate.
  – Changes in stroke volume.

- *Systemic vascular resistance, and the effects should it become deranged:*
  – Tissue perfusion.
  – Systolic and diastolic blood pressure.
  – Pulse pressure.

- *Microcirculation, and how changes of the aforementioned principles have a positive or negative effect on it.*

- *Blood pressure, and how it becomes deranged from disturbances in the aforementioned principles.*

- *How the autonomic nervous system (sympathetic and parasympathetic) can alter cellular perfusion through manipulation of the aforementioned principles.*

INTRODUCTION

*P*erfusion is the delivery of oxygenated blood and glucose to the cells and removal of carbon dioxide and other waste products. For perfusion to be adequate, oxygen must enter the alveoli, cross over the alveolar–capillary membrane, attach to hemoglobin, and be transported via the blood to cells. The blood volume and composition, cardiac function, and vascular resistance all contribute to the movement of oxygenated blood out of the alveolar capillaries and to cells throughout the body.

BLOOD VOLUME

One of the determinants of adequate blood pressure and perfusion is blood volume. An adult has approximately 70 mL of blood for every kilogram (2.2 lb) of body weight. Thus, a patient who weighs 154 lb (70 kg) would have approximately 4,900 mL, or 4.9 liters, of blood volume. Blood volume correlates with body mass; therefore, a larger patient would normally have a greater blood volume. The loss of 1 liter of blood in a 100-lb patient would be much more significant than in a 200-lb patient.

Composition of Blood

Blood is composed of formed elements and plasma. The formed elements, which are cells and proteins, make up approximately 45 percent of blood composition. Plasma is the fluid component that accounts for the remaining 55 percent. The primary function of plasma is to suspend and carry the formed elements.

Plasma is made up primarily of water and plasma proteins. Water comprises 91 percent of plasma. The plasma proteins consist of albumin, antibodies, and clotting factors. *Albumin* is a large molecule that does not pass easily through a capillary. It plays a major role in maintaining the fluid balance in the blood, as is explained in this chapter's section on plasma oncotic pressure. Antibodies are produced by the lymphatic system and are responsible for the defense against infectious organisms. The clotting factors are key in coagulation of blood from damaged vessels. Fibrinogen is the most plentiful clotting factor and is the precursor to the fibrin clot.

The formed elements in the blood are red blood cells (RBCs), white blood cells (WBCs), and platelets. RBCs (erythrocytes) make up approximately 48 percent of the blood cell volume in men and 42 percent in women. The RBCs, which contain hemoglobin, are primarily responsible for carrying oxygen and delivering it to cells for metabolism. The WBCs (leukocytes) protect the body against infection and eliminate dead and injured cells and other debris. The platelets (thrombocytes) are not actual cells but, rather, fragments that play a major role in blood clotting and the control of bleeding.

TABLE 9-1	Distribution of Blood in the Cardiovascular System
Veins	64%
Arteries	13%
Pulmonary vessels	9%
Capillaries	7%
Heart	7%

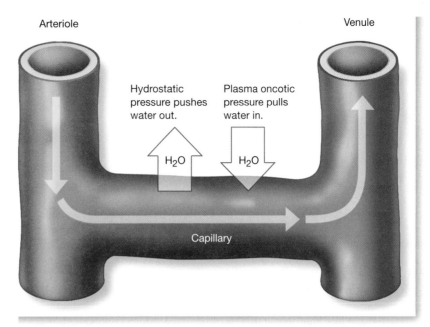

Figure 9-1 Hydrostatic pressure pushes water out of the capillary. Plasma oncotic pressure pulls water into the capillary.

Distribution of Blood

Blood is distributed throughout the cardiovascular system (Table 9-1). The majority of blood is housed within the *venous system*, which is also known as a *reservoir* or *capacitance* system. The venous system is capable of enlarging or reducing its capacity in response to increases or decreases in blood volume. As a patient bleeds, the venous volume is continuously reduced regardless of whether the bleeding is from a vein, an artery, or a capillary.

The venous system is responsible for supplying the right side of the heart with an adequate volume of blood. If the volume entering the right side of the heart is decreased, the amount ejected from the left ventricle, through the arteries, and to the cells is also reduced. Thus, the venous volume plays a major role in maintaining blood pressure and adequate perfusion of the cells. This is discussed in more detail later in this topic. The capillary network is the site of gas exchange occurring with the alveoli or cells.

Hydrostatic Pressure

Hydrostatic pressure is the force inside the vessel or capillary bed generated by the contraction of the heart and blood pressure. Hydrostatic pressure exerts a "push" inside the vessel or capillary—that is, it wants to push fluid out of the vessel or capillary, through the vessel wall, and into the surrounding interstitial space. A high hydrostatic pressure would force more fluid out of the vessel or capillary and promote edema—swelling from excess fluid outside the vessels (▶ Figure 9-1).

For example, if a patient has a left ventricle that is failing and unable to pump blood effectively, the volume and pressure in the left atrium, pulmonary vein, and pulmonary capillaries rise. This occurs because the pulmonary capillaries,

pulmonary vein, and left atrium are the pathways by which blood enters the left ventricle.

When the left ventricle fails to empty effectively, blood backs up into the left atrium and pulmonary vessels, which increases the pressure within them. This increased hydrostatic pressure inside the pulmonary capillaries forces fluid out of them. The extruded fluid has a tendency to collect in the spaces between the alveoli and capillaries and around the alveoli, which reduces the ability of oxygen and carbon dioxide to be exchanged across the alveolar/capillary membrane.

This disturbance reduces the blood oxygen content, leading to cellular hypoxia, and also causes the blood to retain carbon dioxide. The fluid will eventually begin to collapse and fill the alveoli, further diminishing gas exchange. This condition is known as *pulmonary edema*.

Plasma Oncotic Pressure

Plasma oncotic pressure, also known as *colloid oncotic pressure* or *oncotic pressure*, is responsible for keeping fluid inside the vessels. A force is generated inside vessels by large plasma proteins, especially albumin, that attract water and other fluids. Opposite to hydrostatic pressure, oncotic pressure exerts a "pull" inside the vessel. A high oncotic pressure would pull fluid from outside the vessel, through the vessel wall, and into the vessel (review Figure 9-1).

A balance between hydrostatic pressure and plasma oncotic pressure must be maintained for equilibrium of fluid balance. The effects of high and low hydrostatic and oncotic pressures are summarized as follows:

- A *high* hydrostatic pressure will push fluid out of a capillary and promote edema.
- A *low* hydrostatic pressure will push less fluid out of the vessel.
- A *high* oncotic pressure will draw excessive amounts of fluid into the vessel or capillary and promote blood volume overload.
- A *low* oncotic pressure will not exert an adequate pull effect to counteract the push of hydrostatic pressure and will therefore promote loss of vascular volume and promote edema (as seen in patients who are malnourished and have low albumin levels).

PUMP FUNCTION OF THE MYOCARDIUM

To have adequate blood pressure and perfusion, the myocardium must work effectively as a pump. The heart is capable of varying its output to meet a wide range of physiologic demands. It can drastically increase its pump function, up to sixfold. The pump function is typically expressed as the cardiac output. Cardiac output is defined as the amount of blood

> **Direct neural stimulation provides an immediate response in the heart rate and force of ventricular contraction.**

ejected by the left ventricle in 1 minute. The cardiac output has a major influence on blood pressure and perfusion, as discussed in the following sections.

Cardiac Output

A normal cardiac output for an adult at rest is 5 to 7 liters/minute. This means that the ventricles will pump nearly the entire blood volume through the vascular system in 1 minute. If a drop of blood left the left ventricle, in 1 minute it should be back at the left ventricle. The cardiac output is determined by the heart rate and the stroke volume. Cardiac output is expressed by the following equation:

$$\text{Cardiac output} = \text{Heart rate} \times \text{Stroke volume}$$

Heart Rate

The *heart rate* is defined as the number of times the heart contracts in 1 minute. The heart has the property of *automaticity*, meaning it can generate its own impulse. This is achieved through the conduction system with the *sinoatrial (SA) node* being the primary pacemaker.

> **A decrease in myocardial contractility will lead to a decrease in stroke volume and a resulting decrease in cardiac output.**

The heart rate can also be influenced to increase or decrease its rate of firing by several factors outside the heart, primarily hormones and the autonomic nervous system composed of the sympathetic and parasympathetic systems. The influence of the autonomic nervous system on the heart rate is summarized as follows:

- An *increase* in stimulation by the sympathetic nervous system *increases* the heart rate.
- A *decrease* in stimulation by the sympathetic nervous system *decreases* the heart rate.
- An *increase* in stimulation by the parasympathetic nervous system *decreases* the heart rate.

- A *decrease* in stimulation by the parasympathetic nervous system *increases* the heart rate.

The sympathetic and parasympathetic nervous systems exert control over the heart rate through the cardiovascular control center located in the brainstem. The cardiovascular control center is composed of the cardioexcitatory center and the cardioinhibitory center. The cardioexcitatory center increases the heart rate by increasing sympathetic stimulation and decreasing parasympathetic stimulation. The cardioinhibitory center decreases the heart rate by decreasing sympathetic stimulation and increasing parasympathetic stimulation.

Direct neural stimulation provides an immediate response in the heart rate and force of ventricular contraction. In addition, stimulation of the sympathetic nervous system may cause the release of epinephrine and norepinephrine from the adrenal gland located on top of the kidney. The release of these hormones may take a few minutes; however, the response will be sustained as long as the hormones are continuously released and circulating. The beta$_1$ properties in the epinephrine will cause an increase in the heart rate and force of contraction.

Stroke Volume

Stroke volume is defined as the volume of blood ejected by the left ventricle with each contraction. Stroke volume is determined by preload, myocardial contractility, and afterload.

PRELOAD *Preload* is the pressure generated in the left ventricle at the end of diastole (the resting phase of the cardiac cycle). Preload pressure is created by the blood volume in the left ventricle at the end of diastole. The available venous volume, which determines the volume of blood in the ventricle, consequently plays a major role in determining preload. An increase in preload generally increases stroke volume, which in turn increases the cardiac output. Preload determines the force necessary to eject the blood out of the ventricle.

MYOCARDIAL CONTRACTILITY As blood fills the left ventricle, the muscle fibers stretch to house the blood. The stretch of the muscle fiber at the end of diastole determines the force available to

eject the blood from the ventricle. This is known as the *Frank–Starling law of the heart*. As the blood volume increases in the left ventricle, the increased stretch in the muscle fibers generates a commensurate increase in contraction force. In short, the volume of blood in the ventricle automatically generates a contraction forceful enough to eject it. The effectiveness of fiber stretch is limited, however. In the case of a severely dilated ventricle where the fibers are overstretched, the Frank–Starling law no longer applies, and the heart begins to fail.

To have an adequate stroke volume, the left ventricle must be able to generate enough force to effectively eject its blood volume. An increase in myocardial contractility will increase the stroke volume and improve cardiac output. Conversely, a decrease in myocardial contractility will lead to a decrease in stroke volume and a resulting decrease in cardiac output.

For example, a patient with congestive heart failure will have a decrease in contractile force of the left ventricle that is likely to result in diminished cardiac output. A patient who has suffered a heart attack will have a deadened portion of cardiac muscle that will no longer contribute to the contractile force. If the area of necrosis is large, the contractile force will be significantly reduced, with a proportional decrease in stroke volume and cardiac output.

AFTERLOAD *Afterload* is the resistance in the aorta that must be overcome by contraction of the left ventricle to eject the blood. The force generated by the left ventricle must overcome the pressure in the aorta to move the blood forward. A high afterload places an increased workload on the left ventricle. A chronically elevated diastolic blood pressure will create a high afterload, generating an increased myocardial workload that could lead to left ventricular failure over time.

In general, a decrease in either the heart rate or stroke volume will decrease the cardiac output:

- A *decrease* in heart rate causes a *decrease* in cardiac output.
- A *decrease* in stroke volume causes a *decrease* in cardiac output.

The effects of heart rate, blood volume, myocardial contractility, autonomic nervous system stimulation, hormone release, and diastolic blood pressure on cardiac output are these:

- A *decrease* in heart rate will *decrease* cardiac output.
- An *increase* in heart rate, if not excessive, will *increase* cardiac output.
- A *decrease* in blood volume will *decrease* preload, stroke volume, and cardiac output.
- An *increase* in blood volume will *increase* preload, stroke volume, and cardiac output.
- A *decrease* in myocardial contractility will *decrease* stroke volume and cardiac output.
- An *increase* in myocardial contractility will *increase* stroke volume and cardiac output.
- Neural stimulation from the sympathetic nervous system will *increase* heart rate, myocardial contractility, and cardiac output.
- Neural stimulation from the parasympathetic nervous system will *decrease* heart rate, myocardial contractility, and cardiac output.
- Beta$_1$ stimulation from epinephrine will *increase* heart rate, myocardial contractility, and cardiac output.
- Beta$_1$ blockade (e.g., a patient on a beta blocker) will block beta$_1$ stimulation and *decrease* heart rate, myocardial contractility, and cardiac output.
- An extremely high diastolic blood pressure will *increase* the pressure in the aorta, requiring a more forceful contraction to overcome the aortic pressure and a higher myocardial workload, and it may weaken the heart and decrease the cardiac output over time.
- A *decrease* in the diastolic blood pressure will *decrease* the pressure in the aorta, require a less forceful contraction to overcome the aortic pressure, and reduce the myocardial workload, which may improve the cardiac output in a weakened heart.

A faster heart rate may increase cardiac output; however, if the rate is extremely fast, the cardiac output may actually decrease. With excessively fast heart rates, usually greater than 160 beats per minute (bpm) in the adult patient, the time between beats is so short that there is not enough time for the ventricles to fill. This reduces the preload, which in turn reduces the cardiac output.

SYSTEMIC VASCULAR RESISTANCE

Systemic vascular resistance is the resistance that is offered to blood flow through a vessel. As a vessel constricts (decreases its diameter), resistance inside the vessel increases, which typically increases pressure inside the vessel. Conversely, as a vessel dilates (increases its diameter), resistance inside the vessel decreases, which typically decreases pressure inside the vessel.

Vessel size influences blood pressure. *Vasoconstriction* decreases vessel diameter, increases resistance, and increases blood pressure. *Vasodilation* increases vessel diameter, decreases resistance, and decreases blood pressure.

Pressure within the vessels is greatest during cardiac contraction (systole) and least during cardiac relaxation (diastole). The basic measure of systemic vascular resistance is the diastolic blood pressure because it is assessed during the relaxation phase, indicating the resting pressure within the vessels. Systolic blood pressure, created by the wave of blood ejected from the left ventricle during contraction, increases the pressure within the vessels beyond their resting pressure.

An abnormally high diastolic blood pressure is not a desirable condition. The diastolic blood pressure is the pressure inside the arteries and the aortic root immediately prior to contraction of the left ventricle. The higher the diastolic blood pressure, the greater the resistance to blood being ejected from the left ventricle. That means the left ventricle has to work harder to pump the blood out against a higher diastolic pressure. If the diastolic blood pressure is chronically elevated, it will eventually cause the heart to fail. It is all related to resistance of flow and harder workloads.

For example, a person is given two weights to lift simultaneously. The weight in the right hand weighs only 1 lb, whereas the weight in the left hand weighs 10 lb. Which extremity and muscle would become fatigued and fail first if the person were asked to continuously lift the weights? Obviously the left arm lifting the 10-lb weight would fatigue and fail first because the muscle is working against a greater resistance.

Relate this example to the heart of a patient with a chronically elevated diastolic blood pressure. The high resistance to blood flow causes the left ventricle to work harder to pump the blood out. If the left ventricle has to contract chronically against the high resistance, it eventually weakens and fails. This condition is known as *left ventricular failure* or *congestive heart failure*.

The autonomic nervous system influences the systemic vascular resistance. Direct neural stimulation from the sympathetic nervous system causes the vessels to constrict, increasing vessel resistance and pressure. Parasympathetic nervous system stimulation causes the vessels to dilate, reducing resistance and pressure. In addition, the epinephrine and norepinephrine that are released by the adrenal gland in response to sympathetic stimulation have alpha properties. Alpha$_1$ receptor stimulation causes the vessels to constrict, increasing the vessels' resistance and pressure.

If the volume of blood inside a vessel decreases, one way to maintain the pressure is to decrease vessel size and increase resistance. When blood is being lost and overall volume is decreasing, vessels will usually compensate for this loss by continuing to constrict to raise resistance and pressure. Blood pressure may thus be maintained at a normal level, making it appear as if no volume has been lost. That is why it is so important not only to evaluate the vital signs in a patient with blood loss, but also to look for signs of poor perfusion. A drop in pressure is a late finding as blood is lost.

> It is important not only to evaluate the vital signs in a patient with blood loss, but also to look for signs of poor perfusion.

Think back to preceding topics and the discussion of cellular metabolism. As vessels decrease in size to maintain blood pressure, they do so at the expense of cellular perfusion. As the vessels constrict, less blood flows through them, and less oxygen is delivered to the cells. As oxygen delivery decreases, the cells change from aerobic to anaerobic metabolism.

The loss in energy is often noted in the patient's general appearance at the scene. The patient with poor perfusion is typically quiet and reserved and may actually appear sleepy. The patient who is screaming, yelling, and constantly moving about must have a great deal of energy to do so. Adequate delivery of oxygen and glucose to the cells is necessary to produce this amount of energy. Be careful not to mistake this high level of patient energy with the agitation and aggression experienced by patients whose brain cells are hypoxic.

The effects of the autonomic nervous system on systemic vascular resistance are summarized as follows:

- Sympathetic stimulation causes vasoconstriction, which *decreases* vessel diameter and *increases* systemic vascular resistance.
- Parasympathetic stimulation causes vasodilation, which *increases* vessel diameter and *decreases* systemic vascular resistance.
- The alpha$_1$ properties in epinephrine and norepinephrine, released in response to sympathetic stimulation, cause vasoconstriction, which *decreases* vessel diameter and *increases* systemic vascular resistance.

Systemic Vascular Resistance Effect on Pulse Pressure

Systolic blood pressure is a relative indicator of cardiac output, whereas diastolic blood pressure measures the systemic vascular resistance. If the systolic blood pressure is decreasing, it is an indication of diminishing cardiac output. The following describes the effect of systemic vascular resistance on diastolic blood pressure:

- An *increase* in the systemic vascular resistance will *increase* the diastolic blood pressure.
- A *decrease* in the systemic vascular resistance will *decrease* the diastolic blood pressure.

The *pulse pressure* is the difference between the systolic and the diastolic blood pressure readings. If the patient has a blood pressure of 132/74 mmHg, for example, the pulse pressure would be derived by subtracting the diastolic from the systolic. In this case, the pulse pressure would be 58 mmHg (132 − 74 = 58). A *narrow* pulse pressure is defined as being less than 25 percent of the systolic blood pressure reading. In this case, a narrow pulse pressure would be less than 33 mmHg (132 × 25% = 33 mmHg).

In the patient with blood or fluid loss, a narrow pulse pressure is a significant sign.

As a patient loses blood, the following occurs:

- Blood loss *decreases* venous volume, which *decreases* preload, which *decreases* stroke volume, which *decreases* cardiac output.

The systolic blood pressure begins to decrease from the drop in cardiac output. One way the body attempts to compensate for the decrease in blood pressure is by increasing the systemic vascular resistance, which elevates diastolic blood pressure. You will see the following in the blood pressure reading:

↓
Systolic blood pressure | **Narrow pulse pressure**
Diastolic blood pressure |
↑

Although blood pressure may appear to be within normal limits, the narrow pulse pressure may warn you of a dropping cardiac output from blood or fluid loss and a rising systemic vascular resistance as an attempt to compensate for the decreasing pressure.

For example, a patient with suspected bleeding in the abdomen presents with a blood pressure of 108/88 mmHg. Based on normal blood pressure ranges, this blood pressure falls well within a normal range and may not alarm you. However, if you look at the pulse pressure, it is only 20 mmHg (108 − 88 = 20 mmHg).

A normal pulse pressure would be greater than 25 percent of the systolic blood pressure. In this case, a normal pulse pressure would be 27 mmHg or greater (108 × 25% = 27 mmHg). Thus, this patient has a narrow pulse pressure, which may be an indication of a dropping cardiac output from a decrease in venous volume and preload and an increasing systemic vascular resistance to compensate for the decrease in pressure.

By just looking at the patient's blood pressure, you could easily say it is normal. When considering the pulse pressure, as well as other signs of perfusion—such as skin color, temperature, condition, and mental status—you might reclassify it as abnormal.

MICROCIRCULATION

Microcirculation is the flow of blood through the smallest blood vessels: arterioles, capillaries, and venules (▶ **Figure 9-2**).

As mentioned previously, the veins and venules primarily serve a capacitance function by pooling blood as needed and supplying it to the heart as necessary to maintain cardiac output. Arteries branch into arterioles, which are at the terminal ends of the arteries. The arterioles, which are made up of almost all smooth muscle, control the movement of blood into the capillaries.

- Vasoconstriction *decreases* the flow of blood into the capillaries, and vasodilation *increases* the capillary blood flow.

The true capillaries are the sites of exchange between the blood and the cells of nutrients, oxygen, carbon dioxide, glucose, waste products, and metabolic substances. *Metarterioles* are often described as thoroughfares or channels that connect the arterioles and venules. True capillaries branch from the metarterioles. Precapillary sphincters control the movement of blood through the true capillaries. If the precapillary sphincter is relaxed, blood moves through the capillary. If the precapillary sphincter is contracted, the blood is shunted away from the true capillary. The precapillary sphincters help to maintain arterial pressure and control the movement of blood through the capillary beds.

Three regulatory influences control blood flow through the capillaries: local factors, neural factors, and hormonal factors. Local factors are found in the immediate environment around or within the capillary structure—for example, temperature, hypoxia, acidosis, and histamine. A cold temperature would cause the peripheral arterioles to constrict and precapillary sphincters to close, shunting blood away from the capillaries in an attempt to reduce the blood exposure to the cold environment. The opposite would be true in a warm environment, in which the arterioles would dilate, and the precapillary sphincters would open to shunt the blood to the periphery, where it can cool.

Neural factors are associated with the influence of the sympathetic and parasympathetic nervous systems on the arterioles and precapillary sphincters. Sympathetic nervous stimulation would cause the arterioles to constrict and precapillary sphincters to close. Parasympathetic nervous stimulation would cause the arterioles to dilate and the precapillary sphincters to open.

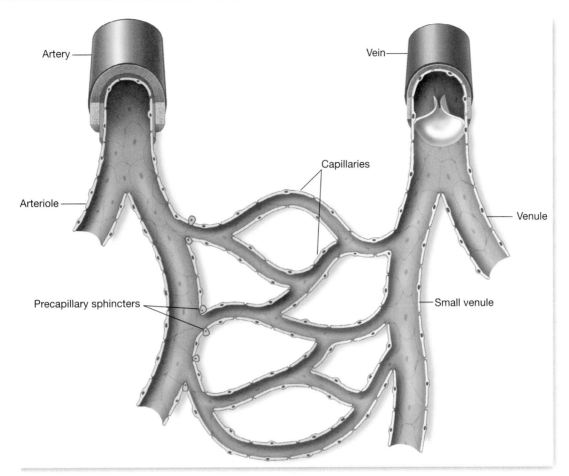

Figure 9-2 Microcirculation is the flow of blood through the smallest blood vessels: arterioles, capillaries, and venules. Precapillary sphincters control the flow of blood through the capillaries.

Hormonal factors are associated with control of the movement of blood through the capillaries. For example, the alpha$_1$ stimulation from epinephrine causes the arterioles to constrict and the precapillary sphincters to close.

In a resting state, the local factors predominantly control blood flow through the capillaries. When adaptation is necessary, the neural factors will change the capillary blood flow. Hormones are usually responsible for a sustained effect on the arterioles and capillaries.

BLOOD PRESSURE

As previously noted, the systolic blood pressure is a measure of cardiac output. The diastolic blood pressure is a measure of systemic vascular resistance. The body's compensation mechanisms are geared toward maintaining pressure inside the vessel and perfusion of the cells.

Blood pressure (BP) is derived by multiplying two major factors: cardiac output (CO) and systemic vascular resistance (SVR).

$$BP = CO \times SVR$$

Both the cardiac output and systemic vascular resistance have a direct effect on blood pressure, which is summarized as follows:

- An *increase* in cardiac output will *increase* blood pressure.
- A *decrease* in cardiac output will *decrease* blood pressure.
- An *increase* in the heart rate will *increase* the cardiac output, which will *increase* blood pressure.
- A *decrease* in the heart rate will *decrease* the cardiac output, which will *decrease* blood pressure.
- An *increase* in the stroke volume will *increase* the cardiac output, which will *increase* blood pressure.
- A *decrease* in the stroke volume will *decrease* the cardiac output, which will *decrease* blood pressure.
- An *increase* in systemic vascular resistance will *increase* blood pressure.
- A *decrease* in systemic vascular resistance will *decrease* blood pressure.

Perfusion of cells is linked to blood pressure. To maintain adequate perfusion, the blood must be pushed with enough force to constantly deliver oxygen and glucose to the cells and remove carbon dioxide and other waste products. The general effect of blood pressure on perfusion is as follows:

- An *increase* in blood pressure will *increase* cellular perfusion.
- A *decrease* in blood pressure will *decrease* cellular perfusion.

Regulation of Blood Pressure by Baroreceptors and Chemoreceptors

Blood pressure is monitored and regulated by both baroreceptors and chemoreceptors.

BARORECEPTORS *Baroreceptors,* located in the aortic arch and carotid sinuses, are stretch-sensitive receptors that detect changes in blood pressure. As the pressure inside the vessels changes, it decreases or increases the stretch of the

> **Vasodilation increases the vessel diameter and decreases the systemic vascular resistance, which decreases blood pressure.**

fibers of the baroreceptors. The baroreceptors, having thus detected the change in blood pressure, send impulses to the cardioregulatory and vasomotor centers in the brainstem to make compensatory alterations in blood pressure. The cardioregulatory center consists of the cardioexcitatory (cardioacceleratory) center and the cardioinhibitory center, which control heart rate and force of cardiac contraction. The vasomotor center controls the vessel size and resistance through vasoconstriction and vasodilation.

An increase in blood pressure prompts the baroreceptors to signal the brainstem to alter heart function and vessel size to decrease blood pressure. The cardioinhibitory center responds by sending parasympathetic nervous system impulses that cause the heart to decrease heart rate and myocardial contractility. A decrease in myocardial contractility decreases stroke volume. A decrease in stroke volume and heart rate decreases cardiac output. A decrease in cardiac output decreases blood pressure. The vasomotor center responds by parasympathetic impulses to dilate the blood vessels. Vasodilation increases the vessel diameter and decreases the systemic vascular resistance, which decreases blood pressure.

A decrease in blood pressure prompts the baroreceptors to signal the brainstem to alter heart function and vessel size to increase blood pressure. The cardioexci-

tatory and vasomotor centers send out sympathetic nervous system impulses to increase the heart rate and myocardial contractility and to constrict the vessels. The increase in heart rate increases the cardiac output. The increase in myocardial contractility increases the stroke volume, which increases the cardiac output. An increase in cardiac output increases blood pressure. Vasoconstriction decreases blood vessel diameter and increases the systemic vascular resistance, which increases blood pressure.

CHEMORECEPTORS As discussed previously, the chemoreceptors monitor the content of oxygen, carbon dioxide, and hydrogen ions, as well as the pH of blood. The greatest stimulation to change blood pressure occurs when the oxygen content in arterial blood decreases. An increase in the carbon dioxide level and a decrease in the pH (more acid) have a much lesser effect on increasing blood pressure. When the oxygen content in the arterial blood falls, the carbon dioxide level increases or pH decreases (more acid in the blood), and the brainstem triggers the sympathetic nervous system through the cardioexcitatory center and vasomotor centers to increase blood pressure by increasing the heart rate, myocardial contractility, and vasoconstriction.

The increase in blood pressure is intended to improve the delivery of oxygen to the brain cells and to remove more carbon dioxide. These changes account for the signs you may observe as an AEMT. An early sign of hypoxia is pale, cool, clammy skin and an increase in heart rate. The pale, cool skin is from vasoconstriction, and the increase in heart rate is from sympathetic stimulation of the SA node.

A decrease in blood pressure and oxygen content in the blood will also trigger the release of a cascade of hormones from different endocrine organs. This is discussed in greater detail in Topic 38, "Shock."

Maintaining aerobic metabolism is essential for the cells, the organs, and the patient to survive. In summary, to maintain aerobic metabolism of cells, the following must be adequate:

- Oxygen content in ambient air
- Patency of the airway
- Minute ventilation
  - Ventilatory rate
  - Tidal volume
- Alveolar ventilation
  - Ventilatory rate
  - Tidal volume
- Perfusion in the pulmonary capillaries
  - Venous volume
  - Right ventricular pump function
- Gas exchange between the capillaries and the alveoli
- Content of blood
  - Red blood cells
  - Hemoglobin
  - Plasma
- Cardiac output
  - Heart rate
  - Preload
  - Stroke volume
  - Myocardial contractility
  - Afterload
- Systemic vascular resistance
  - Sympathetic nervous system stimulation
  - Parasympathetic nervous system stimulation
  - Gas exchange between the capillaries and the cells

TRANSITIONING

REVIEW ITEMS

1. A dramatic increase in the pressure and blood volume in the pulmonary capillaries would likely lead to _____.
   a. bronchospasm
   b. pulmonary edema
   c. a decrease in heart rate
   d. hypotension

2. Which of the following clinical signs would you expect the patient to exhibit in response to a decrease in the plasma oncotic pressure?
   a. hypertension
   b. bradycardia
   c. peripheral edema
   d. jugular venous distention

3. Preload is primarily determined by _____.
   a. venous blood volume
   b. pressure in the aortic root
   c. cellular uptake of glucose
   d. alveolar ventilation

4. Your patient has just received albuterol by nebulizer for bronchospasm. As a side effect of the medication, you would likely see an increase in the heart rate owing to _____.
   a. parasympathetic stimulation
   b. reduction in the oxygen content in the blood
   c. beta$_2$ stimulation of the sinoatrial node
   d. trace amounts of beta$_1$ in the nebulized drug

5. Which of the following signs would directly indicate an increase in systemic vascular resistance?
   a. a decrease in heart rate
   b. a decrease in systolic blood pressure
   c. a widened pulse pressure
   d. pale, cool skin

APPLIED PATHOPHYSIOLOGY

1. Define hydrostatic pressure and plasma oncotic pressure.

2. List, define, and describe the factors that determine the cardiac output, systemic vascular resistance, and blood pressure.

3. Describe the influence of the sympathetic nervous system and parasympathetic nervous system on the cardiac output and blood pressure.

4. Define microcirculation, and describe how it affects blood pressure and perfusion.

5. Identify the location and describe the role of the baroreceptors.

6. Discuss how the chemoreceptors influence changes in blood pressure.

CLINICAL DECISION MAKING

You arrive on the scene and find a 46-year-old man who fell while bicycling for exercise. He has an open midshaft femur fracture. Blood is spurting from the wound. The patient responds slowly when you call out his name. His respiratory rate is 24/minute. His radial pulse is very weak. His skin is extremely pale, cool, and clammy. His blood pressure is 94/76 mmHg, and heart rate is 131 beats per minute.

1. Following scene safety, what is your first immediate action after approaching this patient?

2. What are the life threats to this patient?

3. Why is the patient's mental status deteriorating, and why is he responding so poorly?

4. How is the spurting blood affecting the perfusion of the cells?

5. What is causing a decrease in the systolic blood pressure?

6. Is the pulse pressure narrow? If so, describe why.

7. Why is the skin pale, cool, and clammy?

8. Why is the heart rate 131 bpm?

9. Are this patient's cells likely undergoing aerobic or anaerobic metabolism? Why?

10. Why does the patient have such a lack of energy?

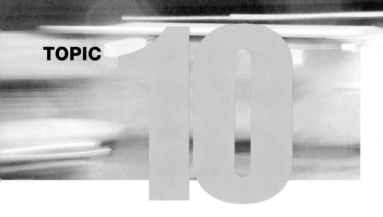

Standard Life Span Development

Competency Applies fundamental knowledge of life span development to patient assessment and management.

LIFE SPAN DEVELOPMENT

- *Brief overview of how understanding life span development can help the Advanced EMT when dealing with differing age brackets.*

- *Identification of the revised age brackets when discussing life span development.*

- *Explanation of the common characteristics of each developmental age bracket:*
  - *Physiologic development.*
  - *Psychological maturation.*
  - *Normal vital signs.*
  - *Assessment tips.*

TABLE 10-1	Stages of Development
Stage of Development	**Age Range**
Neonate	Birth to 1 month
Infant	1 month to 1 year
Toddler	1 to 3 years
Preschooler	3 to 6 years
School age	6 to 12 years
Adolescence	12 to 19 years
Early adulthood	20 to 40 years
Middle adulthood	41 to 60 years
Late adulthood	61 years and older

INTRODUCTION

Many physical and psychosocial changes occur to people throughout their lifetimes. Even though all individuals experience these changes at their own pace, certain benchmarks should be achieved during specific periods. An individual who is not capable of performing certain tasks during the appropriate time frame should be evaluated by a physician. It is important for the Advanced EMT (AEMT) to understand what to expect during each developmental stage (see Table 10-1) and to apply that knowledge when assessing and treating patients (▶ Figure 10-1).

NEONATES AND INFANTS

Some of the most rapid growth and development occur during the neonate and infant period in a child's life. As the child ages, changes will continue to occur in every system of his body.

At birth, the neonate usually weighs around 3 kg, 25 percent of which is the head. The infant cranium has fontanels, which allow room for rapid growth of the brain during this time. Some of the birth weight is lost during the first week of life, but with

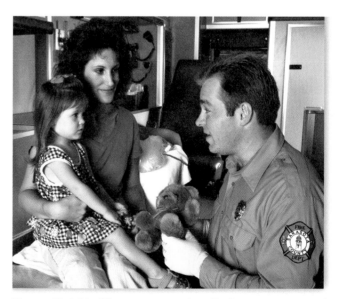

Figure 10-1 Modify your approach to fit the patient's stage of development.

proper breast or formula feedings it is quickly regained. After this initial period, the weight will continue to increase as the infant is able to consume soft, then solid, foods after the primary teeth emerge.

The neonate is primarily a nose breather. An infant's airways are shorter and narrower than those of adults, making the infant more susceptible to airway obstruction. The immune system is immature, and the passive immunity acquired from the mother will be retained for only about the first six months. Immunizations normally are administered after birth and continue to be provided throughout childhood.

The infant's nervous system allows for normal movement and sensation, but at this age the infant is not capable of localizing pain. Reflexes such as blinking, rooting, sucking, and grasping are present at birth and allow for the infant's survival.

Infants also experience psychosocial changes during this period. Their primary relationships involve those who fulfill their needs. By the end of this stage, the infant will be able to recognize the faces of parents and family. The infant will usually cry when separated from caregivers. An infant will also cry in response to pain, a basic need, or anger. Some of the developmental milestones for an infant appear in Table 10-2.

TABLE 10-2 Developmental Milestones for Infants

Age	Gross Motor	Visual–Motor and Problem Solving	Language, Social, and Adaptive
1 month	Raises head slightly from prone position, makes crawling movements	Birth: visually fixes 1 month: has tight grasp, follows to midline	Alerts to sound Regards face
2 months	Holds head in midline, lifts chest off table	No longer clenches fist tightly, follows object past midline	Smiles socially (after being stroked or talked to) Recognizes parent
3 months	Supports on forearms in prone position, holds head up steadily	Holds hands open at rest, follows in circular fashion, responds to visual threat	Coos (produces long vowel sounds in musical fashion) Reaches for familiar people or objects Anticipates feeding
4 months	Rolls front to back, supports on wrists and shifts weight	Reaches with arms in unison, brings hands to environment midline	Laughs, orients to voice Enjoys looking around
5 months	Rolls back to front, sits supported	Transfers objects	Says "ah-goo" Orients to bell (localizes laterally)
6 months	Sits unsupported, puts feet in mouth in supine position	Unilateral reach, uses raking grasp	Babbles Recognizes strangers
7 months	Creeps	7–8 months: inspects objects 7–9 months: finger-feeds	Orients to bell (localizes indirectly)
8 months	Comes to sit, crawls		Says "Dada" indiscriminately
9 months	Pivots when sitting, pulls to stand, "cruises"	Uses pincer grasp, probes with forefinger, gestures, waves bye-bye, holds bottle, throws objects	Says "Mama" indiscriminately Understands "no" Starts to explore environment, plays gesture games (e.g., patty-cake)
10 months			Says "Dada" and "Mama" discriminately Orients to bell (directly)
11 months			Says one word other than "Dada" and "Mama" Follows one-step command with gesture
12 months	Walks alone	Uses mature pincer grasp, releases voluntarily, marks paper with pencil	Uses two words other than "Dada" and "Mama," immature jargoning (runs several unintelligible words together) Imitates actions, comes when called, cooperates with dressing
13 months			Uses three words
14 months			Follows one-step command without gesture

Note: Milestones vary and are designed to provide a general guideline.

Source: Developmental Milestones, in Gunn KL, Nechyba C (eds.). The Harriet Lane Handbook, 16th ed. Copyright © Elsevier (2003).

Tips for Assessment of Neonates and Infants

- The infant's fontanels (when sunken) may provide an indirect estimate of hydration.
- Look at both the chest and abdomen when assessing an infant's respirations.
- Look for symmetrical movement of the extremities during your assessment.
- Keep the infant warm and dry.
- Suspect an underlying cause if the infant continues to cry excessively after needs have been met.
- Keep the parent calm. The infant is an expert in body language.
- Distractions such as toys and penlights are useful tools to help provide emotional control of the infant during the assessment.
- Smile to help reassure the infant.

TODDLERS AND PRESCHOOLERS

Toddlers continue to grow physically throughout this period. The musculoskeletal system increases in density, and the child's weight will taper by the end of this period. The brain is the fastest-growing part of the child's body and will reach 90 percent of its adult weight by the end

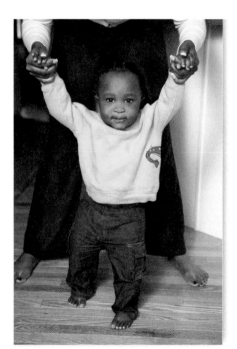

Figure 10-2 A young toddler begins to exhibit improved motor skills and problem-solving abilities.

TABLE 10-3	Developmental Milestones of Toddlers	
Physical Skills	**Social Skills**	**Cognitive Thinking**
Walks alone	Imitates behavior of others	Finds objects even when hidden two or three levels deep
Pulls toys behind when walking	Aware of self as separate from others	Sorts by shape and color
Begins to run	Enthusiastic about company of other children	Plays make-believe
Stands on tiptoe		
Kicks a ball		

Adapted from American Academy of Pediatrics, "Toddler Growth & Development." www.healthychildren.org (accessed November 1, 2010).

TABLE 10-4	Developmental Milestones of Preschoolers	
Physical Skills	**Social Skills**	**Cognitive Thinking**
Climbs well	Imitates adults and playmates	Makes mechanical toys work
Walks up and down stairs	Shows affection for familiar playmates	Plays make-believe
Kicks balls	Can take turns in games	Sorts objects by shape and color
Runs easily	Understands "mine" and "his/hers"	Completes three- and four-piece puzzles
Pedals tricycle		Understands concept of "two"
Bends over without falling		

Adapted from American Academy of Pediatrics, "Preschool Growth & Development." www.healthychildren.org/English/ages-stages/preschool/Pages/default.aspx (accessed November 1, 2010).

of this period. Toddlers acquire some fine motor skills during this period. These children acquire active immunity, as they are exposed to various pathogens. It is during this period that toddlers will be potty trained.

Children in this age group are able to communicate through language. They can form sentences and tend to take each word literally. They develop friendships and participate in playtime. Playing allows a child to engage in new activities, solve problems, and develop social skills (▶ **Figure 10-2**).

Toddlers will often experience separation anxiety about their parents. These children frequently have misconceptions about illnesses and injuries, and many believe their behavior may have caused the problems. Some developmental milestones for toddlers and preschoolers appear in **Tables 10-3** and **10-4**.

Tips for Assessment of Toddlers and Preschoolers

- Speak softly and use language the child can understand.
- Allow the child to touch the equipment before you use it.
- Allow the parent to stay with the child if possible.
- Praise and reassure the child. This will help build a positive rapport.
- Allow the child to have some control over his experience, such as picking which ear you examine first.
- Use a toy or favorite object to help calm the child.

SCHOOL-AGE CHILDREN

Children in school continue to grow and change. Many experience some discomfort as their bones increase in size and density.

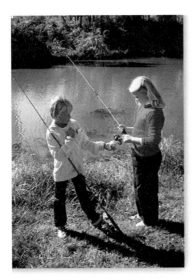

Figure 10-3 School-age children participate in a wide variety of activities and use their experiences to develop skills to solve problems.

They lose their primary teeth and begin to replace them with permanent ones. Their brain function continues to increase.

Children in this age group are able to communicate in various forms. They can read and write. During this period, they develop their own self-concept and begin to compare themselves with their peers. Many participate in a wide variety of extracurricular activities and use their experiences to develop skills to solve problems (▶ Figure 10-3). They understand concepts of pain, death, and illness but usually are afraid when such events occur.

Tips for Assessment of School-Age Children

- A child may have misconceptions about how much you can do. Answer and address the child's concerns and fears honestly.
- Communicate with the child at his level.
- Explain procedures to the child before doing them.
- Gain information from both the child and parent. Make sure you include the child in your conversation.
- Continue to provide choices for the child as long as it does not impede emergency care.

ADOLESCENTS

Adolescents continue to grow—usually in spurts—during this period. Usually this growth ends at age 16 for girls and 18 for boys. It is during this stage that the adolescent will go through puberty and experience significant sexual development. The female adolescent will begin menstruation, her breasts will enlarge, she will grow pubic and axillary hair, her hips will widen, and her waist will get smaller. The male adolescent will grow facial, pubic, and axillary hair, his voice will deepen, his shoulders will broaden, his muscles will increase in size, and his penis and testicles will grow. Both genders will experience hormonal changes during this time.

Adolescents desire to be treated as adults, and they value their privacy. They are capable of making many types of decisions, but they still require parental consent for treatment. Many adolescents participate in risky behaviors during this period and view themselves as invulnerable. Conflicts in family relationships, especially with parents, are common during this time. Adolescents' sense of identity and self-esteem are influenced drastically by their body image and peer relationships (▶ Figure 10-4).

Tips for Assessment of Adolescents

- Begin by interviewing the parent and adolescent together, then gain consent from the parent to finish the interview and assessment in private with the adolescent.
- Conduct the interview and assessment as you would for an adult
- Remain unbiased and nonjudgmental.

EARLY ADULTHOOD

During early adulthood, peak physical condition is obtained; then the physical condition begins to slow down. Fat is stored, weight is gained, and muscle tone is decreased in the adult body. The habits and routines established during this period affect the quality of health and life.

It is during early adulthood that many individuals complete school, adopt

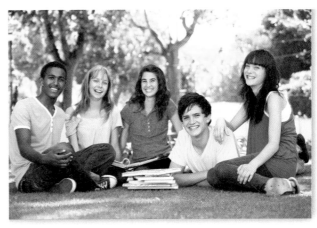

Figure 10-4 Adolescents' sense of identity and self-esteem are influenced by their body image and peer relationships. (© Monkey Business Images/Shutterstock)

careers, and leave their parents' homes. Many adults will choose to marry and begin families of their own. These adults typically have the highest levels of job stress but are usually more capable of coping with the stress than they were when they were younger.

MIDDLE ADULTHOOD

During middle adulthood, the body experiences varying amounts of degradation but is usually capable of functioning at high levels. Chronic illnesses, vision and hearing changes, and cardiovascular concerns are common during this time. Women experience menopause during this period, and many will lose height because of osteoporosis.

Most adults during this period accomplish their personal goals. Some delay seeking help for their own health issues so they can help their parents or children. They are aware of time, and tend to create goals for the remainder of their lives. It is during this period that their children usually leave home, and they become grandparents.

LATE ADULTHOOD

During late adulthood, the rate of occurrence of disease and illness increases, and body systems continue to deteriorate. The workload and size of the heart increase, and the functional blood volume decreases. The lung capacity and diffusion of gases in the alveoli are diminished. The loss of neurons in the brain can result in problems with memory

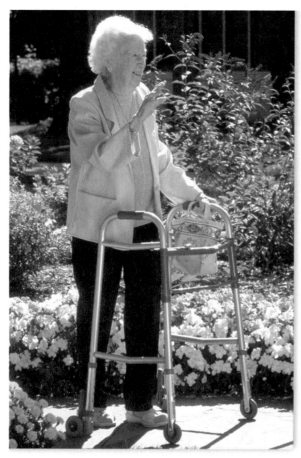

Figure 10-5 Many older adults face new challenges, but the ability to learn and adjust continues throughout life.

and movement. Sensory functions also decrease, and many individuals will require aids to help compensate for the loss. The gastrointestinal system functions less effectively; problems with absorption, constipation, and hydration are common in this age group. Adults during this period have decreased metabolism and renal functions. Many older adults will have underlying chronic conditions that may exist outside the current emergency.

Older adults face challenges that they may have not experienced before (▶ Figure 10-5). They reflect on their lives and consider their death or those of their loved ones. Some older adults have difficulty finding self-worth. Many are forced into retirement and have to make difficult housing and living decisions. Finances may influence the ability of some of these adults to receive certain health care benefits and remain compliant with their medications.

Tips for Assessment of Adults in Middle or Late Adulthood

- Speak in a normal tone unless you are certain that the patient has a hearing problem.
- Allow extra time for the patient to formulate a response to your questions.
- Do not assume that every elderly patient has cognitive or physical problems.
- Show respect for the patient and listen attentively to the patient's needs.

NORMAL VITAL SIGNS

It is very important to assess vital signs on every patient multiple times to identify trends and obtain a more accurate physiologic assessment of the patient. The Advanced EMT should know the common ranges of vital signs for every age group. By knowing the usual values for each group, it is possible to identify when they are not within the norm and incorporate that knowledge into your emergency care.

Table 10-5 shows the normal vital sign ranges during each stage of development.

TABLE 10-5 Normal Vital Signs

Stage of Development	Pulse (beats per minute)	Respirations (breaths per minute)	Blood Pressure (average mmHg)	Temperature (degrees Fahrenheit)
Infancy: at birth	100–180	30–60	60–90 systolic	98–100
Infancy: at 1 year	100–160	30–60	87–105 systolic	98–100
Toddlers	80–110	24–40	95–105 systolic	98.6–99.6
Preschoolers	70–110	22–34	95–110 systolic	98.6–99.6
School age	65–110	18–30	97–112 systolic	98.6
Adolescence	60–90	12–26	112–128 systolic	98.6
Early adulthood	60–100	12–20	120/80	98.6
Middle adulthood	60–100	12–20	120/80	98.6
Late adulthood	Depends on patient's physical and health status	Depends on patient's physical and health status	Depends on patient's physical and health status	98.6

Modified from Bryan E. Bledsoe, Robert S. Porter, and Richard A. Cherry, *Paramedic Care Principles & Practice,* 3rd ed. Upper Saddle River, NJ: Pearson/Prentice Hall, 2009.

REVIEW ITEMS

1. You are assessing a toddler. You expect his pulse rate to be between _____ times a minute.
   - a. 80 and 110
   - b. 60 and 100
   - c. 100 and 160
   - d. 65 and 110

2. By what age should an infant be able to sit unsupported?
   - a. 2 months
   - b. 4 months
   - c. 6 months
   - d. 8 months

3. During which stage does significant sexual development occur?
   - a. school age
   - b. adolescence
   - c. early adulthood
   - d. middle adulthood

4. Which of the following occurs during late adulthood?
   - a. The blood volume increases.
   - b. The blood volume decreases.
   - c. The size of the heart decreases.
   - d. The lung capacity increases.

5. A neonate's head weighs about _____ percent of the entire body weight.
   - a. 10
   - b. 40
   - c. 15
   - d. 25

APPLIED KNOWLEDGE

1. List the stages of development and their corresponding ages.

2. Explain the significance of knowing the milestones for each age group.

3. What physical changes occur to adolescents during puberty?

4. Why is it important to use age-appropriate language during your assessment?

CLINICAL DECISION MAKING

You arrive at a residence for a child who fell. You are met by an adolescent, who states she was babysitting her 2-year-old niece. She says she put the child down for a nap in her crib about an hour earlier. She says she was talking to her boyfriend on the telephone when she heard a loud thump. When she ran into the room she saw the child on the floor crying.

1. What types of responses to your questions should you expect from the adolescent?

2. Is the mechanism of injury described by the teen a reasonable one based on the child's age?

The teen states she picked up the child and tried to comfort her, but it didn't work. She says she just kept calling for Mama and holding her arm. She called the parents, who were out of town, and then called the ambulance.

3. How should you approach the child?

4. What techniques can you use to establish a good rapport with the toddler?

You talk to the parents on speakerphone as you approach the child. You perform your primary and secondary assessments.

5. What vital signs do you expect your patient to have?

6. What do you know about the bones of a toddler?

7. How do you expect the patient to respond to you?

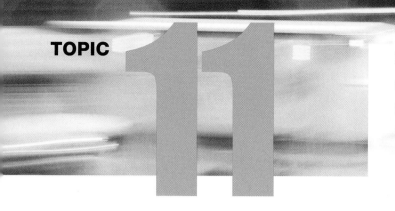

Standard Public Health

Competency Uses simple knowledge of the principles of the role of EMS during public health emergencies.

PUBLIC HEALTH AND EMS

TRANSITION *highlights*

- Introduction to public health and its determining components, and what it means to the Advanced EMT.

- Differences between public health and individual patient care.

- Important milestones public health has achieved, identifying many of those that have directly affected EMS.

- Interface between EMS and public health principals.

INTRODUCTION

Public health is a complex, diverse field composed of people from different backgrounds. Because of its complexity, public health is hard to define. According to the world-renowned public health leader C. E. A. Winslow, who wrote in 1920, public health is

> The science and art of preventing disease, prolonging life, and promoting health and efficiency through organized community effort for the sanitation of the environment, the control of communicable infections, the education of the individual in personal hygiene, the organization of medical and nursing services for the early diagnosis and preventive treatment of disease, and for the development of the social machinery to insure everyone a standard of living adequate for the maintenance of health, so organizing these benefits as to enable every citizen to realize his birthright of health and longevity. *(Winslow 1920)*

Winslow's definition was also referenced in the seminal report, "The Future of Public Health" (Institute of Medicine 1988), which outlined the mission and functions of public health. The mission of public health, according

The core functions of public health include assessment, policy development, and assurance.

to the Institute of Medicine (IOM), is "fulfilling society's interests in assuring [*sic*] conditions in which people can be healthy." Then, in 1994, the U.S. Public Health Service (USPHS) released the document "Public Health in America" with the intent to provide a consensus on definition, vision, and function for public health professionals as well as the public.

According to the USPHS document, the mission of public health is to "promote physical and mental health and prevent disease, injury, and disability" by preventing epidemics and the spread of disease, protecting against environmental hazards, preventing injuries, promoting and encouraging healthy behaviors, responding to disasters and assisting communities in recovery, and ensuring the quality and accessibility of health services (U.S. Public Health Service 2008).

These definitions reflect the core concepts of public health, with an emphasis on prevention. To perform the missions given by the IOM and the USPHS, governmental agencies and private organizations must lead organized efforts to do so. However, government agencies are charged with a major role in ensuring that the mission, core functions, and essential services of public health are achieved.

The core functions of public health addressed at all levels of government include assessment, policy development, and assurance, which are carried out through public health's multiple arms: epidemiology, biostatistics, health policy and management/health administration, behavioral or social science/health education, and environmental health.

Assessment, including epidemiology and biostatistics first and foremost, is the systematic collection, assembly, analysis, and availability of information on the health of the community. *Policy development* entails the development of policies and plans that support individual and community health efforts, enforcement of laws and regulations, and research for new solutions; it involves all arms of government and public health. *Assurance*, generally led by the health policy and management/health administration arm, ensures the provision of health services through the involvement of policy makers and the public in the decision-making process (Institute of Medicine 1988). These core functions are executed through the 10 essential public health services shown in Table 11-1.

TABLE 11-1 Core Functions of Public Health and Essential Public Health Services

Core Functions	Essential Public Health Services
Assessment	Monitor health status to identify community health problems
	Diagnose and investigate health problems and health hazards in the community
	Inform, educate, and empower people about health issues
Policy Development	Mobilize community partnerships to identify and solve health problems
	Develop policies and plans that support individual and community health efforts
	Enforce laws and regulations that protect health and ensure safety
Assurance	Link people to needed personal health services and ensure the provision of health care when otherwise unavailable
	Ensure a competent public health and personal health care workforce
	Evaluate effectiveness, accessibility, and quality of personal and population-based health services
Assessment Policy Development Assurance	Research for new insights and innovative solutions to health problems

Source: Centers for Disease Control and Prevention, National Public Health Performance Standards Program, www.cdc.gov/od/ocphp/nphpsp/index.htm.

PUBLIC HEALTH VERSUS INDIVIDUAL PATIENT CARE

Public health is a unique field in that it partners with many health professions to ensure a healthy population. As a result, public health is often confused with many other professions that may have similar goals and missions. One of the most frequent partnerships occurs between public health and the medical profession.

Although public health and the medical profession work closely to ensure healthy individuals, and both are grounded in science (Afifi and Breslow 1994), the two entities view health differently (see Table 11-2). Public health centers on the prevention of disease, injury, or disability *before* diagnosis of a condition in an entire population. Public health views disability or health conditions as a consequence of numerous factors, including behavioral, biological, social, economic, cultural, environmental, and psychological issues (Institute of Medicine 2003).

In contrast, the medical profession deals with the acute care of ill individuals *after* the onset of symptoms and/or disease. The medical profession views disease or disability as a result of an issue within the body or mind of the individual (Byock 1999). In recent years, however, the medical profession has begun to discourage these views and instead has sought to incorporate aspects of disease prevention into the medical practice. In addition, public health continually uses the expertise of the medical profession in dealing with disease epidemics, including cancer, obesity, influenza, and others.

ACHIEVEMENTS OF PUBLIC HEALTH

Many major improvements in health have been accomplished through public health measures. An excellent way to understand the influence that public health has had on the lives of many is to review the greatest achievements of public health. According to the *Morbidity and Mortality Weekly Report* (Centers for Disease Control and Prevention 1999), the following are the greatest public health achievements:

- Vaccination, resulting in the eradication or elimination of smallpox and poliomyelitis, and control of measles, rubella, tetanus, diphtheria, chickenpox, and human papillomavirus (HPV), among others
- Motor vehicle safety, resulting in a decrease in fatalities owing to laws regulating seat belt use, child safety seats, and alcohol consumption
- Safer workplaces, decreasing worker injury fatalities as a result of improved safety equipment, machinery, and devices, ventilation, and other regulatory efforts
- Control of infectious diseases, through improved water and sanitation practices and advanced scientific and technological advances
- Decline in deaths from coronary heart disease and stroke, from health education and promotion efforts targeting risk factor reduction, increased numbers and better trained emergency medical providers
- Safer and healthier foods, the consequence of handwashing, sanitation, decreased microbial contamination, refrigeration, pasteurization, and pesticides
- Healthier mothers and babies, owing to improved prenatal care, nutrition practices, hygiene, and vaccinations
- Family planning, providing options allowing men and women to better

TABLE 11-2 Public Health versus Medicine

Public Health	Medicine
Population health	Individual health
Disease, condition, or disability = consequence of multiple factors	Disease, condition, or disability = problem within the body or mind
Emphasis on prevention through health education and health promotion	Emphasis on diagnosis and treatment of the patient
Health professionals from various backgrounds working in many settings	Physicians with various specialties working primarily in health care settings

Sources: Byock 1999; Institute of Medicine 1988.

control family size and pregnancies through contraception and fertility measures

- Fluoridation of drinking water, preventing tooth loss and decay
- Recognition of tobacco use as a health hazard, resulting in increased health education and promotion efforts and laws to prevent smoking

Further explanation of public health achievements is shown by the trends in leading causes of mortality in the 21st century in the United States. The leading causes of death in 1900 are a stark contrast to the leading causes of death today. In 1900, the top three causes of death were pneumonia and influenza, tuberculosis, and diarrheal diseases, and the average life expectancy at birth was 47.3 years of age (National Center for Health Statistics n.d.; Arias 2007). In 2006, however, heart disease, cancer, and stroke were the top three causes of death, and the average life expectancy at birth had increased by 30 years to 77.7 years of age, with 20 of those years attributed to public health measures (Heron et al. 2009).

PUBLIC HEALTH LAWS, REGULATIONS, AND GUIDELINES

Although health is viewed as a right of all individuals, it was not a part of the U.S. Constitution. Health was viewed as a primary responsibility of the states. Thus, most public health activities are implemented by state and local governments, although all levels—national, state, and local—are responsible for ensuring a healthy population. Therefore, state and local governments have developed mechanisms to prevent disease, promote health, and protect the health status of their residents by ensuring organized community efforts through enforcement of public health laws, regulations, and guidelines (Institute of Medicine 2003; Kocher 2009; Mensah et al. 2004a, 2004b).

These mechanisms include disease surveillance to monitor disease, injuries, and disability; health screenings and testing; health education and promotion; access to and quality of health care services; vaccinations; and ensuring safe and sanitary conditions (Institute of Medicine 2003).

EMS INTERFACE WITH PUBLIC HEALTH

Preventing, promoting, and protecting the health of a population is no small undertaking; it requires the collective responsibility of all public, private, and voluntary organizations, in addition to individuals and informal associations. As such, public health functions as an intersectoral system in which all organizations and entities contribute and work together to deliver essential public health services within communities (Centers for Disease Control and Prevention 2005).

In 1996, the *EMS Agenda for the Future* envisioned EMS being fully integrated with health care providers, public health, and public safety in treatment and surveillance activities (National Registry of Emergency Medical Technicians 1996). In 2002, the National Public Health Performance Standards Program (Centers for Disease Control and Prevention 2007) unveiled a diagram demonstrating the interrelationships in the public health system. ▶ Figure 11-1 shows the role of the EMS along with other organizations

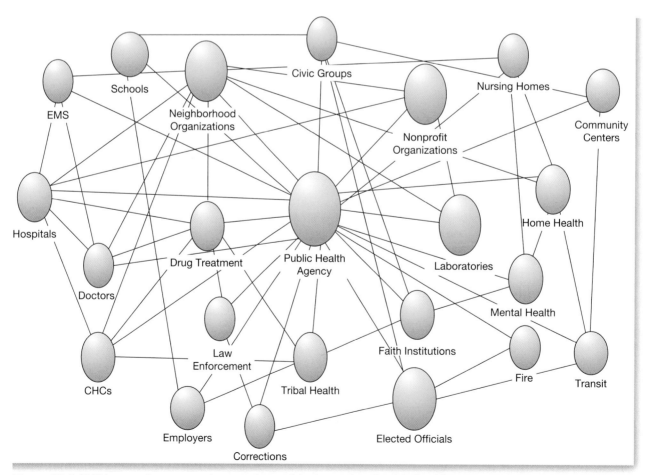

Figure 11-1 EMS has a role among other members of the interrelated public health system.

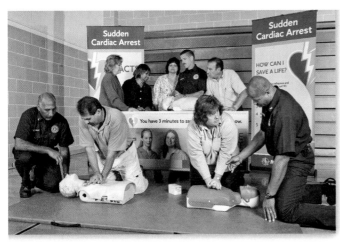

Figure 11-2 The roles of EMS in public health include participation in public education programs and health screenings.

driving under the influence; inform about risk factors for chronic disease; prevent falls; educate about fire injury prevention; promote seat belt, car seat, and helmet use campaigns; and provide correct, relevant, and timely information to communities (▶ Figure 11-2).

During prevention of disease progression, or *secondary prevention*, the role of EMS includes screening to identify those at risk and to minimize disease complications; reporting any potential public health concerns; maintaining safe home environments for children; ensuring public access to automated external defibrillators (AEDs) to help those at high risk for heart attacks; and, of particular and growing importance in recent years, emergency management planning. For example, EMS has been identified by states and local public health agencies to assist with

surveillance, mitigation, and response activities in pandemic influenza planning (Centers for Disease Control and Prevention 2009).

In addition, in disease management and rehabilitation, or *tertiary prevention*, EMS provides treatment and acute care to the community.

In summary, the mission of ensuring the health of the population can be undertaken only through collaborative resources and the efforts of multiple agencies, or the public health system, in which EMS personnel play a vital function. EMS supports public health not only through providing individual treatment and acute patient care but also through surveillance activities and by assisting in the prevention of diseases and disability and reducing the need for further medical care. Continued integration of public health efforts is necessary for responding appropriately to the threats of chronic and infectious disease.

> **Public health functions as an intersectoral system in which all entities work together to deliver essential public health services within communities.**

and entities in the local public health system.

Public health and EMS are partners in ensuring the health of the public. EMS assists public health through multiple functions, both in treatment of the public and in monitoring health and the conditions in which people live. The role of EMS is essential in all levels of prevention. In *primary prevention*—prevention of disease and disability within the community—EMS helps with health promotion and public health education efforts to prevent

TRANSITIONING

REVIEW ITEMS

1. A primary role of EMS that relates directly to the mission of public health is _____.
   a. preventing epidemics through vaccination programs
   b. preventing consumer injuries through education programs
   c. adhering to strict medical direction
   d. implementing quality improvement programs

2. Providing run sheet data on the incidence of gunshot wounds in a particular geographic area would most likely be used directly by which of the following public health arms?
   a. policy development
   b. epidemiology
   c. health administration
   d. behavioral health education

3. The difference between public health and the medical profession is that public health focuses on _____.
   a. prevention of a disease, injury, or disability before diagnosis of a condition in an entire population

   b. treatment of a disease or injury after the onset of signs and symptoms or the diagnosis of the condition
   c. prevention of illness or injury, focusing on individuals in a particular group
   d. the disease or disability as a result of an issue within the body or mind of the individual

4. To which of the following greatest public health achievements has EMS contributed significantly?
   a. elimination of smallpox through vaccination
   b. control of infection through sanitation
   c. decline in coronary heart disease and stroke deaths
   d. healthier mothers and babies through prenatal care

5. Most public health activities are governed by _____.
   a. the U.S. Constitution
   b. the executive branch of the government
   c. federal agencies
   d. state and local laws

REFERENCES

Afifi, A. A., and Breslow, L. 1994. The maturing paradigm of public health. *Annu Rev Public Health*, 15:223–235.

Arias, Elizabeth. 2007. United States Life Tables, 2004. Centers for Disease Control: *National Vital Statistics Reports*, 56:9. www.cdc.gov/nchs/data/nvsr/nvsr56/nvsr56_09.pdf.

Byock, I. R. 1999. Conceptual models and the outcomes of caring. *J Pain Symptom Manage*, 17(2):83–92.

Centers for Disease Control and Prevention. 1999. Ten great public health achievements—United States, 1900–1999. *MMWR*, 48(12):241–243.

_____. 2005. *Building Our Nation's Health System: National Public Health Performance Standards Program*. www.cdc.gov/od/ocphp/nphpsp/PDF/FactSheet.pdf.

_____. 2007. *National Public Health Performance Standards Program: User Guide*. www.cdc.gov/od/ocphp/nphpsp/PDF/UserGuide.pdf.

_____. 2009. *Interim guidance for emergency medical services (EMS) systems and 9-1-1 public safety answering points (PSAPs) for management of patients with confirmed or suspected swine-origin Influenza A (H1N1) infection*. www.cdc.gov/h1n1flu/guidance_ems.htm.

Heron, M. Hoyert, D. L., Murphy, S. L., et al. 2009. *National vital statistics reports. Deaths: Final Data for 2006*. National Center for Health Statistics. www.cdc.gov/nchs/data/nvsr/nvsr57/nvsr57_14.pdf.

Institute of Medicine. 1988. *Future of Public Health*. Washington, DC: National Academy Press.

_____. 2003. *Future of Public Health in the 21st Century*. Washington, DC: National Academy Press.

Kocher, P. 2009. Key concepts of U.S. law in public health practice. PowerPoint Presentation. www2.cdc.gov/phlp/NCCDPHP_Workshop/materials.asp.

Mensah, G. A., Goodman, R. A., Zaza, S., et al. 2004a, January. Law as a tool for preventing chronic diseases: Expanding the spectrum of effective public health strategies, part 1. *Prev Chronic Dis*. www.cdc.gov/pcd/issues/2004/jan/03_0033.htm.

_____. 2004b, April. Law as a tool for preventing chronic diseases: Expanding the spectrum of effective public health strategies, part 2. *Prev Chronic Dis*. www.cdc.gov/pcd/issues/2004/apr/04_0009.htm.

National Center for Health Statistics. n.d. *Leading causes of death, 1900–1908*. www.cdc.gov/nchs/data/dvs/lead1900_98.pdf.

National Registry of Emergency Medical Technicians. 1996. *EMS agenda for the future*. www.nremt.org/nremt/about/emsAgendaFuture.asp.

U.S. Public Health Service. 2008. *Public Health in America*. www.health.gov/phfunctions/public.htm.

Winslow, C. E. A. 1920. The untilled fields of public health. *Science*, 51:23.

Standard Principles of Pharmacology

Competency Applies to patient assessment and management fundamental knowledge of the medications carried by Advanced EMTs that may be administered to a patient during an emergency.

TOPIC

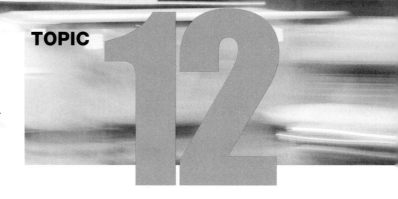

EMS PHARMACOLOGY

INTRODUCTION

As prehospital care has advanced in the 21st century, so has the use of pharmacology in the prehospital environment. Advanced EMTs (AEMTs) have the ability to administer a core group of medications that can have a profound effect in reversing a variety of medical conditions. Therefore, staying current with new pharmacologic treatments in the care of the critically ill or injured patient now presents a tremendous task for the AEMT.

Although understanding a drug's indications, dose, and route of administration are all important, the understanding of how a drug works in the body (on a cellular level) is essential knowledge the AEMT must have.

AEMTs should not (and cannot) become complacent and rely exclusively on charts or pocket references to guide drug therapy during patient management. Books and charts cannot interpret special circumstances that exist in every patient encounter, nor can they offer all the differential approaches to drug therapy that may be required. That is not to say that having reference material immediately available is inappropriate, just that relying solely on a reference chart to make drug therapy decisions is *not* the intended purpose of these guides.

Proper patient management will occur only when the AEMT understands the pathophysiology behind the patient's condition, understands the physiologic actions of the drugs, and then integrates this information to provide the appropriate drug therapy for the patient. A reference chart or book should be used to augment this decision-making process, not replace it.

To aid in the learning process, the information contained within this topic is presented in a logical, concise, and easy-to-read format. It will take an investment of time on the part of the reader, however, to comprehend and apply the information. One word of caution is essential. Do not simply try to memorize drug indications, side effects, contraindications, and so forth. Information learned by rote memory is often lost because of a lack of use, or, during the stress of an emergency, it cannot be recalled. Instead, take the time to thoroughly understand how a drug works. If you are familiar with the way a drug works in the body, the indications, contraindications, and side effects become

obvious. Thus, the only thing left to memorize is the specific drug dose—and there is no shortcut to memorizing drug doses.

The drugs that are discussed here include oxygen, oral glucose, aspirin, nitroglycerin, epinephrine, activated charcoal, naloxone, and bronchodilators.

Note: Although the National EMS Education Standards and the Scope of Practice documents provide a framework for the AEMT's practice, we still expect there to be some state-by-state variation in the medications that are administered by the AEMT. Always follow your local protocols for specific information on medications and dosing strategies.

AEMTs should not become complacent and rely exclusively on charts or pocket references to guide drug therapy during patient management.

PREVENTING MEDICATION ERRORS

As an AEMT, you will have greater responsibility with each of the advanced modalities you use. Studies in the hospital setting have shown that errors are surprisingly common. This likely carries over to EMS. There are many types of errors, but few of these are more dangerous than medication errors.

> The decision to administer a drug is only half the picture; the other half is the decision of when *not* to use a drug.

A medication error may be an error in dose, route, pace of administration, or administering a medication to an allergic patient. A medication may also be administered to a patient whose condition does not match what the drug is intended for. The following points will help you reduce medication errors in your practice as an AEMT.

- Be familiar with all medications you carry and the relevant information for each (indications, contraindications, dose, route, etc.). Carry a reference or have reference information available in the ambulance. Know your protocols.
- Many medication containers look similar. Be sure you have obtained the correct medication from the drug box.
- When speaking with medical direction, verify all medication orders back to the physician and wait for confirmation. Write down the medication, dose, route, and time of the order.
- Verify the amount and concentration of all medications before you administer them.
- Work as a team. Monitor all actions going on around the patient. Your partner or crew should do the same. Good teamwork can help prevent errors. Many AEMTs verify the medication, dose, and route again with a partner before administration.
- Do not practice while fatigued. Fatigue is a significant contributing factor in many medical errors.
- Errors should be prevented. If an error does occur, however, be sure to report it immediately to the emergency department and to a supervisor within your organization. You should also follow your department's guidelines for documenting errors.

EPIDEMIOLOGY

Appreciating the commonality of drug administration in the prehospital setting would certainly help the AEMT understand how often it occurs. However, perhaps what is more important than how often a drug is given (because this is a skill) is how often the situation presents in which a drug may be necessary. To medicate or not is a clinical decision that must be approached logically. To best describe this, one needs to look at the frequency in which these disease processes and emergencies occur. In essence, the decision to administer a drug is only half the picture; the other half is the decision of when *not* to use a drug.

Oxygen is a drug commonly used in the prehospital setting for tissue hypoxia, although hypoxia is a common finding in almost any medical or traumatic emergency—and thus, it is not an emergency in and of itself. No research has looked at the incidence of hypoxia in general; rather, hypoxia has been studied in light of other medical and traumatic conditions. As a result, no statistics speak to the frequency of hypoxia in general; there is, however, the potential for hypoxia in every patient cared for by the AEMT. This makes oxygen the drug most frequently administered by the AEMT.

Recent research has focused on the harmful effects of high oxygen concentration in certain diseases (e.g., post–cardiac arrest, acute coronary syndrome, and stroke). This has caused many systems to base oxygen delivery route and flow on pulse oximetry readings and, in some cases, limit oxygen delivery. It appears that oxygen may not be the benign drug it was once considered.

Hypoglycemia, for which the AEMT may administer glucose (orally or as D_{50}), occurs more frequently in adults and less frequently in children. Approximately 1 in 1,000 people will experience a hypoglycemic episode for which EMS may be summoned. In these situations, the AEMT will need to determine whether oral glucose may be safely administered or whether the patient's condition or situation precludes its use. Overall, of patients who present with signs and symptoms similar to hypoglycemia, 10 percent will actually be hypoglycemic.

Opiate overdose is responsible for 11 percent of ED visits nationwide. The trend has increased since the 1990s, with prescription opiate abuse believed to be the cause. Heroin is a common drug of abuse. Deaths from heroin are most common in men from 20 to 23 years old who have used heroin for 5 to 10 years. Newer users account for only about 15 percent of heroin deaths. Abstinence resulting in a decline in tolerance is believed to be responsible for many of these deaths. An example is recently released prison inmates, for whom the rate of death from heroin overdose is 12 times greater than that for the general population. Naloxone (Narcan) is an opioid antagonist that may be administered IV, IM, SQ, or nasally.

The use of aspirin and nitroglycerin for a patient with cardiac chest pain also occurs frequently. The overall hospital incidence rate for the presentation of chest pain to the emergency department is just over 12 percent (or approximately 7 to 8 million people per year). For 4 million of these people, this chest pain is from a cardiac event. The use of oxygen, aspirin, and nitroglycerin will occur often in this category of patient.

It is estimated that almost 41 million people in the United States have a severe allergy disorder. In the ongoing management of these patients, the physician will often prescribe an epinephrine auto-injector (EpiPen) for use at home should the patient be exposed to the allergen. The AEMT can assist with the administration of the patient's device and, in most cases, will have some sort of epinephrine carried on the ambulance either in auto-injector form or in ampules for IM delivery with a syringe. The AEMT should be well versed in its actions and indications to prevent accidental or inappropriate use that can easily lead to heightened patient morbidity and mortality. Anaphylactic reactions kill more than 1,500 people per year, although the number of people susceptible to an anaphylactic reaction nears 15 percent of the total U.S. population.

Activated charcoal is used for certain ingested poisons. Death from ingesting a poison (intentionally and unintentionally) occurs to more than 35,000 Americans per year. Although activated charcoal may not be used for all ingested poisons, it can be beneficial to some, and the AEMT will have to delineate between the two when the situations arise.

AEMTs will respond to many calls for respiratory distress. This is a type of call in which the bronchodilators available to the AEMT will be very beneficial, both in reversing bronchospasm and relieving a patient's anxiety and distress. The most commonly used medication, albuterol, is often administered by the AEMT via small-volume nebulizer (SVN), but the metered-dose inhaler (MDI) is also effective and may be used. These devices are used when a patient suffers from a respiratory problem in which bronchoconstriction limits airway movement. The most common reason for MDI usage is asthma, which has been on the rise for the past several years. Bronchoconstriction from chronic lung conditions may also be reversed with albuterol.

PATHOPHYSIOLOGY

As discussed in the pathophysiology section of this book, all disturbances of the body—resulting from trauma, illness, or otherwise—occur because of some disturbance that affects normal cellular activity. For example, the patient who is hypoxic because of a chest injury does not have the available oxygen in the bloodstream to maintain normal metabolism and energy production. The body quickly slips into anaerobic metabolism, and a detrimental cascade of events occurs, resulting in acid production and cellular death. With this death, critical masses of tissues and organs begin to fail, eventually resulting in system dysfunction and patient death.

Thus, as the AEMT assesses for findings of dyspnea, the underlying hypoxia has already started to alter cellular functioning, and this in turn is what creates the signs and symptoms the AEMT recognizes.

As such, the administration of appropriate drugs in these (and other) situations is done to *alter* cellular activity—not to make a cell do something it cannot normally do. A drug alters cellular activity by manipulating the target cell's receptor sites. This manipulation then alters intracellular activity.

There are basically two categories of cellular receptor sites—agonists and antagonists—that influence intracellular activity. Agonist receptor sites (and hence agonist drugs) are those that stimulate the receptor sites on the cells to cause an effect, whereas antagonist receptor sites (and drugs) block the receptor sites to inhibit certain cellular functions. This alteration of cellular activity, in turn, affects the action of the tissues and organ systems they are part of, culminating in the desired clinical effect.

Although Table 12-1 does not illustrate a pathologic process per se, it does illustrate how the medications used by the AEMT can have an effect on the pathophysiology of a disease process and help move the body back toward homeostasis. For a more thorough discussion of these drugs, the AEMT should refer to the sections of this book that correspond to the medical emergencies for which these drugs are indicated.

ASSESSMENT FINDINGS

The medical emergencies discussed in this section are found throughout the rest of this book under their own respective topics. As such, the AEMT can refer to those sections for a more enhanced discussion on the pathophysiology, assessment findings, drug therapy, and treatment guidelines. However, for purposes of completeness, Table 12-2 provides an overview of common assessment findings for each of the medical emergencies the AEMT may encounter that may result in drug therapy. (Please note that oxygen should be used for all the medical conditions listed in the table.)

Remember that no drug can be given to the patient by the AEMT without proper authorization by either offline or online medical control. For all medications, ensure that the patient's "five rights" (right dose, route, patient, time, and medication) exist first.

EMERGENCY MEDICAL CARE

Regardless of the specific etiology causing the medical emergency, salient assessment steps and interventions must always be performed for the patient, especially when drug therapy is warranted. Time is always of the essence for an unstable patient, so interventions that the AEMT employs must be completed efficiently and expediently. Remember also to repeat your assessment and assess the effectiveness of interventions that you are using to ensure that they are appropriate and working as well as possible.

1. **Ensure an open airway.** Use common airway techniques to guarantee this.

2. **Provide oxygen.** If the patient is breathing inadequately, provide positive pressure ventilation (PPV) at 10 to 12/min with high-flow supplemental oxygen. Use pulse oximetry as a guide in determining the oxygen required for patients breathing adequately.

3. **Position the patient as appropriate.** If the patient has an altered mental status, a lateral recumbent position will help maintain the airway should the patient regurgitate.

4. **For chest pain patients:**
   a. *Administer 160 to 325 mg aspirin if local protocol allows.*
   b. *Administer 0.3 to 0.4 mg of nitroglycerin if local protocol allows.*

5. **For hypoglycemic patients:** *Administer 1 25g D_{50} IV or 1 tube of oral glucose if the patient is able to maintain his own airway and local protocol allows.*

6. **For anaphylactic patients:** *Administer 0.3 mg of epinephrine (0.15 mg for children) IM or via prescribed autoinjection pen if local protocol allows.*

7. **For patients who recently ingested poison:** *Administer 1 gram per kilogram activated charcoal if the patient is able to swallow and local protocol allows.*

8. **For dyspneic patients with asthma or a chronic pulmonary disease:** *Administer albuterol via SVN or MDI if the patient is breathing adequately and local protocol allows. Also keep the patient in a semi- or high Fowler's position to help ease breathing.*

9. **Provide rapid transport to emergency department.** Notify the receiving emergency department as early as possible. If the patient becomes pulseless and apneic (no pulse, no respirations), immediately apply the automated external defibrillator.

Administration of medications to patients is a very serious responsibility for any level of EMS provider. As much as a medication may help alleviate a patient's condition, it may also be harmful or fatal should the medication be used inappropriately or given to the wrong patient or for the wrong condition. Before administering any medication, be sure you fully understand how the medication works, how the medication is administered, the

TABLE 12-1 Some Medications Commonly Used by AEMTs

Generic Name	Common Trade Name(s)	Mechanism of Action	Indications and Administration
Oxygen (▶ Figure 12-1)	None	Oxygen allows the body to extract the maximum amount of energy from glucose molecules during aerobic metabolism. When supplemented, it allows the bloodstream and red blood cells to carry more oxygen for cellular metabolic activity. Without oxygen, waste products accumulate and the cell will die, so its proper use is extremely important.	Indicated in any patient who has objective or subjective respiratory distress. Given by mask (12–15 lpm) or cannula (1–6 lpm), it should be used when indications of respiratory distress are present, the pulse oximeter is < 95%, the patient complains of dyspnea, or the patient has a medical condition or injury that may lead to hypoxemia.
Dextrose, oral glucose (▶ Figure 12-2)	50% Dextrose, Glutose, Insta-Glucose	Simple sugar obtained by the body through diet that serves as the primary source of energy for the cells. In the presence of oxygen, the mitochondria of the cells convert glucose into ATP, which is the actual energy source used by the body. Without adequate glucose, energy levels will be depleted, and the cells will die.	IV dextrose (25g) is administered in hypoglycemia (blood glucose < 60 mg/dL). It is administered carefully to prevent extravasation (which can cause tissue necrosis). Oral glucose is administered by placing the gel in the mucous membranes of the mouth, where it is absorbed into the bloodstream and distributed to the body.
Aspirin (acetylsalicylic acid) (▶ Figure 12-3)	Bayer, Ecotrin, Bufferin, Buffex	This drug causes rapid antiplatelet activity that prevents the platelets from clumping together during a clotting cascade, thereby inhibiting or limiting the formation of a thrombus at the site of coronary artery occlusion. As such, aspirin may help to maintain sufficient coronary artery perfusion.	Specifically, baby aspirin is used so the patient can easily chew up and swallow the dose (160–325 mg). The drug should be administered to the patient displaying chest pain that is suggestive of an acute coronary event. This drug is typically administered prior to nitroglycerin.
Nitroglycerin (▶ Figure 12-4, bottle at right)	Nitrostat	Nitroglycerin is a medication that will promote both coronary and peripheral vasodilation. The coronary vasodilation improves coronary perfusion, whereas the peripheral vasodilation drops preload and afterload, which in turn diminishes myocardial workload and oxygen requirements. Thus, as it improves coronary perfusion and oxygen delivery, it also diminishes the amount of work the heart has to perform.	Nitroglycerin should be administered to a patient suffering from chest pain characteristic to an acute coronary event. Each dose is 0.3 mg or 0.4 mg, administered sublingually. Do not use nitroglycerin if blood pressure is low, the patient has taken erectile dysfunction (ED) drugs in the past 24 to 48 hours, or you lack proper medical direction to do so.
Nitroglycerin spray (Figure 12-4, bottle at left)	Nitrolingual spray	Same mechanism of action as nitroglycerin tablets; the only difference is how the drug is packaged.	Same indications and dose as nitroglycerin tablets, but this is a sublingual spray.
Epinephrine (▶ Figure 12-5)	Adrenalin	Epinephrine is a drug that has both alpha and beta adrenergic properties. The alpha properties promote vascular constriction to raise blood pressure and inhibit tissue edema, the $beta_1$ properties increase cardiac output, and the $beta_2$ properties promote bronchial smooth muscle relaxation. This helps to correct the laryngeal edema, bronchoconstriction, and hypotension (this is primarily an alpha effect) seen in anaphylaxis.	Epinephrine is administered in the form of an "epi" auto-injector pen. The dose of 0.3 mg (pediatric dose is 0.15 mg) is injected into the lateral thigh of the patient experiencing a moderate to severe anaphylactic reaction. The drug must be prescribed to the patient, and the EMT needs medical direction orders to use it. The dose may be repeated if necessary.
Activated charcoal (▶ Figure 12-6)	Super-Char, InstaChar, Actidose, LiquiChar, Charcoaid	This is a black powder that is very porous. When ingested, it will adsorb poisons in the stomach, prevent absorption by the GI tract, and enhance elimination in the body. As such, the poison can be eliminated from the body with less-extensive damaging effects.	Activated charcoal should be administered to a patient who has ingested a poison by mouth, only on specific orders from medical direction. It is most effective if administered within 1 hour of ingestion. The dose is 1 g/kg of premixed medication.
Small-volume nebulizers (SVNs) (▶ Figure 12-7) Metered-dose inhalers (MDIs) (▶ Figure 12-8)	Proventil, albuterol	$Beta_2$ specific medications, which, on inhalation and deposition on the smooth muscle of the bronchioles, promote relaxation, allow better airflow, and relieve dyspnea.	Albuterol 2.5 mg in 3 mL nebulized. May repeat per protocol. Albuterol MDI, 2 puffs using spacer device when possible. May repeat per protocol. NOTE: Various medications (other bronchodilators, steroids) are prescribed to patients as inhalers. Bronchodilators are administered to a patient who displays dyspnea (subjective and objective); often this includes wheezing on auscultation.

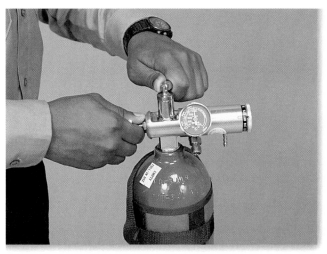

Figure 12-1 Oxygen gas is considered a medication. It is the most commonly used medication in EMS and is carried on the EMS unit.

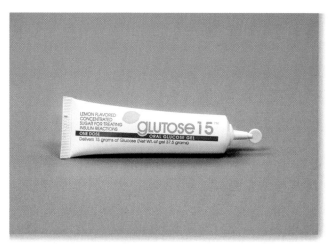

Figure 12-2 Oral glucose is a viscous gel used in acute diabetic emergencies. It is carried on the EMS unit.

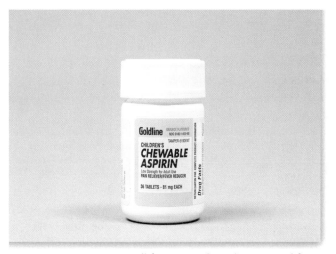

Figure 12-3 Aspirin, in pill form, may be administered for chest pain when a heart attack is suspected.

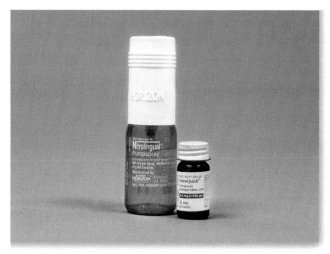

Figure 12-4 Nitroglycerin tablets are one common form of nitroglycerin. Nitroglycerin spray is another form.

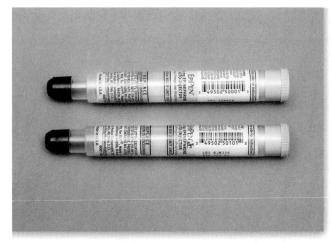

Figure 12-5 An epinephrine auto-injector, such as the EpiPen, may be prescribed for patients with a history of severe allergic or anaphylactic reactions.

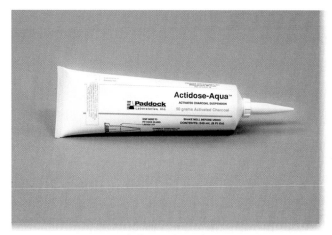

Figure 12-6 Activated charcoal is administered in suspension form and is carried on some EMS units. It may be used in poisoning and overdose emergencies.

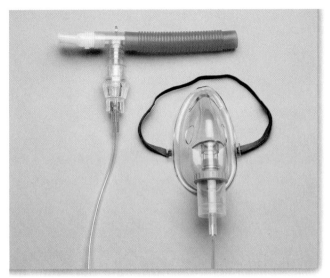

Figure 12-7 Nebulized medications may be administered by a small-volume nebulizer, through either a mouthpiece or a face mask. (© *Carl Leet, YSU*)

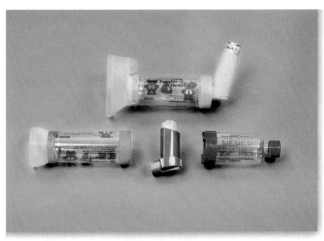

Figure 12-8 A metered-dose inhaler or a metered-dose inhaler with a spacer may be prescribed for respiratory conditions.

TABLE 12-2 Drugs to Be Used in Medical Emergencies

Medical Emergency	History Findings	Assessment Findings	Drug Name and Dose
Myocardial infarction (MI)	Coronary artery disease, hypertension, previous MI, angina, prescribed cardio-vascular drugs	Substernal chest pain, typically dull; radiation to arm, back, neck; possible dyspnea; possible abnormal breath sounds; nausea and vomiting; diaphoresis	Chewable baby aspirin should be given orally at 160–325 mg. This usually amounts to 2–4 baby aspirins. Nitroglycerin tablets or spray can be given at 0.3 to 0.4 mg sublingually.
Hypoglycemic episode	Altered mental status, rapid onset, history of diabetes, insulin injection without eating, physical exertion	Changes in mental status, possible seizures, tachycardia, diaphoresis, low blood sugar (< 60 mg/dL)	25 g D_{50} IV. Oral glucose may be given orally (between cheeks and gums) to responsive patients with an intact gag reflex. Typical dose is the full contents of one tube.
Acute anaphylaxis	History of known allergies, history of exposure to allergen, prescription of EpiPen	Mild to severe dyspnea, itching and hives on skin, warm and reddened skin, wheezing to auscultation, stridor, possible change in mental status, pulse ox diminished, tachycardia and hypotension	0.3 mg of epinephrine IM or via EpiPen (0.15 mg for children). Epi auto-injector is injected in the lateral thigh region for moderate to severe anaphylaxis. Consider redosing with ongoing symptoms.
Ingested poison	Known or suspected ingestion of caustic substance; possible psychiatric history or history of attempted suicide (activated charcoal is not used with caustics)	Visible burns (to mouth, lips and pharynx), abdominal pain, nausea and vomiting, diarrhea, possible change in mental status and changes in vital signs	For certain types of ingested poisons, activated charcoal may be administered at 1 g/kg orally. It may be necessary to mix drug in cold water.
Respiratory distress	Asthma, emphysema, chronic bronchitis, MOI or NOI to chest, possible physical exertion, subjective respiratory distress.	Tripod positioning, nasal flaring, diminishing pulse oximetry, abnormal breath sounds (rales, wheezing, ronchi, or diminished), retractions, tachypnea, vital sign changes	Oxygen should be administered based on pulse oximetry reading in responsive patients—especially those experiencing acute coronary syndromes and suspected stroke. Oxygen should not be withheld from patients in significant distress. If the patient is breathing inadequately, administer oxygen during PPV. MDI (2 puffs) or SVN with inhaled beta$_2$ agonists for reactive airway conditions, as indicated by protocol.

Medical Emergency	History Findings	Assessment Findings	Drug Name and Dose
Hypoxemia	Altered mental status, changes in vital signs, diminished pulse oximetry, history of significant illness or injury, cyanosis	Tachycardia, low pulse oximetry (<95%), changes in skin color (cyanosis), anxiety or mental depression, general objective signs of respiratory distress	High-flow oxygen (>12 lpm) should be given via nonrebreather if the patient is breathing adequately. If breathing inadequately, administer oxygen during PPV.
Opioid overdose (▶ Figure 12-9)	History of opioid use or prior overdose	Lethargy, depressed respirations, track marks of other evidence of drug injection, pinpoint pupils (not in Demerol and some other semisynthetic narcotics)	Naloxone 0.4–2.0 mg IV, IM, or intranasally titrated to attain adequate respirations. NOTE: Additional doses may be required, as the effect of opioids may outlast the antagonist effect of naloxone.

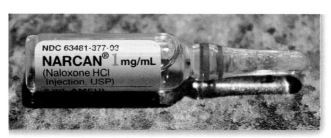

Figure 12-9 Naloxone is used in opioid overdoses and may be administered IV, IM, SQ, or intranasally.

appropriate dose, contraindications to the medications, and potential side effects.

Always operate within your local medical directives (whether offline or online); if a situation arises in which you are not sure whether a medication should be administered or not, always consult medical direction at the receiving facility for additional guidance. In addition, following the administration of any medication, complete a reassessment of the patient to determine whether any changes exist in the patient's clinical status that may necessitate a change in your treatment goals.

TRANSITIONING

REVIEW ITEMS

1. If a drug causes a stimulatory effect on the body, thereby increasing its normal metabolic cellular activity, what type of effect is being provided to the receptor sites in the cellular wall?
   a. agonist
   b. antagonist
   c. stimulatory
   d. depressant

2. What drug characteristic causes the blood vessels of the body to constrict, thereby raising blood pressure?
   a. indication
   b. side effect
   c. contraindication
   d. mechanism of action

3. A patient you are caring for needs activated charcoal administered. The patient weighs 240 pounds. What would be the total dose of medication?
   a. 87 grams
   b. 109 grams
   c. 120 grams
   d. 240 grams

4. A patient with emphysema presents to EMS. He is extremely dyspneic and has an altered mental status as well as minimal breath sounds in the bases of the lungs bilaterally, and the pulse oximeter is dropping. What drug would be most warranted in this situation?
   a. MDI
   b. oxygen
   c. EpiPen
   d. mechanical ventilation

5. Nitroglycerin is a medication that will typically cause what type of side effect in the body?
   a. rapid breathing
   b. slowing of the pulse
   c. dropping of blood pressure
   d. diminishment in mental status

APPLIED PATHOPHYSIOLOGY

You are caring for an elderly female patient with respiratory distress. The patient has a history of emphysema. Currently she is speaking in full sentences and has a respiratory rate of 26/minute, the pulse oximeter reads 94 percent on room air, bilateral breath sounds are present but diminished, and blood pressure is 149/86 mmHg.

1. Given this presentation, list two drugs that may be appropriate for this patient.

2. Beyond oxygen, what other medications (and their respective doses) could be administered to a patient complaining of chest pain that is consistent with an acute coronary event?

CLINICAL DECISION MAKING

You encounter a 59-year-old male patient sitting on the front porch of his residence. As you approach the patient, you see that he is struggling very hard to breathe. On the ground beside him is a yard rake and a can of aerosolized hornet/bee killer. After determining that the scene is safe, you approach the patient. He is sitting upright in a tripod position and appears to be in significant respiratory distress.

1. Based on what you observe in the scene size-up, list the possible conditions you suspect the patient is experiencing.

The primary assessment reveals that the patient is anxious and confused. You hear stridorous sounds on inhalation, and you determine that he has a respiratory rate of 38/minute with minimal chest rise and fall. The peripheral pulses are absent, and his heart rate is 116 beats per minute. The skin is warm and flushed, and you note reddened hives on the body. The SpO$_2$ reading is 84 percent.

2. What are the life threats to this patient?

3. What immediate emergency care should you provide based on the initial assessment?

4. What conditions have you ruled out from your initial consideration in the scene size-up?

During the secondary assessment, inspection of the mouth reveals the mucous membranes are swollen and breath sounds are becoming distant, and you note both inspiratory and expiratory wheezing bilaterally. The patient also states that he feels a "tightness" in his chest that seems to spread down both arms. The abdomen is unremarkable, the

pelvis is stable, and there are no deformities or evidence of trauma to the extremities. The extremities are warm, flushed, and diaphoretic. The peripheral pulses are barely palpable. The patient states that he has mild asthma and is allergic to certain bee stings, for which he carries an EpiPen. His medical history also includes mild asthma, for which he takes albuterol as needed. His last food intake was three hours ago and consisted of a fast-food hamburger and fries. His blood pressure is 80/62 mmHg, heart rate is 138 beats per minute, and his respirations are 36 per minute and increasingly labored.

5. What conditions have you ruled out in your differential field diagnosis? Why?

6. What conditions are you considering as a probable cause? Why?

7. Based on your differential diagnosis, what are the next steps in emergency care? Why?

8. Based on the history, what type of reaction is this patient experiencing?

9. For the following pathophysiologic changes, list the drug and its corresponding dose that would best correct the underlying disturbance:
   a. SpO$_2$ 84 percent
   b. Inspiratory stridor
   c. Bilateral wheezing
   d. Hypotension

Standard Airway Management, Respiration, and Artificial Ventilation

Competency Applies knowledge (fundamental depth, foundational breadth) of additional upper airway anatomy and physiology to patient assessment and management in order to ensure a patent airway, adequate mechanical ventilation, and respiration for patients of all ages.

TOPIC

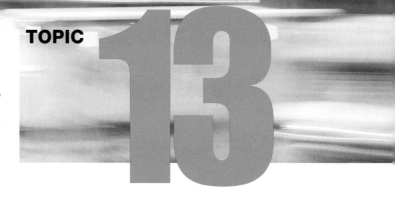

ISSUES IN AIRWAY MANAGEMENT, OXYGENATION, AND VENTILATION

INTRODUCTION

Hypoxia kills. This is a fact that every Advanced EMT should understand. Whether the hypoxia is caused by a primary breathing problem or associated with a larger illness or injury, assessment and treatment must focus on reversing this disorder.

The diagnosis of airway and respiratory dysfunction can be a complicated and difficult process. Many very different illnesses can present with similar signs and symptoms. Thankfully, however, the immediate assessment and treatment of a patient in respiratory failure remain consistent, regardless of the nature of the illness. Although differential diagnosis is important, early recognition and immediate action are more important, especially when the overall cause is unclear.

EPIDEMIOLOGY

According to the Centers for Disease Control and Prevention, respiratory distress accounts for roughly 2 percent of all emergency department visits. Although this may seem like a small percentage, the absolute numbers are, in fact, very high, considering how many patients use the EMS system overall. This means that as AEMTs, we see a significant number of respiratory distress patients in the field.

PATHOPHYSIOLOGY

Respiratory dysfunctions are typically the result of either an obstruction of air movement, such as something in the way, or changes in the respiratory structures that affect the movement of oxygen and carbon dioxide. Occasionally both issues play a role. Respiratory dysfunctions can be further classified as either upper or lower airway problems. Upper airway issues affect the airway structures above the glottic opening (▶ Figure 13-1), and lower airway disorders affect the structures found from the trachea to the alveoli.

Upper Airway Dysfunction

The classic upper airway problem is the obstructed airway. When we think of this, we often picture a child choking on a small toy. However, far more commonly, upper airway obstruction

TRANSITION *highlights*

- *Frequency with which respiratory distress disorders occur in the United States.*

- *Thorough overview of the pathophysiological changes that occur with the following disorders:*
  - *Upper airway dysfunction.*
  - *Lower airway dysfunction.*

- *Delineating between respiratory distress and respiratory failure.*

- *Signs and symptoms that illustrate ventilatory adequacy or inadequacy.*

- *Core treatment interventions for a patient suffering from a disturbance to the airway.*

- *How to determine when or when not to ventilate, based on signs and symptoms.*

- *New ventilator rates for a patient with a pulse and a patient without a pulse.*

- *Use of continuous positive airway pressure (CPAP) during prehospital management of a patient with respiratory distress.*

is the result of poor airway muscle tone resulting from altered mental status. When the brain is not functioning properly, the muscles and nerves that protect the airway fail. This failure frequently results in an inability to keep an airway open. For example, when lying supine, a patient with an altered mental status may relax the muscles of the upper airway too much and allow the epiglottis to fall back and cover the glottic opening (▶ Figure 13-2).

The upper airway can also be affected by structural changes. Airflow can be impeded by swelling in and around the larynx. Conditions such as burns, infection, anaphylaxis, and even direct trauma can cause laryngeal edema and inflammation and

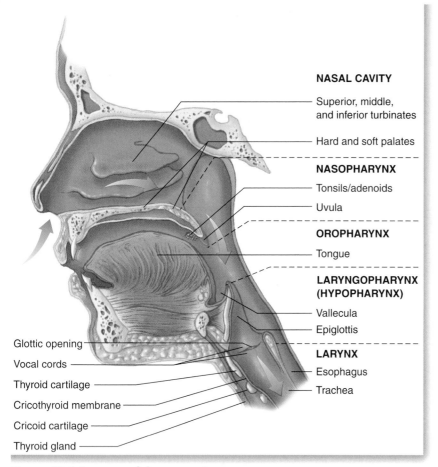

Figure 13-1 Anatomy of the upper airway.

NASAL CAVITY
- Superior, middle, and inferior turbinates
- Hard and soft palates

NASOPHARYNX
- Tonsils/adenoids
- Uvula

OROPHARYNX
- Tongue

LARYNGOPHARYNX (HYPOPHARYNX)
- Vallecula
- Epiglottis

LARYNX
- Esophagus
- Trachea

Glottic opening
Vocal cords
Thyroid cartilage
Cricothyroid membrane
Cricoid cartilage
Thyroid gland

result in a rapid decrease in the size of the glottic opening, thus significantly obstructing airflow.

Lower Airway Dysfunction

The most common cause of lower airway dysfunction is bronchoconstriction. A number of diseases and disorders, such as asthma and anaphylaxis, can cause the bronchiole passages to spasm and constrict. Even small changes in the diameter of these tubes can cause tremendous resistance to airflow that can seriously decrease the movement of air.

In addition to bronchoconstriction, other disorders can structurally change how gas is exchanged in the alveoli. Problems such as congestive heart failure, near drowning, and even altitude sickness can cause the fluid portion of the blood to cross the alveolar membrane and inter-

> When assessing breathing, always keep minute ventilation and alveolar ventilation in mind.

fere with the diffusion of oxygen and carbon dioxide. This pulmonary edema thickens the alveolar membrane, collapses some alveoli, and even (in late stages) can fill the alveoli themselves. Infections such as pneumonia can cause similar dysfunction. In these cases, the alveoli can be obstructed by pus and other byproducts of infection, causing a similar gas exchange issue.

ASSESSMENT FINDINGS

When assessing a patient with respiratory distress, the most important goal may not be to determine the exact nature of the disorder. Far more important may be the need to recognize respiratory failure and support ventilation.

The primary assessment is a critical component of the assessment in any patient. It is even

more important in a patient with respiratory distress. It begins by ensuring patency of the airway: "Is it open?" Of course, if the answer is no, you must take steps to open it. Beyond the immediate moment, you must consider the future: "Will it stay open?" Is the ongoing patency of this airway threatened, and if so, what steps are necessary to reverse that course?

When assessing breathing, you also must consider multiple elements. First, you must ensure that the patient actually is breathing; but second, you must further ensure that the patient's breathing is adequate to meet the needs of his body. "Look, listen, and feel" will quickly provide an answer to the first question, but for the second question you must engage in some critical thinking.

Always keep minute ventilation and alveolar ventilation in mind when assessing breathing. You must ask yourself continually how much air is actually reaching the alveoli each minute. Remember that minute volume is comprised of both rate and volume. Breathing within an acceptable rate is important, but again, you must consider how much volume is being moved down to the alveoli in each breath. In addition, keep in mind the concept of dead space.

In the primary assessment, you need to look at breathing (▶ Figure 13-3). How fast or slow is the patient breathing? Quickly listen to both sides of the patient's chest. This is the time not for a thorough examination of lung sounds but, rather, for a quick assurance that air is moving in and out on both sides. It takes only seconds to determine that volume is inadequate. Sounds of dysfunction are also rapidly identified with even a quick listen. For example, are there wheezes that might

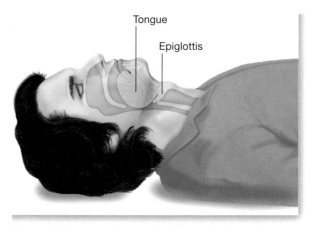

Tongue

Epiglottis

Figure 13-2 Loss of control of the upper airway may occur, for example, when the muscles of the upper airway relax too much and the epiglottis is allowed to fall back and cover the glottic opening.

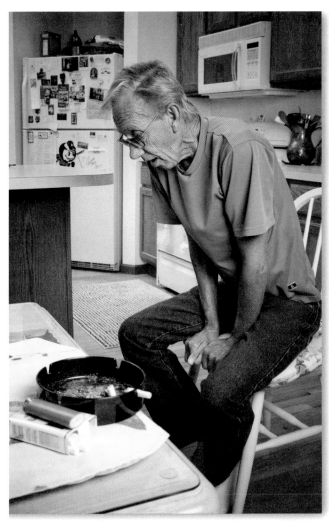

Figure 13-3 Patient suffering respiratory distress, indicated by his tripod position.

The sympathetic nervous system tells the heart to beat faster and stronger.

These compensatory mechanisms can be easily identified in your assessment of breathing. What is the respiratory rate? How hard is the patient working to breathe? Look at the patient's chest: Is the patient using accessory muscles? All these findings indicate the body's effort to compensate. As with compensated shock, often these measures can temporarily sustain normal body function and hold off the challenge.

When respiratory compensation works, we deem the patient to be in respiratory *distress*—that is, he is challenged, but the compensatory efforts are sustaining normal function despite the problem. A patient in respiratory distress will exhibit signs of the challenge, such as tripod positioning (see **Figure 13-3**), accessory muscle use, and increased respiration rate, yet he should also be showing signs that these measures are allowing normal function. The patient's brain should be oxygenated, and therefore he should have a normal mental status. He should not be showing signs of profound hypoxia, such as cyanosis. The key to differentiating respiratory distress from respiratory failure is identifying that normal function.

occurs when compensation fails. At this point, the challenge continues and the body may be attempting to compensate, but function has been affected. Oxygen may not be getting distributed, carbon dioxide is being retained, and the muscles of respiration tire. As an AEMT, you must be ever vigilant to recognize respiratory failure because it demonstrates that what the patient is doing on his own is not enough.

A patient in respiratory failure exhibits signs and symptoms similar to those of a patient in respiratory distress. He will have a challenge, he will be compensating, but he will not be meeting his needs. Look for signs that compensation has failed. Altered mental status is a key indicator. Anxiety, combativeness, somnolence, and even unconsciousness all point to hypoxia and hypercapnia. Look for additional signs of hypoxia, such as cyanosis and low oxygen saturation. These findings are especially worrisome if they occur despite supplemental oxygen. Look for other signs of failure, including signs of respiratory fatigue. Respiratory muscles need oxygen and eventually fail as they become hypoxic. Look for slowing rates, irregular patterns, and gasping as indicators of respiratory failure (▶ **Figure 13-5**).

> Respiratory *failure* occurs when compensation fails.

identify bronchoconstriction? Consider also the patient's ability to speak. If he must take a breath after every word, his minute volume has been seriously challenged.

Finally, as an advanced provider, you may be tempted to move on to advanced modalities such as airway and intravenous lines. Resist this temptation until the primary assessment is complete and all immediate life threats have been addressed.

Respiratory Distress

When a person experiences a challenge to respiratory system function, the body responds in a predictable manner: It compensates. As in shock, the brain takes specific steps to help overcome the deficit caused by the offending issue. When the brain senses increasing carbon dioxide and low oxygen, the respiratory center in the medulla increases the respiratory rate. Additional muscles in the neck, chest, and abdomen (accessory muscles) are engaged to assist with breathing (▶ **Figure 13-4**).

Respiratory Failure

Unfortunately, the body's compensation is limited. Some respiratory challenges exceed the body's ability to compensate. Other times, compensation simply fails over time. Keep in mind that when we ask muscles to do more work, more oxygen is required. If hypoxia is already a challenge, the muscles of compensation can help for only a short time. Respiratory *failure*

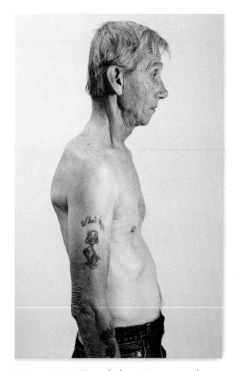

Figure 13-4 Barrel chest in an emphysema patient.

Adequate breathing:
Speaks full sentences;
alert and calm

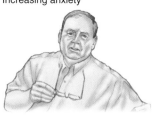

Nonrebreather mask or nasal cannula

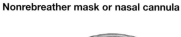

Increasing respiratory distress:
Visibly short of breath;
Speaking 3–4 word sentences;
Increasing anxiety

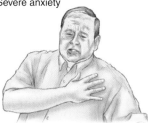

Nonrebreather mask

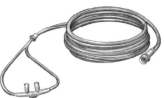

Key decision-making point:

Recognize inadequate breathing
before respiratory arrest
develops.

**Assist ventilations
before they stop altogether!**

Severe respiratory distress:
Speaking only 1–2 word sentences;
Very diaphoretic (sweaty);
Severe anxiety

Assisted ventilations
Pocket face mask (PFM),
bag-valve mask (BVM), or
flow-restricted, oxygen-powered
ventilation device (FROPVD)

Assist the patient's own
ventilations, adjusting the
rate for rapid or slow
breathing

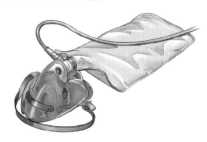

Continues to deteriorate:
Sleepy with head-bobbing;
Becomes unarousable

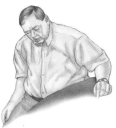

Artificial ventilation
Pocket face mask (PFM),
bag-valve mask (BVM), or
flow-restricted, oxygen-powered
ventilation device (FROPV)

Assisted ventilations at
12/minute for an adult or
20/minute for a child or infant

Respiratory arrest:
No breathing

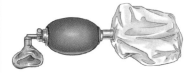

Figure 13-5 The continuum of breathing ranges from normal, adequate breathing to no breathing at all. It is essential to recognize the need for assisted ventilations even before severe respiratory distress develops.

Remember that a patient in respiratory failure may indeed be breathing. Consider the following example:

You are assessing a 14-year-old asthma patient. He has been having an attack for roughly an hour now. You assess his airway and find that he has a patent airway, but he has difficulty speaking. He is breathing at a rate of 54 breaths per minute. You find him in tripod position; when you look at his chest you note retractions and other accessory muscle use. When you listen to his chest you can barely hear any air movement at all. His fingernails are blue. When you attempt to engage him with questions, you note that he has a very sleepy affect.

This young man is in respiratory failure. He is compensating for his asthma, as evidenced by his respiratory rate, his use of accessory muscles, and his position, but those compensatory mechanisms are not working, as demonstrated by his altered mental status and cyanosis. This patient needs immediate help.

It is important to also remember that identifying respiratory distress does not require diagnosing a specific respiratory dysfunction. You may identify failure (and take action) long before you have time to accurately complete a differential diagnosis. Luckily, the treatment for respiratory failure is, for the most part, the same regardless of what disorder is causing it.

EMERGENCY MEDICAL CARE

Different respiratory dysfunctions will require different treatments. Discussion of all the specific treatments for individual respiratory dysfunctions is beyond the scope of this topic. However, some general treatment philosophies are common despite the etiology of the respiratory dysfunction. Those common treatments are presented in the following sections.

Airway

Ensuring an open airway is essential to all other respiratory treatments. If the patient does not have an open airway, give him one. If that airway is threatened, take steps to protect it. When appropriate, consider oropharyngeal and nasopharyngeal airway adjuncts to help keep an airway open.

Respiratory Distress

The treatment goal when dealing with a patient in respiratory distress is to support

the compensatory efforts of the patient and work on reversing the challenge. Remember, a patient in respiratory distress is compensating for a respiratory challenge and—at least so far—this compensation is successful. Supplemental oxygen to increase saturation is important. After you ensure that the status is *distress* and not *failure*, you should use your assessment to better determine the nature of the dysfunction. In this case, you have time to investigate and focus treatment.

For example, you might listen more carefully to lung sounds in the secondary assessment. You might hear wheezes and recognize them as the sound of bronchoconstriction. Knowing this, you might discuss with medical control the option of assisting the patient with his home nebulizer treatment. Overall, the key purpose of treating respiratory distress is preventing it from becoming respiratory failure. A nonrebreather mask delivering high concentrations of oxygen is one option for treating respiratory distress (▶ Figure 13-6; also see Figure 13-5).

Respiratory Failure

When you recognize respiratory failure, you no longer have time for lengthy assessment and investigation. Remember that, by nature, respiratory failure means that what the patient is doing alone is not working. Respiratory failure requires immediate outside intervention to prevent the next stage: respiratory arrest.

With few exceptions, respiratory failure requires assisting the patient with a bag-valve mask. You must now take over for where

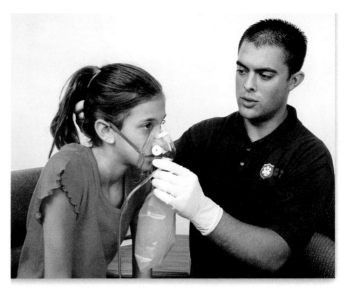

Figure 13-6 Provide oxygen via a nonrebreather mask to the patient who is breathing adequately but with difficulty (respiratory distress).

the patient's own respiratory system has failed. There are two goals for this assisted ventilation: improving oxygenation and improving ventilation. Once again, consider minute volume. In a patient breathing exceptionally fast, your goal is not to slow down the rate but rather to increase a diminished tidal volume. Every third, fourth, or even fifth breath, you will deliver a positive pressure breath with a tidal volume greater than the patient is able to achieve on his own.

A bag-valve mask delivers high-concentration oxygen, and in a state of fatigued respiratory muscles, it may be the only way oxygen will enter the system effectively (▶ Figure 13-7).

Choosing to ventilate a breathing patient is a very difficult decision. Keep in mind that it is better to be aggressive in this situation than to allow prolonged hypoxia. Although positive pressure

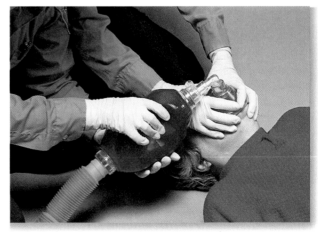

Figure 13-7 Two rescuers deliver bag-valve-mask ventilation.

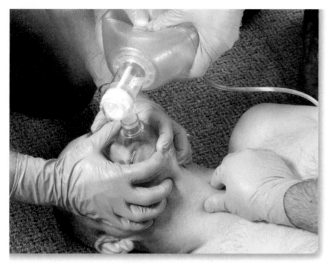

Figure 13-8 Applying cricoid pressure (Sellick maneuver) with positive pressure ventilation.

ventilation has negative side effects, the costs of hypoxia typically outweigh the risks of using a bag-valve mask. Remember also that you will continually reassess the patient. Often a quick decision to ventilate a patient may be enough to replace respiratory failure with respiratory distress. Positive pressure ventilation can always be stopped if the patient improves.

Positive Pressure Ventilation

The body normally uses negative pressure to bring air into the chest. The diaphragm contracts, the intercostal muscles flex, and negative pressure is created in the chest cavity to pull air in through the glottis opening. With a bag-valve mask, an opposite mechanism is used to move air into the lungs: Positive pressure is applied externally to force air in.

Positive pressure ventilation sometimes disrupts normal body functions. For example, the heart uses the negative pressure of breathing to assist with filling. When positive pressure is applied, the heart can no longer rely on the negative pressure, and often filling is decreased. This can drop cardiac output. The esophagus is also not designed for positive pressure air entry. Because it is an expandable tube, positive pressure ventilation often drives air into the stomach. This gastric insufflation can lead to pressure on the diaphragm and decreased lung capacity.

Despite these difficulties, positive pressure ventilation is essential for a patient who is not breathing or is in respiratory failure. Keeping the following side effects in mind will help you improve your positive pressure ventilation technique.

- **Minimize the effect of positive pressure.** Ventilate with only enough volume to raise the chest wall. Doing this helps minimize the effects of positive pressure on the heart and can increase cardiac filling.

- **Keep gastric insufflation in mind.** Always use an airway adjunct (when possible). Airway adjuncts help create better channels for air and help avoid forcing air into the esophagus. Although you may consider also using cricoid pressure (the Sellick maneuver) to compress the esophagus during ventilation (▶ Figure 13-8), recent evidence has cast some doubt on the value of this procedure, and the American Heart Association (AHA) has significantly limited its recommendations for cricoid pressure in its 2010 guidelines.

- **Hyperventilation kills.** Ventilate at appropriate rates (12–20/minute for children and 10–12/minute for adults). This helps prevent gastric insufflation as well as preventing the unnecessary removal of too much carbon dioxide, which can lead to cerebral vasoconstriction and reduced blood flow to the brain.

The cost–benefit analysis of positive pressure ventilation is an important one. Your ability to effectively identify respiratory failure is essential. Even more essential, however, is your decision to act on that problem. Far too often, respiratory failure is identified but allowed to worsen because of indecision. Always remember that your assessment is more than just a gathering of information; it is a very important element of making critical decisions.

Continuous Positive Airway Pressure

Continuous positive airway pressure (CPAP) is a technology that uses positive pressure in a different manner than a bag-valve mask. The positive pressure created by a CPAP system does not force air in but, rather, creates a constant, slight flow of air against which the patient will breathe. This "wall of resistance" will often make the work of breathing easier, keep alveoli open, and make breathing more effective (▶ Figure 13-9).

A variety of CPAP systems are available. In general, CPAP systems create a higher flow of air by mixing oxygen with room air (although some systems use just room air). For years, sleep apnea patients used positive pressure to keep open the soft tissues of the hypopharynx and prevent snoring. In EMS, that pressure is used to "pneumatically splint" open lower airways and the alveoli.

USES OF CPAP CPAP is most commonly used to treat acute pulmonary edema (APE). By pressurizing the inside of the alveoli, the fluid of pulmonary edema is prevented from crossing the alveolar membrane. It also helps prevent the collapse of alveoli under the weight of the edema. CPAP has been proven to rapidly improve APE in some patients and, in many cases, to prevent the need for intubation.

CPAP is also used to treat other forms of respiratory distress. Keeping small airways open via the pneumatic splint tends to increase oxygenation and decrease the sensation of difficulty breathing. Keeping the alveoli from collapsing also leads to

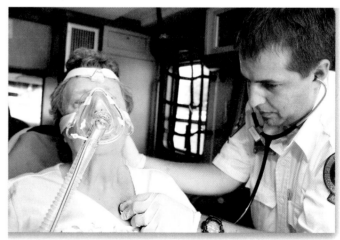

Figure 13-9 Continuous positive airway pressure (CPAP) is used for the awake and spontaneously breathing patient who needs ventilatory support. (© Ken Kerr)

increased surface area for gas exchange. These effects can help a variety of respiratory disorders, including bronchospasm and pneumonia. Indications for CPAP vary from system to system, so always follow local protocol.

APPLYING CPAP   CPAP is *not* artificial ventilation. If the patient cannot maintain an airway or breathe on his own, he is *not* a candidate for CPAP. Many patients will need more aggressive treatments. Always use a thorough patient assessment to make the correct treatment choice.

Just as with a bag-valve mask, the positive pressure of CPAP can also drop cardiac output by counteracting the negative filling pressure of the heart. Therefore, you should never apply CPAP to a hypotensive patient. Follow local guidelines for minimum systolic blood pressure values.

CPAP can also be difficult psychologically for a patient. A mask is strapped to the face of a patient who is already having difficulty breathing. Often a patient will not tolerate this treatment. CPAP should never be forced. Consider allowing the

patient to hold the mask on his face before strapping it on. Often, when the patient feels the effects, he will be more likely to allow the strap.

CPAP can be rapidly beneficial, but not every patient will get better after its application. Reassessment is critical. Many times CPAP will be applied to patients who are close to respiratory failure. These patients sometimes progress to respiratory failure and will need more aggressive treatment. Remember also that hypotension can be a side effect.

TRANSITIONING

REVIEW ITEMS

1. Which of the following problems would be designated as an upper airway disorder?
   a. laryngeal edema caused by anaphylaxis
   b. bronchoconstriction caused by asthma
   c. destruction of the alveoli caused by emphysema
   d. pulmonary edema caused by congestive heart failure

2. You are assessing a patient who has a hoarse voice after being struck in the throat by a baseball. Given the primary assessment, which of the following would be your most important next step?
   a. Request ALS for fear of a potentially threatened airway.
   b. Apply a cold pack to the neck for pain management.
   c. Ask the patient to sip cool water.
   d. Continue on to your secondary assessment.

3. Which of the following signs would help you differentiate respiratory distress from respiratory failure?
   a. altered mental status
   b. increased respiratory rate
   c. accessory muscle use
   d. increased heart rate

4. You are treating a patient in respiratory failure. Which of the following treatments should you complete first?
   a. Deliver positive pressure ventilations with a bag-valve mask.
   b. Deliver supplemental oxygen with a nasal cannula.
   c. Begin chest compressions.
   d. Complete a thorough secondary assessment.

5. Which of the following vital signs would rule out the use of CPAP?
   a. respiratory rate of 4/min
   b. respiratory rate of 40/min
   c. blood pressure of 198/100 mmHg
   d. heart rate of 140

APPLIED PATHOPHYSIOLOGY

1. List three ways in which the body compensates for a respiratory challenge.

2. Explain how these compensatory methods may be recognized in an assessment.

3. Discuss why compensation might fail in a hypoxic respiratory distress patient.

4. Describe how positive pressure ventilation is different from the way a person normally breathes.

CLINICAL DECISION MAKING

You are assessing a 65-year-old female patient with COPD. Her family says that she has had shortness of breath for three days, but "she is much worse today." You find the patient sitting upright, looking scared, and unable to speak.

1. What indications does your general impression give you that this woman's condition may be critical?

Your patient has a patent airway and is breathing 48 times per minute. She has lung sounds bilaterally but is moving little air, with a prominent wheeze. Her radial pulse is 128, her skin is wet, and she is confused (this is not her normal state).

2. Is this patient in respiratory distress or respiratory failure? Please discuss why you feel this way.

3. Based on your primary assessment, are any immediate interventions necessary? If so, what are they?

4. Explain the pathophysiologic cause for the following:
   a. Confusion
   b. Wheezing
   c. Increased heart rate

The family reports to you that the patient also has a history of acute pulmonary edema secondary to CHF.

5. Based on your primary survey, is it important to determine whether this patient is currently in APE or exacerbated COPD? Why or why not?

6. If you determined that this patient was in APE, how would it change your immediate interventions?

Standard Patient Assessment

Competency Applies scene information and patient
assessment findings (scene size-up, primary and
secondary assessment, patient history, reassessment)
to guide emergency management.

TOPIC

14

CRITICAL THINKING

INTRODUCTION

The ability to think critically is desired by EMS providers at every level—and may largely be a measure of clinical success. However, the concept is not easily defined, quantified, or taught.

Your initial EMT class presented a patient assessment process to you that looked like a neat diagram. You likely thought that was the way assessment would go. Experience has taught you that those guides were just that—guides—and that many variables are considered in assessment. Your Advanced EMT class honed your assessment skills and added a series of new medications and skills to your toolbox. With each of these new modalities, however, new and different clinical decisions must be made for each patient.

When it comes to assessment, many different AEMTs could assess the same cardiac patient, and there would be just as many ways to ask the history questions and do a physical assessment. The only steadfast rule is to address life threats first.

As an introduction, consider the following example of how you may use critical thinking in everyday life. It is not limited to medicine.

When you were trying to start your car, it did not want to start. When the car finally started, it ran rough. It bucked and sputtered. Then the "check engine" light came on. You were about to go on a long drive, so you had to make a decision or two.

The car was relatively new and well maintained. There were no odors, no unusual sounds, and no stains on the garage floor indicating leaking fluids. The gas gauge was between one-quarter full and empty. The weather had been rainy for weeks.

You questioned whether you should take the car on the trip or bring it to the shop. You decided that driving it would not cause damage. Bringing it to the shop would cost hundreds in diagnostics, which you did not want if they were unnecessary.

You decide to drive your car to a gas station, put in some dry gas, and fill the tank. After doing that, you drive it around town for a few minutes to see if the car runs better. It does. The "check engine" light turns off, and you go to your destination uneventfully.

This real-life example demonstrates the components of a critical thinking process: identifying a problem (chief complaint), gathering facts (history and physical exam), identifying possibilities and narrowing these possibilities to probabilities (differential

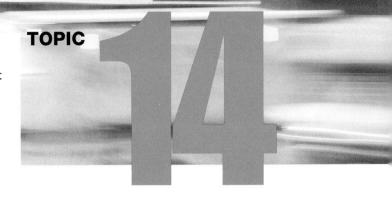

TRANSITION *highlights*

- Definition of critical thinking and how it relates to the Advanced EMT.

- *Difference between clinician and technician as it pertains to the role of critical thinking in the prehospital environment.*

- *Importance of determining patient life threats.*

- *Developing a differential diagnosis based on assessment phases and assessment findings:*
  - Scene size-up.
  - Primary assessment.
  - Secondary assessment.
  - Reassessment.
  - Monitoring devices.

- *Constructing care plans based on the Advanced EMT's assessment findings and differential diagnoses.*

diagnosis), developing a plan, evaluating risks versus benefits, and implementing the plan.

This topic focuses on the thinking process—that is, how to get to the treatment choices, rather than on the treatment itself.

CRITICAL THINKING DEFINED

Chapman et al., in *Rosen's Emergency Medicine* (Elsevier, 2001), describe the critical thinking process as having three parts: medical inquiry (history, physical exam, and diagnostic testing), clinical decision making (a cognitive process that evaluates information to diagnose or manage a patient's condition), and clinical reasoning, which involves both medical inquiry and clinical decision making.

In fact, proper decisions are made only after evaluating necessary, accurate information. The relationship between decision making and reasoning is a continuous process—a feedback loop, rather than a straight line from assessment to care. New

TECHNICIAN VERSUS CLINICIAN

EMS is summoned by a 73-year-old woman who is having difficulty breathing. The crew arrives to see the woman sitting in the tripod position, with her feet dangling over the side of her bed. She states that she suddenly developed difficulty breathing.

While obtaining a pertinent history and administering oxygen, the patient's medications of Duo-vent and Nasonex are discovered. The patient responds that her doctor recently gave her the medications for allergies. She said that she went to the doctor for wheezing about 10 days ago. Her only history is that of hypertension, for which she has not refilled her prescription in some time.

She does, in fact, have some scattered wheezes, and her blood pressure is on the high side.

From this point on, the technician and clinician take different approaches.

The technician hears wheezes, notes that there is a treatment for recently diagnosed wheezes, and either administers the inhaler or provides albuterol by small-volume nebulizer.

The clinician uses a differential diagnostic process to identify causes for the patient's condition. Through this process, and the accompanying respiratory and cardiac workup, it is determined that the patient has had a recent weight gain, complained about abdominal fullness, had difficulty breathing when walking up stairs at home, and began sleeping in her chair because of orthopnea. She quit smoking many years ago and denies occupational or other exposure to respiratory toxins.

This information, combined with the history of hypertension—a risk factor for heart failure—led the clinician to correctly determine that the patient was experiencing congestive heart failure and to begin appropriate therapy. The earlier diagnosis of allergies was made based on the early presence of wheezing—which is also an early sign of congestive heart failure. Knowledge of pathophysiology is a crucial foundation to an effective differential diagnostic process.

Note that the technician-versus-clinician discussion is not an attack on any specific level of provider. In fact, technicians and clinicians are both found within each level of provider.

An AEMT who is a thinking clinician is able to identify patients who are stable or unstable and require prompt transport. The AEMT/clinician also makes decisions such as when to call for support or air-medical evacuation, when to perform a rapid extrication, and when to immobilize the patient before removing him from the vehicle.

In most cases, clinicians are not created in class—they are developed on the street through experience, continuing education, and clinical mentoring.

Regardless of your level of training, strive to be a clinician.

---

information is evaluated as it is obtained and applied to the body of knowledge about the patient's condition and filtered through practicality, risks, and benefits.

The concept of critical thinking is more than a process; it is a mind-set. As part of this discussion, it is a good time to revisit the difference between a technician and a clinician. In the context of this topic, the ability to apply clinical reasoning to a patient problem belongs exclusively to the clinician.

A technician is not expected to use high levels of reasoning skills. Technicians are strictly protocol driven and respond in a specific way when a certain group of signs and symptoms appears.

Clinicians, however, gather pertinent information from many sources, evaluate that information carefully, and develop a treatment plan from protocols or a series of protocols that will benefit the patient (see sidebar, Technician versus Clinician).

THE ADVANCED EMT AS A CLINICIAN

There is a difference between a clinician and a technician in EMS. Part of the difference involves the amount of training and experience possessed by a provider. The second, and perhaps the most important, is the mind-set of the clinician.

The clinician is not satisfied by observing superficial information or apparent patterns. Clinicians look at each patient as a challenge or puzzle and seek pertinent assessment information, even about patients who appear to have an obvious presenting problem.

Consider a challenging patient presentation and a decision you may have to make as an AEMT. You are called to a patient with respiratory distress. The patient has a history of congestive heart failure (CHF) and chronic obstructive pulmonary disease (COPD). You have the ability to administer a small-volume nebulizer for one of these conditions. But how will you know which condition to treat? Assessment and thinking will get you there.

Look at this from another perspective: yours, as a patient. Who would you want for your primary care provider? Would you want someone who came in, did a few perfunctory tests, and made an assumption and a treatment decision based on this scant information? Or would you prefer the person who listened to you, considered a variety of possibilities (differential diagnosis, discussed later), looked to find the most likely cause of your condition, and tested and treated you accordingly? Like most people, you would choose the latter, the clinician.

TREAT LIFE THREATS FIRST

The primary assessment is vitally important. EMT class does not prepare students for the critical patients who will be seen and the immediate interventions necessary for their survival. Advanced training now adds other modalities, such as advanced airways, that can distract from these vital initial steps of ABC. In fact, opening the airway, checking for breathing, and looking for and controlling bleeding are a small portion of this initial process.

The primary assessment (▶ Figure 14-1) is a foundation for the entire call and cannot be completed without touching the patient. Something as simple as noticing cool, moist skin and a rapid pulse early in the call alerts you to shock long before taking vital signs.

During the primary assessment, you should also be able to identify breathing

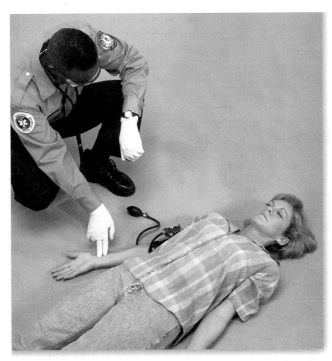

Figure 14-1 The primary assessment must be completed before any diagnostic steps are taken.

problems (this requires exposing the patient, a stethoscope, and, in some cases, palpation or percussion), including pneumothorax, open chest injury, and inadequate breathing; identify shock (by a quick note of skin condition, pulse rate, and quality); and decide whether the patient is a load-and-go priority.

Patient care is part of this early process, including oxygen, ventilation, bleeding control, and care for shock if necessary.

THE DIFFERENTIAL DIAGNOSTIC PROCESS

Even though we are not given the full spectrum of diagnostic modalities that in-hospital clinicians have, we do have an ever-expanding toolbox and a significant arsenal of treatments to employ based on our assessment findings. Sometimes called a *presumptive* or *field diagnosis*, differential diagnosis is an important responsibility because the clinician makes treatment decisions based on it.

The differential diagnostic approach is a hallmark of advanced-level providers. The modalities you are allowed to perform are based on sound assessment and decisions leading to a valid differential diagnostic process. This process is fueled by solid initial training, quality continuing education, field experience, and clinical

mentoring at any level of EMS certification or licensure.

Consider the following case: You are called to a patient who complains of chest pain (▶ **Figure 14-2**). The 55-year-old man has a history of angina and hypertension. He describes the pain as slightly to the left of center of his chest, tearing in nature, and radiating to his throat. It is different from any angina he has had in the past. He took one nitroglycerin tablet without relief. You complete his vital signs and find that his pulse is 104, blood pressure 180/104 mmHg, and respirations 20 and slightly labored. His skin is warm and slightly moist.

Following protocol, you would likely have the ability to administer a second and a third nitroglycerin tablet.

But is this truly cardiac pain?

The clinician listens to the patient and gets a thorough description of the pain. Although it appears to be cardiac because of the radiation to the throat, it is atypical for the patient and thus worthy of additional assessment.

To be most effective, the provider—at any level—uses a differential diagnostic approach. In this approach, the provider develops a list of possible causes of the chest pain. This might include myocardial infarction, pneumonia, pneumothorax, pulmonary embolus, proximal aortic dissection, and trauma (rib fracture, muscle pull).

With the exception of ECG monitoring or diagnostic 12-lead ECG (which may be available to some AEMTs), methods of evaluating and narrowing possibilities down to probabilities exist at all levels of EMS practice for those who think like clinicians. Even if treatment options for each condition are not available, the information obtained from the examination will allow you to promptly alert the hospital about potentially serious conditions.

The goal of the differential diagnostic process is to narrow a wide range of possibilities down to probabilities. Consider the following to either rule out or include any of the following in this patient's differential diagnosis:

> The differential diagnostic process is fueled by solid initial training, quality continuing education, field experience, and clinical mentoring

Differential Diagnosis	Include in or Exclude from Presumptive Diagnosis by
Cardiac event (ischemia, infarct)	Detailed history Absence of finding other conditions during assessment process
Pneumonia	Fever, chills, malaise Cough, may be productive Gradual onset
Pneumothorax	Sudden onset (spontaneous pneumothorax) Lung sounds Pain may be pleuritic
Proximal aortic dissection	Pain characteristic (location, description) Difference in radial pulse strength, quality Blood pressure differences between arms
Pulmonary embolus	Recent immobilization Pain or discomfort in legs (deep vein thrombosis)
Trauma	History of injury (fall, lifting) Description of pain Pain on palpation or movement

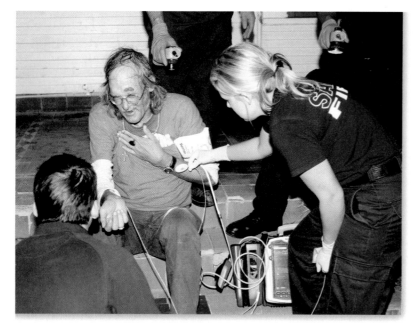

Figure 14-2 Chest pain is one complaint for which a differential diagnostic approach is important.

After development of the list of differentials, the actual exams and history items do not add significant initial time and are clinically very relevant.

The patient denies trauma. The area is nontender to palpation. He denies immobilization, fever, cough, or other illness. Lung sounds are present, clear, and equal bilaterally. The exam reveals a radial pulse deficit, with a blood pressure in the left arm now at 180/100 mmHg, whereas the pressure in the right arm is 130/80 mmHg.

Your presumptive diagnosis now shifts to an ascending aortic aneurysm. Suddenly, aspirin and a second nitroglycerin tablet are not looking as appealing as they did a few minutes ago.

This process is not without pitfalls, of course. The clinician must also know the pitfalls and balance risk versus benefits appropriately (the clinical reasoning process). For example, it has been reported that 10 percent to 15 percent of patients who have myocardial infarction have pain that is reported as pleuritic or affected by movement. It would be unwise to rule out any condition or to advise against treatment and transport based on any single finding. The clinician should also realize that ascending aneurysms occur in an extremely small percentage of the population. One should not expect to see that a lot—but it is crucial to be able to identify it when it is present.

ASSESSMENT: AN ONGOING PROCESS

An experienced provider realizes that rarely will the first planned assessments be enough. The finding from the first assessments will bring up additional questions—or even take the provider in an entirely different direction (▶ Figure 14-3).

New AEMTs like it when a question is answered. Experienced AEMTs like it when a question brings about two more questions.

In fact, the assessment process is dynamic and directly linked to the differential diagnostic process described previously. Although it is not the scope of this topic to discuss every possible history and assessment technique, the following are some high-yield favorites:

- In the SAMPLE history, look for key information—especially in "events." It is last in the old SAMPLE sequence but among the first in importance. Especially valuable in cases involving altered mental status, the events can be an important piece of the puzzle in building a clinical case for seizure versus simple fainting versus more serious pathologies. Specifically, probe for prodromal signs and symptoms such as dizziness, weakness, palpitations, changes in skin color, temperature, and condition before the episode, and whether the patient was able to lower himself to the ground or dropped like a rock. Often, patients will be able to describe a feeling of their vision closing in, described as a blackout or "whiting out."

- Listen to lung sounds properly and in a setting where it is possible to hear them. Although we wish to make diagnostic decisions based on these sounds, the assessment performed is often inadequate. Many providers listen to lung sounds over one or two locations (often only anteriorly), and that is all. Lung sounds must be listened to for a full cycle and in multiple

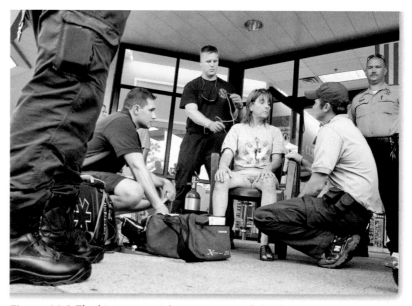

Figure 14-3 The history provides a majority of the diagnostic clues in the medical emergency.

locations. The patient should breathe in and out deeply with the mouth open. With wheezes and other lung sounds, it is incomplete to note merely that they are present; it should also be noted where in the respiratory cycle these sounds are heard. Because of the structure of the lungs, if you have not auscultated posteriorly, you have not heard the lower lobes.

- Use orthostatic vital signs—safely. Orthostatic vital signs are somewhat misunderstood and are often misapplied. The general concept is to take the vital signs of a supine patient. Ideally, the patient should have been supine for about 10 minutes prior to the exam. Have the patient stand, and take the vital signs immediately. Take them again 2 minutes later. Pulse elevation of 10 to 20 beats per minute or blood pressure decrease of 10 to 20 mmHg may indicate blood or other significant volume loss. Be sure to support the patient. If the patient feels dizzy or faint, stop the test and consider it positive. Rates indicating hypovolemia may vary in the elderly and in those taking medications that slow the pulse, such as beta blockers.

- Consider risk factors. This is a standard practice for in-hospital clinicians but is used less in the field. Smoking, diabetes, obesity, hypercholesterolemia, and hypertension are all significant risk factors for myocardial infarction and stroke. Even though these are not the definite smoking gun we would like for diagnosis, when weighted properly they may make the difference in some precautionary treatment and transport decisions.

EMBRACE CONTRADICTIONS AND CHALLENGES

If every patient came with a diagnosis, EMS would be boring. Patients often throw us curves—and only the clinicians among us are there to catch them. Remain open to the fact that patients may have coexisting conditions. Pneumonia and urinary tract infections are common causes of sepsis. Medications mask the reactions to illness and injury. Geriatric patients present differently in many disease states. Occasionally the patient's complaint is not even the most serious problem you uncover. It is up to the clinician to determine what findings are important—and in what proportion.

DEVELOP CAREFUL, STRATEGIC, DYNAMIC CARE PLANS

To many providers, especially those new to their level of certification, care is about performing modalities. Experienced providers, however, know that care is a carefully balanced event. It is balanced between need and risk, standing order and online consult, and present need at the scene versus consideration of hospital care down the line. In some cases, oxygen and calming are prudent, powerful treatments.

Care plans fit into the continuum of clinical reasoning in that constant monitoring for therapeutic benefit or adverse reaction is necessary—and that the patient's response to a particular modality may be diagnostic.

Each patient contact is a clinical mystery waiting to be solved and an educational experience that builds the foundation of a true clinician.

TRANSITIONING

REVIEW ITEMS

1. The concept of differential diagnosis is best described as narrowing _____.
   a. probabilities to probabilities
   b. possibilities to probabilities
   c. chief complaint to differentials
   d. differentials to di agnostics

2. Which of the following is *not* part of the clinical thinking process?
   a. clinical reasoning
   b. medical inquiry
   c. clinical decision making
   d. ethical inquiry

3. The difference between a technician mind-set and a clinician mind-set is best described as follows:
   a. The clinician identifies a narrow pattern of signs and symptoms and provides scripted treatment protocols, whereas the technician synthesizes information from various sources and applies treatments from protocol or protocols as necessary.
   b. The technician identifies a narrow pattern of signs and symptoms and provides scripted treatment protocols, whereas the clinician synthesizes information from various sources and applies treatments from protocol or protocols as necessary.
   c. Technicians rarely use online medical direction, largely depending on protocols and assessment findings to determine care plans. Clinicians are driven mostly by online medical direction.
   d. Clinicians are most closely related to the Advanced Practice Paramedic concept and have skills and knowledge similar to those of physician extenders.

4. Differential diagnosis possibilities for respiratory distress would likely include all of the following *except* _____.
   a. myocardial infarction
   b. pulmonary embolus
   c. cerebrovascular accident
   d. COPD exacerbation

5. Orthostatic hypotension is defined as a(n) _____ of _____ beats per minute in pulse.
   a. increase; 5–10
   b. decrease; 5–10
   c. increase; 10–20
   d. decrease; 10–20

6. To auscultate the lung bases you must listen _____.
   a. anteriorly
   b. laterally
   c. medially
   d. posteriorly

7. How are risk factors used as part of differential diagnosis?
   a. To confirm that a condition is present
   b. As backup to differential diagnosis
   c. As a factor to weigh into the differential diagnosis
   d. Risk factors are not a significant factor in differential diagnosis.

8. Which of the following should be performed as part of a primary assessment/life threat determination?
   a. obtaining a blood pressure
   b. palpating the femur
   c. obtaining a history of current events
   d. administering oxygen

9. Determining the exact details around a syncopal episode would be done during which part of the SAMPLE history?
   a. signs and symptoms
   b. allergies
   c. pertinent past history
   d. events

10. Differential diagnosis for chest pain might include all of the following *except* _____.
    a. hypertension
    b. aortic aneurysm
    c. pulmonary embolus
    d. pneumonia

APPLIED PATHOPHYSIOLOGY

You are called to a patient with an altered mental status. You begin a differential diagnostic process and come up with the possible causes listed in the following table. For each cause, list the pathophysiologic processes that could cause altered mental status. Hypoglycemia is included as an example in the first row.

Potential Cause of Altered Mental Status	Pathophysiology
Hypoglycemia	The brain cannot tolerate a lack of glucose as a fuel even for a short time. Hypoglycemia causes brain cell dysfunction.
Stroke	
Sepsis	
Seizure	
Head injury	
Hypoxia	

CLINICAL DECISION MAKING

Your ambulance is called to a motor vehicle collision in which a car has been T-boned while turning left. You are presented with three occupants between the two cars. Two are reporting injury. After performing a scene size-up and requesting an additional ambulance and personnel, your triage leads you to an approximately 20-year-old woman who is lying on the ground. She was the restrained passenger who took the impact directly into her door.

You noted between 12 and 15 inches of intrusion into her passenger space. Your primary assessment reveals a rapid pulse and respirations. Your crew administers oxygen and gets vital signs, while you perform a rapid secondary exam. You note no signs of injury during your exam (the patient denies pain, she has adequate respirations without chest pain or tenderness, her abdomen is soft and nontender, and no bone or spine injury is noted). The patient is upset about the crash but rational and not anxious.

Vital signs are reported as pulse 124 and regular, respirations 28, blood pressure 118/68 mmHG, pupils equal and reactive, skin cool and dry.

1. What role does mechanism of injury play in your decision making in reference to the patient's initial priority and status determination?

2. How does your knowledge of anatomy help you to predict injury patterns and organ involvement?

3. What do the vital signs tell you about the patient's status? Do you believe the patient is in shock? Why or why not?

4. If you had a local hospital 10 minutes away and a trauma center 30 minutes away, to which would you choose to transport this patient? What factors affect your decision?

15

Standard Patient Assessment

Competency Applies scene information and patient assessment findings (scene size-up, primary and secondary assessment, patient history, reassessment) to guide emergency management.

ASSESSMENT OF THE TRAUMA PATIENT

TRANSITION *highlights*

- *Update of assessment terminology to meet National EMS Education Standards nomenclature.*
- *Increased importance of patient physiologic status rather than mechanism of injury in determining patient instability or potential instability.*
- *Primary assessment process for the trauma victim.*
- *Comparison of the secondary assessment for a stable versus an unstable trauma patient.*
- *How vital sign trending can help identify types of traumatic conditions.*
- *Importance of performing a reassessment of the injured or traumatized patient.*

INTRODUCTION

The next two topics discuss patient assessment: Trauma assessment is the focus of this topic, and the next topic is medical assessment. This split is done because the ways trauma patients and medical patients are assessed are significantly different. These topics will also introduce you to the patient assessment process as outlined in the National EMS Education Standards because it will differ from the way you were taught in your initial EMS training.

Trauma assessment is a hands-on process (▶ Figure 15-1). A medical axiom states that 80 percent of the key information you will obtain to care for your trauma patient comes from a hands-on exam, and 20 percent comes from the history. You will later learn that the opposite is true for medical patients. This is not to say there is no value in the history; it is just that a hands-on exam is likely to produce more finite and applicable results.

If you took your initial EMT-B class after 1994, you learned a scripted approach to assessment. You likely learned a scene size-

up, initial assessment, and rapid trauma exam or focused assessment, followed by a detailed, then an ongoing, assessment. Your Advanced EMT class and subsequent practice refined this model.

The National EMS Education Standards do not provide this scripted approach. The standards do include a scene size-up, which is very similar to the existing size-up, and a primary assessment, which is similar to the existing initial assessment. Missing from the standards is the detailed information on executing the subsequent hands-on assessments. The standards do include a reassessment, which is similar to the existing ongoing assessment.

As an experienced provider, you will notice new EMTs, AEMTs, and reference sources using this new assessment terminology. It will not affect your assessment or your ability to work with newly trained providers. Table 15-1 compares the prior EMS curricula terms with the education standards.

SCENE SIZE-UP

The scene size-up comprises the following components for the trauma patient:

- Scene safety
- Standard Precautions
- Mechanism of injury
- Number of patients
- Hazards/resources needed

The only area with a change to the science is mechanism of injury. In the past, mechanism of injury was used as a significant predictor of injury and was a formative part of the early decisions EMS providers made in reference to the trauma patient.

Now, although mechanism of injury is still part of the puzzle, it is considered of less prognostic value than in prior years. In the past, mechanism of injury was a singular factor in determining

If you took your initial EMT-B class after 1994, you learned a scripted approach to assessment. The National EMS Education Standards do not provide this scripted approach.

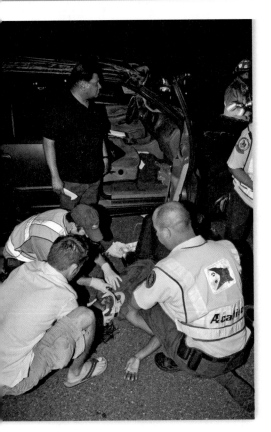

Figure 15-1 Trauma assessment.

TABLE 15-1	Comparison of the Assessment Flow in Prior Curricula and National EMS Education Standards (Trauma Assessment)
Prior Curricula	**National EMS Education Standards**
Scene size-up	Scene size-up
Initial assessment	Primary assessment
Rapid trauma exam	Secondary examination assessment
Focused exam	Secondary examination assessment
Detailed assessment	Secondary examination assessment
Ongoing assessment	Reassessment

whether a patient should receive a rapid examination and be expedited from the scene. Under new trauma triage guidelines issued by the Centers for Disease Control and Prevention (CDC), mechanism of injury is actually the third consideration in trauma triage. Examples of the guidelines are as follows (the complete CDC trauma triage decision scheme can be found in ▶ **Figure 15-2**):

1. **Physiologic criteria.** Does the patient have physiologic signs of instability, including a diminished Glasgow Coma Scale (GCS; <14), a decreased systolic blood pressure (<90 mmHg), or respirations <10 or >29 per minute? If so, the patient should be transported to a trauma center.

2. **Anatomic criteria.** Does the patient have anatomic signs of serious injury? These include penetrating injuries to the head and torso, flail chest, multiple long bone fractures, and other significant injuries. These injuries indicate the need for transport to a trauma center.

3. **Mechanism of injury.** Has the patient experienced a fall (adult >20 feet, child >10 feet or two to three times the child's height), ejection from a vehicle, or a death in the same passenger compartment or significant intrusion of dam-

age into the passenger compartment? In many cases you will have already decided to transport to a trauma center, but if not, these mechanisms will indicate a trauma center is warranted.

4. **Special patient or scene considerations.** These include the age of the patient, pregnancy, some additional specific injuries, and the judgment of the EMS provider.

Although the significance of mechanism of injury has been reduced, it has not been eliminated. The decision scheme simply places it in a more practical place—and more in line with the way we work in the field. Mechanism of injury still has a primary role in initially determining whether cervical spine stabilization should be maintained.

If your assessment reveals an unstable patient (altered mental status or hypotension), the patient is clearly injured. The same holds true for specific injuries found during assessment. When a patient has a significant mechanism of injury, he may or may not be injured. Research has yet to show a definitive correlation between mechanism of injury and actual injury.

PRIMARY ASSESSMENT

The primary assessment remains the step during which we identify and treat threats to life. The primary assessment will differ among patients, based on their needs. An alert and oriented patient is less likely to need an aggressive primary assessment than a patient with an altered mental status.

Traditionally guided by the mnemonic ABC—except in the case of an apparently lifeless person, when CAB is recommended by the American Heart Association—the primary assessment

proceeds as follows. Remember that A-B-C may be altered depending on the patient's presentation, injuries, and priority (e.g., a patient with exsanguinating hemorrhage would receive bleeding control first).

General Impression: How does the patient look?

This initial step helps to determine whether the patient appears responsive or not and provides a first glance at patient positioning (e.g., holding c-spine, clenched fist to chest) and general appearance (e.g., pale, anxious). Based on these observations alone, you can begin to determine the criticality of the patient and the pace with which you will assess and treat this patient.

Begin cervical spine stabilization if spine injury is suspected.

Airway: Is it open, and will it remain open if I divert my attention elsewhere?

If the patient is alert, oriented, and breathing, it is likely that you will need to take no action here. When a patient has an altered mental status or noisy (sonorous or gurgling) breathing, you must open the airway and suction as necessary. This is especially important in trauma patients who have facial trauma or direct laryngeal trauma that may bleed into the airway.

Interventions:
Positioning
Oral or nasal airway
Suction

Breathing: Is the patient breathing? Is the patient breathing enough to support life?

As with the airway step, the assessment and care you give will depend on the patient's

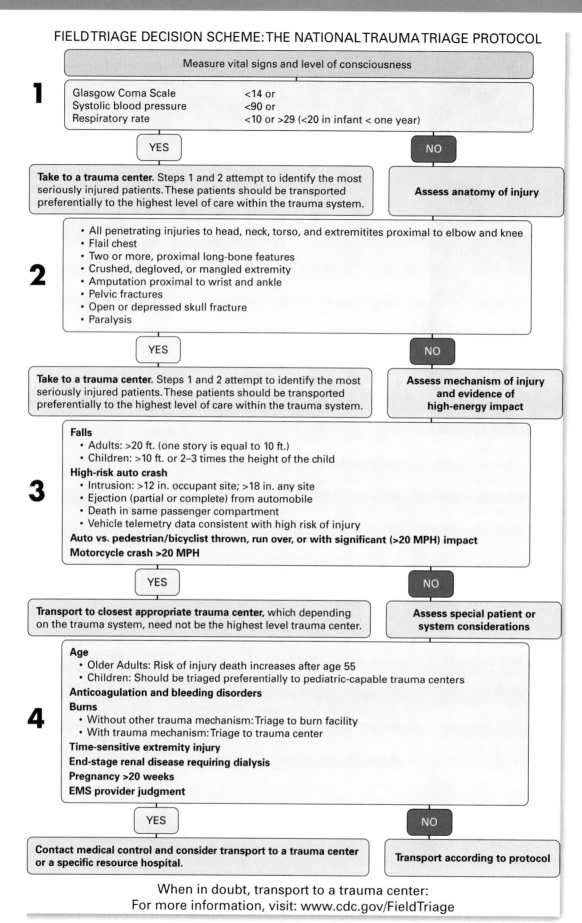

FIELD TRIAGE DECISION SCHEME: THE NATIONAL TRAUMA TRIAGE PROTOCOL

Measure vital signs and level of consciousness

1

Glasgow Coma Scale	<14 or
Systolic blood pressure	<90 or
Respiratory rate	<10 or >29 (<20 in infant < one year)

YES → **Take to a trauma center.** Steps 1 and 2 attempt to identify the most seriously injured patients. These patients should be transported preferentially to the highest level of care within the trauma system.

NO → **Assess anatomy of injury**

2

- All penetrating injuries to head, neck, torso, and extremitites proximal to elbow and knee
- Flail chest
- Two or more, proximal long-bone features
- Crushed, degloved, or mangled extremity
- Amputation proximal to wrist and ankle
- Pelvic fractures
- Open or depressed skull fracture
- Paralysis

YES → **Take to a trauma center.** Steps 1 and 2 attempt to identify the most seriously injured patients. These patients should be transported preferentially to the highest level of care within the trauma system.

NO → **Assess mechanism of injury and evidence of high-energy impact**

3

Falls
- Adults: >20 ft. (one story is equal to 10 ft.)
- Children: >10 ft. or 2–3 times the height of the child

High-risk auto crash
- Intrusion: >12 in. occupant site; >18 in. any site
- Ejection (partial or complete) from automobile
- Death in same passenger compartment
- Vehicle telemetry data consistent with high risk of injury

Auto vs. pedestrian/bicyclist thrown, run over, or with significant (>20 MPH) impact
Motorcycle crash >20 MPH

YES → **Transport to closest appropriate trauma center,** which depending on the trauma system, need not be the highest level trauma center.

NO → **Assess special patient or system considerations**

4

Age
- Older Adults: Risk of injury death increases after age 55
- Children: Should be triaged preferentially to pediatric-capable trauma centers

Anticoagulation and bleeding disorders

Burns
- Without other trauma mechanism: Triage to burn facility
- With trauma mechanism: Triage to trauma center

Time-sensitive extremity injury
End-stage renal disease requiring dialysis
Pregnancy >20 weeks
EMS provider judgment

YES → **Contact medical control and consider transport to a trauma center or a specific resource hospital.**

NO → **Transport according to protocol**

When in doubt, transport to a trauma center:
For more information, visit: www.cdc.gov/FieldTriage

Figure 15-2 CDC Trauma Triage Guidelines.
Source: Morbidity and Mortality Weekly Report, Vol. 58, No RR-1 (2009).

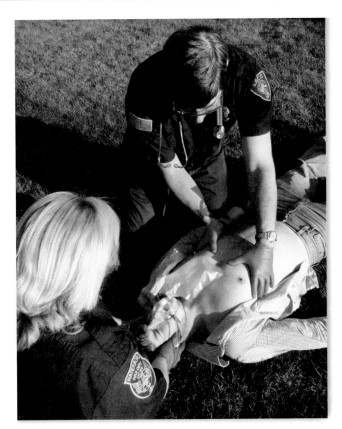

Figure 15-3 **Assess the chest during the primary assessment.**

the bleeding is severe, stop it during the primary assessment. If it is not severe, it will be treated later. Then check the patient's pulse and skin color, temperature, and condition. If the patient is in shock, you should know that now rather than waiting until later in the assessment.

Interventions:

Control of severe bleeding

Treatment for shock

At this point you will begin to consider the need for vascular access en route to the hospital. *Note:* Science is constantly evolving about the value of prehospital fluid resuscitation. Follow your local protocols in this regard.

If a patient appears to have a minor, isolated injury (such as an ankle injury), it is acceptable to assess and treat only that one injury or location.

History

Although the hands-on examination of a trauma patient offers the highest yield of information, there is still definitely a place for the history.

In addition to obtaining the signs and symptoms from the responsive patient, the history can serve to identify factors that may have caused the trauma or may be relevant to the patient's presentation or to identifying complications to his treatment. For example:

- You may find that a patient had a medical episode (syncope, seizure, hypoglycemia) that caused the patient's fall or motor vehicle collision.
- Medications may mask signs of shock. Beta blockers may prevent an increase in pulse, which will mask the progression of shock.
- The patient may have had a prior stroke, which has caused some weakness on one side of the extremities that could be mistaken during tests of grip strength.

Speaking to the patient, family, and bystanders who may have witnessed the event may provide significant information on the events surrounding the trauma.

Vital Signs

Vital signs—or, more important, *trends* in vital signs (see Table 15-3)—are crucial in determining the severity and progression of your patient's condition. The traditional vital signs include the following:

- Pulse
- Respirations
- Skin color, temperature, and condition
- Blood pressure
- Pupils

Pulse oximetry is in such common use that it is frequently considered a sixth vital sign. Use caution when obtaining pulse oximetry readings on patients who are hypoperfusing, however, as the readings are frequently inaccurate. The hemoglobin in the blood may be 100 percent saturated, but this is of minimal value diagnostically when the patient is severely hypovolemic.

mental status. Patients who are alert, oriented, and not anxious likely have adequate breathing. Those who have an altered mental status or injury to any part of the face, neck, or chest will need further evaluation (▶ Figure 15-3).

In the trauma patient:

- Assess the chest to determine if it is intact and to examine for flail segments.
- Look for penetrating injuries and open wounds.
- Listen for lung sounds on both sides to determine whether a pneumothorax or tension pneumothorax is present.

Interventions:

Oxygen via cannula or mask

Positive pressure ventilation via BVM, FROPVD, or pocket face mask

Treating critical chest injury (e.g., occlusive dressing, stabilize flail segment)

Advanced airway devices (when allowed by protocol and clinically appropriate)

Circulation: Does the patient have a pulse? Is the patient bleeding severely? Is the patient in shock?

Patients who are talking have a pulse, but they may be in shock. The fact that a patient is responsive does not eliminate the need for further assessment in this step. If the patient is responsive, continue to talk to him and ask where he is hurt. Look for obvious bleeding. If

Priority Determination: What is my patient's status and his transport priority?

Is my patient stable, potentially unstable, or unstable? At this point, you will decide on your patient's general status and make decisions based on that status. If your patient is unstable, he will be rapidly assessed and transported from the scene, with spinal considerations, to an appropriate destination. Stable patients will be assessed, fully immobilized, and transported routinely to the hospital. The wide range of potentially unstable patients will be treated more expediently than stable patients, who will receive more care on scene than unstable patients.

SECONDARY ASSESSMENT

The secondary assessment (▶ Figure 15-4) is one head-to-toe exam, but it may be done in at least two ways, depending on the status of the patient determined at the end of the primary assessment. Patients who are unstable will receive this head-to-toe exam more quickly, whereas those who appear to be more stable (some of whom are potentially unstable) will receive the secondary exam proportionally more slowly (see Table 15-2).

FIRST TAKE STANDARD PRECAUTIONS

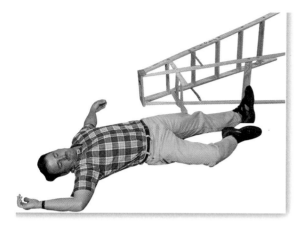

Reassess mechanism of injury (MOI). If it is not significant (e.g., patient has a cut finger), focus the physical exam only on the injured part. If the MOI is significant:

- Continue manual stabilization of the head and neck.
- Consider requesting ALS personnel.
- Reconsider transport decision.
- Reassess mental status.
- Perform a trauma assessment.

TRAUMA ASSESSMENT

Rapidly assess each part of the body for the following problems (say "Dee-cap B-T-L-S" as a memory prompt):

Deformities   Burns
Contusions   Tenderness
Abrasions   Lacerations
Punctures/Penetrations   Swelling

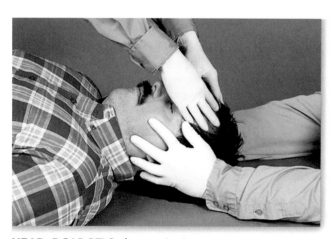

HEAD: DCAP-BTLS plus crepitation.

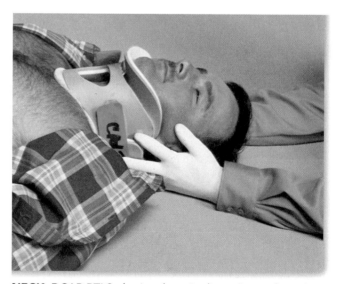

NECK: DCAP-BTLS plus jugular vein distention and crepitation (then apply cervical collar).

Figure 15-4 Secondary assessment is a head-to-toe examination.

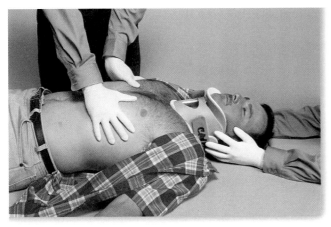

CHEST: DCAP-BTLS plus crepitation, paradoxical motion, and breath sounds (absent, present, equal).

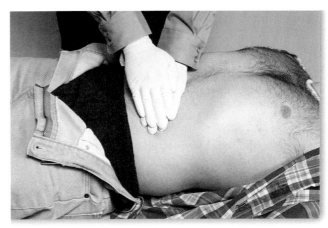

ABDOMEN: DCAP-BTLS plus firm, soft, distended.

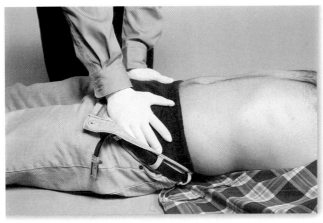

PELVIS: DCAP-BTLS with gentle compression for tenderness or motion.

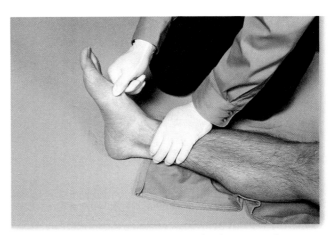

EXTREMITIES: DCAP-BTLS plus distal pulse, motor function, and sensation.

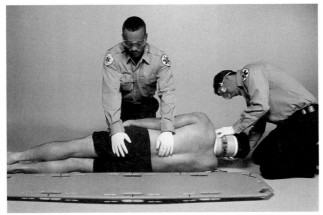

POSTERIOR: DCAP-BTLS. (To examine posterior, roll patient using spinal precautions.)

Figure 15-4 (Continued)

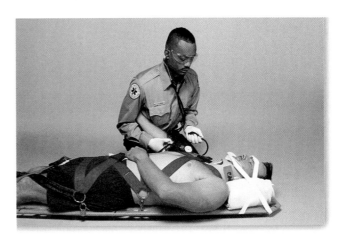

VITAL SIGNS

VITAL SIGNS

Assess the patient's baseline vital signs:

- Respiration
- Pulse
- Skin color, temperature, condition (capillary refill in infants and children)
- Pupils
- Blood pressure
- Oxygen saturation (if directed by local protocol)

SAMPLE HISTORY

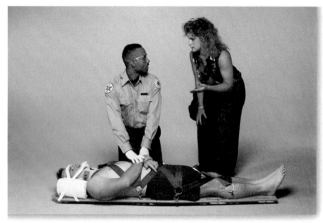

Interview patient or (if patient is unresponsive) interview family and bystanders to get as much information as possible about the patient's problem.

Ask about:

Signs and symptoms
Allergies
Medications
Pertinent past history
Last oral intake
Events leading to problem

INTERVENTIONS AND TRANSPORT

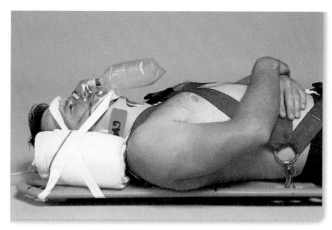

Contact online medical direction and perform interventions as needed.

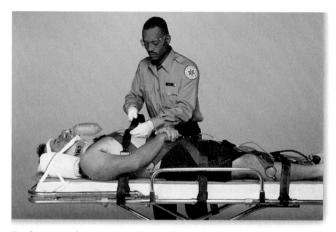

Package and transport the patient.

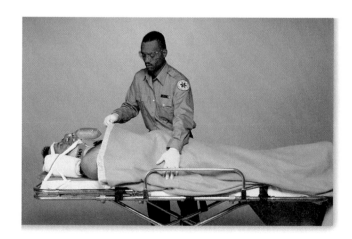

Figure 15-4 (Continued)

TABLE 15-2   Secondary Assessments of Unstable and Stable Patients

Secondary Assessment—Unstable Patient	Secondary Assessment—Stable Patient
Purpose: To perform a rapid exam that will help identify major injuries and end with the patient being placed on a spine board.	*Purpose:* To perform a head-to-toe assessment on a stable patient to determine a full picture of the patient's injuries. -or- To assess a single injured area on a patient if the mechanism of injury and chief complaint indicate the injury is isolated.
Further examination can be done en route if time permits.	
Maintain c-spine stabilization throughout.	Maintain c-spine stabilization if indicated.
Rapidly examine the following: • Head • Neck • Chest • Abdomen • Pelvis • Extremities • Posterior	Examine in detail (when indicated): • Head • Face • Neck • Shoulders/clavicles • Chest • Abdomen • Pelvis • Lower extremities • Upper extremities • Posterior

TABLE 15-3   Vital Sign Trends in Traumatic Conditions

	Pulse	Respirations	Blood Pressure	Pulse Pressure	Skin
Shock	Increase	Increase	Decrease (late)	Narrows	Becomes cool and clammy
Increasing intracranial pressure (late)	Decrease	Irregular	Increase	Widens	Varies
Anxious, uninjured patient calming down	Decrease	Decrease	May decrease or remain the same	No significant change	Becomes warm and dry

Pulse oximetry will likely have a greater role in patient assessment and care, as more protocols specify oxygen delivery amounts and devices based on oximetry readings. Unstable trauma patients and any patient suspected of being hypovolemic will still receive high-concentration oxygen via nonrebreather mask when breathing adequately, as well as positive pressure ventilation with oxygen when necessary for inadequate or absent breathing.

Vital signs are monitored frequently, depending on the patient's status. Generally, the patient's vitals are rechecked approximately every 15 minutes (and at least twice) when the patient is stable and every 5 minutes when the patient is unstable—transport time and priorities permitting.

Noninvasive blood pressure (NIBP) devices (▶ Figure 15-5) are being used more frequently in the field and are specifically mentioned in the education standards. NIBP devices are convenient in that they automatically measure the patient's blood pressure at preselected intervals.

You should always take one manual blood pressure during the call—preferably at the beginning—to compare with the NIBP reading. Because the NIBP is a mechanical device, it may occasionally dis-play an incorrect or erroneous reading. Obtaining an occasional manual blood pressure will help reduce the impact of

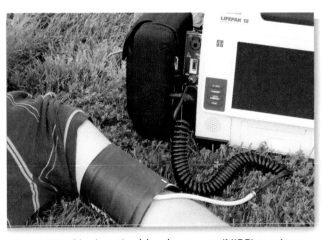

Figure 15-5 Noninvasive blood pressure (NIBP) monitor.

the erroneous readings, especially in hypotensive patients.

REASSESSMENT

You should reassess your patient frequently while he is in your care. This will help to observe trends in the patient's condition. In the absence of higher priorities (e.g., suction or ventilating your patient), your reassessment will cover the following components when applicable and time permits:

- Reevaluate components of the primary assessment.

- Reevaluate the chief complaint and/or injuries.
- Recheck vital signs.
- Verify that all interventions (splinting, spinal immobilization) are still effective.

Reassessment should be performed approximately every 15 minutes for stable patients and every 5 minutes for unstable patients when time and priorities permit (▶ Figure 15-6).

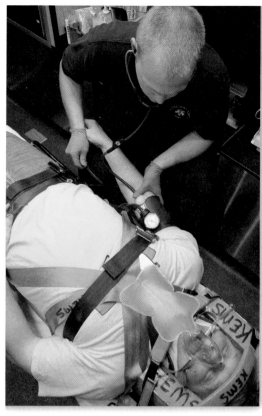

Figure 15-6 Reassessment is done en route to the hospital—every 5 minutes for the unstable patient, every 15 minutes for the stable patient.

TRANSITIONING

REVIEW ITEMS

1. Your patient's blood pressure has increased, his pulse has decreased, and his pulse pressure has widened. He likely has _____.
   a. sepsis
   b. spinal shock
   c. hypovolemic shock
   d. increasing intracranial pressure

2. Pulse oximetry may not be relevant in trauma cases because _____.
   a. hemoglobin no longer carries oxygen when the patient is in shock
   b. the hemoglobin is saturated but the patient has reduced volume
   c. the hemoglobin will be saturated with carbon dioxide instead of oxygen
   d. a special probe is necessary to detect carboxyhemoglobin in trauma cases

3. Your trauma patient is unstable. En route to the hospital, he began bleeding into his airway. You were unable to reassess the patient after 5 minutes because you were performing suction almost constantly. You are concerned because your run report will not contain a second set of vital signs. What should you do?
   a. Note the reason for the single set of vitals in your narrative.
   b. Because you saw that the pulse oximeter reflected a pulse, you should use that number and use the other vital signs from the initial set you took.
   c. Make up a set of vitals that match the patient's declining condition.
   d. Do nothing. It was not your fault.

4. Which of the following would *not* be included in the primary assessment for a trauma patient?
   a. stabilizing a flail segment
   b. listening for lungs sounds bilaterally
   c. applying a tourniquet
   d. taking a pulse

5. What is the primary difference in secondary assessment between a stable and an unstable patient?
   a. location the exam is performed
   b. speed of the exam
   c. thoroughness of the exam
   d. level of responsiveness of the patient

APPLIED KNOWLEDGE

For each assessment task, label the assessment step in which it would be first performed:

_____ 1. Checking for a pulse

_____ 2. Palpating the tibia

_____ 3. Obtaining a second blood pressure

_____ 4. Sealing an open chest wound

_____ 5. Placing the patient on a backboard

_____ 6. Observing mechanism of injury

_____ 7. Forming a general impression

_____ 8. Administering oxygen

a. scene size-up

b. primary assessment

c. secondary assessment

d. reassessment

CLINICAL DECISION MAKING

You are called to a patient who was stabbed by his wife. You drive to the patient's neighborhood while the EMS dispatcher is trying to determine whether police have arrived on scene yet. As you round a corner, you observe what appears to be the patient out on the sidewalk. He is clutching his chest, his hand bloody.

1. What are the risks of approaching the scene?

2. What do you do to remain safe?

The police arrive on scene quickly and secure it. There is no sign of the wife. Because the patient is standing at the street, you bring him into your ambulance. He looks anxious and pale. His breathing is labored. He is still clutching at his chest with a bloody hand.

3. Assuming the wound to his chest is the only injury, what would you expect to find in the primary assessment?

4. What care would you perform in the primary assessment?

After your assessment and care in the primary assessment, you perform a secondary assessment, which reveals no further injuries. During transport to the hospital, you perform an initial set of vital signs and then reassess the patient on a regular basis.

5. If the patient were to have a worsening of his chest injury, how would you expect his vital signs to trend?

6. How would you balance any advanced life support care versus assessment and transport? What are your priorities?

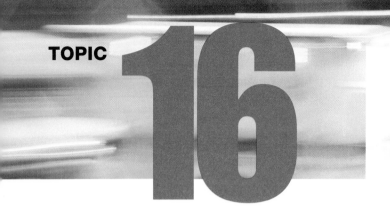

Standard Patient Assessment

Competency Applies scene information and patient assessment findings (scene size-up, primary and secondary assessment, patient history, reassessment) to guide emergency management.

ASSESSMENT OF THE MEDICAL PATIENT

TRANSITION *highlights*

- *Importance for the Advanced EMT to assess a medical patient with a body system approach.*

- *Reinforcement of the critical thinking and differential diagnosis processes for the Advanced EMT while completing a medical assessment and developing a patient care plan.*

- *Illustration of body systems the Advanced EMT should assess when confronted with a patient with one of several common complaints.*

- *Important questions to ask the patient when assessing a certain body system given the patient's complaint(s).*

INTRODUCTION

Medical emergencies can be looked at as a mystery that must be solved. To solve the mystery, you will gather facts in your assessment.

The assessment of the medical patient is focused on the patient history. As mentioned in Topic 15, "Assessment of the Trauma Patient," trauma patient assessment centers on the hands-on exam. The opposite is true here. You will gain a majority of your information about the medical patient from the history. This is not to say that the physical examination is unimportant, just that experience has demonstrated the importance of this history.

Again, as with trauma assessment, the EMS Education Standards have done away with a detailed process. Instead, you will perform examinations on body systems. For example, if a patient has chest pain or discomfort, you will assess the cardiac and respiratory systems. A patient with an altered mental status will require the examination of several systems to determine the potential cause and choose the correct interventions. This more closely resembles the assessment processes and patterns used by advanced providers.

ASSESSMENT OF THE MEDICAL PATIENT

The processes used when assessing the medical patient are similar to the steps in trauma patient assessment (see Table 16-1), but within each of the examinations are some differences.

Scene Size-Up

The scene size-up remains a foundational part of the assessment. You will ensure scene safety and determine what Standard Precautions are necessary. You will determine how many patients are present and what resources are necessary. There are rarely multiple medical patients (although it can happen), and the resources you need often center around lifting assistance for bariatric patients or advanced life support for critical patients.

You will also determine the nature of illness (NOI). This takes the place of mechanism of injury in the trauma patient. The NOI is your first impression of the kind of medical problem your patient has. You will determine this from a variety of sources. Dispatch will begin this process with the information it relays to you. You may also get information from family members or bystanders as you approach. Finally, as you approach the patient

| TABLE 16-1 | Differences Between Prior EMS Curricula and National EMS Education Standards |
Prior EMS Curricula	National EMS Education Standards
Scene size-up	Scene size-up
Initial assessment	Primary assessment
Focused history and physical exam	Secondary assessment
Ongoing assessment	Reassessment

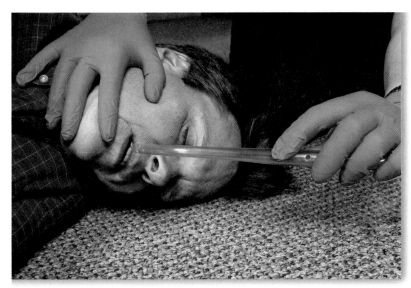

Figure 16-1 The primary assessment focuses on identifying and treating life threats.

and arrive at his side, you will get this information and bridge into the primary assessment.

Primary Assessment

The primary assessment (▶ Figure 16-1) begins with a general impression and then revolves around the ABCs—namely, identifying and correcting life threats.

The discussion that follows deals with a patient experiencing a medical emergency. If you encounter a patient who appears lifeless on first impression and does not appear to be breathing, you will begin the CAB sequence recommended by the American Heart Association. Remember that multiple rescuers may be present, so tasks may be handled simultaneously.

Beginning with the general impression, observe your patient as you approach (see Table 16-2). This will be formative in how you continue the primary assessment. If you see an alert patient, your primary assessment will be much different than if you see an unresponsive patient on the floor.

There are other clues, though—and there are many types of patients between alert and unresponsive. You may observe patients who are clutching their chest, in the tripod position, profoundly anxious, or have such poor skin color you can see it from across the room. As an experienced AEMT, you have likely seen some or all of these patients and realize that these are all important clues that, when observed and responded to properly, help to make your care more efficient and intuitive.

AIRWAY The patient's airway must be open and clear of secretions (a patent airway) and remain that way. Responsive patients usually do this for themselves, whereas patients with an altered mental status may require a head-tilt, chin-lift to open the airway, and suction. Measure and insert an oral airway if the patient does not have a gag reflex. A nasal airway may also be an option if the patient will not accept the oral airway.

Unresponsive patients may require nearly continuous airway care throughout the call.

BREATHING Your patient must be breathing—and breathing adequately. You will carefully assess the patient to ensure adequate breathing. If the patient is breathing inadequately, you must provide positive pressure ventilation with a pocket face mask, bag-valve mask, or flow-restricted, oxygen-powered ventilation device (FROPVD).

Patients breathing adequately will receive oxygen based on their physical appearance, complaint, and pulse oximetry readings. In most systems, the days of giving all patients 12 to 15 liters via nonrebreather mask are over. Although you must follow your local protocols, many systems now recommend a nasal cannula, or even no oxygen, when patients have adequate signs of perfusion and normal pulse oximetry readings. It is believed that too much oxygen may actually cause harm to some patients (e.g., myocardial infarction [MI], stroke).

You should not, however, withhold oxygen from patients in significant respiratory distress or with signs of hypoxia.

CIRCULATION Circulation is the part of the primary assessment in which you continue to assess circulation (your general impression began this process). Assess the patient's skin color, temperature, and condition as indicators of shock. Check the patient's pulse. If the patient is unresponsive, quickly check the carotid pulse and evaluate for signs of life; if the patient is responsive, check the radial pulse. Note the general pulse rate (do not take the time to get an actual rate). Pay attention for abnormally fast or slow rates as indicators that the patient has a more serious

If the pulse is absent, begin the CPR with chest compressions and defibrillation sequence as prescribed by the American Heart Association.

TABLE 16-2	General Impressions
If you see . . .	It may mean . . .
Patient clutching closed fist to chest: Levine's sign	Chest pain or discomfort usually high on the 1–10 scale and potentially severe
Tripod position	Significant respiratory distress
Anxious or restless patient	Hypoxia
Poor skin color (pale) and condition (moist)	Shock, hypoglycemia

condition. If the pulse is absent, begin the CPR with chest compressions and defibrillation sequence as prescribed by the American Heart Association.

The circulation portion of the primary assessment is also the place to look for bleeding. Although external bleeding is primarily a trauma issue, examine the scene in the early parts of the call for vomited blood, melena, or hematochezia, indicating gastrointestinal bleeding.

PRIORITY DETERMINATION The priority determination is the point at which you synthesize all the information you learned in the primary assessment and decide on a patient priority and status. A properly performed primary assessment will give you enough information to make this determination and will help you decide how quickly you should pace your call. As an advanced provider, you will have likely begun to form some ideas about your differential diagnostic possibilities and considered the possibility of the need for advanced modalities such as airway control, vascular access, and medication administration.

Secondary Assessment

The secondary assessment is where the major changes are found when assessing the medical patient. In addition to collecting a detailed history and vital signs, you will perform body system exams. These exams involve system-specific questions and a physical exam when appropriate.

Perhaps most significant is the fact that the AEMT must understand enough about the specific complaint and possible causes to choose the correct body system exam or exams to perform. In medicine, this is called a *differential diagnostic approach* (discussed in Topic 14, "Critical Thinking"). The clinician thinks of all the possible causes for a patient complaint (within reason), performs examinations to either rule in or tentatively rule out causes, and makes a treatment decision based on the findings. This is also referred to as going from *possible* to *probable* causes.

The way you perform a secondary exam will depend on a number of factors, the most important of which is the patient's overall status. Patients who have an altered mental status, problems with the ABCs, any condition that could

lead to instability (e.g., cardiac or respiratory difficulties), or any condition that requires prompt transport to appropriate facilities (e.g., patients with MI or stroke) will be expedited from the scene after a primary assessment and a quick history and physical exam (▶ Figure 16-2). The remainder of the history and physical examination will be provided en route.

In stable patients—and those without critical complaints—you will take more time on the scene to do a complete history and examination.

The medical assessment is especially important because the AEMT has a significant toolbox available to treat a variety of medical conditions. Your assessment and the differential diagnostic process will provide the ability to determine which medication, if any, will be of benefit to the patient.

HISTORY The history is a dynamic process—and arguably the most important for the medical patient (▶ Figure 16-3). It is not the intent of this text to reteach the entire process and repeat simple mnemonics. Instead, this section will focus on insights that experienced providers use to make their history more effective and insightful.

Events: Because it is at the end of the SAMPLE mnemonic, many do not use this important concept to its fullest. Patients do not always know the things they should tell you. For example, with patients who suddenly passed out, it is important to know whether they were active or sitting. Patients may report that they were standing when they actually just went from a sitting to a standing position suddenly.

The patient's activities and observations about the onset are also significant. Patients may recall specific feelings before an event (e.g., "whiting out" or an aura before a seizure). Carefully explore the events.

Onset: There is a significant difference in medical diagnosis between gradual and sudden onset. Using respiratory distress as an example, patients who have respiratory distress with a slow onset, pleuritic pain, and fever likely have a condition such as pneumonia. Patients who have a history of COPD often have a respiratory infection for a day

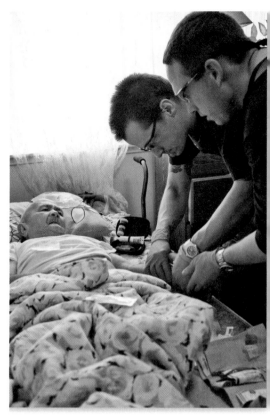

Figure 16-2 The on-scene secondary assessment is expedited when the patient is unstable.

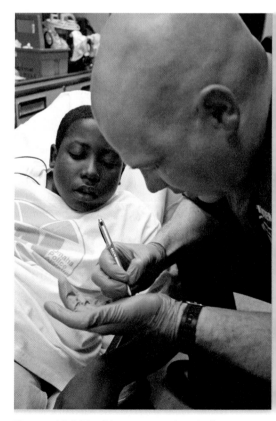

Figure 16-3 The history provides vital information for the medical patient.

or several days, which triggers an acute exacerbation. Patients who have a sudden onset are more likely to have an acute condition such as an asthma attack, aortic dissection, or an MI.

The classic presentation of a patient experiencing a worsening of congestive heart failure is a patient who calls because he suddenly cannot breathe. A careful history usually reveals weight gain, increasing orthopnea, dyspnea on exertion, and edema for days or even weeks before the call to EMS. (It is worth noting, though, that a rapid change in blood pressure can rapidly precipitate congestive heart failure or "flash pulmonary edema.")

Medications: It is not enough to ask about medications or copy down the names from containers you find. Medications themselves often play a role in the patient's condition, for a number of reasons. Patients often self-adjust their medication dose because of side effects or financial concerns. A recent change in medication, especially with antihypertensives and cardiac medications, can cause syncope or other medical problems. Remember to ask about over-the-counter medications.

BODY SYSTEM EXAMS Even though body system exams (Table 16-3) are new to the education standards, you already do this in your current practice as an AEMT.

The body system exams are a combination of the history and targeted physical examination (Table 16-4). Subsequent topics in this text will supplement your knowledge about the pathophysiology and assessment of specific conditions.

VITAL SIGNS An initial set of vital signs followed by repeated sets for trending are important in the assessment of the medical patient. If you use noninvasive blood pressure or other mechanical devices, be sure to check vital signs manually at least once to verify the noninvasive readings and more frequently if the patient is hypotensive.

Again, it is not the intent here to reteach basic skills, but the following insights into vital signs will help your assessment of the medical patient.

TABLE 16-3 Body System Approach to Common Medical Complaints

Complaint/Presenting Problem	Body Systems to Examine
Difficulty breathing	Respiratory Cardiac
Chest pain or discomfort	Cardiac Respiratory
Altered mental status	Endocrine Neurologic Scene evaluation
General malaise	Will require more focused history to determine systems
Syncopal episode	Cardiac Respiratory Endocrine Neurologic
Abdominal pain or discomfort	Gastrointestinal
Seizure	Neurologic If patient does not come out of the seizure or has an ongoing altered mental status, add endocrine and cardiac

TABLE 16-4 Examples of Physical Exam Elements and History Questions by Body System

Respiratory	Chest shape and symmetry
	Presence/absence of lung sounds
	Abnormal lung sounds
	Work of breathing (effort)
	Body position
	Pedal edema or ascites
	Cyanosis
	History: OPQRST to include:
	    Medications
	    Dyspnea on exertion
	    Orthopnea

Cardiac (note overlap with respiratory)	Pulse
	Compare pulse in upper extremities
	Blood pressure
	Skin color, temperature, and condition
	History: OPQRST to include:
	    Medications
	    Detailed description of pain/discomfort
	    Dyspnea on exertion
	    Orthopnea

Neurologic	Mental status Ability to follow commands Prehospital stroke scale Mental status exam (thoughts, perception, mood, affect) History: OPQRST to include: Onset/events (gradual or rapid onset)

Endocrine	Mental status
	Blood glucose monitoring
	Skin color, temperature, and condition
	History: OPQRST to include:
	    Focus on oral intake and medications
	    Recent illness?
	    Change in medications?

Note: Specifics may vary by patient and presentation.

Watch vital signs for shock. Although it is easy to think of shock and trauma going together, medical patients can also experience shock. GI bleed, late sepsis, anaphylaxis, and MI are potential causes of medical shock.

Pay attention to the respiratory rate. It is easy to gravitate more toward pulse, blood pressure, and skin color. Respirations are a key vital sign and one of the earliest changes in shock—but respirations will also be an indication of acid–base balance. Patients with diabetic ketoacidosis and those who have overdosed on aspirin (acetylsalicylic acid) will have rapid, deep respirations in an attempt to rid the body of acids.

Check pupils. Pupils may be the only indicator of a narcotic overdose (although not every narcotic causes pinpoint pupils) and may also help alert you to intracranial bleeds that occur spontaneously (as opposed to those from trauma).

Trends are best. Always take and evaluate multiple sets of vital signs.

Reassessment

As with trauma, reassessment is performed about every 15 minutes for stable patients and about every 5 minutes for unstable patients (unless other priorities prevent it) (▶ Figure 16-4).

The components of the reassessment include the following:

- Repeating the primary assessment
- Repeating vital signs
- Reassessing the chief complaint
- Reassessing the effect of interventions performed and ensuring that ongoing interventions are working properly

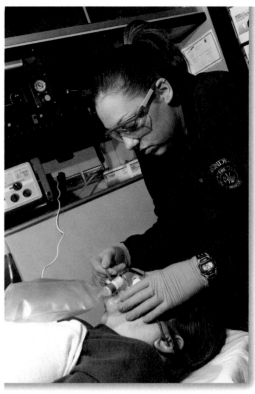

Figure 16-4 Reassessment is done en route to the hospital and performed every 5 minutes for the unstable patient and every 15 minutes for the stable patient.

TRANSITIONING • • • • • • •

REVIEW ITEMS

1. The best description of the body system exam is _____.
   a. the patient history
   b. the detailed hands-on portion of the assessment
   c. the rapid history and vital signs
   d. the targeted history and physical exam

2. Observing skin color, temperature, and condition in the primary assessment _____.
   a. helps identify shock early
   b. is primarily a sign of myocardial infarction
   c. is of little value in a medical patient
   d. is primarily used for identifying patients with heat emergencies

3. An elderly patient who complains of suddenly passing out would receive an assessment of which body systems?
   a. cardiac
   b. cardiac and respiratory
   c. cardiac, respiratory, and neurological
   d. cardiac, respiratory, neurological, and endocrine

4. The presence of dark, tarry blood in the stool is called _____.
   a. hematochezia
   b. melena
   c. frank blood
   d. hemoccult

5. You have arrived at a patient's side and are completing the primary assessment. The patient had chest pains, which have subsided, and he complains of a little difficulty breathing. His oxygen saturation is 92 percent. How would you administer oxygen to this patient?
   a. 2 lpm via cannula
   b. 4 lpm via cannula
   c. 6 lpm via Venturi mask
   d. 12 lpm via nonrebreather

APPLIED PATHOPHYSIOLOGY

For each of the following body systems, choose one complaint or patient presentation that would cause you to examine it. Looking at things from a different angle helps learning and application.

Body System	Patient Presentation or Complaint
Respiratory	
Cardiac	
Endocrine	
Neurologic	

CLINICAL DECISION MAKING

You are called to a patient who passed out at the mall. You arrive to find the patient alert, sitting upright on a bench, and a little pale. The patient is a 68-year-old woman who was shopping with her daughter and grandchildren. The family members are gathered around the patient and look worried.

The patient states she is fine now. She tells you that she had felt a little dizzy and then apparently passed out, although she remembers nothing past the dizziness. She denies injury from the fall and would really just like to leave the mall and go home to rest.

The patient has a history of hypertension and hypercholesterolemia and sees her physician regularly. She denies chest pain and difficulty breathing. Her color seems to have returned in the few minutes you have been talking with her.

1. For each of the following body systems, list three things you would want to examine or ask:
   a. Respiratory
   b. Cardiac
   c. Neurologic
   d. Endocrine

2. What questions will you ask in the onset and events portion of the history to gain additional insight into the cause of the patient's syncope?

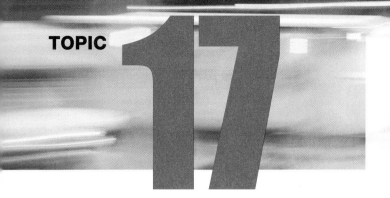

Educational Standard Medicine

Competency Applies fundamental knowledge to provide basic and selected advanced emergency care and transportation based on assessment findings for an acutely ill patient.

NEUROLOGY: ALTERED MENTAL STATUS

TRANSITION highlights

- **Overview of the necessary components that determine consciousness and normal orientation.**

- **Frequency of occurrence of altered mental status.**

- **Specific central nervous system structures that influence body homeostasis and contribute to a patient's mental status:**
  - Cerebral hemispheres.
  - Cerebrum.
  - Brainstem (medulla, midbrain, pons).
  - Reticular activating system.

- **Major categories of altered mental status that can help the assessment and management for the Advanced EMT:**
  - Structural.
  - Metabolic.

- **Assessment approach for a patient with an altered mental status, focusing on differentiating structural versus metabolic causes.**

INTRODUCTION

*A*ltered mental status is defined as any state of awareness that differs from the normal awareness of a conscious person. A state of general wakefulness, consciousness involves being aware of and responsive to the environment. It relies on specific portions of the brain to work together and function properly. To be conscious, the patient must have a fully intact brainstem and one functioning cerebral hemisphere. Injury to either of these structures leads to an alteration in consciousness, or altered mental status.

The portion of the brainstem accountable for maintaining consciousness is the reticular activating system (RAS), also known as the ascending reticular activating system (ARAS). A network of

specialized nerve cells, the reticular activating system controls states of arousal and consciousness, including wakefulness, attentiveness, and sleep. For a person to be awake, the RAS and one cerebral hemisphere must be intact.

An altered mental status arises from a lesion or injury that causes a dysfunction to the RAS or to both cerebral hemispheres. Therefore, a unilateral lesion to one of the cerebral hemispheres usually does not induce impaired consciousness. On the other hand, even the smallest focal lesion to the RAS can affect mental status.

EPIDEMIOLOGY

Alterations in mental status affect many age groups. In particular, the elderly are susceptible to varying drug–drug interactions and alterations of therapeutic medication dosages. This accounts for an average of 30 percent of altered mental status in the elderly. In this age group, minor infections, such as an upper respiratory tract infection or urinary tract infection, and even fever, can cause an altered mental status.

Also, immunocompromised patients, such as those suffering with AIDS or undergoing chemotherapy, are prone to opportunistic infections. These infections can cause an altered mental status as well.

Just as an infectious process can affect the elderly and immunocompromised patients, it can affect children too. Infection is the most common cause of impaired consciousness in infants (see Table 17-1).

TABLE 17-1	Common Age-Related Etiology of Altered Mental Status
Infants	Infection, trauma, abuse, metabolic lesion
Toddlers	Toxic ingestion, trauma
Adolescents/ young adults	Toxic ingestion, recreational drug use, trauma
Elderly persons	Medication alterations, alterations in living environment, stroke, infection, trauma, fever

PATHOPHYSIOLOGY

The brain is an intricate organ of the human body that has several working parts. When looking down at the top of the brain, the *cerebral cortex* is observed. It is the outermost layer of the brain that covers the cerebrum. The *cerebrum* is the home for higher mental functions, such as memory, learning, judgment, and emotions, all of which make individuals unique. When the cerebrum is split down the middle, it is separated into the left and right cerebral hemispheres. The cerebral hemispheres include the frontal lobe, parietal lobe, temporal lobe, and occipital lobe. Movement, speech, sensation, and conscious thought processes are housed within the cerebral hemispheres (▶ Figure 17-1).

The *cerebellum* is located just beneath the cerebral hemispheres. It is the portion of the brain that plays an important role in motor control. It is also involved in some cognitive functions, such as attention and language. Most important, the cerebellum contributes to coordination, balance, precision, and accurate timing. Injury or damage to the cerebellum does not cause paralysis but instead impairs posture, fine motor movement, and motor learning.

The *brainstem* is seated beneath the cerebellum and joins the spinal cord to the brain. The brainstem regulates the autonomic responses of the body, such as heart rate, breathing, and blood pressure, and it maintains alertness. The brainstem is the pathway for the fiber tracts connecting the peripheral nerves and spinal cord to the higher portions of the brain. The three portions of the brainstem that relay these functions are the medulla oblongata, the midbrain, and the pons.

The *medulla oblongata* functions primarily as a relay station for the motor tracts crossing between the brain and spinal cord. It contains the regulatory center of the respiratory, vasomotor, and cardiac systems. It also affects mechanisms that control swallowing, coughing, gagging, and vomiting.

The *midbrain* serves as the pathway of the cerebral hemispheres, containing the auditory and visual reflex centers. One of its most important roles is eye movement.

The *pons* is the main housing for the respiratory center within the brain. It is a bridgelike structure that links different parts of the brain. The pons serves as the communication station between the

> Injury or damage to the cerebellum does not cause paralysis but instead impairs posture, fine motor movement, and motor learning.

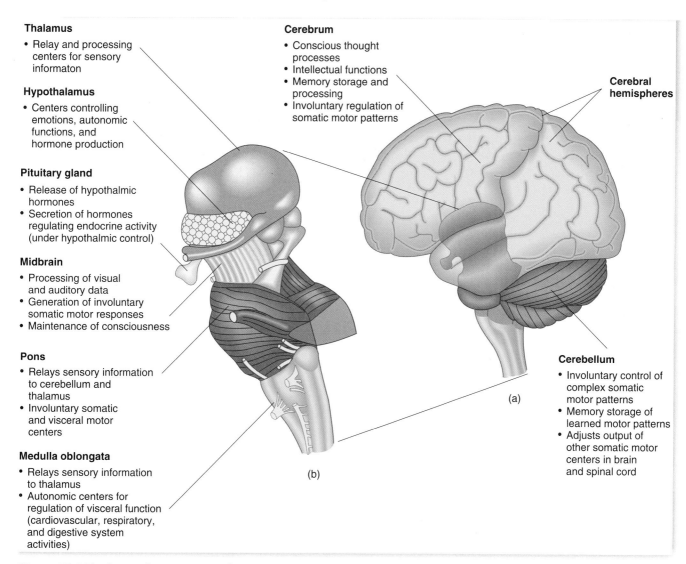

Thalamus
- Relay and processing centers for sensory informaton

Hypothalamus
- Centers controlling emotions, autonomic functions, and hormone production

Pituitary gland
- Release of hypothalmic hormones
- Secretion of hormones regulating endocrine activity (under hypothalmic control)

Midbrain
- Processing of visual and auditory data
- Generation of involuntary somatic motor responses
- Maintenance of consciousness

Pons
- Relays sensory information to cerebellum and thalamus
- Involuntary somatic and visceral motor centers

Medulla oblongata
- Relays sensory information to thalamus
- Autonomic centers for regulation of visceral function (cardiovascular, respiratory, and digestive system activities)

Cerebrum
- Conscious thought processes
- Intellectual functions
- Memory storage and processing
- Involuntary regulation of somatic motor patterns

Cerebral hemispheres

Cerebellum
- Involuntary control of complex somatic motor patterns
- Memory storage of learned motor patterns
- Adjusts output of other somatic motor centers in brain and spinal cord

(a)

(b)

Figure 17-1 The human brain: (a) Superficial view of the brain. (b) Components of the brainstem.

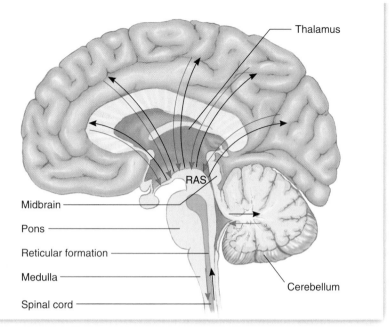

Figure 17-2 The reticular activating system (RAS) sends and receives messages from various parts of the brain.

medulla and the higher cortical structures of the brain.

Found within the brainstem is the RAS (▶ Figure 17-2). The RAS is the main "on/off switch" for the brain. It is made up of both cholinergic and adrenergic components to control activity and the appropriate behavioral state. During sleep, the neurons in the RAS fire at a much slower rate than they do during the waking state. The RAS also mediates transitions from relaxed wakefulness to periods of high attention.

Increased blood flow allows for increased alertness and attention when necessary. However, a general decline of reactivity in the reticular activating system occurs with age. Disruption in the system has been implicated in disorders such as schizophrenia, Parkinson disease, post-traumatic stress disorder, narcolepsy, depression, autism, Alzheimer disease, and many others.

Often, loss of consciousness stems from hypoperfusion to the RAS. A reduction in cerebral blood flow of 35 percent or more results in a loss of consciousness. Mechanisms that can adversely affect the components of perfusion are cardiac output, systemic vascular resistance, and blood volume.

The causes of altered mental status are divided into two major categories: structural and metabolic. *Structural* or *primary lesions* include brain tumor, hemorrhage within the skull but not within the brain, hemorrhage within the brain, hydrocephalus, brain abscess or infection, degenerative brain disease, and direct trauma to the brain. Thus, a structural lesion or insult causes damage to the brain tissue.

A *metabolic* or *secondary lesion* is a result of circulating metabolites or toxins causing a lack of necessary substances in blood, such as glucose and oxygen. These lesions can result from severe hypoxia or anoxia, liver or kidney failure, poisoning or drug overdose, hyper- or hypoglycemia, and even electrolyte imbalance (▶ Figure 17-3). It is imperative that you manage the life-threatening conditions and continue to monitor for further deterioration in patients with altered mental status, regardless of the etiology.

ASSESSMENT FINDINGS

As an Advanced EMT, on dispatch and arrival at the scene you can begin to determine the etiology of an altered mental status. For example, when you arrive on scene and find the patient at the bottom of the basement steps, you can immediately begin to suspect an altered mental status stemming from a traumatic event. Do not develop tunnel vision and discard any other possibilities for the alteration in mental status, however. Remember that it is possible that the

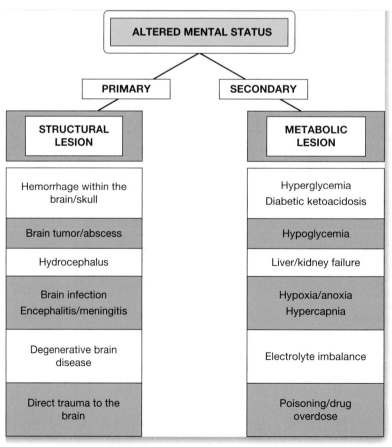

Figure 17-3 Structural and metabolic lesions as causes of altered mental status.

patient had a medical event, such as a syncopal episode, while walking down the stairs. In this case, the altered mental status would be the result of a medical condition masked by a secondary traumatic event.

During your scene size-up, ensure that you assess the scene as thoroughly as you assess your patient. The patient's environment can tell a story to help you determine the cause of altered mental status. Drug paraphernalia, liquor or beer bottles, home oxygen tanks, and even the patient's medications can provide a wealth of knowledge. If the patient's medications are not in plain sight, have a family member, police officer, or emergency medical responder check for them in the kitchen, bathroom, and bedroom. Ensure that they check the refrigerator as well, as some medications, especially insulin, must stay cool. Gather all the medications and keep them with the patient. Further important information can be obtained from these medications and the packaging after you arrive at the emergency department.

The primary assessment, as always, focuses on the ABCs. Provide initial manual spinal stabilization followed by full immobilization if a spinal column or spinal cord injury is suspected or the patient has evidence of trauma and an altered level of consciousness. If a spine injury is suspected, open the airway using a jaw-thrust maneuver; otherwise use a head-tilt, chin-lift technique. Assess the airway to ensure that it is clear of obstruction, and suction as needed. Commonly, unresponsive patients do not have an intact gag reflex, so be certain to maintain an open airway at all times. Use a nasopharyngeal or oropharyngeal airway when necessary.

It is possible that the breathing rate and depth may be inadequate in the patient with altered mental status. Maintain an SpO$_2$ reading above 94 percent to prevent hypoxia and to ensure an adequate supply of oxygen to the brain at all times. If the breathing is inadequate, provide positive pressure ventilation with high-concentration oxygen delivered via the ventilation device. After all, the cause for the altered mental status could be hypoxia resulting from an airway occlusion or respiratory problem.

In your secondary assessment, your partner may obtain the vital signs as you begin to gather further information from the family and bystanders. During your evaluation of the patient's history, you want to ask the following questions:

- What was the patient doing prior to the alteration in mental status?
- Did the patient have any complaints prior to the event? Examples include shortness of breath, chest pain, weakness, dizziness, or numbness.
- Did anything make the symptoms worse or better? Was the onset of the symptoms gradual or sudden?
- How long has the patient had the complaints? When was the patient last known to be well?
- What are the patient's drug allergies?
- What prescription and nonprescription (e.g., acetaminophen) medications is the patient taking? Include dosages and how many times a day the patient is taking them. When able, take the prescription bottles or packaging with you to the emergency department.
- What is the patient's past medical history? Why is the patient taking prescription medications? What physicians has the patient seen in the past?
- When was the patient's last oral intake? What was it? Was alcohol ingested?

It is important to assess the blood glucose level very early in the assessment of a patient with an altered mental status. In addition, if allowed by local protocol, collect a blood sample for evaluation in the laboratory at the hospital, prior to the administration of 50 percent dextrose or glucagon.

On arrival at the emergency department, be sure to accurately relay the information you obtained from your primary and secondary assessments. The emergency department staff relies heavily on your assessment of the patient's last known well. (The patient's last known well is the most exact time family or bystanders witnessed the patient at his normal mentation.) This key piece of information guides the emergency department staff in further treatment and evaluation of the patient. As an AEMT, you are the link between the patient's previous environment and the emergency department; therefore, the staff values your knowledge.

When determining level of consciousness, the Glasgow Coma Scale (GCS) is frequently used (see Table 17-2). GCS is a widely accepted numerical schema for defining the depth of coma. It is an initial evaluation of consciousness but does not

> **Drug paraphernalia, liquor or beer bottles, home oxygen tanks, and even the patient's medications can provide a wealth of knowledge.**

TABLE 17-2	Glasgow Coma Scale	
Area Assessed	**Response**	**Points**
Eye opening	Eyes are open spontaneously	4
	Eye opening in response to verbal stimuli: verbal command, speech, or shout	3
	Eye opening in response to painful stimuli: pain applied to the sternum or extremities	2
	None	1
Verbal response	Oriented	5
	Confused conversation, disoriented	4
	Inappropriate responses to questions, discernable words	3
	Incomprehensible speech	2
	None	1
Motor response	Moves appropriately to command	6
	Responds to pain with purposeful movement	5
	Withdraws from painful stimuli	4
	Responds to pain with abnormal flexion (decorticate posturing)	3
	Responds to pain with abnormal extension (decerebrate posturing)	2
	None	1

aid in diagnosing the cause for altered mental status. When you are evaluating the patient's eye opening, ensure that you are looking at the eyes when approaching the patient. Are the patient's eyes open as you approach (spontaneous), or do they open because the patient heard you approach (verbal stimuli)?

EMERGENCY CARE

Differential diagnosis and primary assessment should occur simultaneously in patients with an altered mental status. Management of airway, breathing, and circulation should occur concurrently with the attainment of a blood glucose level. If trauma is involved, maintenance of spinal immobilization should be done as well. Check the scene for possible clues that might provide the etiology of the altered mental status, such as an empty prescription bottle of benzodiazepines that was filled the previous day. Also assess for a MedicAlert® tag for identifying information. For further emergency care of the patient with an altered mental status, do the following:

- Provide spinal immobilization if you suspect a vertebral or spinal cord injury.
- Maintain a patent airway.
- Suction secretions and potential obstruction from the airway.
- Provide oxygen therapy based on the patient's oxygenation status. If the SpO₂ reading is less than 94 percent, or if signs or symptoms of hypoxia, complaint of dyspnea, or signs of shock or heart failure are present, administer supplemental oxygen.
- Provide positive pressure ventilation if the tidal volume or respiratory rate is inadequate.
- Evaluate and monitor the vital signs.
- Initiate an intravenous line of normal saline at a to-keep-open rate. Draw blood if allowed by your local protocol.
- If the blood glucose reading is less than 60 mg/dL and the patient has signs and symptoms of hypoglycemia (altered mental status is the primary indicator), administer 25 grams of 50 percent dextrose in water. If an intravenous line cannot be established, administer 1 mg of glucagon intramuscularly.
- Position the patient and initiate transport.
- Reassess the patient and the vital signs every 5 minutes.

TRANSITIONING

REVIEW ITEMS

1. The reticular activating system is responsible for _____ .
   a. pupillary reaction
   b. wakefulness
   c. blood pressure
   d. heart rate

2. A unilateral lesion to the reticular activating system will not cause impaired consciousness.
   a. True
   b. False

3. Which of the following can cause an alteration of mental status in the elderly patient?
   a. hypoxia
   b. fever
   c. new medication therapy
   d. low potassium
   e. all of the above

CLINICAL DECISION MAKING

You are dispatched to a local nursing home for an 81-year-old male patient. Staff reports he has had an altered mental status for the past 24 hours and a rectal temperature of 104°F.

1. List 10 questions you would ask the nursing home staff regarding the patient's altered mental status.

2. How would you expect the patient to present? Choose one answer with each system.

Integumentary	Cool	Warm	Hot	Varies
Respiratory	Slow	Normal	Fast	Varies
Cardiovascular	Slow	Normal	Fast	Varies

Your primary assessment reveals the patient to be lethargic; he opens his eyes to a sternal rub and attempts to grab your hand as you rub his

chest. He has a respiratory rate of 28 breaths per minute with adequate chest rise and fall. There is no cyanosis, but the pulse rate is 140 beats per minute. The SpO₂ reading is 97 percent on 4 liters/minute via nasal cannula. The blood glucose level is 92 mg/dL.

3. Whatt are the life threats to this patient?

4. What emergency care would you provide to this patient?

5. What is the patient's Glasgow Coma Scale score?

6. What would you consider to be the cause of the altered mental status in this patient?

7. How frequently would you reassess this patient?

Educational Standard Medicine

Competency Applies fundamental knowledge to provide basic and selected advanced emergency care and transportation based on assessment findings for an acutely ill patient.

TOPIC 18

NEUROLOGY: STROKE

INTRODUCTION

Stroke is an emergency involving the disruption of blood flow through a cerebral vessel within the brain. It may result in significant motor (movement), sensory, or cognitive (thought or perception) dysfunction, or even death. It is also commonly referred to as a "brain attack," as immediate recognition and management can reduce the amount of disability or death associated with stroke. Most recently, stroke is being referred to as an *acute cerebrovascular syndrome*.

EPIDEMIOLOGY

Stroke is the third-leading cause of death in the United States. It is also a major cause of permanent disability and results in billions of dollars in medical costs and lost productivity. According to the American Stroke Association, 700,000 people in the United States suffer a stroke each year, which is approximately one case every 45 seconds. Every 3 minutes, a person will die from a stroke. African Americans and Hispanics/Latinos have a higher risk of suffering a stroke. Women suffer about 40,000 more strokes per year than men.

PATHOPHYSIOLOGY

Often, the signs or symptoms of stroke are subtle and go unrecognized for a period of time by the patient and family. As with a heart attack, though, immediate recognition of the stroke condition and initiation of treatment can reduce the amount of disability and death. There is a very narrow window within which thrombolytic drugs can be used to dissolve a clot and restore circulation to the brain tissue. It is imperative that the responding EMS personnel be completely aware of and able to recognize the signs and symptoms of stroke; gain information regarding the time of onset of the first signs and symptoms from family, relatives, friends, or bystanders at the scene; initiate stroke treatment; begin rapid transport; and accurately report the stroke findings to the receiving medical facility.

Types of Stroke

A *stroke* is defined as acute impairment of neurologic function that results from an interruption of cerebral blood flow to a

TRANSITION *highlights*

- *Overview of the frequency that strokes occur in the United States.*
- *Types and pathophysiology of strokes that occur that inhibit blood flow to distal brain tissue and cause permanent damage:*
  – Ischemic.
  – Embolic.
- *Types of "mini-strokes" that typically do not cause permanent damage:*
  – TIA.
  – RIND.
- *Type of stroke caused by hypoperfusion, rather than occlusion of blood pressure.*
- *Relating the location of the stroke with the cerebral artery.*
- *Incorporating the stroke scale assessment tools into the patient assessment format.*
- *Primary assessment and management principles for a stroke.*

specific area in the brain. The two broad categories of stroke are ischemic and hemorrhagic. *Ischemic strokes* result from the occlusion of a cerebral artery by a blockage or a clot. *Hemorrhagic strokes* occur from a cerebral vessel that ruptures and disrupts the blood flow and allows bleeding in and around the brain (▶ Figure 18-1).

ISCHEMIC STROKE Approximately 80 percent to 85 percent of all strokes are *ischemic strokes*. The primary etiology of these strokes is from blockage of a cerebral artery that obstructs blood flow to an area

There is a very narrow window within which thrombolytic drugs can be used to dissolve a clot and restore circulation to the brain tissue.

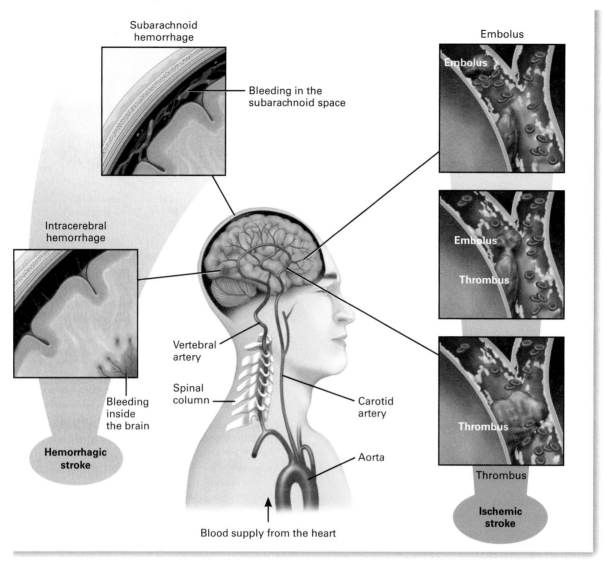

Subarachnoid
hemorrhage

Bleeding in the
subarachnoid space

Intracerebral
hemorrhage

Bleeding
inside
the brain

**Hemorrhagic
stroke**

Vertebral
artery

Spinal
column

Carotid
artery

Aorta

Blood supply from the heart

Embolus

Embolus

Embolus

Thrombus

Thrombus

Thrombus

**Ischemic
stroke**

Figure 18-1 Causes of stroke. Blood is carried from the heart to the brain via the carotid and vertebral arteries, which form a ring and branches within the brain. An *ischemic stroke* occurs when a thrombus is formed on the wall of an artery or when an embolus travels from another area until it lodges in and blocks an arterial branch. A *hemorrhagic stroke* occurs when a cerebral artery ruptures and bleeds into the brain (examples shown: subarachnoid bleeding on the surface of the brain and intracerebral bleeding within the brain).

of the brain. The most common underlying cause of ischemic strokes is atherosclerosis, the process in which fatty deposits collect and line the walls of vessels. This fat will continue to build up inside the vessel wall and may eventually lead to a blockage (thrombus) at the site of the buildup, or a piece of the fatty plaque can break off and travel down the bloodstream (embolus), causing a blockage in a smaller vessel distal to the fatty buildup.

About 60 percent of ischemic strokes are thrombotic.

Ischemic strokes are further classified as thrombotic stroke, embolic stroke, transient ischemic attack (TIA), reversible ischemic neurologic deficit (RIND), and hypoperfusion stroke.

Thrombotic Stroke   A *thrombotic stroke* results from an acute blockage of a cerebral artery at the site of the buildup of fatty deposits, where the internal diameter (lumen) of the vessel is narrowed. This type of clot, a *cerebral thrombosis*, is often referred to as a "stationary clot" because the site of blockage is at the same site at which the clot has formed. About 60 percent of ischemic strokes are thrombotic.

The signs and symptoms of thrombotic stroke may be progressive. As clot formation progresses, blood flow is reduced to areas supplied by the affected cerebral artery, and ischemia to the brain cells worsens, producing signs and symptoms that may gradually develop and progress. During thrombus formation, as the artery narrows, the surrounding smaller cerebral arteries may begin to dilate in an attempt to deliver more blood to the brain tissue distal to the diseased artery. This collateral circulation, which is similar to that found in the coronary vessels in the heart, may reduce the extent of brain tissue ischemia and death following the stroke.

Embolic Stroke *Embolic strokes*, which account for approximately 40 percent of ischemic strokes, result from a *cerebral embolism*, which is a clot or a piece of intravascular material that commonly forms in a proximal artery or in the heart and travels through the cerebral circulation until it becomes lodged. If a piece of material breaks off a thrombus forming in a vessel and begins to travel downstream, it is referred to as a *thromboembolus*. This type of clot is often referred to as a "traveling clot," as it is not formed at the site of blockage.

Embolic strokes may present with more sudden onset of signs and symptoms, as the blockage is a sudden event, and the surrounding cerebral vessels have no chance to dilate and produce a collateral circulation effect. The most common site for thromboembolus formation is in the carotid arteries and in the heart during periods of atrial fibrillation. Atrial fibrillation causes the atria to dilate and blood to stagnate, promoting the formation of clots. An embolism does not have to be a piece of clot or plaque; it can also be an air bubble, tumor tissue, or fat tissue.

Transient Ischemic Attack A *transient ischemic attack* (TIA) is a condition in which the patient suffers a temporary interruption of blood flow to an area of the brain from either an embolism that arises from another proximal vessel and lodges in a cerebral artery or a disruption in a plaque in an area of atherosclerosis in the vessel. The interrupted flow resolves itself after the clot is either dislodged or dissolves. Remember that the entire clotting process is in a constant state of clot formation and lysis.

TIAs produce sudden onset of the signs and symptoms of stroke; however, the signs and symptoms typically last for only a few minutes to, usually, no more than one hour. The signs and symptoms of TIA will resolve within 24 hours following onset. TIAs are often referred to by laypeople as "mini-strokes." It was once thought that no permanent neurologic damage was associated with a TIA; however, more recent evidence indicates that actual brain tissue damage occurs.

In addition to atherosclerosis and emboli, TIAs may also occur as a result of the following:

- Arterial dissection
- Inflammation of the arteries (arteritis)
- Sympathomimetic drugs such as cocaine

TIAs are highly predictive of impending stroke in patients; thus, they are also referred to as "warning strokes." Approximately 30 percent of patients who have TIAs will suffer a stroke in the future. Thus, it is imperative that EMS personnel be aggressive in assessing and managing the patient who has suffered a TIA.

Because the signs and symptoms resolve very quickly, the TIA patient may refuse emergency care and transport. Even though prehospital care for a TIA that has resolved is completely supportive, it is extremely important for Advanced EMTs to educate the patient about the high risk of suffering a true stroke in the near future that may result in permanent disability.

Reversible Ischemic Neurologic Deficit *Reversible ischemic neurologic deficit* (RIND) is very similar to a TIA in etiology. It produces the same signs and symptoms of stroke; however, a RIND typically resolves within 24 to 72 hours after onset. Likewise, RIND is also a significant predictor of an impending stroke.

Hypoperfusion Hypoperfusion may cause a state in which low perfusion causes the brain to receive an inadequate flow of blood through the cerebral arteries. The entire brain becomes ischemic and is subject to brain infarction (death). Unlike thrombotic and embolic stroke, the etiology of a hypoperfusion state is not due to an isolated event of occlusion of a cerebral artery by a thrombus or embolism that produces focal ischemia and brain tissue necrosis. Instead, hypoperfusion states are associated with very poor cerebral blood flow conditions that arise from cardiac arrest, acute myocardial infarction with a decrease in cardiac output from pump dysfunction, and hemodynamically significant cardiac dysrhythmias that create poor perfusion states.

Because hypoperfusion affects the entire brain, the signs and symptoms are typically global in nature and do not result in focal neurologic deficits.

Classification of Ischemic Stroke by Supplying Vessel Ischemic strokes can be further classified by the vessel and the area of the brain supplied by that respective blood vessel. The anterior portion of the brain blood supply originates from the carotid arteries. The anterior circulation is responsible for perfusing about 80 percent of the brain tissue. Occlusion of the carotid artery typically will disrupt blood flow to the cerebral hemispheres. The posterior area of the brain is supplied by the vertebrobasilar artery, which makes up the remaining 20 percent of brain perfusion. An occlusion to the vertebrobasilar artery or its branch will usually involve the brain stem. The presentation of the patient will vary based on which vessel was occluded and what area of the brain becomes ischemic and eventually infarcted.

Pathophysiology of Thrombus Formation in Ischemic Stroke The concept of a ruptured plaque typical of the myocardial infarction patient leading to vessel occlusion is also true of the ischemic stroke; however, the occlusion is occurring in a cerebral vessel instead of a coronary vessel. Fatty deposits inside the cerebral vessel lead to fatty streaks. The fatty streaks promote the formation of an *atheroma* (a buildup of atherosclerotic plaque inside the vessel). The atheroma hardens and causes narrowing of the diseased artery. The atheroma becomes inflamed, and ulceration occurs. The plaque ruptures inside the vessel.

The body views the internal rupture as an injury to the vessel and begins the cascade of physiologic events to clot the injured artery. The chain starts with platelet deposits, which explains why aspirin is commonly used in this condition. This is followed by formal clot formation, which is why early administration of thrombolytic or "clot-busting" agents is effective. This chain of events is actually a protective process to stop a bleeding vessel that ends up occluding the cerebral artery and blocking the blood supply to the distal area of the brain, leading to ischemia and eventually infarction. If the occlusion occurs at the site of the thrombus formation, it becomes a thrombotic stroke.

This process explains the progressive nature of the signs and symptoms seen in thrombotic stroke. A piece of the clot can break off, travel distally in the cerebral artery or a branch until it becomes lodged, and create an embolic stroke.

HEMORRHAGIC STROKE A *hemorrhagic stroke* is caused by a rupture of a cerebral vessel with resultant bleeding into brain tissue or areas surrounding the brain. Approximately 10 percent to 15 percent of all strokes are hemorrhagic in nature. When a vessel ruptures, the blood leaks from the vessel, accumulates in the brain, and causes the brain tissue to become compressed. Brain damage from a ruptured vessel may result from direct trauma to the brain cells, the compression of the brain from increasing intracranial pressure, release of chemical mediators, spasm of local blood vessels, loss of blood flow distal to the ruptured cerebral vessel, and edema formation from the expanding blood and its compressive effects.

Two common causes of a ruptured vessel leading to hemorrhagic stroke are aneurysms and arteriovenous malformations (AVMs). An *aneurysm* is a weakened area in a blood vessel that balloons out. It may continue to weaken and eventually rupture and bleed into the brain or its surrounding tissue.

> **An aneurysm may continue to weaken and eventually rupture and bleed into the brain or its surrounding tissue.**

An *arteriovenous malformation* is an abnormal formation of blood vessels that diverts blood away from the brain tissue and connects the arteries directly to the veins. The abnormal vessels of AVMs are weakened and dilate over a period of time. The vessels are prone to rupture from the high pressure contained within the arteries. AVMs are most often caused by congenital defects and are not easily detected prior to rupture. AVMs may be found within brain tissue or within the subarachnoid space in the meningeal layers above the brain tissue.

Types of Hemorrhagic Stroke   The two major types of hemorrhagic stroke are intracerebral hemorrhage and subarachnoid hemorrhage. An *intracerebral hemorrhage* (ICH) is caused by a cerebral vessel that ruptures and bleeds directly into the brain tissue. The ruptured vessels are usually small arterioles that have been damaged over time by chronic hypertension.

In a *subarachnoid hemorrhage* (SAH), the vessel ruptures into the subarachnoid space located above the actual brain tissue. Aneurysms are more often the cause of SAH, whereas AVMs are less likely the etiology. When an aneurysm ruptures, it bleeds into the subarachnoid space at the systemic arterial pressure. This produces the sudden onset of severe and dramatic signs and symptoms.

ICH is more common than SAH. Both ICH and SAH carry a higher acute mortality rate than does ischemic stroke. Remember that the vast majority of ICH is caused by spontaneous hemorrhage in vessels damaged by chronic hypertension.

Pathophysiology of Neurologic Dysfunction and Damage in Stroke

Brain cells need two critical elements for normal function: oxygen and glucose. Without these two elements, brain cells begin to dysfunction and will eventually die. When an artery becomes occluded from thrombus formation, collateral circulation will assist with the maintenance of blood flow to the areas of the brain distal to the occluded artery. This may prevent a larger area of brain tissue death; however, the area surrounding the dead tissue will continue to receive some blood flow but may become ischemic from a low blood flow state.

When cerebral blood flow to an area of brain tissue drops below its normal level, it may cause the cells to become "electrically silent." The brain cells are still intact and retain the ability to function; however, they cease the transmission of electrical impulses. Thus, the cells are not dead but act as if they are and will not transmit electrical impulses. This causes the patient to present with neurologic deficits such as motor, sensory, or cognitive dysfunction.

If the blood flow is restored to these ischemic cells, they will become electrically active, continue to function, and once again transmit electrical impulses. This may be evident in the patient who initially presents with what seems to be a severe stroke with significant neurologic dysfunction but who then later regains function in many of the previously dysfunctional areas.

If the cerebral blood flow drops drastically, the brain cells begin to fail. Brain cells are particularly vulnerable due to the fact that, unlike many other cells in the body, they do not store glucose and rely completely on glucose delivered via the bloodstream. Calcium levels within the cells and potassium levels outside the cells increase. Because of a reduction of glucose delivery to the cells, the production of energy (adenosine triphosphate [ATP]) is severely depleted. With the loss of ATP, the sodium–potassium pump fails and allows potassium to remain outside the cell, whereas sodium is no longer pumped out of the cell. Because sodium attracts water, the cells begin to swell and will eventually rupture and die. This process is known as *cytoxic edema*.

The area of the brain surrounding the primary stroke site that continues to receive cerebral blood flow from collateral circulation is termed the *ischemic penumbra* or *ischemic shadow*. Because the tissue is receiving a lower cerebral blood flow than normal, the brain cells become "electrically silent." Irreversible brain cell damage in this area has not yet occurred, though, and the function of these brain cells can be reversed. This is the area of brain that can possibly be salvaged and the extent of the brain injury limited. Neuroprotective agents are being researched that can protect the ischemic penumbra and preserve the brain cells.

ASSESSMENT OF THE STROKE PATIENT

Time is paramount in the management of a stroke patient. It may mean the difference between a patient who suffers significant permanent disability and one who recovers completely or with only minor deficits. A very narrow window of 3 to 4.5 hours is available for the administration of thrombolytic drugs that can destroy a clot and restore circulation to the ischemic brain tissue. (Mechanical methods of clot removal may increase this window.) It is imperative that EMS personnel be able to recognize even the most subtle signs and symptoms of stroke so rapid and aggressive stroke treatment can be provided.

Signs and Symptoms of Stroke

The signs and symptoms of stroke may be subtle and unrecognized as significant by the patient, relatives, or bystanders. Simple numbness of the arm may be downplayed as insignificant by the patient for a long period of time until the signs and symptoms progress to a more severe condition. The patient may then seek EMS assistance; however, several hours may have passed, during which the chance for reversal of the stroke may have been eliminated.

It is imperative that in your history taking you attempt to determine the precise time of onset of the first sign or symptom of stroke, no matter how subtle. This is vital information that must be reported to the receiving medical facility. It is often referred to by the American Stroke Association as time "last normal." That is, what was the specific time the patient was last seen as "normal" with no neurologic deficits? This is extremely important information for the AEMT to collect and report to the receiving medical facility.

General signs and symptoms of stroke include the following:

- Facial droop (▶ Figure 18-2)
- Slurred speech
- Difficulty in speaking (dysphasia) or inability to speak (aphasia)
- Numbness to the face, arm, or leg, especially on one side of the body
- Headache (may not be severe in ischemic stroke)

- Weakness (paresis) or paralysis (plegia), especially to one side of the body (hemiparesis and hemiplegia) (▶ Figure 18-3)
- Confusion, agitation, or other severe altered mental status
- Gait disturbance, noted by trouble walking
- Dizziness associated with vomiting
- Loss of balance or coordination

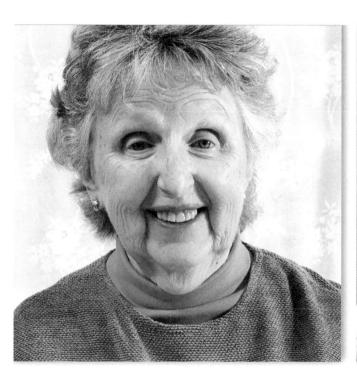
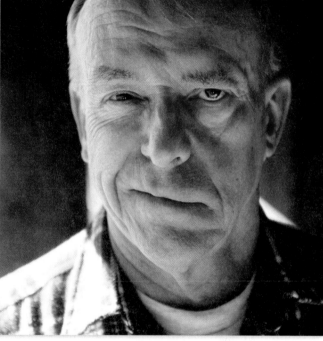

Figure 18-2 (a) The face of a nonstroke patient has normal symmetry. (b) The face of a stroke patient often has an abnormal, drooped appearance on one side. (© Michal Heron)

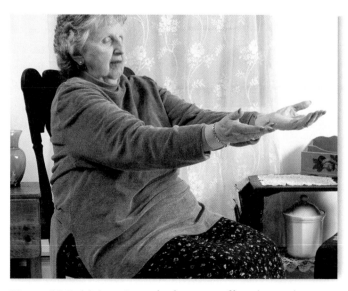
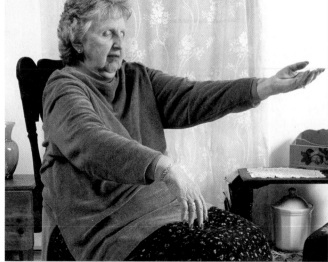

Figure 18-3 (a) A patient who has not suffered a stroke can generally hold the arms in an extended position with eyes closed. (b) A stroke patient will often display "arm drift" or "pronator drift"—one arm will remain extended when held outward with eyes closed, but the other arm will drift or drop downward and pronate (palm turned downward).

Cincinnati Prehospital Stroke Scale

Sign of Stroke	Patient Activity	Interpretation
Facial droop	Have patient look up at you, smile, and show his teeth.	*Normal:* Symmetry to both sides. *Abnormal:* One side of the face droops or does not move symmetrically.
Arm drift	Have patient lift arms up and hold them out with eyes closed for 10 seconds.	*Normal:* Symmetrical movement in both arms. *Abnormal:* One arm drifts down or asymmetrical movement of the arms.
Abnormal speech	Have the patient say,"You can't teach an old dog new tricks."	*Normal:* The correct words are used and no slurring of words is noted. *Abnormal:* The words are slurred, the wrong words are used, or the patient is aphasic.

Kothari R. U., Pancioli A., Liu T., Broderick J. Cincinnati Prehospital Stroke Scale: Reproducibility and validity. *Annals of Emergency Medicine.* 1999; 33:373–378.

Figure 18-4 The Cincinnati Prehospital Stroke Scale (CPSS).

Los Angeles Prehospital Stroke Screen (LAPSS)

Considerations	Yes	Unknown	No
Age **greater than** 45 years			
No history of seizures or epilepsy			
Duration of symptoms is **less** than 24 hours			
Patient is **not** wheelchair bound or bedridden			
Blood glucose level **between 60 and 400 mg/dL**			

Physical exam to determine unilateral asymmetry	Equal	R Weakness	L Weakness
A. Have patient look up, smile, and show teeth		Droop	Droop
B. Compare grip strength of upper extremities		Weak grip	Weak grip
		No grip	No grip
C. Assess arm strength for drift or weakness		Drifts down	Drifts down
		Falls rapidly	Falls rapidly

Kidwell C. S., Saver J. L., Schubert G. B., Eckstein M., Starkman S. Design and retrospective analysis of the Los Angeles Prehospital Stroke Screen (LAPSS). *Prehospital Emergency Care.* 1998;2:267–273.
Kidwell C. S., Starkman S., Eckstein M., Weems K., Saver J. L. Identifying stroke in the field: Prospective validation of the Los Angeles Prehospital Stroke Screen (LAPSS). *Stroke.* 2000; 31:71–76.

Figure 18-5 The Los Angeles Prehospital Stroke Screen (LAPSS).

- Loss of vision or disturbed vision in one or both eyes
- Inability to understand
- Incontinence

Patients who experience an ICH or SAH may present with many of the aforementioned signs and symptoms. However, ICH and SAH patients typically complain of a sudden onset of the "worst headache they have ever experienced" with pain that may radiate to the face and neck. The headache may be accompanied by nausea, vomiting, intolerance to light and noise, and an altered mental status. These signs and symptoms, especially deterioration in the mental status, may continue to progress as the bleeding continues within the brain. Patients with ICH and SAH will typically present with more severe depressed mental status and headache as compared with ischemic stroke patients.

Stroke Assessment Scales

Two common stroke assessment scales with high predictive value used in the prehospital setting are the Cincinnati Prehospital Stroke Scale (CPSS) (▶ Figure 18-4) and the Los Angeles Prehospital Stroke Screen (LAPSS) (▶ Figure 18-5). Either of these scales should be included in your assessment of the stroke patient and reported to the medical facility. A Glasgow Coma Scale score should also be obtained on the suspected stroke patient. It is imperative for EMS personnel to collect and report this information to ensure adequate and aggressive assessment and management of the stroke patient.

EMERGENCY MEDICAL CARE FOR THE STROKE PATIENT

The emergency care provided to a stroke patient is primarily supportive; however, it must be geared to reverse any hypoxemia and hypoperfusion. It is vital to ensure an adequate airway, adequate ventilation, adequate oxygenation, and adequate circulation in the primary assessment. Provide the following emergency care:

- **Airway:** Stroke patients are at an increased risk of loss of airway control and aspiration. Ensure that an adequate airway is established and maintained. To prevent aspiration, place the patient in a lateral recumbent position. If vomiting is severe and the airway is severely compromised, it may be necessary to use an advanced airway device to protect the patient from aspiration.
- **Ventilation:** Assess the tidal volume and rate of ventilation. If either the tidal volume or rate is inadequate, immediately begin ventilation at a rate of 10 to 12 per minute.
- **Oxygenation:** Apply a pulse oximeter to monitor the oxygen saturation levels. If the patient exhibits signs of hypoxia, shock, or heart failure; complains of dyspnea; or has an SpO_2 reading of < 94 percent, or if no SpO_2 reading is available, provide supplemental oxygen via a nasal cannula at 2 to 4 lpm. Titrate the oxygen to the signs and symptoms and SpO_2 reading.

  Be sure to respond immediately to declines in oxygen saturation by reassessing the adequacy of the airway or ventilation, managing the airway or ventilating if necessary, or increasing the oxygen concentration. If the SpO_2 reading continues to decline, does not increase above 94 percent, or the signs of hypoxia are not subsiding, place the patient on a nonrebreather mask at 15 lpm. If the tidal volume or respiratory rate becomes inadequate, immediately begin bag-valve-mask ventilation.

- **Circulation:** Initiate an intravenous line of normal saline. Obtain a blood sample if your protocol allows. Run the IV at a to-keep-open rate. If the systolic blood pressure drops below 90 mmHg, increase the rate of fluid administration. It is important to keep the systolic blood pressure at a level that is normal for the patient, as the brain develops very specific ranges in which it autoregulates cerebral perfusion. Be careful not to provide excessive amounts of fluid. Hypertension in the stroke patient is not treated in the prehospital setting.
- **Blood Glucose Level:** Obtain a blood glucose level (BGL), as hypoglycemia can mimic stroke. If the BGL is < 50 mg/dL, administer 25 grams of 50 percent dextrose in water. *Do not* administer glucose or glucose-containing solutions if the patient has a normal or high BGL reading.
- **Transport:** Protect and rapidly transport an acute stroke patient to the most appropriate medical facility for proper medical management.

TRANSITIONING

REVIEW ITEMS

1. A 58-year-old male patient presents with a sudden onset of left facial droop, slurred speech, and hemiparesis to the left arm. The patient states he has a headache when questioned during the history. You should suspect _____.
   a. an embolic stroke
   b. a subarachnoid hemorrhage
   c. an intracerebral hemorrhage
   d. a reversible ischemic neurologic deficit

2. You are assessing a patient who presents with confusion and is drooling. The family states that she was watching television and began to act confused. Her blood pressure is 298/132 mmHg, radial pulse is 112 bpm, and respirations are 19 with adequate chest rise. The skin is warm and dry to touch. The SpO_2 reads 98 percent on room air. You should _____.
   a. apply a nonrebreather mask at 15 lpm
   b. administer a tube of oral glucose
   c. suction the airway and begin bag-mask ventilation
   d. place the patient in a lateral recumbent position

3. What assessment finding would indicate that the neurons have become "electrically silent" from a decrease in cerebral perfusion and subsequent cerebral ischemia?
   a. an SpO_2 reading that is less than 95 percent
   b. loss of motor and sensory function
   c. an increase in systolic blood pressure
   d. an irregular heart rate

4. One of the most vital pieces of information for EMS to pass on to the receiving facility when managing a suspected ischemic stroke patient is _____.
   a. the last oral intake
   b. the event prior to the stroke
   c. the exact time of onset of signs or symptoms
   d. whether the patient is complaining of a headache

5. An ominous sign that the patient is experiencing a hemorrhagic stroke is _____.

    a. severe systolic hypertension

    b. a continuous deterioration in mental status

    c. an irregular heart rate with a weak radial pulse

    d. facial droop and slurred speech

APPLIED PATHOPHYSIOLOGY

1. List and describe the pathophysiology of the two general types of stroke.

2. Explain how to differentiate between a transient ischemic attack and a thrombotic stroke.

3. Explain why neurons become "electrically silent" and the associated clinical patient presentation.

4. Explain the pathophysiology associated with an acute clot formation within a cerebral artery, leading to an ischemic stroke.

5. Describe what type of stroke would typically cause a presentation in which the patient appears sicker and continues to deteriorate.

CLINICAL DECISION MAKING

You find a 68-year-old female patient who is awake and alert but is not responding appropriately to your questions or commands. Her husband states that the patient was in the kitchen cooking dinner and suddenly began to pour water into the oven. When questioned, she responded inappropriately. She is seated on a chair in the kitchen.

1. Based on the scene size-up, list the possible conditions you should suspect.

The primary assessment reveals that that patient is alert but not responding appropriately to your questions and commands. Her respiratory rate is 16/minute with adequate chest rise. Her radial pulse is irregular, at a rate of 80 bpm. Her skin is warm and dry. Her SpO$_2$ reading is 97 percent on room air.

2. Are there any immediate life threats to the patient?

3. What emergency care would you provide based on the primary assessment?

Following the secondary assessment, you note that the patient's pupils are equal and reactive to light, there is no evidence of trauma to the head, and the oral mucosa is pink and moist. There is no jugular venous distention, the breath sounds are equal and clear bilaterally, and the abdomen is soft. When assessing the extremities, you note that the patient is not moving her left arm or leg. She freely moves the right side of the body. She does not respond appropriately when you attempt to perform a neurologic exam of the extremities.

The blood pressure is 188/108 mmHg, the heart rate is 82/minute, and the respirations are 16/minute with adequate chest rise. The blood glucose is 114 mg/dL. She takes warfarin (Coumadin) and atenolol (Tenormin) and has a history of an "irregular heartbeat," according to her husband. She last ate at lunch, approximately three hours earlier. She has no known allergies.

4. What conditions have you ruled out in your differential diagnosis? Why?

5. What condition do you suspect? Why?

6. Why is the heart rhythm significant in this patient?

7. What further emergency care would you provide?

8. What vital information would you relay to the receiving medical facility?

Educational Standard Medicine

Competency Applies fundamental knowledge to provide basic and selected advanced emergency care and transportation based on assessment findings for an acutely ill patient.

TOPIC

NEUROLOGY: SEIZURES

INTRODUCTION

A seizure is defined as excessive electrical discharges in a group of cells within the cerebral cortex of the brain. A seizure results from an imbalance of excitatory and inhibitory impulses in the cortical neurons. The signs and symptoms of a seizure vary drastically and depend on the location and pattern of those discharges. This can be evidenced by brief episodes of inattention, muscle jerking, involuntary muscle contractions, or convulsions. A convulsion is the most dramatic manifestation of a seizure; however, it is important to understand that it is only one sign, and it does not occur in many types of seizures.

A person's experiencing one seizure does not lead to a diagnosis of epilepsy. Epilepsy is defined as two or more unprovoked seizures that occur 24 hours apart. It is a chronic brain disorder that has caused fear, discrimination, and social stigma for centuries. A comprehensive understanding of the various types of seizures and the respective clinical manifestations is imperative to recognizing a seizure condition and providing appropriate emergency care.

EPIDEMIOLOGY

About 6 percent of the U.S. population will experience one seizure in a lifetime. Epilepsy, on the other hand, plagues approximately 50 million people worldwide, or 7 out of every 1,000 people in the population. Epilepsy affects men slightly more than women, but it involves all ages. Fifty percent of seizures leading to epilepsy begin in childhood or adolescence. The highest incidence overall involves children under 2 years of age and adults older than 65 years of age. Those with a family history also have a higher incidence of the condition.

Thirty percent of those suffering from epilepsy are unable to obtain control of their seizures, even with the best medication available. The goal of treatment is to have no further seizures and no unwanted side effects. Treatment is effective 70 percent of the time in patients who are compliant with their medication therapy.

The risk for premature death of those suffering from epilepsy is increased by 2 to 3 percent compared with the general population. Patients who reach status epilepticus have a 20 percent

TRANSITION *highlights*

- *Frequency, types, and morbidity associated with seizures in the United States.*
- *Etiology of a seizure from a pathophysiologic point of view.*
- *Phases of a seizure (preictal, ictal, postictal).*
- *Types of seizures seen by Advanced EMTs:*
  - Simple and complex partial seizures.
  - Generalized and absence seizures.
  - Tonic and clonic seizures.
  - Myoclonic seizures.
  - Atonic seizures.
  - Status epilepticus.
- *Common antiepileptic drugs taken by patients with seizure disorders.*
- *Assessment findings presented in a way to help isolate the type of seizure the patient is presenting with.*
- *Treatment steps when confronted with a patient having a seizure.*

mortality rate. Patients over 75 years of age have the highest mortality rate because of predisposing factors related to age, such as degenerative disease and vascular pathologies.

PATHOPHYSIOLOGY
Causes of a Seizure

The two general categories of seizures are primary (idiopathic) and secondary (symptomatic). *Primary* or *idiopathic seizures* appear suddenly, without an underlying cause, and typically involve generalized seizures. *Secondary* or *symptomatic seizures* stem from

Epilepsy is defined as two or more unprovoked seizures that occur 24 hours apart.

> **The preictal (aura) phase is short and represents changes in behavior or actions just seconds before the seizure.**

an acquired insult, such as head injury or stroke, or can be an indication of an underlying medical condition. A large number of causes of secondary or symptomatic are seizures (see Table 19-1).

Approximately 5 percent of those diagnosed with trauma, cerebrovascular disease, or infectious brain injuries have symptomatic or secondary seizures. The incidence for posttraumatic seizures is 2 percent for the general population.

Febrile Seizures

A *febrile seizure* is caused by an elevated body temperature that is not associated with a central nervous system infection. These seizures occur during the low seizure threshold in a child's life. They occur most commonly in children aged six months to five years and in males more frequently than in females. An average of 3.5 percent of children will have a febrile seizure by their fifth birthday. Upper respiratory infections, ear infections (otitis media), and viral syndromes all predispose a child to fever.

Simple febrile seizures are generalized, lasting less than 15 minutes, and do not recur in a 24-hour period. Complex febrile seizures are focal, are prolonged, and recur within a 24-hour period. A complex febrile seizure requires prompt emergency care. Prophylactic fever reduction and treatment of the underlying cause of fever can help prevent febrile seizures.

PHASES OF A SEIZURE

Seizures typically present in three phases: preictal, ictal, and postictal. The *preictal (aura) phase* is short and represents changes in behavior or actions just seconds before the seizure. These can be very subtle changes in posture and auditory (hearing), olfactory (smell), or visual disturbances experienced by the patient. The *ictus (ictal) phase* is the actual seizure. Muscle stiffening, contractions, and even convulsions can occur during this phase. Signs and symptoms, as well as length of the ictus, depend on the type of seizure.

TABLE 19-1	Common Causes of Seizures
Brain injuries/diseases	Degenerative tissue disease, cerebrovascular disturbances, stroke, space-occupying lesions, tumors, intracranial hemorrhage
Metabolic causes	Fever, critical variations in blood glucose, electrolytes, or oxygenation levels in the blood, heat stroke
Toxins	Drug abuse, alcohol abuse, poisonous or toxic substance abuse, alcohol withdrawal
Infections	Encephalitis, meningitis, central nervous system infections, infectious brain injury
Posttraumatic head injury	Intracranial hemorrhage, skull fractures, craniotomy, other brain surgeries
Pregnancy	Eclampsia

Immediately following the seizure, the *postictal phase* occurs. The patient may present with lethargy or confusion for a short period of time. In many situations the postictal phase resolves quickly; however, the duration and manifestations may vary from seizure to seizure in the same patient. Strokelike findings may also be seen.

Types of Seizures

There are several types of seizures with differing patient presentations. The two major categories of seizures are *partial* and *generalized*. Partial seizures are further categorized as *simple* and *complex*. The category itself can explain some of the expected signs and symptoms. For example, a partial seizure implies that only one cerebral hemisphere is involved; thus, an awake state is preserved. "Simple" indicates that the patient will be not only awake but also alert and oriented.

PARTIAL SEIZURES

Simple Partial Seizure The abnormal electrical activity of *simple partial seizures* is localized in one area or focus of the cerebral cortex of the brain. Only one cerebral hemisphere is involved, and the ascending reticular activating system is not involved; thus, consciousness is preserved. Each region of the brain is responsible for a specific function; therefore, noting and reporting the specific motor activity and sensory response during a simple partial seizure may assist with the determination of the area of brain affected. These seizures are also referred to as *focal motor* or *Jacksonian motor seizures*. Generally, they last a few seconds to a few minutes.

Complex Partial Seizure A *complex partial or psychomotor seizure* is commonly triggered by agitation in the temporal lobe and is often preceded by an aura and impaired consciousness. Asking the patient if he can remember the seizure event is a common way to evaluate whether consciousness was preserved or not. The patient typically exhibits signs of restlessness and automatisms (involuntary repetitive behaviors such as lip smacking, chewing, finger rolling, fidgeting, or walking).

This type of seizure usually lasts 60 to 90 seconds and is followed by a postictal period of confusion that typically lasts much longer. Generalized weakness and fatigue may last for several days following this type of seizure.

GENERALIZED SEIZURES

Generalized seizures involve six subtypes: absence or petit mal seizures, tonic seizures, clonic seizures, myoclonic seizures, atonic seizures, and tonic–clonic seizures.

Absence Seizure *Absence seizures* (previously called petit mal seizures) are brief episodes of impaired consciousness, typically without a loss of motor function. Neither an aura prior to the seizure nor a period of postictal confusion afterward occurs. These seizures present with a sudden cessation of activity for approximately 5 to 15 seconds in duration. The patient appears to be staring off, blinking, or rolling the eyes, with no vocalization or apparent hearing at the time. The patient then continues on where he previously left off before the seizure, with no aftereffects. This type of seizure occurs more frequently in children and adolescents.

Tonic Seizure In *tonic seizures*, consciousness is usually preserved. Muscle tone is markedly increased, causing stiffening muscle movements. Extension or flexion of the head, neck, trunk, and/or extremities is involved. A precipitating factor leading up to this seizure is drowsiness, typically occurring on falling asleep or awakening. The onset of these seizures is sudden and lasts for around 20 seconds.

Clonic Seizure *Clonus* is defined as rapid alternating patterns of contraction and relaxation of the muscles. Clinical manifestations of a *clonic seizure* include rhythmic motor movements evidenced by muscle jerking. Typically the upper and lower extremities jerk rhythmically and simultaneously, sometimes involving both sides of the body. These seizures may have a focal origin; therefore, they may or may not impair consciousness. Clonic seizures occur in various age groups, including newborns, but are a fairly rare occurrence.

Myoclonic Seizure *Myoclonic seizures* are characterized by a sudden onset of very brief muscle spasms or jerks that last a second or two. They affect the same side of the body at the same time. These seizures may occur once or several times in a short time frame. A typical example is a sudden muscle jerk that wakes a person up while he is falling asleep. Myoclonic seizures occur more often in childhood, can present at any age, and can occur in epileptics or nonepileptics. The frequency of myoclonic seizures is increased by environmental factors such as triggering lights, drugs, alcohol, stress, and fatigue.

Atonic Seizure *Atonic*, literally meaning without tone, is another type of generalized seizure, in which the patient remains conscious but has a sudden cessation of muscle tone. These patients often suddenly fall to the ground. The sudden fall is known as a *body attack* or *drop seizure*. Many patients injure themselves during the seizure and may choose to wear a hel-

met for protection. These seizures, which are very short in duration—typically lasting less than 15 seconds—affect both children and adults.

Generalized Tonic–Clonic Seizure A generalized *tonic–clonic seizure*, previously called a *grand mal seizure*, is the most common type of generalized seizure (▶ Figure 19-1). Because this type of seizure involves a convulsion, it is the one most recognized by Advanced EMTs (AEMTs) and the general public.

The seizure onset involves both cerebral hemispheres and the ascending reticular activating system (ARAS); thus, both sides of the body are involved, and the patient loses consciousness. The patient typically presents with severe muscle rigidity and a loss of consciousness that evolves to a generalized uncontrolled muscular jerking. The tonic phase takes place first, causing severe generalized muscle contraction. When the respiratory muscles of the thorax suddenly contract,

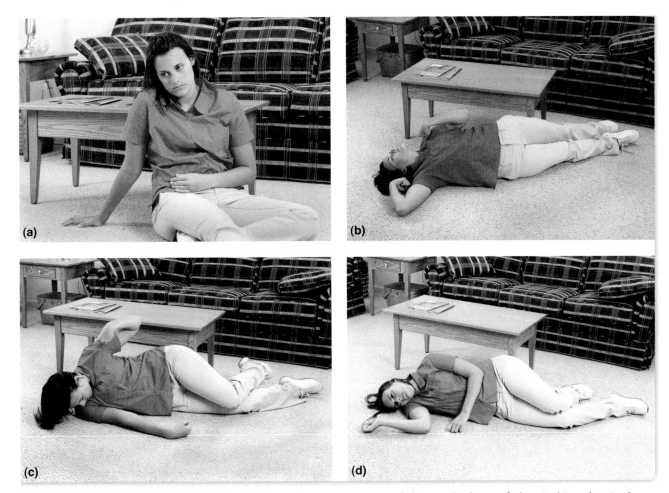

Figure 19-1 A generalized tonic–clonic, or grand mal, seizure is a sign of abnormal release of electrical impulses in the brain: (a) Aura. (b) Loss of consciousness followed by tonic phase. (c) Clonic phase. (d) Postictal phase.

> **It is recommended that status epilepticus be treated aggressively after 5 minutes of continuous seizure activity.**

air is forced through the vocal cords, causing a groan or cry. The patient then loses consciousness, often causing him to fall to the floor.

During the clonic phase, the muscular contraction alternates with relaxation, causing the typical rapid and uncontrolled jerky movement. Patients typically have foamy oral secretions, become tachycardic, have pupil dilation, and undergo bowel and/or bladder incontinence. Commonly, the patient bites the tongue, causing the foamy oral secretions to be tinged with blood.

This type of seizure generally lasts 1 to 3 minutes and is followed by a postictal state that often lasts up to 30 minutes. The postictal state is evidenced by a slow return of consciousness and may be accompanied by drowsiness, agitation, and confusion. The duration for recovery and patient presentation during the postictal state changes from seizure to seizure, not only in different patients but also in the same patient.

Should the patient have two or more seizures without regaining consciousness, or seize for longer than 5 minutes, the patient is classified as being in status epilepticus, a dire emergency.

Status Epilepticus

Status epilepticus occurs in 25 percent of patients diagnosed with epilepsy. Men and women are affected equally by status epilepticus, and it is more prevalent in children and the elderly.

Literally meaning "continuous state of seizure," status epilepticus initiates a catecholamine surge, causing significant physiologic changes in the body. These changes include, but are not limited to, hypertension and tachydysrhythmia (rapid heart rate), as well as increases in temperature, blood glucose levels, and cerebral metabolic demand.

It is recommended that status epilepticus be treated aggressively after 5 minutes of continuous seizure activity. Typically the patient will present with persistent, rhythmic tonic–clonic convulsions with impairment of consciousness. Associated injuries include head and facial trauma,

tongue lacerations, and even shoulder dislocations.

Overall, the mortality rate of status epilepticus is 20 percent, mostly related to the underlying cause of the seizure activity. Elderly patients with ischemic or hypoxic central nervous system injuries experience an even higher mortality rate. Status epilepticus is a life-threatening emergency that requires rapid and aggressive airway and ventilatory management and oxygenation to prevent hypoxemia and subsequent brain injury.

ANTIEPILEPTIC DRUG THERAPY

An average of 7 of every 1,000 people have a continuous issue with seizures requiring treatment. The goal of treatment is to completely eliminate seizures without any unwanted side effects. Broad-spectrum antiepileptic drugs are effective for a wide variety of seizures. On the other hand, narrow-spectrum antiepileptic drugs work specifically for absence, partial, focal, and myoclonic seizures. Medications found at the scene or on the patient's body may cause you to suspect a history of epilepsy or seizure disorder (see Table 19-2).

The narrow therapeutic range associated with these drugs (and their generic equivalents) or a poorly compliant patient may result in breakthrough seizures or unwanted side effects. Antiepileptic drugs are not a cure for epilepsy; they simply suppress seizure activity.

ASSESSMENT FINDINGS

When you arrive on the scene for a seizure patient, assess the environment for drugs, alcohol, and other toxic substances that

may be the cause for the seizure. Ask yourself the following questions:

- Are the patient's medications visible or available for you to examine?
- Is the patient taking any antiepileptic drugs?
- Is the proper amount of medication contained in the bottles?

The environment may help in determining a possible cause of the seizure, including epilepsy or a secondary etiology.

Not all seizures are medical in nature; they can also be secondary to a traumatic event. Assess the scene for a possible mechanism of injury and, during the physical exam, inspect and palpate for evidence of trauma. To help you determine the patient's positioning prior to the seizure, look for items he may have knocked over. As you approach the patient, make certain he is in a location in which you are able to provide care. If necessary, move the patient.

During the primary assessment, focus on airway management, the need for ventilatory support, and oxygenation. Gather information about the seizure from family or bystanders at the scene. The patient may have had a complaint prior to the seizure or might have indicated that he was about to have a seizure. Determine the answer to these questions during the history:

- Was the patient standing, and did the patient then fall to the ground once the seizure started?
- Was the patient's entire body involved or just a specific body part?
- How long did the seizure last? (Remember, though, that time estimates during such events are often inaccurate.)
- How did the patient present immediately following the seizure?

TABLE 19-2	Antiepileptic Drug Therapy
Broad-Spectrum Antiepileptic Drugs	**Narrow-Spectrum Antiepileptic Drugs**
Valproic acid (Depakote, Depakene)	Phenytoin (Dilantin)
Lamotrigine (Lamictal)	Phenobarbital
Levetiracetam (Keppra)	Carbamazepine (Tegretol)
Clonazepam (Clonopin)	Oxcarbazepine (Trileptal)
Topiramate (Topamax)	Gabapentin (Neurontin)
Zonisamide (Zonegran)	Pregabalin (Lyrica)
Diazepam rectal gel (Diastat)	Vigabatrin (Sabril)

TABLE 19-3	Seizure Assessment Findings Based on Seizure Type			
Type of Seizure	Aura	Consciousness	Amnesia	Postictal
Simple partial	Yes	Not affected	No	No
Complex partial	Yes	Impaired	Yes	Yes
Absence/petit mal	No	Impaired	No	No
Tonic	No	Not affected	No	No
Clonic	No	Varies	No	No
Myoclonic	No	Not affected	No	No
Atonic	No	Not affected	No	No
Tonic–clonic	Yes	Impaired	Yes	Yes

Based on the assessment findings, you can attempt to determine the type of seizure the patient may have experienced (see Table 19-3).

EMERGENCY CARE

Emergency care focuses on the airway, breathing, oxygenation, and circulation. Determine whether the patient is still having seizures. Seizure activity may present as tremorlike activity, as the muscles fatigue in a prolonged seizure.

Ensure that no objects nearby may cause further injury to the patient (▶ Figure 19-2). Protect the patient's head until the convulsions subside. Do not attempt to restrain the patient or force an oral airway into the patient's mouth, as you may cause more harm than good. Bite blocks are no longer recommended. If necessary, remove any restrictive clothing or collars. Further emergency care includes the following:

- Establish a patent airway. If you suspect trauma, open the airway using a jaw-thrust maneuver; otherwise use a head-tilt, chin-lift technique.
- Suction the airway until it is clear of any obstruction. Commonly, seizure patients will have foamy oral secretions in the airway. Should you see blood within those secretions, it is likely that the patient bit down on the buccal mucosa or the tongue. Ensure that the airway is clear of these secretions and prevent the risk of aspiration to the patient (▶ Figure 19-3).
- Observe the patient's rate and depth of respirations. If the respiratory effort is adequate, provide supplemental oxygen. Should the patient's respiratory effort be insufficient, such as shallow respirations or bradypnea, support with positive pressure ventilation using a bag-valve mask and high-concentration supplemental oxygen.
- Patients who are grossly cyanotic or have continuous seizures for more than 5 minutes require immediate and aggressive ventilatory support and oxygenation. Ventilate the patient with a bag-valve-mask device with supplemental high-concentration oxygen.
- Check the patient's peripheral and central pulses and perform a skin assessment. A finding of warm moist skin is common; however, hot skin may indicate a febrile seizure. If heat stroke is suspected, cool the patient according to your heat stroke protocol. A febrile etiology of seizure does not require cooling.
- Assess the blood glucose level (BGL). If the BGL is less than 60 mg/dL, initiate an intravenous line, draw blood if allowed by local protocol, and administer 25 grams of 50 percent dextrose in water.
- Seizure activity may precede a cardiac arrest. If this is the case, start immediate compression of the chest.
- The patient's mental status and recovery can vary significantly during the postictal period. Determine whether consciousness was regained between seizures. Recovery may take minutes to hours.
- In the case of a patient who has epilepsy or a recurrent seizure disorder, consult with medical direction to determine whether transport to the emergency department is necessary.
- In cases of status epilepticus, establish an intravenous line of normal

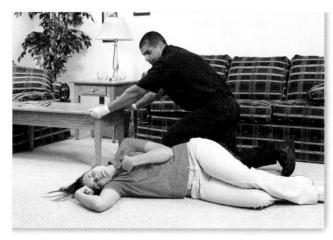

Figure 19-2 Protect the patient from injury by moving furniture and other objects away from the patient.

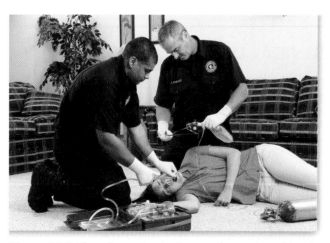

Figure 19-3 Clear the patient's airways of secretions, blood, and vomitus.

saline. Quickly assess the blood glucose level. If the BGL is <60 mg/dL, administer 25 grams of 50 percent dextrose in water. If the patient continues to seize after administration of dextrose or the BGL is >60 mg/dL, administer a benzodiazepine if your protocol allows. Diazepam (Valium) is often used as the first-line intravenous medication at a dose of 5 to 10 mg and can be repeated every 10 minutes up to a total dose of 30 mg. In pediatric patients, it may be administered rectally at 0.3 to 0.5 mg/kg. Acceptable alternative medications are lorazepam (Ativan) at a dose of 0.1 mg/kg or midazolam (Versed) at a dose of 0.2 mg/kg. Some systems may allow the AEMT to administer midazolam via the intranasal route at 0.2 mg/kg.

TRANSITIONING

REVIEW ITEMS

1. A 67-year-old man presents with seizurelike activity. You observe a MedicAlert tag on the patient's neck that indicates "allergy to penicillin, patient is on Coumadin, and patient is a diabetic." Which of the following is most likely the cause of the seizure?
   a. allergic reaction to penicillin
   b. cardiac dysrhythmia
   c. hypoglycemic event
   d. clotting disorder

2. A 14-year-old with a history of a seizure disorder was witnessed to be staring at the ground and blinking frequently for a 10-second period. How would you expect the patient to present immediately after the brief period of abnormal activity?
   a. fully awake and oriented   b. lethargic
   c. unresponsive   d. fully awake but confused

3. You are transporting an unresponsive 27-year-old female patient who experienced a seizure 10 minutes prior to transport. You observe her muscles stiffen and her extremities begin to jerk rhythmically. You would suspect _____.
   a. a recurrent tonic–clonic seizure
   b. an atonic seizure

   c. a petit mal seizure
   d. status epilepticus

4. An unresponsive 7-month-old boy presents with clonic activity, has white froth coming from his mouth, and has hot skin. You would _____.
   a. let the mother hold the child to comfort him
   b. provide high-flow supplemental oxygen via a nonrebreather mask
   c. suction the airway
   d. immobilize the patient

5. What type of seizure would you suspect that the unresponsive 7-month-old is experiencing?
   a. absence   b. febrile
   c. simple partial   d. myoclonic

6. In what phase is the patient aware of an impending seizure?
   a. ictus   b. preictal
   c. tonic   d. postictal

APPLIED PATHOPHYSIOLOGY

1. List 10 possible causes of a seizure.

2. List five examples of antiepileptic drugs. You may use either generic or brand names.

CLINICAL DECISION MAKING

Your EMS unit responds to for a call about a 37-year-old woman having a seizure in a bar. After a 2-minute response time, you and your partner arrive on scene along with the police department. You are taken inside the establishment and find a woman lying supine on the floor next to a barstool, convulsing. Her purse is open on top of the bar, with a bottle of Keppra in sight.

1. What are possible concerns during your scene size-up?

2. What are the possible causes of her seizure?

3. Why is this seizure *probably* medical in nature?

4. Why is this seizure *probably* traumatic in nature?

After another minute, the patient's seizures stop. She is lying supine with foamy, blood-tinged secretions noted in the oral cavity and slow, snoring respirations. You note that the front of her pants is wet and she is not responding to your questions.

5. What are the immediate life threats for this patient?

6. What emergency care should you take immediately, based on your primary assessment?

7. What will you assess for during your secondary assessment?

Standard Medicine

Competency Applies fundamental knowledge to provide basic and selected advanced emergency care and transportation based on assessment findings for an acutely ill patient.

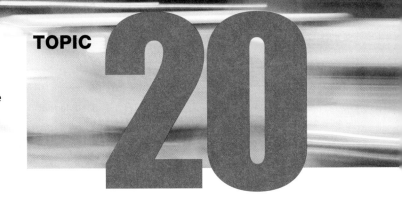

ABDOMINAL EMERGENCIES AND GASTROINTESTINAL BLEEDING

INTRODUCTION

Acute abdominopelvic pain can have any number of causes and may often signal a very serious medical condition. Despite the cause, it is important for you to assess for life-threatening conditions, make the patient as comfortable as possible, administer oxygen, initiate an intravenous line, and transport rapidly.

EPIDEMIOLOGY

Acute abdominal pain is a common condition, accounting for 10 percent of all emergency department visits. Medical texts cite approximately a hundred different causes of abdominal pain. Acute abdominal pain may arise from the cardiac, pulmonary, gastrointestinal, genital, urinary, reproductive, or other body systems. Gastrointestinal bleeding is a condition encountered prehospitally and has an incidence of 100 per 100,000 in the population.

PATHOPHYSIOLOGY

The abdominal cavity contains three types of structures that may contribute to a patient's pain (▶ Figure 20-1).

- **Hollow organs.** The appendix, bladder, common bile duct, fallopian tubes, gallbladder, intestines, stomach, and uterus are all hollow organs located within the abdominal cavity. Each of these organs contains some type of substance that may leak out into the abdominal cavity if it is perforated or injured. This may cause chemical or bacterial peritonitis.
- **Solid organs.** The kidneys, liver, ovaries, pancreas, and spleen are solid abdominal organs. These organs are very vascular and tend to bleed more than hollow organs if they are injured or ruptured. Some of them are covered by a thick fibrous capsule that, when stretched, can cause abdominal pain.
- **Vascular structures.** Portions of the descending aorta and the inferior vena cava are located in the abdominal cavity. Rupture or injury to either vessel will result in major bleeding, rapid blood loss, and death.

TRANSITION highlights

- *Overview of the frequency of abdominal and gastrointestinal bleeding emergencies.*
- *Types of organs present in the abdominal cavity to help illustrate how they may present with pain:*
  - Solid organs.
  - Hollow organs.
  - Vascular organs.
- *Types of pain the patient with an abdominal emergency may be experiencing:*
  - Visceral pain.
  - Parietal pain.
  - Referred pain.
- *How to relate the type of pain with the organ affected:*
  - Distention.
  - Inflammation.
  - Ischemia.
- *Common abdominal emergencies causing pain.*
- *Primary assessment and management principles for a patient experiencing abdominal pain or gastrointestinal bleeding.*

Types of Abdominal Pain

Abdominal pain can be classified as visceral pain, parietal pain, or referred pain.

- *Visceral pain* occurs when the organ itself is involved. Most organs do not have a large number of highly sensitive nerve fibers; therefore, the pain is usually less severe, poorly localized, dull, or aching and may be constant or intermittent. Visceral pain is commonly associated with nausea, vomiting, diaphoresis, and tachycardia. Even if the pain may not appear to be severe, this does not mean that the patient is not suffering from a severe condition.

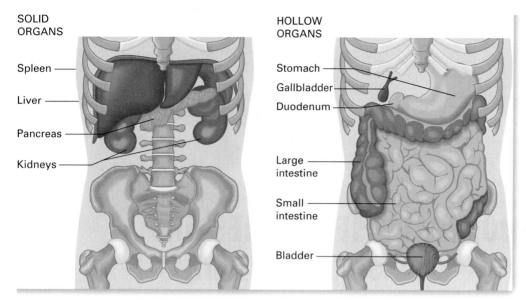

SOLID ORGANS

- Spleen
- Liver
- Pancreas
- Kidneys

HOLLOW ORGANS

- Stomach
- Gallbladder
- Duodenum
- Large intestine
- Small intestine
- Bladder

Figure 20-1 Organs in the abdominal cavity.

walls of the organ, causing a crampy type of pain.

- **Ischemia.** Pain associated with ischemia to an abdominal organ will be steady and severe and will continue to worsen as the organ becomes more hypoxic.

Abdominal pain usually does not create a perception of cutting or tearing, except with certain aortic complications. If an organ is torn, the pain usually results from the blood irritating the peritoneum.

- *Parietal pain*, also called *somatic pain*, is associated with irritation of the peritoneal lining. The peritoneum has a larger amount of highly sensitized nerve endings than abdominal organs do; therefore, the pain is more localized, intense, sharp, and typically constant.
- *Referred pain* is actually visceral pain that is felt elsewhere in the body. It is usually poorly localized but is felt consistently in the part of the body to which it is referred. Referred pain occurs when organs share a nerve pathway with a skin sensory nerve. The brain becomes confused in the interpretation of the impulse and causes the patient to feel pain at a location that may be totally unrelated to the organ involved (▶ Figure 20-2).

Causes of Abdominal Pain

Abdominal pain usually results from one of the following three mechanisms: distention, inflammation, or ischemia.

- **Distention.** If an organ is stretched out or inflated, it can result in pain. If the distention of the organ occurs rapidly, the patient's pain will be acute; if the onset is gradual, the patient may

experience little or no pain. When a solid organ is stretched, it usually results in a steady pain. The peritoneum may also be stretched and result in pain if an organ tugs on it, if there are adhesions from surgery, or if a forceful movement of the small intestine associated with a bowel obstruction occurs. Pregnant women in their third trimester usually do not experience this type of pain because their peritoneum is stretched so far that it is no longer sensitive.

- **Inflammation.** Inflammation of a hollow organ may irritate the lining of the

Conditions Causing Acute Abdominal Pain

The following are some common conditions that may cause abdominal pain. Definitive care for almost all these conditions is hospitalization and, possibly, surgical intervention. It is not necessary to try to isolate the exact cause of the pain or distress in the field; however, it is imperative that you accurately assess and manage your patient with an abdominal emergency.

GASTROINTESTINAL BLEEDING *Gastrointestinal (GI) bleeding* can occur anywhere within the gastrointestinal tract and can be attributed to numerous causes. Most bleeds are classified by their location,

Signs and symptoms of gastrointestinal bleeding vary and may include hematemesis, melena, and hematochezia.

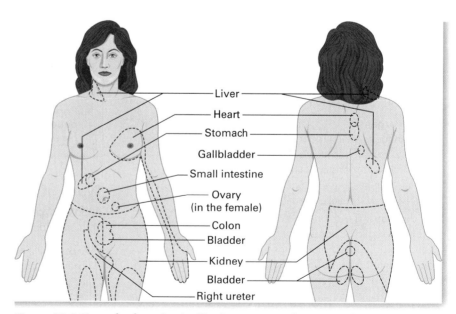

- Liver
- Heart
- Stomach
- Gallbladder
- Small intestine
- Ovary (in the female)
- Colon
- Bladder
- Kidney
- Bladder
- Right ureter

Figure 20-2 Sites of referred pain. The lines point to locations where pain may be felt when there is disease of or injury to the named organ.

in either the upper tract or lower tract. The most common causes of upper GI bleeding are ulcers and esophageal varices. Lower GI bleeds are frequently caused by diverticulosis and tumors. Other conditions that may cause lower GI bleeding are polyps and tumors, hemorrhoids, Crohn disease, arteriovenous malformations, and colitis.

Signs and symptoms of gastrointestinal bleeding vary and may include hematemesis (vomiting blood), melena (dark foul-smelling tarry stools), and hematochezia (bright red blood in the stools). The color of the blood is important to note. If the blood is bright red, it may signify a rapid onset; if it is dark, it can indicate that the blood has been partially decomposed and digested. Abdominal pain, tachycardia, altered mental status, and signs of shock may occur if gastrointestinal bleeding exists.

PERITONITIS Irritation and inflammation of the peritoneum is called *peritonitis*. Peritonitis occurs when blood, pus, bacteria, or chemical substances leak into the peritoneal cavity. The severity of the pain depends on the quantity and type of substance that is leaked. Patients with peritonitis usually resist any movement, as a result of their pain.

APPENDICITIS *Appendicitis* is the inflammation of the appendix. It is usually caused by a blockage in the intestines. Pain is initially felt as poorly localized periumbilical pain that becomes more distinct and localized to the right lower quadrant. Unusual presentations are more common in the young and the elderly. If left untreated, the tissue may die and rupture, which could result in abscess formation, peritonitis, or shock.

PANCREATITIS *Pancreatitis* is the inflammation of the pancreas. It may cause severe pain in the middle of the upper quadrants of the abdomen, which may radiate to the mid- to lower back. Pancreatitis may be triggered by a variety of causes, including ingestion of alcohol, gallstones, or infection. Complications that may result from pancreatitis include abscesses, sepsis, hemorrhage, tissue death, hypoglycemia or hyperglycemia, and organ failure.

CHOLECYSTITIS *Cholecystitis* is the inflammation of the gallbladder. It is commonly associated with the presence of gallstones that may actually block the opening of the gallbladder to the small intestine.

This blockage causes an increase in pressure inside the gallbladder that can cause severe pain and, if left untreated, may cause tissue death, perforation, or pancreatitis.

ESOPHAGEAL VARICES *Esophageal varices* are bulging, engorged, or weakened blood vessels in the lining of the lower part of the esophagus. They are caused by increased pressure in the venous blood supply system of the liver, stomach, and esophagus. The most common cause is chronic heavy alcohol use, although any cause of cirrhosis can also cause varices. Varices are usually identified by painless bleeding that can be profuse, which can make managing a patient's airway and breathing difficult.

GASTROENTERITIS *Gastroenteritis* is the inflammation of the stomach and small intestines. It is commonly associated with a sudden onset of vomiting and diarrhea. Chronic gastroenteritis is most commonly a result of an infection. Acute gastroenteritis is normally caused by a viral or bacterial infection and is commonly diagnosed in children. If left untreated, it may result in the breakdown of the mucosal layers in the gastrointestinal tract and can lead to dehydration, hemorrhage, ulceration, and perforation.

ULCERS *Ulcers* are open wounds or sores within the digestive tract that are associated with a breakdown of the protective lining of the gastrointestinal tract (▶ **Figure 20-3**). The type of abdominal pain associated with an ulcer is affected by its location and severity. Most ulcers are located in the stomach or the beginning of the small intestines. If left untreated, bleeding, peritonitis, perforation, hemorrhage, or shock may occur.

INTESTINAL OBSTRUCTION An *intestinal obstruction* is a blockage that interrupts the normal flow of the intestinal contents within the intestines. Blockages occurring in the small intestines are usually the result of an adhesion or a hernia. Blockages of the large intestines are commonly caused by a tumor, fecal impaction, or volvulus (a twisting of the intestine). If left untreated, intestinal obstruction may lead to sepsis, perforation, infarction, or peritonitis.

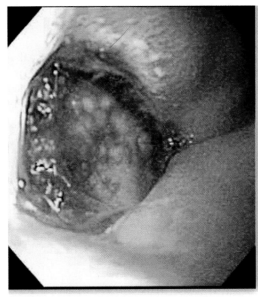

Figure 20-3 Endoscopic view of a duodenal ulcer.

HERNIA A *hernia* is a protrusion or thrusting forward of a portion of the intestine through an opening or weakness in the abdominal wall. Hernias are most commonly associated with increased pressure in the abdominal cavity during heavy lifting or straining, causing the peritoneum to be pushed into the weakness or opening. Most are not life threatening but, if left untreated, may lead to tissue death or perforation.

> If left untreated, intestinal obstruction may lead to sepsis, perforation, infarction, or peritonitis.

ABDOMINAL AORTIC ANEURYSM An *abdominal aortic aneurysm* is a weakened, ballooned, and enlarged area of the wall of the abdominal aorta. Pain from an aneurysm may be felt in the abdomen, back, and groin. The aneurysm may eventually rupture and is one of the most lethal causes of abdominal pain. Death may occur from massive blood loss into the abdominal cavity or retroperitoneum.

VOMITING, DIARRHEA, CONSTIPATION *Vomiting*, *diarrhea*, and *constipation* can all cause abdominal pain. Rarely are they emergencies by themselves; however, if the vomiting has persisted for hours or if diarrhea has persisted for days, the patient may become dehydrated.

Significant fluid loss, electrolyte imbalances, shock, cardiac dysrhythmias, or other conditions may occur if these conditions are left untreated.

ASSESSMENT FINDINGS

All patients with abdominal pain should be considered to have a life-threatening condition until proven otherwise. This is especially true if the pain lasts for six hours or longer, regardless of its intensity. Priority transport should be provided if the patient has a poor general appearance, is unresponsive, or has an altered mental status, severe pain, or signs of shock.

Begin your assessment by securing a safe scene. Face and eye protection should be used if the patient is vomiting. Look for any mechanism of injury to rule out trauma. Note any distinct smells, emesis in wastebaskets or garbage cans, and over-the-counter medications that may have been used to help alleviate the abdominal pain before your arrival.

As you approach the patient, form a general impression. Stabilize the spine if injury is suspected. A person with an acute abdomen generally appears very ill and will assume a guarded position (▶ Figure 20-4). You may find a patient experiencing parietal pain lying supine with the knees flexed up toward the chest. This position limits the stretch of the abdominal muscles and puts less pressure on the peritoneum. The patient in this position is usually very still and breathing shallowly so the diaphragm does not push on the peritoneum and abdominal organs and cause more pain.

Ensure a patent airway and suction if needed. Apply high-concentration oxygen therapy and assist the patient's ventilations if necessary. Assess circulation by checking the pulse for rate and regularity, identifying and controlling major bleeding, and noting skin color, temperature, and condition. Look for signs of shock.

In addition to SAMPLE and OPQRST questions, you should ask whether the patient has a history of abdominal pain, surgeries, appetite changes, nausea or vomiting, color and type of stools or emesis, difficulty urinating, or other any other associated complaints.

The physical exam will focus on the abdomen; however, you should still assess the rest of the body for associated signs and symptoms. Begin by inspecting the abdomen. Palpate each quadrant, beginning with the area of the abdomen that is the least painful and farthest from the site of pain. The abdomen should be soft and nontender. Note any rigidity, guarding, or masses. Obtain and document the patient's baseline vital signs.

Signs and Symptoms

The following signs and symptoms may be associated with acute abdominal pain:

- Pain or tenderness—can be diffuse or localized; crampy, sharp, aching, or knifelike
- Rapid and shallow breathing and tachycardia
- Pulsating masses
- Nausea, vomiting, and/or diarrhea
- Rigid abdomen (involuntary reflex that produces a boardlike abdomen) or guarding (voluntary contraction of the abdominal muscles)
- Distended abdomen
- Fever or chills
- Belching or flatulence
- Changes in bowel habits or urination
- Other signs and symptoms associated with shock

EMERGENCY MEDICAL CARE

The following procedures should be following when caring for a patient with an abdominal emergency:

1. **Keep the airway patent.** Be prepared to suction. Insert an oropharyngeal or nasopharyngeal airway if necessary.

2. **Place the patient in the position of comfort if no spinal injury is suspected.** If the patient is vomiting or has an altered mental status, place him in a lateral recumbent position to protect the airway. If hypovolemic shock is suspected or evident, place the patient in a supine position.

3. **If breathing is adequate, administer oxygen based on the SpO$_2$ reading and patient signs and symptoms.** If the SpO$_2$ reading is greater than 95 percent and no signs or symptoms of hypoxia, shock, or respiratory distress are present, you may choose to apply oxygen via a nasal cannula at 2 to 4 lpm. If signs of hypoxia, shock, or respiratory distress are present, or if the SpO$_2$ reading is less than 95 percent, place the patient on a nonrebreather mask at 15 lpm.

4. **Never give anything by mouth.**

5. **Calm and reassure the patient.** Provide emotional support.

6. **Initiate an intravenous line of normal saline or lactated Ringer's with a large-bore catheter.** Draw blood according to your local protocol. If signs of shock are present or the patient is hypotensive, administer fluid to maintain a radial pulse or the systolic blood pressure above 90 to 100 mmHg. Be sure to monitor the patient's breath sounds for an indication of fluid overload, especially in the

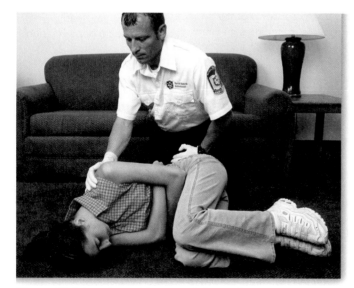

Figure 20-4 A patient with acute abdominal pain may be found in a guarded position.

elderly and those with heart disease. If the patient begins to complain of dyspnea and crackles (rales) are heard in the posterior lower lobes, reduce the amount and rate of fluid being infused.

7. **Initiate a quick and efficient transport.** Perform reassessment during transport. Document and record all vital signs. Communicate all findings to the receiving facility. Reassess the patient every 5 minutes.

TRANSITIONING

REVIEW ITEMS

1. A patient presents with copious amounts of bright red hematemesis. Based on that initial finding, you suspect the patient may have _____.
   a. ruptured esophageal varices
   b. acute appendicitis
   c. cholecystitis
   d. a bowel obstruction

2. Which of the following is a common cause of lower gastrointestinal bleeding?
   a. appendicitis
   b. hepatitis
   c. diverticulosis
   d. pancreatitis

3. Abdominal pain lasting more than _____ hours should be considered an emergency.
   a. 4   b. 6
   c. 8   d. 12

4. Patients complaining of severe abdominal pain are commonly found in what position?
   a. supine
   b. prone
   c. guarded
   d. high Fowler

5. The presence of melena indicates _____.
   a. partially digested blood in the vomit
   b. undigested blood in the vomit
   c. partially digested blood in the stool
   d. undigested blood in the stool

APPLIED PATHOPHYSIOLOGY

1. List the three primary causes of visceral pain.

2. Explain the difference between visceral and somatic pain.

3. Explain why referred pain is felt in other areas of the body.

4. Explain why palpation of the most painful abdominal quadrant should be performed last.

5. List five illnesses that can cause a patient to present with gastrointestinal bleeding.

CLINICAL DECISION MAKING

You are dispatched to the residence of a 33-year-old female patient complaining of abdominal pain. On arrival, you ensure that the scene is safe. You are escorted into the residence by a teenage boy who identifies himself as the patient's son. As you approach the patient, you notice that she appears to be in severe pain and is lying in a fetal position on the living room floor. She has a wastebasket on the floor next to her with greenish-colored vomit in it.

1. Based on the scene size-up characteristics, list the possible conditions you suspect the patient is experiencing.

The primary assessment reveals that the patient is anxious, alert, and disoriented, and she is complaining that her stomach hurts; she denies any trauma. She is breathing adequately with a respiratory rate of 20/minute. Her heart rate is 114 beats/minute, and her radial pulses are rapid and strong. Her skin is pale, cool, and diaphoretic. The SpO_2 reading is 94 percent.

2. What are the life threats to this patient?

3. What immediate emergency care should you provide based on the primary assessment?

4. What conditions have you ruled out from your initial consideration in the scene size-up?

5. What conditions are you still considering as the possible cause?

During the secondary assessment, your patient states that she has been in pain for the past three hours. She says the pain, which is severe and colicky, began about 30 minutes after eating spicy fajitas at a Mexican restaurant. She states that she is nauseated and vomited three times after she took Tums and Pepto-Bismol. She denies any allergies, past medical problems, or taking any other medications. Her abdomen is soft, and tenderness is noted to the upper right side and under the right costal margin. Her pelvis is stable, and no deformities or trauma are evident. Her blood pressure is 106/68 mmHg.

6. What conditions have you ruled out in your differential field diagnosis? Why?

7. What conditions are you considering as a probable cause? Why?

8. Based on your differential diagnosis, what are the next steps in emergency care? Why?

9. Explain how you came to a differential field diagnosis based on specific history and physical assessment findings.

Standard Medicine

Competency Applies fundamental knowledge to provide basic and selected advanced emergency care and transportation based on assessment findings for an acutely ill patient.

TOPIC

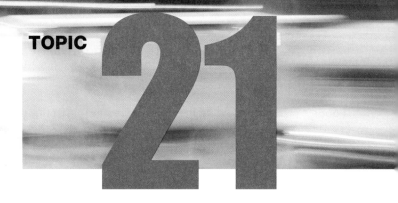

IMMUNOLOGY: ANAPHYLACTIC AND ANAPHYLACTOID REACTIONS

INTRODUCTION

An *allergic reaction* is an immunologic or nonimmunologic response to an allergen or antigen resulting in the release of chemical mediators from specific cells within the body. Allergic reactions can occur on a continuum from mild to severe. Anaphylaxis, in the simplest sense, is an allergic reaction on the severe end of the continuum. However, it is important to understand that the condition of anaphylaxis can present with a multitude of clinical manifestations. Thus, anaphylaxis itself has its own continuum of criticality, from mild to severe, which is not well agreed on in the medical literature.

EPIDEMIOLOGY

Anaphylaxis is not a reportable disease; therefore, the morbidity and mortality rates are not well established. Studies suggest that the lifetime risk of an individual experiencing an anaphylactic reaction is between 1 percent and 3 percent, with a mortality rate of 1 percent. It is estimated that 20,000 to 50,000 persons suffer an anaphylactic reaction in the United States each year. The incidence rate has been reported to be increasing, especially in individuals under 20 years of age.

Penicillin (0.7% to 10%), insect stings (0.5% to 5%), radiocontrast media (0.22% to 1%), and food (0.0004%) remain the most common triggers. Food is the most common trigger in children, adolescents, and young adults, whereas medications, insect venom, and idiopathic (unknown) causes are more often seen in middle-aged and older individuals.

PATHOPHYSIOLOGY

Classically, *anaphylaxis* can be best defined as a systemic, misdirected, immune-mediated hypersensitivity reaction resulting in the release of chemical mediators from mast cells and basophils, affecting multiple organ systems. Historically, anaphylaxis was thought to occur only in patients who were previously sensitized and subsequently reexposed to an allergen.

TRANSITION *highlights*

- *Overview of the frequency of immunologic emergencies to include frequency, types, and death rates.*

- *Pathology underlying important types of immunologic emergencies:*
  - *Anaphylactic reaction.*
  - *Anaphylactoid reaction.*
  - *Vascular organs.*

- *Chemical mediators that result in detrimental changes to body physiology during anaphylactic and anaphylactoid reactions:*
  - *Increased capillary permeability.*
  - *Decreased vascular smooth muscle tone.*
  - *Increased bronchial smooth muscle tone.*
  - *Enhanced mucus secretion in the respiratory tree.*

- *Illustration of the relationship between pathophysiologic changes by body system and the types of signs or symptoms that would be present.*

- *Review of how to distinguish between a mild and severe anaphylactic or anaphylactoid reaction.*

- *Why epinephrine is the drug of choice with a moderate to severe anaphylactic or anaphylactoid reaction.*

Anaphylactic Reaction

In an anaphylactic reaction, the patient must be sensitized. Sensitization occurs when an antigen is introduced into the body and viewed as a foreign substance. Antigens may include venom, foods, pollen, medications, latex, and other substances (see Table 21-1). The body responds by producing antibodies, specifically immunoglobulin E (IgE), to fight off the antigen.

TABLE 21-1 Common Causes of Anaphylactic Reactions

Venom	Wasps, hornets, yellow jackets, fire ants, deer flies, gnats, horseflies, mosquitoes, cockroaches, miller moths, snakes, spiders
Foods	Peanuts, Brazil nuts, macadamia nuts, other nuts, milk, eggs, shellfish, white fish, food additives, chocolate, cottonseed oil, berries
Pollen	Plants, ragweed, grass
Medications	Antibiotics, local anesthetics, vitamins, seizure medication, muscle relaxants, insulin, tetanus and diphtheria toxoids
Other substances	Latex, glue

The IgE antibodies attach to mast cells, which are found in connective tissue, and basophils, which are immature mast cells found circulating in the blood. These antibodies could remain attached to the mast cells and basophils for seconds, minutes, days, weeks, months, or years.

As long as the antibodies remain attached, the patient is considered to be sensitized and primed for an allergic reaction if the antigen is reintroduced in the body. On reexposure, the antigen physically attaches itself to the antibodies on the mast cells and basophils and creates a condition that is often referred to as the classic antigen–antibody induced reaction. This reaction causes the mast cells and basophils to degranulate (break down), releasing chemical mediators (substances) into the interstitial fluid surrounding the cells.

Common chemical mediators that are released are histamine, leukotriene, prostaglandin, and tryptase. These mediators are absorbed by capillaries, enter the blood, and begin to circulate throughout the body, producing systemic multiorgan effects. Thus, for this type of classic anaphylactic reaction to occur, the patient must have been exposed to the antigen previously, antibodies must have been produced, and the antibodies must attach to the mast cells and basophils and remain attached. On reexposure to the antigen, the antigen must attach to the antibodies, the mast cells and basophils must break down, and chemical mediators must be released.

> **The anaphylactoid reaction presents with the same pathologic conditions and signs and symptoms as the classic anaphylactic reaction.**

For the patient to experience the systemic and multiple-organ pathologic response and exhibit the typical signs and symptoms, a large enough quantity of mediators must be released from the mast cells and basophils. If the reaction remains localized or only a small amount of mediators are released, the patient may present with minor signs and symptoms. Likewise, if the organs and vascular structures do not respond to the chemical mediators, the signs and symptoms will not likely be significant.

Anaphylactoid Reaction

Previously, EMS education materials addressed only the classic type of anaphylactic reaction. Thus, when EMS providers arrived on scene to treat a patient suspected of having an anaphylactic reaction, the history gathering focused on an attempt to identify what the potential antigen was and when the reexposure occurred. If the patient presented with signs and symptoms of a classic anaphylactic reaction but had never been exposed previously to the substance that was thought to be the antigen, the question arose as to whether the patient was truly experiencing an anaphylactic reaction.

Consider this example: A patient has received a prescription for a narcotic to treat pain. He has never taken any narcotic in any form. After taking the narcotic for the first time, he develops typical signs and symptoms of an anaphylactic reaction. Based on the classic antigen–antibody reaction, he could not be experiencing a true anaphylactic reaction because he never took the narcotic previously, and his body would not have produced the antibodies to fight off the introduced antigen (narcotic). He would not be sensitized, and no antibodies

would be attached to the mast cells and basophils to initiate the reaction.

Such a situation could cause conflicting and confusing information for the EMS provider, and in some cases treatment might be altered or withheld because of the lack of evidence of sensitization and reexposure. In this example, the patient was experiencing what is known as an *anaphylactoid reaction*. The patient undergoes basically the same pathologic processes and exhibits the same signs and symptoms of the classic anaphylactic reaction.

The anaphylactoid reaction is not the typical immunologic antigen–antibody reaction, however. The anaphylactoid substance that the patient ingests, injects, absorbs, or inhales causes the mast cells and basophils to break down and release chemical mediators. Because the anaphylactoid substances are "direct" chemical mediator-releasing agents, antibodies do not have to be produced or attached to mast cells and basophils, the patient does not have to be sensitized, and reexposure to the substance does not have to occur (see Table 21-2).

The first-time exposure may cause a direct release of a mass of chemical mediators and create a life-threatening condition, with signs and symptoms that appear to be a full-blown anaphylactic reaction. Thus, even though the patient in our example has never ingested a narcotic before in his life, this first-time ingestion has stimulated the direct release of chemical mediators and produced a life-threatening anaphylactoid reaction.

The anaphylactoid reaction presents with the same pathologic conditions and signs and symptoms as the classic anaphylactic reaction. Thus, other than history of exposure and the underlying mechanism, the conditions are indistinguishable and are treated exactly the same.

TABLE 21-2 Common Causes of Anaphylactoid Reactions

Radiopaque contrast media
Nonsteroidal antiinflammatory drugs (NSAIDs)
Aspirin
Opiates
Thiamine

EFFECTS OF CHEMICAL MEDIATORS

The antigen or substance triggering the anaphylactic reaction itself is harmless and does not have any real effect on the tissues or organs; however, it does cause the release of chemical mediators from mast cells and basophils. Histamine, the primary chemical mediator, along with leukotriene, prostaglandin, and tryptase, is released when the mast cell or basophil membrane breaks down in response to the antigen in an anaphylactic (or direct chemical-releasing substance in an anaphylactoid) reaction. The chemical mediators circulate and produce the abnormal cell, tissue, organ, and organ system response.

Almost all fatal episodes, signs displayed, and symptoms experienced by the patient experiencing an anaphylactoid reaction are related to one of the following more common effects of the chemical mediators (▶ Figure 21-1):

- Increased capillary permeability
- Decreased vascular smooth muscle tone (vasodilation)
- Increased bronchial smooth muscle tone (bronchoconstriction)
- Increased mucus secretion in the tracheobronchial tract

Increased Capillary Permeability

An increase in capillary permeability allows fluid to leak from the capillary bed and collect in the interstitial space around the cells. This is commonly seen as edema in the patient. Often the edema is noted around the face, tongue, and neck because of the large number of vessels in that area of the body, and in the hands, feet, and ankles, caused by gravity pulling the fluid downward (▶ Figure 21-2).

The increased capillary permeability in the mucous membranes can lead to edema in the airway structures, including the oropharynx, hypopharynx, larynx, and tracheobronchial tract. The swelling occurs inward, reducing the internal diameter of the airway structures; this leads to an increase in resistance to airflow, making it difficult for the patient to move air into and out of the lungs. The swelling could lead to complete airway closure, a common cause of death in severe allergic reactions.

The fluid loss creates a decrease in plasma volume, thereby reducing the overall blood volume in the vascular space. This loss could produce hypotension from a decrease in cardiac preload, leading to poor perfusion. When hypotension and poor perfusion are present, the patient is categorized as being in *anaphylactic shock*.

Decreased Vascular Smooth Muscle Tone (Vasodilation)

A decrease in vascular smooth muscle tone causes vessels to dilate. This creates an increase in the internal diameter of the vessel. When the vessel size increases, the resistance to blood flow inside the vessel decreases. A decrease in vascular resistance leads to a decrease in blood pressure, which may result in poor perfusion. As the vessel dilates, more blood volume is needed to fill the vascular space. If the space is not filled, the pressure inside drops, leading to hypotension. In anaphylaxis, both vasodilation and fluid loss from an increase in capillary permeability can produce severe hypotension and extremely poor tissue and organ perfusion.

ANAPHYLAXIS
Life-threatening responses to release of chemical mediators

Bronchoconstriction
Normal bronchiole   Constricted bronchiole

Capillary permeability
H_2O H_2O H_2O
Normal bronchiole   Edema of the bronchiole
Normal upper airway   Edema of the upper airway

Vasodilation
Normal vessel   Dilated vessel

Acute respiratory compromise
Occluded upper airway
Labored respirations

Acute circulatory compromise
Falling blood pressure
Weak pulse
Poor tissue perfusion

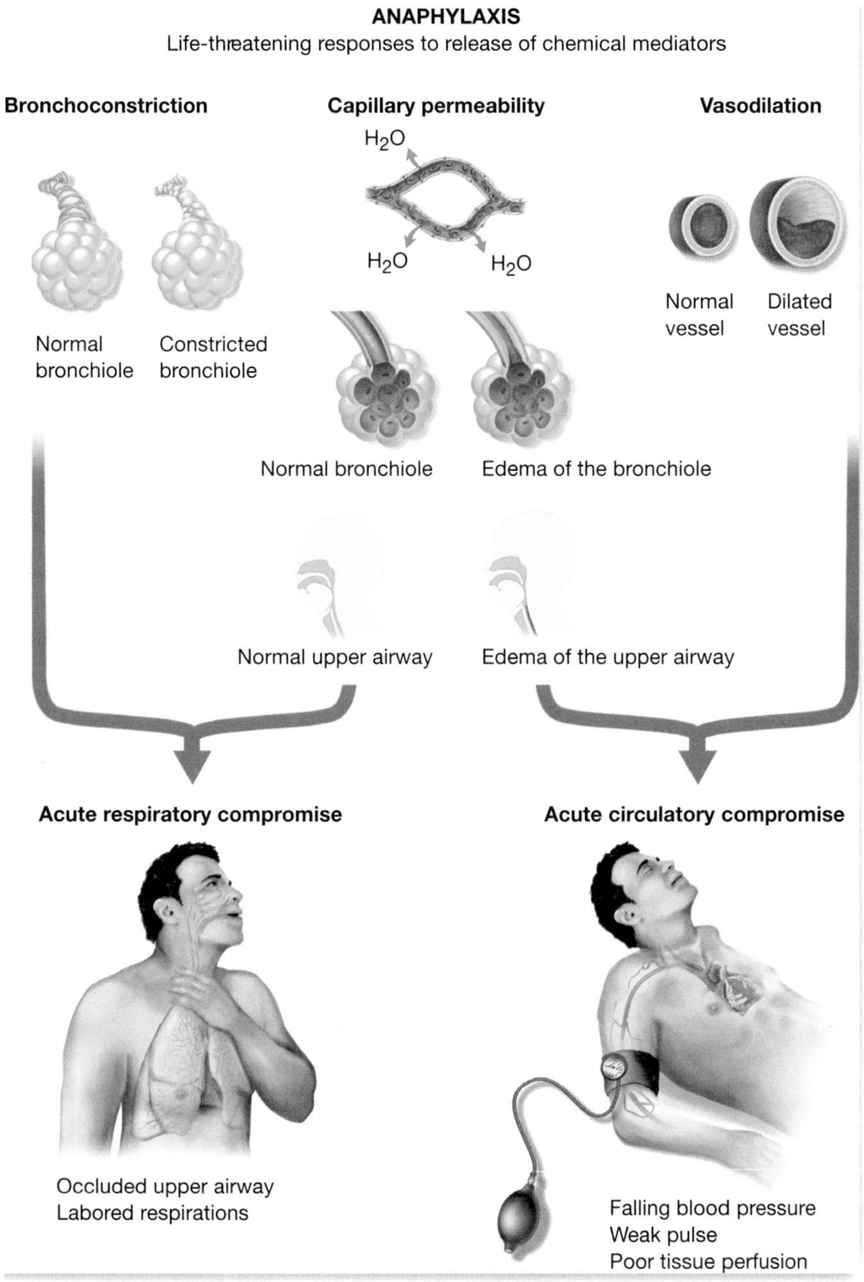

Figure 21-1 Life-threatening responses in anaphylactic reaction: bronchoconstriction, capillary permeability, vasodilation, and an increase in mucus production.

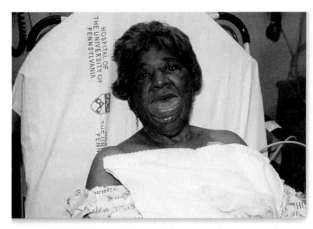

Figure 21-2 Localized angioedema to the tongue from an anaphylactic reaction. (© *Edward T. Dickinson, MD*)

Increased Bronchial Smooth Muscle Tone (Bronchoconstriction)

The chemical mediators may cause the bronchial smooth muscle to constrict, leading to an increase in airway pressure. The higher airway pressure makes it more difficult for the patient to move air into and out of the alveoli. The lower airway could be further narrowed by swollen mucous membranes from an increase in capillary permeability. This may cause a reduction in the amount of air moved into and out of the lungs (tidal volume) and alveoli (alveolar ventilation), leading to severe hypoxia and the retention of carbon dioxide.

Patients with bronchoconstriction will likely present with wheezing and signs of respiratory distress. Signs of hypoxia, such as a poor SpO$_2$ reading and anxiety, may also be present.

Increased Mucus Secretion in the Tracheobronchial Tract

An increase in mucus secretion can lead to plugging of the smaller airways. The mucus is thick and sticky and difficult for the patient to expectorate. The patient often presents with an unproductive cough that is an attempt to expel the mucus.

These pathophysiologic responses related to chemical mediator effects on cells, tissue, organs, and organ systems produce the signs and symptoms seen in the patient. Hemodynamic instability and airway and ventilatory compromise are also a result of the mediators. If the chemical mediator effects can be reversed, the signs, symptoms, airway and ventilatory compromise, and hemodynamic instability will be eliminated. Thus, emergency care is geared toward reversing the pathophysiologic effects of the chemical mediators.

ASSESSMENT FINDINGS

During the scene size-up, you may find evidence of the actual antigen or direct chemical mediator-releasing substance or route of introduction into the body. As with poisoning, the route may include injection, ingestion, inhalation, or absorption. Injection is the route most often associated with anaphylactic reactions.

Fatal episodes of anaphylaxis are associated with airway occlusion, respiratory failure, severe hypoxia, and circulatory collapse. Thus, it is imperative to pay particular attention to the airway, ventilation, oxygenation, and circulatory status during the primary assessment. It may be necessary to be very aggressive with airway management if stridor or other evidence of airway occlusion is present.

Carefully assess for an adequate tidal volume and respiratory rate. If either respiratory rate or tidal volume is inadequate, immediately initiate positive pressure ventilation. In the spontaneously breathing patient, deliver a high concentration of oxygenation via a nonrebreather mask, or deliver it via the ventilation device in a patient with inadequate breathing.

Assess the circulatory status by checking peripheral and central pulses and skin color, temperature, and condition. Weak or absent peripheral pulses are an indication of poor perfusion. Warm, flushed skin is an indication of vasodilation, whereas edema and urticaria (hives; ▶ Figure 21-3) indicate an increase in capillary permeability. Both contribute to hypotension and poor perfusion.

When gathering a history, in addition to the standard information collected, be sure to inquire about the following:

- Are the signs and symptoms getting worse?
- Does the patient have a history of allergic reaction or anaphylaxis? If so, how severe was the reaction? Was the patient hospitalized?
- Has the patient ever been exposed to the suspected triggering substance previously?
- Has the patient taken any medications in an attempt to relieve the signs and symptoms?
- How quick was the onset of the signs and symptoms?

The signs and symptoms of the reaction typically involve the skin, respiratory tract, cardiovascular system, gastrointestinal system, central nervous system, and genitourinary system. Common signs and symptoms of anaphylactic reactions by body system are listed in Table 21-3.

> **Patients with bronchoconstriction will likely present with wheezing and signs of respiratory distress.**

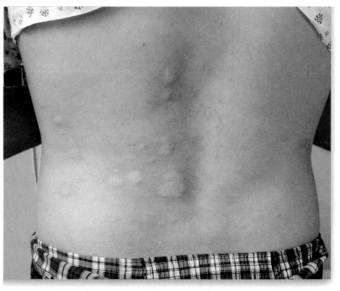

Figure 21-3 Urticaria (hives) from an allergic reaction to a penicillin-derivative drug. (© *Charles Stewart, MD & Associates*)

TABLE 21-3   Common Signs and Symptoms of Anaphylactic Reactions

Sign or System	Pathophysiology
Integumentary System (Skin)	
Warm, tingling feeling in the face, mouth, chest, feet, and hands	Vasodilation and increased capillary permeability
Intense itching (pruritis), especially of the hands and feet	Increased capillary permeability
Urticaria (hives)	Increased capillary permeability
Flushed or red skin	Vasodilation causing blood to pool in peripheral vessels
Swelling of the face, lips, neck, hands, feet, and tongue	Increased capillary permeability causing fluid to leak into interstitial spaces
Cyanosis	Bronchoconstriction and increased capillary permeability reducing alveolar ventilation and gas exchange
Respiratory System	
Complaint of "lump," "tightness," or obstructed feeling in throat	Increased capillary permeability causing swelling of laryngeal tissue
Cough	Increased mucus production producing a cough in an attempt to expel mucus
Tachypnea	Bronchoconstriction and increased capillary permeability recucing alveolar oxygenation
Labored breathing and other evidence of respiratory distress or failure	Bronchoconstriction and increased capillary permeability reducing alveolar oxygenation
Wheezing	Bronchoconstriction and increased capillary permeability narrowing the internal diameter of the bronchiole
Stridor	Increased capillary permeability causing swelling of the laryngeal tissue
Hoarseness or inability to talk	Increased capillary permeability causing swelling of the laryngeal tissue
Difficulty in breathing	Bronchoconstriction and increased capillary permeability reducing alveolar oxygenation
Cardiovascular System	
Tachycardia	Increased capillary permeability, vasodilation, and hypoxia from bronchoconstriction
Hypotension	Increased capillary permeability and vasodilation
Absent or weak peripheral pulses	Increased capillary permeability and vasodilation
Central Nervous System	
Increased anxiety and restlessness	Hypoxia associated with bronchoconstriction and hypotension from increased capillary permeability and vasodilation
Confusion to unresponsiveness	Hypercarbia associated with bronchoconstriction
Lightheadedness	Hypoxia associated with bronchoconstriction and hypotension from increased capillary permeability and vasodilation
Headache	Vasodilation
Seizure	Hypoxia associated with bronchoconstriction and hypotension from increased capillary permeability and vasodilation
Gastrointestinal System	
Nausea and vomiting	Increased capillary permeability and smooth muscle contraction
Diarrhea	Increased capillary permeability
Abdominal cramping	Increase in smooth muscle contraction
Difficulty in swallowing	Increase in smooth muscle contraction and increase in capillary permeability, causing swelling of the opening to the esophagus
Genitourinary System	
Urgent need to urinate	Increase in smooth muscle contraction
Uterine cramping	Increase in smooth muscle contraction
Generalized Signs and Symptoms	
Itchy, watery, red eyes	Increased capillary permeability
Runny and stuffy nose	Increased capillary permeability and vasodilation

When assessing the vital signs, the respiratory rate is likely to be elevated with evidence of respiratory distress. As the condition progresses and the patient tires, the respiratory distress may deteriorate to respiratory failure. The respiratory rate may begin to decrease as the patient continues to fail. Tachycardia is typical with weak pulses. In severe cases, the peripheral pulses may be absent. Unlike other types of shock, the skin is red, warm, and dry with urticaria (hives) and pruritus (itching). Hypotension is common in a severe reaction.

The following are other notable characteristics associated with assessment:

- Parenteral (injection) introduction of the antigen or direct chemical-releasing substance typically produces the most severe reactions.
- The faster the onset of signs and symptoms, the more severe the reaction. Most reactions occur within minutes; however, reactions usually occur within 30 minutes. In rare occasions, the reaction may take hours to days to occur.
- Signs and symptoms often peak within 15 to 30 minutes.
- Skin and respiratory signs and symptoms are the most common and earliest to appear.
- Mild signs and symptoms could progress to a severe reaction within minutes and without warning.

- Most fatalities occur within 30 minutes of exposure.
- A biphasic or multiphasic reaction may occur. The patient may respond effectively to the emergency care and appear to be recovering when the signs and symptoms of the reaction recur.

EMERGENCY MEDICAL CARE

One of the initial keys to emergency care is to recognize whether the reaction is mild, moderate, or severe (see Table 21-4).

A mild reaction typically requires only minimal care—most often, only oxygen administration—and close reassessment for deterioration to a moderate to severe reaction. Patients experiencing a moderate to severe reaction require much more aggressive emergency medical care. The emergency care should include the following:

- Establish and maintain a patent airway. Hyperextend the neck and provide a jaw thrust or chin lift to establish an airway. Early signs indicating that the patient might require aggressive airway management, including insertion of an advanced airway device, are hoarseness, edema to the oropharynx, stridor, and edema to the tongue (lingual edema).

- Suction secretions.
- Administer a high concentration of oxygen via a nonrebreather mask to the patient with an adequate tidal volume and respiratory rate. Titrate the oxygen to maintain an SpO_2 reading of greater than 94 percent. If the tidal volume or respiratory rate is inadequate, immediately initiate positive pressure ventilation with a bag-valve-mask device while maximizing supplemental oxygen administration. It may be difficult to ventilate the patient because of the high airway resistance created by the upper and lower airway edema and bronchoconstriction.

- Initiate an intravenous infusion of normal saline or lactated Ringer's with a large-bore (14- to 16-gauge) catheter in a large vein. Infuse the fluid wide open until a minimum systolic blood pressure of 90 mmHg is obtained. Maintain the systolic blood pressure above 90 mmHg. This may require the infusion of large amounts of fluid; therefore, a second intravenous line may be required.

- Epinephrine should be administered to patients with an anaphylactic reaction who present with systemic signs and symptoms, especially those with hypotension, poor perfusion, airway swelling, or difficulty in breathing. Administer epinephrine

TABLE 21-4	Differentiating Between a Mild and a Moderate to Severe Reaction	
Sign or Symptom	**Mild Reaction**	**Moderate to Severe Reaction**
Pruritus (itching)	Present	Present and usually widespread
Urticaria (hives)	Present, localized	Present and usually widespread
Flushed skin	If present, localized	Widespread
Cyanosis	Not present	Present around lips, oral mucosa, and nail beds
Edema	Present but mild to moderate	Severe in face, lips, tongue, neck, and distal extremities
Heart rate	Normal to slight tachycardia	Moderate to severe tachycardia
Blood pressure	Normal	Moderately to severely decreased with signs of poor perfusion
Peripheral pulses	Present and normal amplitude	Weak or absent
Mental status	Anxious but alert and oriented	Decreases to unresponsive
Respirations	Normal or slightly tachypneic; normal tidal volume	Severely tachypneic with evidence of respiratory distress or failure; tidal volume likely decreased
Wheezing	None or slight with good breath sounds	Present in all lung fields to very poor lung sounds with little air movement
Stridor	None	May be present

by auto-injector or intramuscular (IM) injection in the anterolateral aspect of the middle third of the thigh. This location provides the fastest absorption. Epinephrine can be administered subcutaneously (SQ); however, when this route is used the absorbtion is much slower, and epinephrine delivery to the core circulation might be delayed significantly when the anaphylaxis is associated with poor perfusion or hypotension.

The recommended adult dose is 0.2 to 0.5 mg of a 1:1000 dilution administered intramuscularly. The adult epinephrine auto-injector typically delivers a 0.3 mg dose. The pediatric dose is 0.1 mg/kg, not to exceed the adult dose (0.2 to 0.5 mg). The pediatric epinephrine auto-injector delivers a dose of 0.15 mg. The pediatric auto-injector should be used in children less than 66 lbs or 30 kg. If the child is larger than 66 lbs or 30 kg, use the adult epinephrine auto-injector.

Epinephrine can be repeated every 5 to 15 minutes if the patient continues to exhibit evidence of hypotension, airway swelling, and severe respiratory distress or failure.

- Initiate rapid transport.
- If the reaction is associated with a sting or an injection of the antigen to an extremity, apply a loose tourniquet proximal to the site and place the extremity in a dependent position.

- Some EMS systems may allow the Advanced EMT (AEMT) to administer diphenhydramine (Benadryl). A typical dose is 25 to 50 mg IV or IM.

- If the patient continues to present with respiratory distress and diffuse wheezing after the administration of epinephrine and no signs of hypotension or poor perfusion are present, consider the administration of an aerosolized beta-2 agonist delivered via nebulizer or metered-dose inhaler. Albuterol is commonly nebulized at a dose of 2.5 mg diluted to 3 mL of normal saline in both adult and pediatric patients or levalbuterol at 0.625 to 1.25 mg diluted to 3 mL of normal saline in the adult and 0.31 to 0.625 mg diluted to 3 mL of normal saline in the pediatric patient.

- If no signs of respiratory distress or failure are present, and the airway is not compromised by edema and the patient continues to present with hypotension, continue to infuse large amounts of normal saline or lactated Ringer's at a wide-open rate. It may be necessary to establish a second intravenous line.

- If the patient is on beta blockers or remains hypotensive after administration of repeat doses of epinephrine and fluids, consider the administration of glucagon at 1 to 5 mg intravenously over 5 minutes.

Why Epinephrine?—The Drug of Choice

Recall that the etiologies of almost all the signs and symptoms and fatal events—such as airway compromise, respiratory failure, hypoxia, and cardiovascular collapse—associated with an anaphylactic or anaphylactoid reaction are related to increases in capillary permeability, bronchoconstriction, vasodilation, and mucus production. If these can be reversed, the signs and symptoms and chance of a fatal episode also will be reversed. Thus, a focus in the emergency care of the patient is to decrease the permeability of the capillaries, dilate the bronchioles, and constrict the vessels.

Epinephrine becomes the drug of choice because of its ability to stimulate alpha and beta receptors. Alpha stimulation causes vascular smooth muscle contraction, leading to vasoconstriction. Vasoconstriction decreases the vessel diameter and increases resistance to blood flow, leading to an increase in blood pressure and perfusion. The vasoconstriction also tightens the capillaries. This will also reverse hypotension by reducing the leakage of plasma volume to the interstitial space. The beta-2 stimulation dilates the bronchiole smooth muscle and reverses the bronchoconstriction. Thus, epinephrine administration eliminates the capillary permeability, vasodilation, and bronchoconstriction associated with anaphylaxis.

TRANSITIONING

REVIEW ITEMS

1. A patient presents with widespread urticaria covering the majority of his body. Based on that initial finding, you should suspect that the patient is also likely to present with _____.
   a. cardiac dysrhythmias
   b. bradycardia
   c. pale cool skin
   d. hypotension

2. An anaphylactic patient presents with stridor, hoarseness, and an increased effort to breathe. Which property of epinephrine would likely reverse these signs?
   a. alpha stimulation
   b. beta-1 stimulation
   c. beta-2 stimulation
   d. delta stimulation

3. The pathophysiologic response that creates a life-threatening upper airway compromise is related to _____.
   a. an increase in mucus secretion
   b. an increase in capillary permeability
   c. a decrease in vascular tone
   d. an increase in smooth muscle contraction

4. Immediately following the administration of epinephrine, the patient appears to be responding effectively. Which of the following should you suspect may present as a direct result of the emergency care?
   a. an increase in heart rate
   b. an increase in flushing of the skin
   c. a decrease in peripheral pulse amplitude
   d. a widened pulse pressure

5. Following the administration of epinephrine, the hypotension, poor perfusion, stridor, and severe respiratory distress are reversed. However, the patient continues to present with diffuse bilateral wheezing and mild respiratory distress. You should _____.

    a. begin to assist the patient's spontaneous respirations with a bag-valve-mask device

    b. administer a second dose of epinephrine by deep intramuscular injection

    c. continue with oxygen therapy and reassess the respiratory status in 5 minutes

    d. contact medical direction for an order to administer a beta-2 agonist by inhalation

APPLIED PATHOPHYSIOLOGY

1. List the four primary pathophysiologic responses to the release of chemical mediators that produce the life-threatening condition and signs and symptoms in anaphylaxis.

2. Explain the difference in the patient presentation between an anaphylactic and anaphylactoid reaction.

3. Explain the process of sensitization in the IgE-mediated anaphylactic reaction.

4. What triggers the release of the chemical mediators from mast cells and basophils in the IgE-mediated reaction?

5. List the properties of epinephrine and their specific effects on reversing the pathophysiologic responses to the chemical mediators.

6. What property of epinephrine would be considered a side effect?

7. Why?

CLINICAL DECISION MAKING

You encounter a 23-year-old male patient sitting on the front porch of his residence. You note a lawn mower out in the front yard, and the grass is partially cut. As you have determined that the scene is safe, you approach the patient. He is sitting upright in a tripod position and appears to be in significant respiratory distress.

1. Based on the scene size-up characteristics, list the possible conditions you suspect the patient is experiencing.

The primary assessment reveals that the patient is anxious, confused, and disoriented and has stridorous sounds on respiration, a respiratory rate of 28 per minute with chest rise and fall, circumoral cyanosis, absent peripheral pulses, and a heart rate of 128 beats per minute. The skin is warm and flushed. The SpO$_2$ reading is 74 percent.

2. What are the life threats to this patient?

3. What immediate emergency care should you provide based on the primary assessment?

4. Explain the pathophysiologic causes for the following:

    a. Anxiousness

    b. Confusion and disorientation

    c. Stridorous sounds

    d. Warm flushed skin

5. What conditions have you ruled out from your initial consideration in the scene size-up?

6. What conditions are you still considering as the possible cause? Are there any conditions that you would add as a possible cause?

During the secondary assessment, you note an edematous tongue and swollen oral mucosa; urticaria to the face, neck, and upper chest; and diffuse bilateral wheezing. The patient has a new-onset cough that is nonproductive. He also complains of a headache and severe dizziness. His respiratory distress is worsening. The abdomen is soft and nontender, the pelvis is stable, and no deformities or evidence of trauma to the extremities are present. The extremities are warm, flushed, and dry. The peripheral pulses are all absent. The patient has no known allergies, has a history of mild asthma, and takes no prescription medication. He had a diet cola about 20 minutes prior to your arrival. He was cutting the grass when he suddenly began to experience shortness of breath and lightheadedness. He admits to taking 800 mg of ibuprofen for a bad headache with the diet cola. His blood pressure is 76/42 mmHg, his heart rate is now 142 beats per minute, and his respirations are 32 per minute and more labored.

7. What conditions have your ruled out in your differential field diagnosis? Why?

8. What conditions are you considering as the probable cause? Why?

9. Based on your differential diagnosis, what are the next steps in emergency care? Why?

10. Explain how you came to a differential field diagnosis based on specific history and physical assessment findings.

11. What was the trigger for the condition the patient is experiencing?

12. Based on the history, what type of reaction is this patient experiencing?

13. If his circulation is not improved, what skin signs will begin to appear? Why?

Standard Medicine

Competency Applies fundamental knowledge to provide basic and selected advanced emergency care and transportation based on assessment findings for an acutely ill patient.

TOPIC

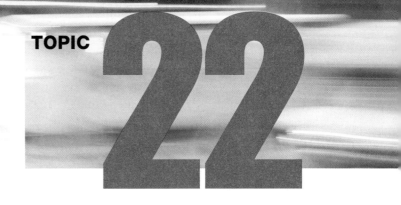

INFECTIOUS DISEASE

INTRODUCTION

From the common cold to the rapidly expanding list of multidrug-resistant organisms, infectious disease is a topic that should be on every emergency medical provider's mind. Unfortunately, infectious disease is not a simple topic. Today's Advanced EMTs are faced with not just how to protect themselves from microorganisms, but also how to prepare for a world in which pandemic outbreaks and medication-resistant diseases are a reality.

EMS has evolved from a world of "gloves and maybe goggles" to a world of assisting with vaccinations and preparing for what seem like doomsday scenarios. We can no longer rely on minimum training to face today's infectious disease threat. What we do not know can assuredly kill us! As an advanced provider, you must have a working knowledge of the threats you are faced with every day, and you must understand your role in mitigating and defending against the spread of, in many cases, life-threatening disease. This topic focuses on the evolving threats that infectious disease poses to emergency medical providers and discusses key concepts in personal protection.

SPREADING INFECTION

The World Health Organization (WHO) defines *infectious disease* as pathogenic microorganisms—such as bacteria, viruses, parasites, or fungi—that can be spread, directly or indirectly, from one person to another. A disease is considered *communicable* when it is transmitted easily from one person to another (Table 22-1). In your basic EMT class you learned about the basics of disease transmission. Diseases that were caused by organisms (or vectors) were discussed, as well as diseases that were bloodborne, airborne, and foodborne. Disease transmission has changed little since the dawn of time, and the concepts you learned remain very important. Threats such as HIV, hepatitis, and tuberculosis are still very real to health care workers, and new threats are evolving every day.

Bloodborne diseases pose a particular threat to you as an AEMT. As an AEMT, you will administer medications and use intravenous therapy. These skills require the use and disposal of needles and other sharps that pose the risk of injury when not

TRANSITION highlights

- *How infection spreads.*
- *Protection from disease.*
- *Multidrug-resistant organisms.*
- *Current infectious diseases prevalent in the community.*
- *Influenza.*
- *The role of EMS in public health.*

used safely. The Centers for Disease Control and Prevention (CDC) estimates that roughly 82 percent of health care worker exposures to bloodborne diseases occur as a result of needle- or sharp-related incidents. Although improved safety strategies have demonstrated a 96 percent decline in the number of these incidents since 1983, the necessity of using needles and other sharps means that this threat is still very real.

A number of pathogens are discussed in the following sections.

Hepatitis

Hepatitis translates to an inflammation of the liver. It is generally caused by a viral infection and can be classified among a series of groupings, with A, B, and C being the most common classifications. Hepatitis A and E are technically contracted through fecal contact and therefore are considered food- and waterborne, but hepatitis B, C, and D are bloodborne. The CDC estimates that there are roughly 80,000 new infections of hepatitis in the United States each year.

The pathophysiology of hepatitis is not simple and depends greatly on the type (classification) of the hepatitis strain.

> A disease is considered communicable when it is transmitted easily from one person to another.

TABLE 22-1 Communicable Diseases

Disease	Mode of Transmission	Incubation
AIDS (acquired immune deficiency syndrome)	HIV-infected blood via intravenous drug use, unprotected sexual contact, blood transfusions, or (rarely) accidental needle sticks; mothers may pass HIV to their unborn children	Several months or years
Hepatitis	Blood, stool, or other body fluids; contaminated objects	Weeks to months, depending on type
Meningitis, bacterial	Oral and nasal secretions	2–10 days
Mumps	Droplets of saliva or objects contaminated by saliva	14–24 days
Pertussis (whooping cough)	Respiratory secretions or airborne droplets	6–20 days
Pneumonia, bacterial and viral	Oral and nasal droplets and secretions	Several days
Rubella (German measles)	Airborne droplets; mothers may pass the disease to unborn children	10–12 days
Staphylococcal skin infections	Direct contact with infected wounds or sore or with contaminated objects	Several days
Tuberculosis	Respiratory secretions, airborne or on contaminated objects	2–6 weeks
Varicella (chickenpox)	Airborne droplets; can also be spread by contact with open sores	11–21 days

In simple terms, however, the hepatitis virus seeks out and invades healthy liver cells. Its reproduction destroys these cells and causes an immune response in the liver. Liver function is damaged both immediately and over time as the disease persists.

Hepatitis symptoms can be chronic, in the form of long-term decline in function and liver failure, or acute, in the form of short-term "flareups." Specific symptoms include fatigue, abdominal pain, nausea, vomiting, and evidence of liver failure such as jaundice (yellowing of the eyes). It is also important to remember that there are roughly 4.4 million Americans living with chronic hepatitis. Many of these chronically infected patients will be essentially asymptomatic.

Hepatitis and its variety of forms pose perhaps the highest risk to EMS providers. Although the incidence of hepatitis transmission among health care workers has decreased in recent years, its *virulence*, or ability of the organism to produce disease, makes it particularly dangerous.

Hepatitis B, C, and D are transmitted through blood and are particularly hardy. Unlike other infectious organisms, the hepatitis virus can survive outside the body much longer than those that cause other diseases. This means that needle-stick injuries and other percutaneous (penetrating the protective barrier of the skin) exposures pose a high risk. As an AEMT, you must take careful steps to protect yourself from the dangers of potential sharp-related injuries and practice appropriate decontamination procedures.

HIV/AIDS

The human immunodeficiency virus (HIV) is a bloodborne pathogen that potentially leads to acquired immune deficiency syndrome (AIDS). AIDS, if developed, is deadly. Although HIV is significantly more difficult to transmit than hepatitis, its potential consequences make it a high-level threat to health care workers.

Recent treatment advances have prevented many HIV-infected patients from developing AIDS. As a result, the true incidence and mortality of HIV and AIDS has become difficult to assess. That said, the CDC estimates that slightly fewer than 700,000 Americans are infected with HIV. The number of confirmed occupational transmissions among health care workers is very low, but given the potential lethality of AIDS, we must consider even one transmission as one too many.

AIDS is characterized by a destruction of the immune system. Over time, essential T cells are destroyed, leaving the body vulnerable to opportunistic infections. As a result, most AIDS deaths are caused by secondary diseases, such as respiratory infections and malignancies.

HIV is a bloodborne disease. Among health care workers, almost all transmissions have occurred through needle-stick and sharp-related injuries. Therefore, the most effective way to protect against occupational transmission of HIV is to promote safe sharp handling and disposal.

It is important to remember that even in the case of an infected patient, not every needle-stick injury will transmit disease. According to the WHO, only about 3 in 1000 of these types of injury will actually transmit disease. Many factors contribute to the probability, including the amount of patient blood on or in the penetrating sharp; how deep the needle penetrated, and whether or not it penetrated a vein or artery; and how high the viral load in the patient is. Nonetheless, any needle-stick or sharp injury is a high-risk exposure and should be handled seriously.

Some occupational transmissions through body fluid contact have also been

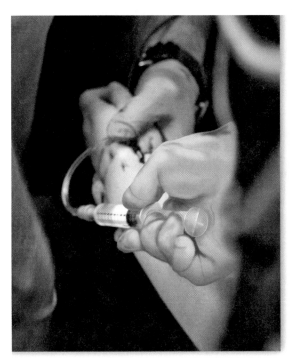

Figure 22-1 Standard Precautions are required to protect you from disease.

reported. Although these are exceptionally rare, body fluid contact to open wounds and mucous membranes can transmit the disease. Standard Precautions are designed to protect us from any patient's body fluids and generally can provide an effective barrier against this type of transmission (▶ Figure 22-1). In some cases, a higher level of personal protective equipment may be necessary. Always assess the specific need of the situation and protect yourself accordingly.

Tuberculosis

Tuberculosis (TB) is spread by a bacterium called *Mycobacterium tuberculosis*. These bacteria are transmitted through respiratory droplets and can pose a risk to emergency providers. Although the incidence of TB in the United States is at its lowest rate in history, the WHO points out that roughly one-third of the world's population is currently infected with the TB bacillus. Although the vast majority of TB infection is *latent* (only 5 percent to 10 percent of those infected will develop symptoms of the disease), the risk of transmission is still very real.

Active TB develops in 5 percent to 10 percent of the people exposed to the TB bacteria and is characterized by a massive immune response in the lining of the airway and the parenchymal tissue. Inflammation and subsequent changes to the

lung cell structure cause poor diffusion and ultimately destruction of the tissue itself.

The signs and symptoms of active TB include persistent cough with blood-tinged sputum, fever, weight loss, and night sweats.

Some populations are considered high risk for developing TB. These include drug users, HIV patients, those living or working in congregate settings (e.g., jails, nursing homes, and shelters), and those in close proximity to TB patients (e.g., health care workers and family members living in the same home), among others.

Contact with patients demonstrating active TB will require respiratory protection to prevent transmission. An N-95 type respirator will protect you from the respiratory droplet transfer of a TB patient; for any respirator to be effective, however, a proper fit test must be completed prior to using the mask in a high-risk environment.

As an AEMT, you learned about respiratory protection and personal protective equipment, but remember that there are many levels of protection against disease. Protective equipment is only one part. Consider now the role of fit testing and proper equipment placement in the context of preventing infection.

MULTIDRUG-RESISTANT ORGANISMS
In most cases, tuberculosis is both preventable and treatable, but in some cases, the bacteria that cause TB have evolved to become resistant to some (and, in rare cases, all) of the medications used to traditionally treat it—especially in HIV-infected patients. Most commonly, this evolution is enhanced by partial and unfinished courses of antibiotic treatment. When a patient takes only a part of the prescribed course of antibiotic therapy, the bacteria are exposed to the medication, but are not completely eradicated. The remaining bacteria reproduce and develop resistance. Drug-resistant TB can still be treated, but the modalities used are far more extensive and invasive.

TB is not the only organism to develop a resistance to standard medications used

for treatment. In recent years, we have witnessed an explosive evolution of microorganisms resistant to traditional therapies. These are commonly referred to as *multidrug-resistant organisms* (MDROs).

METHICILLIN-RESISTANT *STAPHYLO-COCCUS AUREUS* Methicillin-resistant *Staphylococcus aureus* (MRSA) has evolved in much the same way as TB, but at a much more profound pace. MRSA is the drug-resistant variant of the simple *Staphylococcus aureus* bacteria. Staph bacteria are very common. In fact, about one-quarter of the population carries *Staphylococcus* bacteria on their skin and/or in their nose. This type of bacteria causes a variety of different infections, from localized skin infections to respiratory infections. How many of these staph infections involve MRSA is difficult to say. The CDC notes that, in some instances, MRSA can account for more than 40 percent to 60 percent of staph infections.

MRSA can be divided into two groups: hospital acquired (HA) and community acquired (CA). Hospital-acquired MRSA results from transmission of the disease in a health care setting, typically from surgical procedures, catheters, and endotracheal tubes. The rate of MRSA versus simple staph infection is highest in this group. Community-acquired MRSA occurs in otherwise healthy people when the bacteria are passed by contact. This commonly occurs in populations living in close proximity to one another. Children in day care, athletes, and members of the military are common victims of this type of transmission.

EMS members are exposed to staph and MRSA commonly through our patient population. Frequently we transport patients with known (and unknown cases) of MRSA. In one study of an urban ambulance fleet, 10 of 21 ambulances were found to harbor MRSA colonies in the ambulances and on the equipment used. MRSA can be transmitted by skin contact and/or by respiratory contact, and as such, an appropriate level of personal protective equipment should be used to prevent the spread of bacteria. In some cases, patients will be identified as having MRSA. In a known MRSA patient, it will frequently be known whether respiratory protection is necessary. We also likely transport many MRSA patients without knowing it. Standard Precautions will help limit exposure, but quality decontamination procedures are also necessary to prevent transmission to staff members and to other patients. As an AEMT, you learned about Standard Precautions, but now consider the importance of quality decontamination in fighting the spread of infectious disease.

OTHER DRUG-RESISTANT ORGANISMS

Other drug-resistant organisms include vancomycin-resistant enterococci (VRE) and Clostridium difficile (C-Dif). These are similar examples of commonly occurring bacteria developing a resistance to common treatments and are frequently present in otherwise routine infections. Many other MDROs exist; an in-depth discussion of each is far beyond the scope of this chapter. However, as an AEMT, you should continue to educate yourself on the subject of these threats. The CDC is an excellent resource and provides many organism-specific recommendations for personal protection (see the bibliography at the end of this topic). Most important, though, you should protect against the all microorganisms by using Standard Precautions and a higher level of personal protective equipment when necessary. Remember also that appropriate hand washing is your first and best line of defense (see box).

Flu and Pandemic Flu

In 1918, 50 million people around the world died of influenza. Nearly 3 percent of the world's population died of what is typically a relatively minor infection. Influenza (flu) is a viral infection that has multiple different classifications (influenza A, B, C) and subclassifications (e.g., H1N1, H5, N1). Influenza is quite virulent and is spread via airborne droplets and through contact with respiratory fluids (such as in surface contamination). Various strains of influenza strike regionally each year.

The influenza virus targets the airway and respiratory system. An immune response, in an attempt to rid the lungs of the invading pathogen, causes inflammation and changes to the lining of the respiratory tract. Cytokines (specific immune-related proteins) and other chemicals released from infected cells cause fever and fatigue. The most common

HAND WASHING

For a pathogen to be spread, the organism must be transferred from one person to another. As you learned in EMT class, this can be done (among other methods) through the air, through body fluids, or through food. Commonly, humans transfer organisms through touch—for example, a person wipes her nose and then touches a table. The virus on the table is then touched by a second person and transferred into his body when he wipes his own eye. This type of infection can be controlled with simple hand washing (▶ Figure 22-2).

For all the engineering and personal protective equipment you have, there is no more effective strategy in fighting the spread of disease than to simply wash your hands. When washing, remember the key elements:

- Warm flowing water with soap
- At least 15 seconds of scrubbing over all surfaces
- Thorough rinsing

Remember to also avoid reexposure through touching faucet handles and doorknobs. Consider using paper towels to minimize this type of contamination. Alcohol-based hand sanitizers are effective for most organisms and can be used when hand washing is not available (▶ Figure 22-3). However, the MDRO Clostridium difficile is not destroyed by alcohol-based gels and foams.

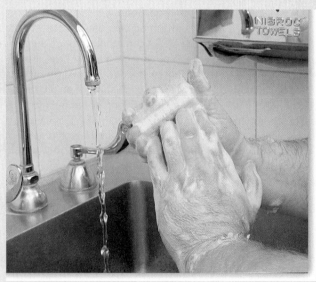

Figure 22-2 Hand washing is vital for preventing the spread of disease.

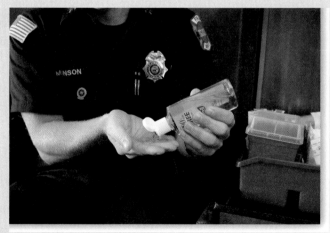

Figure 22-3 Alcohol-based hand cleaner is effective and can be used when soap and water are not available.

strains of flu cause fever, chills, muscle pains, and coughing.

To a healthy person, most influenza is not usually life threatening, but in some cases it can be dangerous. Influenza can create a life-threatening situation in patients who are already compromised by chronic illness, pregnancy, and underlying disease. Older patients and the very young often fall victim. The CDC estimates that influenza kills somewhere between 3,000 and 50,000 people each year in the United States.

In the past several years, the world has seen the rise of particularly virulent strains of influenza. Influenza A H1N1 was an aggressive form of flu that debilitated patients regardless of their previous health status. In 2009 it killed more than 18,000 people and was found in 214 countries. Many of the victims were in good health before the onset of the disease. The WHO designated H1N1 as a *pandemic*. A pandemic occurs when a contagious disease infects and harms people over a wide geographic distribution (in the case of H1N1, over the entire world).

The danger of a pandemic illness is, first and foremost, widespread death, but consider also the other implications of widespread illness. Imagine the consequences of 60 percent of a hospital's staff being sick at the same time. Imagine what would happen if 90 percent of a city's fire department fell ill. Such circumstances would rapidly overwhelm health care services, cripple important infrastructure, and require systems of triage and in-home treatment previously unimagined by current medical systems. In response to the threat of pandemic diseases, the role of EMS would significantly change.

Examples of this changing role can be seen by examining the H1N1 threat. In response to the pandemic threat, a vaccine was developed. In many areas, EMS was enlisted to help deliver the inoculations. As an AEMT, your ability to administer injections may make you a valuable component of the public health system. In addition to your traditional role of responder, you may now be employed in a preventive setting.

EMS is at high risk to be exposed to the flu. Close quarters in the back of an ambulance make for higher probability of respiratory droplet contact. All health care professionals should protect themselves in a suspected case of the flu by using respiratory protection (a mask for you and a mask for your patient) and by being vaccinated each year. Hand washing and decontamination are also essential. Remember also to avoid becoming a vector (an organism that transmits disease) yourself. If you are sick, stay home. If you cough, cough into your elbow and not your hand. These simple procedures are truly effective in stopping even a pandemic event.

Other Contagious Diseases

Pertussis, or whooping cough, is a bacterial infection that attacks the airway and lung tissue. Advanced pertussis is characterized by a destruction of the cilia and epithelial lining of the respiratory tract. This causes an accumulation of mucus and debris in the airways and a reduction of airflow. A violent cough develops in response to these complications.

The cough of pertussis is its hallmark and namesake. Chronic coughing often persists for weeks and even months. A rapid inhalation followed the cough often makes a "whooping" type of sound. Coughing in pertussis patients can also cause barotrauma, such as pneumothorax and pneumomediastinum.

Pertussis is most common in young children less than 6 months of age, but has shown recent increases in incidence among adolescents. Patients in the advanced stages of the disease will display the signature cough and history of respiratory symptoms. Fever and recent history of upper respiratory symptoms are common precursors to the cough. The tetanus, diphtheria, and pertussis (DPT) vaccination protects against the spread of pertussis, but its effects can wane over time. Outbreaks of pertussis have recently been seen in California, New York, and Pennsylvania.

Measles and *mumps* have also seen recent resurgences. Although these diseases are traditionally protected against by childhood vaccinations, noncompliance with vaccination recommendations and poor health infrastructure in developing countries have caused recent regional outbreaks and spikes in incidence of these diseases.

Destruction of public health infrastructure, as in the case of disaster, has led to outbreak and higher incidence of otherwise rare contagious diseases. Outbreaks of cholera and typhoid have occurred following the earthquakes in Haiti and the tsunamis of the Pacific. Both typhoid and cholera are transmitted through contaminated water. The loss of drinking water sanitation capabilities means that areas already crippled by disaster now must contend with infectious disease as well. Although these outbreaks are typically regional in nature, air travel and global relief efforts often lead to spread of the epidemic beyond its primary area.

Infectious diseases will continue to challenge the health care resources of the world. As we find ways to manage one challenge, new and previously unknown threats emerge to tax our capabilities. As health care becomes more sophisticated in its response to the spread of disease, the importance of EMS as a partner in public health becomes clear.

EMS AND PUBLIC HEALTH

We traditionally think of the role of the AEMT as assessing, treating, and transporting patients. However, EMS has developed a significant responsibility within public health, especially in the context of infectious disease. EMS frequently partners with other elements of the health care system (e.g., hospitals, physicians, and state agencies) to develop and enact strategies to prevent and stop the spread of infectious disease (▶ Figure 22-4). Besides the traditional roles, today's EMS provider is responsible for a variety of additional functions in the lager public health partnership. Consider the tactics for fighting disease listed in Table 22-2, and then think about how EMS professionals might play a part.

At all levels, EMS can play an important role. As health care professionals, we must first monitor our own health and adhere to vaccine recommendations. Personal protective equipment must be prepared, allocated, and fit-tested before being used in a high-risk environment. Initial and continuing education must discuss the infectious disease threats to the well-being of providers and to the well-being of our patients. We must be ready to answer the call in times of outbreaks.

EMS frequently partners with other health care agencies to prevent and

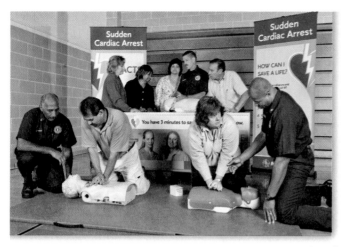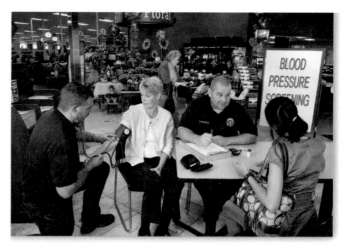

Figure 22-4 EMS in the public health setting.

react to outbreaks of disease. In certain circumstances, AEMTs might be used to screen for diseases, distribute medications, or administer vaccinations to protect a specific catchment area. When hospitals reach their surge capacity (the maximum number of patients they are capable of handling), EMS is tasked with moving the overflow to outlying facilities. Although transport is a traditional role of EMS, consider how this role might change when tasked with transferring infected patients. Consider also the impact of a pandemic disease overwhelming local health resources. Protocols, transport decisions, and hospital destinations all could be altered significantly.

> **Disease surveillance is also an increasing responsibility of EMS.**

Disease surveillance is also an increasing responsibility of EMS. Advanced EMTs often participate in research and in many cases have specific reporting responsibilities (e.g., elder and child abuse or suspicious injuries). In rural and underprivileged areas, EMS may be the most sophisticated health care services that many patients see. Information provided in patient care reports may assist in research and in tracking outbreaks and epidemics.

Just as EMS has played a role in enhancing the response to out-of-hospital cardiac arrest through community CPR classes, AEMTs may also play a role in community education with regard to infectious disease. From prevention to recognition, community education certainly involves EMS and is an important element of fighting infectious disease.

CONCLUSIONS

It is most important that all EMS professionals learn to protect themselves from infectious disease. Understanding the characteristics of the key threats will help tailor your response when faced with a potentially infectious patient. More than personal protection, however, the role of the AEMT has expanded in the fight against contagious pathogens. AEMTs administer vaccinations, conduct disease screenings, and provide community education. As diseases become challenging to fight, partnerships must develop throughout health care to provide an optimal response. EMS plays a vital role in response, and its responsibilities continue to increase.

TABLE 22-2	EMS as an Agent of Public Health
Strategy	**Role of EMS**
Prevention	• AEMTs administering vaccinations • Stringent immunizations and health care monitoring of EMS providers • Dispersal of personal protective equipment • Hand washing • Equipment decontamination • Public education
Recognition	• Continuing education • Public education • Disease reporting • Research
Limiting exposure	• Safety engineering • Personal protective equipment • Safe sharps handling • Safe and sanitary patient transport
Treatment	• Treatment of symptoms • Safe patient handling • Safe and sanitary patient transport • Evaluation/care/referral • Surge mitigation

REVIEW ITEMS

1. Which of the following diseases does not have a vaccination for prevention of the disease?
   a. HIV
   b. hepatitis A
   c. hepatitis B
   d. measles

2. Which of the following is *not* a high-risk group for TB?
   a. prison inmates
   b. children of a TB-infected parent
   c. churchgoers
   d. HIV-infected persons

3. Another name for pertussis is _____.
   a. diphtheria
   b. cholera
   c. epiglottitis
   d. whooping cough

4. A pandemic infects people _____.
   a. with different diseases in the same area
   b. over a large geographic area
   c. of a similar race or sex
   d. of a similar age

5. Which of the following forms of hepatitis is *not* spread through the bloodborne route?
   a. hepatitis A
   b. hepatitis B
   c. hepatitis C
   d. hepatitis D

APPLIED PATHOPHYSIOLOGY

1. Describe how each of the following diseases is spread.
   a. Tuberculosis
   b. Measles
   c. Hepatitis D
   d. Influenza

2. Why is tuberculosis spread more readily in congregate settings?

3. You are told that hepatitis is easier to contract than HIV. Do you agree? Why or why not?

CLINICAL DECISION MAKING

You are called to a nursing home for a patient who has had a productive cough for several days. Staff members report that he has had a fever, chills, and night sweats. They are concerned because the infection has not cleared with the antibiotics he was prescribed.

1. List several conditions you suspect the patient may have.

The staff adds that the patient has lost weight recently and had developed blood-tinged sputum.

2. Has this helped to narrow down the conditions you suspect?

3. What other factors have you considered?

4. What Standard Precautions would you take for this patient?

BIBLIOGRAPHY

Centers for Disease Control and Prevention (CDC). Fact Sheets: HIV/AIDS, Hepatitis, Tuberculosis. www.cdc.gov.

Centers for Disease Control and Prevention (CDC). Pertussis. www.cdc.gov/features/pertussis/.

Centers for Disease Control and Prevention (CDC). (2003, July). Exposure to Blood: What Healthcare Workers Need to Know.

Centers for Disease Control and Prevention (CDC). (2005, December). Guidelines for Preventing the Transmission of

Mycobacterium Tuberculosis in Health-Care Settings. *MMWR* 54/RR-17.

Centers for Disease Control and Prevention (CDC). (2006, January). Healthcare Infection Control Practices Advisory Committee: Management of Multi-Drug Resistant Organisms in Health-care Settings.

Centers for Disease Control and Prevention (CDC). (2006, December). Surveillance of Occupationally Acquired HIV/AIDS in Healthcare Personnel, as of December 2006 (modified September 2007).

Centers for Disease Control and Prevention (CDC). (2007, October). Overview of Community-Associated MRSA.

Centers for Disease Control and Prevention (CDC). (2011, February). Occupational HIV Transmission and Prevention Among Health Care Workers.

Nicolle, L. Community-acquired MRSA: A Practitioner's Guide. *CMAJ* 2006;175:145.

U.S. Department of Health and Human Services (NIOSH). (1988). Guidelines for Protecting the Safety and Health of Health Care Workers, 1988 Publication No. 88-119.

U.S. Department of Health and Human Services. (2008, September). HIV Post-Exposure Prophylaxis: Guidance from the UK Chief Medical Officer's Expert Advisory Group on AIDS (2nd ed.).

World Health Organization (WHO). (2009, April). Priority Interventions: HIV/AIDS Prevention, Treatment and Care in the Health Sector.

World Health Organization (WHO). (2010, November). Tuberculosis Fact Sheet N 104.

Standard Medicine

Competency Applies fundamental knowledge to provide basic and selected advanced emergency care and transportation based on assessment findings for an acutely ill patient.

TOPIC
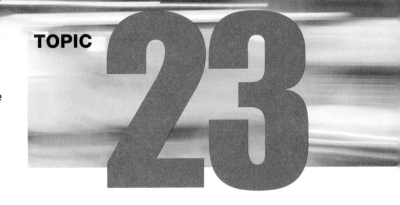

ENDOCRINE EMERGENCIES: DIABETES MELLITUS AND HYPOGLYCEMIA

INTRODUCTION

*D*iabetes mellitus (DM) is a condition in which the patient experiences a chronically elevated blood glucose level. Although EMS frequently responds for those with a low blood glucose level (hypoglycemia), most diabetes mellitus patients struggle on a daily basis to decrease their blood glucose levels to within a normal range. However, the occasional acute hypoglycemic event carries a high risk of morbidity and mortality. Thus, it is imperative that the Advanced EMT quickly recognize the signs and symptoms of hypoglycemia and manage the patient accordingly to prevent any long-term effects from the episode.

EPIDEMIOLOGY

DM is the most common endocrine disorder, with approximately 6 percent of the population afflicted with the disease. Whites are much more likely to have the disease than nonwhites.

Types of Diabetes Mellitus

DM is typically characterized as type 1 or type 2. Type 2 is much more prevalent and makes up approximately 90 percent to 95 percent of cases of DM. Type 1 accounts for the remaining 5 percent to 10 percent of cases.

TYPE 1 DIABETES MELLITUS Type 1 DM results from a chronic autoimmune process that destroys the insulin-producing cells (beta cells) in the pancreas. Interestingly, the cells responsible for secreting other hormones in the pancreas are typically preserved and continue to function. The exact cause of the disorder is not clearly understood; however, theories link genetics, environment, and viruses to the etiology.

Characteristics of type 1 diabetes patients are

- Typically younger than 40 years of age (peak age is 10 to 14 years of age)
- Lean body mass
- May have rapid weight loss
- Polyuria (excessive urination)

TRANSITION *highlights*

- *Frequency of diabetes mellitus and the ethnic predisposition of the disease.*
- *Etiologies of diabetes mellitus (type 1 and type 2).*
- *Roles that the hormones insulin and glucagon play in glucose metabolism.*
- *Cellular metabolism of glucose.*
- *Discussion of how low blood sugar (hypoglycemia) can result from the presence in the body of either too much or too little insulin or from insufficient levels of glucose.*
- *Signs and symptoms seen in hypoglycemia from either the hyperadrenergic or neuroglycopenic pathophysiology.*
- *Emergency medical care for the hypoglycemic patient and the role of oral glucose administration during patient management.*

- Polydipsia (excessive thirst)
- Polyphagia (excessive eating)

Insulin levels in the blood are low to absent; however, glucagon levels are high. (Both hormones are explained in more detail later in this topic.) Because the pancreas is secreting little to no insulin, type 1 patients must take supplemental insulin to manage their blood glucose level. Such patients are more prone to hypoglycemia and diabetic ketoacidosis (DKA).

TYPE 2 DIABETES MELLITUS The pancreas in the patient with type 2 diabetes continues to secrete insulin; however, the blood glucose level is elevated despite the insulin. This is caused by impaired insulin function, an inadequate amount of insulin being released by the pancreas, inability of the insulin to reach

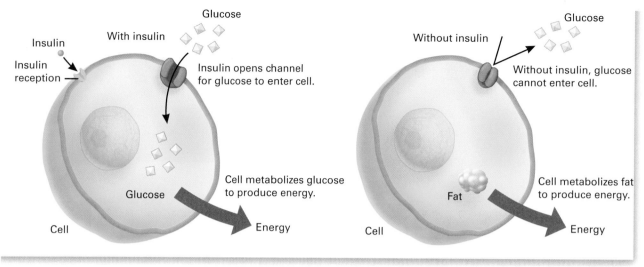

Figure 23-1 Glucose movement into the cell with insulin and the inability of glucose to get into the cell without insulin.

the receptor sites on the cells, or failure of the organ to respond to the circulating insulin.

Characteristics of type 2 diabetes patients are

- Onset usually in middle-age or older adults (however, more children and adolescents are being diagnosed with type 2)
- Obese body mass (however, 20 percent are not obese)
- More gradual onset of signs and symptoms

Type 2 diabetes is usually controlled through diet, exercise, and oral hypoglycemic medications. In some severe cases, the patient may require insulin supplementation. These patients are more prone to developing hyperglycemic hyperosmolar nonketotic syndrome (HHNS).

PATHOPHYSIOLOGY

Hypoglycemia results from a sudden decrease in the amount of glucose circulating in the blood. It is more common in type 1 diabetics who are taking insulin; type 2 diabetics taking oral hypoglycemic drugs can experience a hypoglycemic episode, but it is much more uncommon. Although hypoglycemic episodes are less common in the type 2 diabetic taking oral medications for blood sugar regulation, the longer half-life of the oral medications makes hospitalization necessary—and refusals of care risky, due to the potential for additional blood glucose derangements hours later.

To understand the signs and symptoms of hypoglycemia, one must compre-hend some basic normal physiology and pathophysiology. The primary energy fuel for cells is glucose, a simple sugar that accounts for approximately 95 percent of the sugar in the blood after gastrointestinal absorption. Thus, it is the blood glucose level that AEMTs and other health care practitioners are most interested in determining.

Insulin and Glucagon

Insulin is a hormone secreted by the beta cells in the pancreas. The primary function of insulin is to move glucose from the blood and into the cells, where it can be used for energy. Insulin does not directly carry glucose into the cell; however, it triggers a receptor on the plasma membrane to open a channel allowing a protein helper, through the process of facilitated diffusion, to carry the glucose molecule into the cell (▶ Figure 23-1).

As long as insulin is available in the blood and is active, effective, and able to stimulate the receptor, it will continue to move glucose into cells, even if the blood glucose level falls below the lower level of normal. When this occurs, a large amount of glucose is moved out of the blood, leaving an inadequate supply for the brain cells, which do not store glucose. If the pancreas is functioning normally, insulin secretion will decrease as the blood glucose level drops.

Approximately 60 percent of the blood glucose after a meal will be sent to the liver to be stored in the form of glycogen. *Glycogen* is a complex carbohydrate molecule that will be broken down through a process known as *glycogenolysis* and returned back to the blood as free glucose. This will allow a person to maintain a near-normal blood glucose level between meals. *Glucagon* is a hormone released by the alpha cells in the pancreas that stimulates glycogenolysis and the conversion of noncarbohydrate substances into glucose (*gluconeogenesis*), subsequently raising the blood glucose level. As the blood glucose level decreases to approximately 70 mg/dL, insulin secretion will cease, whereas glucagon will be released to maintain a normal level of glucose and constant supply to the brain cells (▶ Figure 23-2).

Cell Metabolism of Glucose

Once in the cell, glucose is metabolized and produces energy in the form of adenosine triphosphate (ATP). ATP is necessary for cells to maintain a normal function. Without an adequate blood glucose level, alternative energy sources must be used by the cells. As a result, ATP production and cellular function may be altered.

The brain cells, unlike many other cells in the body, cannot effectively use any other energy source but glucose for ATP production. Interestingly, the blood–brain barrier does not require the presence of insulin to move glucose across the brain cell membrane. The brain cannot synthesize glucose, store it for extended periods of time, or concentrate it from the blood. Thus, a decrease in the blood glucose level to below normal may result in brain cell dysfunction from a lack of ATP production, a decrease in oxygen uptake, and a decrease in cerebral blood flow. A prolonged and severe decrease in the

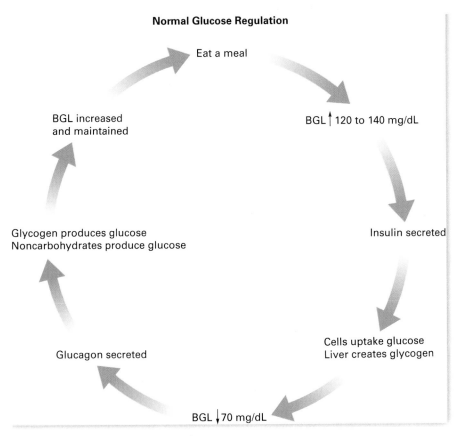

Normal Glucose Regulation

Eat a meal

BGL ↑ 120 to 140 mg/dL

Insulin secreted

Cells uptake glucose
Liver creates glycogen

BGL ↓ 70 mg/dL

Glucagon secreted

Glycogen produces glucose
Noncarbohydrates produce glucose

BGL increased
and maintained

Figure 23-2 Normal glucose regulation.

Hypoglycemia

blood glucose level could result in brain cell death.

A decrease in the blood glucose level below a normal range is known as *hypoglycemia*. Hypoglycemia is precipitated by having either too much insulin or not enough glucose in the blood. This may result from taking too much insulin, missing a meal or not eating enough calories to match the insulin dose, increasing energy output through exercise or work-related activities and not increasing caloric intake, an increased dose of oral hypoglycemic agents (sulphonylureas or meglintides), or unknown causes. Alcohol ingestion inhibits the gluconeogenesis and glycogenolysis, which may predispose the patient to hypoglycemia.

Most DM patients become symptomatic when the blood glucose level decreases to 40 to 50 mg/dL; however, this varies among patients. Patients have different thresholds and may present with severe signs and symptoms with reported blood glucose levels that are higher or lower than 50 mg/dL, which may also vary within the same individual on repeated episodes of hypoglycemia. The onset and severity of signs and symptoms also depend on how quickly the glucose level falls, how low it falls, and the typical level for the patient.

When the blood glucose level decreases beyond the normal range, the body will secrete counterregulatory hormones in an attempt to increase it. Glucagon is secreted from the alpha cells, and epinephrine is released from the adrenal medulla. Both glucagon and epinephrine stimulate gluconeogenesis and glycogenolysis in the liver. Epinephrine will also cause the breakdown of proteins into amino acids for conversion to glucose and will decrease the secretion of insulin from the pancreas. Growth hormone, cortisol, and vasopressin are also secreted as counterregulatory hormones; however, they do not have as significant an effect.

ASSESSMENT FINDINGS

The signs and symptoms exhibited by the hypoglycemic patient are caused by an activated sympathetic nervous system, epinephrine circulating throughout the body in an attempt to increase the blood glucose level, and brain cells that are not functioning properly as a result of the lack of glucose.

Hypoglycemia was once referred to as "insulin shock" because of the similarities of the signs exhibited by both hypovolemic shock and hypoglycemic patients. The primary hormone that produces tachycardia and pale, cool, and clammy skin in the shock patient is epinephrine, which is also released in the hypoglycemic patient, producing similar signs. Because of the stimulation of the sympathetic nervous system and circulating epinephrine, the signs of shock appear in the hypoglycemic patient.

The signs and symptoms of hypoglycemia can be categorized as being either hyperadrenergic, which is associated with an increase in the sympathetic nervous system activity or circulating epinephrine, or neuroglucopenic, which is a result of direct brain cell dysfunction from the lack of glucose (see Table 23-1).

Severe episodes of hypoglycemia may cause hemiplegia, making the patient present as if having a potential stroke. Thus, be sure to assess the blood glucose level in a suspected stroke patient; however, never administer glucose without a confirmed low blood glucose level (BGL), typically less than 60 mg/dL.

EMERGENCY MEDICAL CARE

The hypoglycemic patient needs sugar to raise the blood glucose level as quickly as possible to prevent the brain cells from dying. The AEMT can administer glucose intravenously, which is especially important in the patient with an altered mental status or the potential for the mental status to deteriorate.

Administration of oral glucose may pose a problem if the patient is unable to understand or obey your commands. Placing a substance in the mouth of a patient who has an altered mental status can lead to aspiration, which would complicate the condition. Therefore, initiation of an

> **Most DM patients become symptomatic when the blood glucose level decreases to 40 to 50 mg/dL; however, this varies among patients.**

TABLE 23-1	Signs and Symptoms of Hypoglycemia
Hyperadrenergic (epinephrine release and activation of the sympathetic nervous system)	**Sign or Symptom** Tachycardia Pale, cool, clammy skin Sweating Tremors Weakness Palpitations Irritability Nervousness Tingling or warm sensation Hunger Nausea Vomiting
Neuroglucopenic (inadequate glucose available to brain cells)	**Sign or Symptom** Confusion Drowsiness Amnesia Impaired cognitive function Incoordination Headache Visual disturbance Irritation Aggressive behavior Depressed motor function Seizures Coma Strokelike symptoms

patient in a lateral recumbent position if the mental status is altered. Be prepared to suction.

2. If breathing is adequate, administer oxygen based on the SpO_2 reading and patient signs and symptoms. If the SpO_2 reading is greater than 95 percent and no signs or symptoms of hypoxia or respiratory distress are present, oxygen may not be necessary. If signs of hypoxia or respiratory distress are present, or the SpO_2 reading is less than 95 percent, apply a nasal cannula at 2 to 4 lpm. If breathing is inadequate (inadequate tidal volume or respiratory rate), immediately provide positive pressure ventilation with supplemental oxygen attached to the ventilation device.

3. If the patient is alert and responsive, is exhibiting signs and symptoms of hypoglycemia, has a blood glucose reading of less than 60 mg/dL, is able to obey your commands, and is able to swallow, administer oral glucose. If at any time the patient is unable to obey your commands or unable to swallow, immediately stop the administration of

the oral glucose and proceed with the next step.

4. If the patient has an altered mental status, initiate an intravenous line of normal saline at a to-keep-open rate. Draw blood according to your local protocol. Check the blood glucose level. If the BGL is less than 60 mg/dL, administer 25 grams of 50 percent dextrose in water ($D_{50}W$). In a child less than 8 years of age, administer 25 percent dextrose in water ($D_{25}W$) at a dose of 0.5 to 1 g/kg or 2 to 4 mL/kg. If $D_{25}W$ is not carried, it can be prepared by diluting $D_{50}W$ 1:1 with normal saline. If the patient is not alert following the administration of dextrose, and the BGL remains less than 60 mg/dL, administer a second dose of $D_{50}W$.

If an intravenous line cannot be established rapidly, 1 to 2 mg of glucagon can be administered intramuscularly. The pediatric dose of glucagon is 0.025 to 0.1 mg/kg intramuscularly. It can be repeated in adults and children every 20 minutes. Glucagon should be administered only if an intravenous line cannot be established. The onset of action of glucagon is 10 to 20 minutes, with a peak effect of 30 to 60 minutes.

Liver glycogen must be available for glucagon to be effective. Therefore, if glucagon was administered and then an intravenous line was established, proceed with the administration of intravenous dextrose.

intravenous line and administration of dextrose intravenously is a key component in the management of the patient. The following emergency care should be provided:

1. Establish and maintain a patent airway. Always be alert for vomiting and the potential for aspiration in any patient with an altered mental status. Place the

5. Transport the patient for further evaluation.

TRANSITIONING

REVIEW ITEMS

1. Your patient's blood glucose level is 180 mg/dL; however, there is a decrease in the amount of insulin being released from the pancreas and circulating in the blood. This will result in _____.

    a. an inadequate uptake of glucose by the brain cells

    b. an immediate decrease in the blood glucose level

    c. a reduction in the amount of glucose entering the cell

    d. an increase in the metabolism of glucose by the cell

2. Tachycardia associated with hypoglycemia occurs because of _____.

    a. a reduction in the insulin level in the blood

    b. secretion of epinephrine from the adrenal gland

    c. a reduction in the amount of blood volume

    d. cardiac failure from a low glucose state

3. In a nondiabetic patient, an increase in the blood glucose level will cause _____.

    a. the pancreas to secrete insulin

    b. the sympathetic nervous system to discharge

    c. a decrease in the heart rate

    d. an increase in the amount of circulating glucagon

4. Glucagon secretion will result in _____.

    a. a decrease in the uptake of glucose by the brain

    b. a reduction in the amount of circulating glucose

c. the cessation of metabolism of glucose by the cell

d. an increase in the circulating blood glucose level

5. The signs and symptoms exhibited by the hypoglycemic patient are a direct result of _____.

   a. an attempt by the pancreas to increase the insulin secretion

   b. brain cell dysfunction and the release of epinephrine

   c. an increase in the amount of glucagon circulating in the blood

   d. a reduction in the insulin level and release of glucagon

6. The adult dose of $D_{50}W$ is _____.

   a. 2–4 mL/kg

   b. 0.5–1 g/kg

   c. 10 grams

   d. 25 grams

7. You have confirmed the BGL reading at 38 mg/dL in a 5-year-old patient with an altered mental status. You have an intravenous line established. You should administer _____.

   a. 25 grams of $D_{50}W$

   b. 25 grams of $D_{25}W$

   c. 1 g/kg of $D_{50}W$

   d. 1 g/kg of $D_{25}W$

APPLIED PATHOPHYSIOLOGY

1. Explain the difference between type 1 and type 2 diabetes.

2. Explain the function of insulin and its effect on the blood glucose level.

3. Explain the function of glucagon and its effect on the blood glucose level.

4. Explain how a low blood glucose level affects the brain cells.

5. Explain the difference in the requirement for transport of glucose into a regular cell as compared with the brain cells.

6. Explain the two categories of signs and symptoms of hypoglycemia. List the signs and symptoms based on each category.

CLINICAL DECISION MAKING

You arrive on the scene and find a 23-year-old female patient in the bathroom of a bar. The patrons called 911 because the patient suddenly began to act strangely and became aggressive. She then fled to the bathroom, where she remains. As you approach the patient, she is sitting on the bathroom floor, slumped to her right side and talking incomprehensibly.

1. Based on the scene size-up, list the possible conditions you suspect.

2. What is your major concern when approaching this patient?

As you conduct the primary assessment, you note the patient is making incomprehensible sounds in an attempt to talk. Her airway is clear and her respirations are 18/minute with good chest rise. Her radial pulse is 128 bpm, and her skin is pale, cool, and clammy. Her SpO_2 reading is 98 percent on room air.

3. Are there any immediate life threats?

4. What emergency care should you provide, based on the primary assessment findings?

5. Explain possible causes for the incomprehensible sounds.

6. Explain possible causes for the pale, cool, and clammy skin.

7. Have you ruled out any conditions? What conditions are you still considering?

During the secondary assessment, you note no evidence of trauma to the head, the pupils are equal and reactive to light, and the mouth and nose are clear of any blood, vomitus, or secretions. The oral mucosa is pink. There is no evidence that the patient bit her tongue or oral cavity. There is no jugular vein distention, tracheal deviation, or subcutaneous emphysema. The breath sounds are equal and clear bilaterally, and the chest rise and fall are symmetrical. The abdomen is soft and nontender. You note multiple bruises to the abdomen in different areas. The peripheral pulses are present, and the patient moves all four extremities. The patient does not comply with a sensory test to the extremities. There is no evidence of trauma to the chest, abdomen, posterior thorax, or extremities. The blood pressure is 128/74 mmHg, heart rate is 132 bpm, and respirations are 18/minute with adequate chest rise. Her skin is more pale and cool. The patient is very diaphoretic. The blood glucose is 42 mg/dL. None of the bar patrons knows the patient well enough to provide any history.

8. Based on the assessment findings, what condition do you suspect?

9. Explain the reason for the following findings:

   a. Tachycardia

   b. Pale cool skin

   c. Diaphoresis

   d. Initial aggression

   e. Decrease in mental status

   f. Blood glucose level

10. Which cells are getting glucose, and which cells are being deprived of glucose?

11. What emergency care should you provide?

Standard Medicine

Competency Applies fundamental knowledge to provide basic and selected advanced emergency care and transportation based on assessment findings for an acutely ill patient.

ENDOCRINE EMERGENCIES: HYPERGLYCEMIC DISORDERS

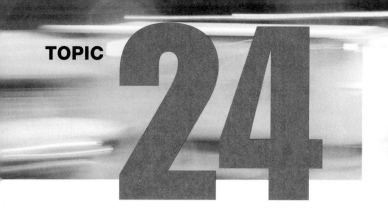

TRANSITION *highlights*

- *Frequency, age and gender distribution, and contributory causes of hyperglycemic episodes.*

- *The major pathophysiologic changes in a hyperglycemic patient with diabetic ketoacidosis:*
  - Metabolic acidosis.
  - Osmotic diuresis.
  - Electrolyte disturbances.

- *Symptomology of diabetic ketoacidosis (DKA).*

- *Major pathophysiologic changes in a hyperglycemic patient with hyperglycemic hyperosmolar nonketotic syndrome (HHNS).*

- *Signs and symptoms associated with DKA and HHNS.*

- *Common emergency care steps for the hyperglycemic patient suffering from either DKA or hyperosmolar hyperglycemic nonketotic coma (HHNC).*

INTRODUCTION

Hyperglycemia refers to conditions in which the blood glucose is excessively elevated beyond a normal level. It is on the opposite end of the continuum of diabetic emergencies as compared with hypoglycemia. Two acute hyperglycemic conditions that Advanced EMTs will encounter in the prehospital environment are diabetic ketoacidosis (DKA) and hyperglycemic hyperosmolar nonketotic *syndrome* (HHNS). HHNS is also frequently referred to as hyperglycemic hyperosmolar nonketotic *coma* (HHNC).

DKA and HHNS must be considered while forming a differential diagnosis when assessing and managing a patient with an altered mental status. This is especially true if the patient has a history of diabetes mellitus (DM). However, be aware that the onset of DKA or HHNS may be the first sign of DM in a patient with no known history. Thus, it is imperative to obtain a blood glucose reading on any patient with an altered mental status, especially if the patient appears to be dehydrated, regardless of a positive or negative history of DM.

In addition to the blood glucose reading, the history—particularly the onset—and physical assessment findings will contribute to the formulation of a differential diagnosis and the appropriate emergency management of the patient.

EPIDEMIOLOGY

Diabetic ketoacidosis most often occurs in type 1 DM. The onset is typically associated with some type of stressor to the body, such as trauma, infection, myocardial infarction, or stroke. Although it is not as common, DKA can occur in type 2 diabetes patients. In approximately 25 percent of cases of DKA, the patient has no known history of DM.

HHNS is most commonly found in elderly patients in their 70s who have type 2 DM; however, it has also been reported in pediatric patients as young as 18 months and in some with type 1 DM. The incidence of HHNS is higher than that of DKA, with 17.5 cases occurring for every 100,000 people. HHNS is slightly more prevalent in female patients than in male patients.

Elderly residents of nursing homes who have preexisting disease or an acute onset of illness—especially if associated with an infection, poor fluid intake, or an increase in urine output—and who are demented are at the highest risk for experiencing HHNS. The dementia typically causes poor fluid intake from a lack of recognition of dehydration. Any condition or illness that results in dehydration increases the risk of HHNS in the patient with type 2 DM, especially in the elderly. The mortality has been reported as high as 10 percent to 20 percent.

Approximately 20 percent to 33 percent of the patients who suffer an acute onset of HHNS have no previous history of DM. These patients are at the highest risk, as they often do not recognize the early warning signs and symptoms of the ensuing severe dehydration. When assessing a patient with signs and symptoms of dehydration, it is imperative to assess the blood glucose level regardless of a known medical history of DM. You may be the first person to initially diagnose the DM condition in the prehospital setting.

DIABETIC KETOACIDOSIS

Because of the variation in the pathology of the condition, the patient experiencing DKA presents significantly differently from one who is hypoglycemic. As with hypoglycemia, by understanding the basic pathophysiology of DKA, there is no need to memorize signs and symptoms to recognize and differentiate between the various conditions.

Pathophysiology of DKA

Unlike hypoglycemia, in which the insulin level is excessive and the blood glucose level is extremely low, diabetic ketoacidosis is associated with a relative or absolute insulin deficiency and a severely elevated blood glucose level, typically greater than 300 mg/dL. Because of the lack of insulin, tissue such as muscle, fat, and liver are unable to take up glucose. Even though the blood has an extremely elevated amount of circulating glucose, the cells are basically starving. Because the blood–brain barrier does not require insulin for glucose to diffuse across it, the brain cells are receiving more than an adequate amount of glucose.

Basically, the general body tissue is starving, whereas the brain has more than an adequate supply of glucose. Thus, the patient does not experience the sudden onset of mental status changes, cognitive and behavioral disturbances, or other brain cell dysfunction (neuroglucopenic) signs and symptoms associated with hypoglycemia.

Three major pathophysiologic syndromes associated with an excessively elevated blood glucose level in DKA contribute to the delay in onset and produce the majority of the signs and symptoms: metabolic acidosis, osmotic diuresis, and electrolyte disturbance.

METABOLIC ACIDOSIS In *metabolic acidosis*, cells are not receiving an adequate fuel source to produce energy because of the lack of insulin. Even though the blood is loaded with glucose, the cells go into a starvation mode. This triggers the release of glucagon and other counterregulatory hormones that promote the breakdown of triglycerides into free fatty acids and initiate gluconeogenesis to produce more glucose for the starving cells. This further elevates the blood glucose level, as the body begins to metabolize protein and fat to produce a source of energy.

Because of the insulin deficiency and release of large amounts of glucagon, free fatty acids circulate in abundance in the blood and are metabolized into acetoacetic acid and B-hydroxybutric acid, both of which are strong organic acids and are referred to as *ketones*. Acetone, produced as acetoacetic acid, is metabolized and begins to accumulate in the blood. Small amounts of acetone are released in the respiration and produce the characteristic fruity breath odor.

In normal metabolism, ketones would be used as fuel in the peripheral tissue; however, because of the starvation state of the cells the ketones are not used. An increase in ketone production and a decrease in peripheral cell use lead to a metabolic acidosis that is referred to as *ketoacidosis*. This is reflected in a decreasing pH value, typically less than 7.40. The patient will also begin to eliminate large amounts of ketones through excretion in the urine.

OSMOTIC DIURESIS *Osmosis* refers to the movement of water (solvent) across a semipermeable membrane from a low particle concentration to a high particle concentration. *Diuresis* refers to urination, which is typically excessive. When the blood glucose level reaches approximately 225 mg/dL, a significant amount of glucose spills over into the urine. A glucose molecule (particle) produces an osmotic effect by drawing water across a semipermeable membrane. As an excessive amount of glucose enters the renal tubules, it draws a large amount of water, which ends up producing a significant amount of urine. This is known as *osmotic diuresis* and leads to volume depletion and dehydration in the patient.

ELECTROLYTE DISTURBANCE Also collecting in the urine is a large amount of ketones. Because ketones are strong organic acids, they must be buffered to be excreted. Sodium is typically used as the buffer. Where sodium goes, water follows. Therefore, the sodium used to buffer the ketones also draws a large amount of water into the renal tubules, producing excessive urine and leading to further volume depletion and dehydration. The loss of large amounts of fluid because of osmotic diuresis leads to further *electrolyte disturbance* and the excretion of other electrolytes, such as potassium, calcium, magnesium, and phosphorus. This produces electrolyte imbalance and disturbances.

The term *diabetic ketoacidosis* literally explains what the patient is experiencing. The term *diabetes* is often thought of as dealing with a glucose derangement or imbalance. However, that is not true. *Diabetes* simply means an increase in urine output. Thus, the *diabetic* in DKA implies an increase in urine output that occurs from osmotic diuresis. The term *ketoacidosis* is fairly self-explanatory. It refers to the metabolic acidosis resulting from ketone production from fat metabolism.

The diabetic ketoacidosis patient is therefore prone to metabolic acidosis from ketone production, severe dehydration from osmotic diuresis, and electrolyte disturbances. These pathophysiologic syndromes produce the signs and symptoms exhibited by the patient.

Assessment Findings Associated with DKA

Unlike the hypoglycemic patient who experiences a sudden onset (within minutes) of signs and symptoms when the supply of glucose to the brain is severely depleted, the DKA patient's brain has a very large and abundant supply of glucose. The slow and gradual onset of signs and symptoms associated with diabetic ketoacidosis is related to the accumulating effect of the dehydration from osmotic diuresis and buildup of acid from ketone production. As the cells slowly become dehydrated and acidotic, the signs and symptoms begin to appear. As the brain cells slowly dehydrate and are affected by the increasing acidic state over hours to days, the mental status slowly begins to become altered.

Osmotic diuresis typically produces the classic signs and symptoms of hyperglycemia:

- Polyuria (excessive urination)
- Polydipsia (excessive drinking of fluids)
- Constant thirst
- Frequent urination at night

Osmotic diuresis leads to dehydration and a potential hypovolemic state from fluid loss, producing the following signs:

- Dry and warm skin
- Poor skin turgor

> **Elderly residents of nursing homes who have preexisting disease or an acute onset of illness and who are demented are at the highest risk for experiencing HHNS.**

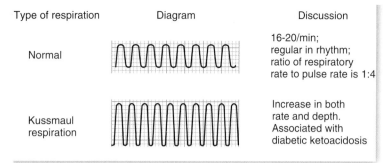

Type of respiration	Diagram	Discussion
Normal		16-20/min; regular in rhythm; ratio of respiratory rate to pulse rate is 1:4
Kussmaul respiration		Increase in both rate and depth. Associated with diabetic ketoacidosis

Figure 24-1 Kussmaul respirations.

- Dry mucous membranes
- Tachycardia
- Hypotension
- Decreased sweating
- Orthostatic vital signs

Other signs and symptoms include the following:

- Nausea and vomiting
- Abdominal pain (especially in children, caused by gastric distention or stretching of the liver capsule)
- Fatigue
- Weakness
- Lethargy
- Confusion

Kussmaul respirations are deep and rapid respirations that are an attempt to compensate for the increasing ketoacidosis (▶ **Figure 24-1**). The deep and rapid respiratory rate blows off carbon dioxide. Carbon dioxide is necessary for the production of carbonic acid. With the decreased availability of carbon dioxide, less carbonic acid is produced, thereby increasing the pH value and allowing more ketoacids to accumulate.

Another common sign is a fruity or acetone odor on the breath. This is a direct result of small amounts of acetone being disposed of through respiration.

ECG changes and dysrhythmias may also result from the electrolyte disturbance.

HYPERGLYCEMIC HYPEROSMOLAR NON-KETOTIC SYNDROME

HHNS is another emergency that the DM patient may experience. Although the condition is also commonly referred to as hyperglycemic hyperosmolar nonketotic coma (HHNC), fewer than 10 percent of patients with HHNS truly become comatose. As the name implies, this condition is associated with an excessively elevated blood glucose level and hyperosmolar extracellular fluid (ECF) without the production and accumulation of a mass amount of ketones in the blood. The primary pathophysiology associated with the condition produces severe dehydration and electrolyte disturbances.

Pathophysiology of HHNS

HHNS is associated with severe elevations in the blood glucose level, often exceeding 600 mg/dL, from an absolute or relative insulin deficiency or from a decreased response of the tissue to the circulating insulin (insulin resistance). This results in glycogenolysis, gluconeogenesis, and a decreased uptake of glucose by the peripheral tissue. A decline in renal function, which is typically found in elderly patients or in patients with renal disease, also contributes to a decrease in glucose clearance. Glycogenolysis may have a limited contribution to the hyperglycemic state, as many of the patients are debilitated or suffering from an acute illness and have a poor diet for several days, causing the glycogen stores in the liver to be depleted over time.

The elevated blood glucose level creates a hyperosmolar extracellular space that begins to pull fluid and dehydrate the intracellular space. Initially, this influx of fluid into the intravascular space will maintain the blood pressure and perfusion. Once the blood glucose level exceeds 180 to 250 mg/dL, a significant amount of glucose spills off into the urine. As the osmotic diuresis continues, the intravascular volume is profoundly depleted, which further decreases renal perfusion and the ability of the kidneys to remove glucose from the blood. The average fluid loss is typically 9 to 10 liters in a 70-kg patient. A common cause of death is circulatory collapse.

Because of a change in the serum osmotic pressure, potassium, sodium, chloride, phosphate, magnesium and bicarbonate may be depleted from the tissues, even though the serum electrolyte levels may appear to be normal or elevated. Sodium, potassium, phosphate, and magnesium are typically lost during the osmotic diuresis, leading to electrolyte imbalances.

Unlike a patient with DKA, the patient with HHNS does not develop ketoacidosis. There are many theories about why there is a lack of ketogenesis; however, the exact cause is not well understood. It is thought that the continued secretion and availability of small amounts of insulin decrease the mass release of counterregulatory hormones and reduce the availability of free fatty acids needed to produce ketones. With no ketoacidosis the patient will not present with Kussmaul respirations or a fruity (acetone) odor on the breath.

Pneumonia, chronic renal insufficiency, gastrointestinal bleeding, urinary tract infection, and sepsis are common precipitating factors of HHNS. Factors that stress the body, such as trauma and burns, will trigger a stress response, releasing a number of hormones (epinephrine, cortisol, and glucagon) that have a tendency to counter the effects of insulin and raise the blood glucose level. Other common underlying causes are

- Stroke
- Myocardial infarction
- Intracranial hemorrhage
- Cushing syndrome
- Poor compliance with oral hypoglycemics or insulin therapy
- Hemorrhage
- Elder abuse or neglect, leading to underhydration
- Renal disease
- Dialysis
- Diuretics
- Beta blockers
- Histamine-2 (H_2) blockers
- Glucocorticoids
- Phenytoin
- Immunosuppressants

Assessment Findings Associated with HHNS

The clinical presentation of HHNS is related to volume depletion and dehydration with a slow onset of the signs and symptoms, usually progressing over a few days. In the early phase of HHNS, the signs and symptoms may be vague, such as leg cramps, weakness, and visual disturbances. As the blood glucose level continues to increase and the patient dehydrates further, the signs and symptoms usually progress in severity to include an alteration in the mental status. Other signs and symptoms include the following:

- Thirst
- Fever (may suggest sepsis or infection as the predisposing factor)
- Polyuria (early)
- Oliguria (often a late sign of a severe dehydrated state)
- Drowsiness, confusion, lethargy, or coma
- Focal seizures that may be continuous (epilepsia partialis continua) or intermittent
- Generalized seizures
- Hemiparesis or sensory deficits
- Tachycardia
- Orthostatic hypotension
- Hypotension (late signs of profound dehydration)
- Poor skin turgor (not a reliable sign in the elderly)
- Dry skin and mucous membranes
- Sunken eyes
- Excessively elevated blood glucose level

EMERGENCY MEDICAL CARE

The signs and symptoms of DKA and HHNS are much more similar to each other than to those of hypoglycemia (see Table 24-1). The focus in emergency care for hypoglycemia is administration of glucose, whereas in DKA and HHNS, the prehospital focus is on rehydrating the patient. Emergency care for both diabetic ketoacidosis and HHNS may include the following:

1. **Establish and maintain a patent airway.** If the patient presents with an altered mental status or is comatose, it may be necessary to establish an airway by a manual maneuver and, in patients with severely altered mental states, potentially with a mechanical device. Altered mental states may lead to aspiration of secretions and warrant the use of an advanced airway.
2. **Establish and maintain adequate ventilation.** If the patient's respiratory rate or tidal volume is inadequate, it is necessary to provide positive pressure ventilation.
3. **Establish and maintain adequate oxygenation.** Assess the patient for evidence of hypoxia. Apply a pulse oximeter and determine the SpO2 reading. If either clinical evidence of hypoxia exists, the patient complains of dyspnea or exhibits signs or respiratory distress, or an SpO2 reading of less than 95 percent on room air is present, administer oxygen via a nasal cannula at 2 to 4 lpm. Titrate the oxygen by increasing the liter flow and possibly changing the delivery device to maintain an SpO2 greater than 95 percent, and abolish the signs of respiratory distress or complaint of dyspnea.
4. **Assess the blood glucose level.** In any patient with preexisting disease who presents with signs and symptoms of dehydration or an altered mental status, especially the elderly, the blood glucose must be checked, regardless of a positive history of diabetes mellitus. DKA and HHNS may be the first indication that the patient has DM. Even though the major complication of the disease is severe dehydration, HHNS carries the highest mortality rate of the diabetic emergencies.

> **Unlike a patient with DKA, the patient with HHNS does not develop ketoacidosis.**

5. **Initiate an intravenous line of normal saline.** Draw blood according to your local protocol. If the patient is hypotensive, administer fluid to maintain the systolic blood pressure above 100 mmHg; otherwise, infuse fluid at a rate of 1 to 2 liters over 1 to 3 hours. In pediatric patients, administer a 20 mL/kg fluid bolus over 1 hour. Be sure to monitor the patient's breath sounds for an indication of fluid overload, especially in the elderly and those with heart disease. If the patient begins to complain of dyspnea, and crackles (rales) are heard in the posterior lower lobes, reduce the amount and rate of fluid being infused.

TABLE 24-1	Signs and Symptoms of Diabetic Emergency Conditions		
Sign or Symptom	**DKA**	**HHNS**	**Hypoglycemia**
Onset	Slow, over days	Slow, over days	Sudden, over minutes
Heart rate	Tachycardia	Tachycardia	Tachycardia
Blood pressure	Low	Low	Normal
Respirations	Kussmaul	Normal	Normal or shallow
Breath odor	Sweet and fruity	None	None
Mental status	Coma (very late)	Confusion	Bizarre behavior, agitated, aggressive, altered, unresponsive
Oral mucosa	Dry	Dry	Salivation
Thirst	Intense	Intense	Absent
Vomiting	Common	Common	Uncommon
Abdominal pain	Common	Uncommon	Absent
Insulin level	Low	Low	High
Blood glucose level	High	Very high	Very low

Emergency care and patient needs	**DKA**	**HHNS**	**Hypoglycemia**
Basic care	Oxygen	Oxygen	Oxygen, oral glucose
ALS care	Fluids	Fluids	IV glucose
Patient needs	More insulin	More insulin	Glucose

TRANSITIONING

REVIEW ITEMS

1. A sign that is common to both DKA and HHNS is _____.
   a. a fruity odor on the breath
   b. warm, flushed skin
   c. Kussmaul respirations
   d. dry oral mucosa

2. Orthostatic hypotension found in both the DKA and HHNS patient is caused by _____.
   a. vasodilation
   b. osmotic diuresis
   c. hyperventilation
   d. cellular hypoxia

3. A large amount of glucose in the vascular space will cause _____.
   a. interstitial fluid to be drawn into the vessel
   b. intravascular fluid to leave the vessel

   c. the vessel to constrict
   d. the vessel to dilate

4. The excessive blood glucose level seen in DKA is typically a result of _____.
   a. too little glucagon production
   b. an excessive amount of insulin
   c. an excessive amount of glucagon
   d. an inadequate amount of insulin

5. Why is metabolic acidosis not typically found in the HHNS patient?
   a. The blood glucose level is not as high as in DKA.
   b. The patient is still producing and secreting some insulin.
   c. Fat cannot be metabolized without insulin available to the cells.
   d. No fat is available for the liver to metabolize.

APPLIED PATHOPHYSIOLOGY

1. Explain the three major pathophysiologic conditions that occur in DKA.

2. Why is glucagon secreted from the pancreas in DKA when the blood glucose level is already significantly elevated?

3. Explain why the onset of the signs and symptoms of DKA occur over days, as compared with minutes in hypoglycemia.

4. Differentiate between the pathophysiology of DKA and HHNS.

5. What causes excessive dehydration in both DKA and HHNS?

6. Why doesn't the HHNS patient experience a severe metabolic acidosis as in the DKA patient?

CLINICAL DECISION MAKING

You are called to a residence and find a 14-year-old male patient lying supine in bed. The parents state that he has not been feeling well for the past week or so. He has gotten much worse over the past two days. The parents thought it was a virus their son picked up from school. As you approach the patient, he is not alert. His breathing appears to be extremely fast and deep.

1. Based on the scene size-up, list the conditions that are possible.

During the primary assessment, you find that the patient responds to verbal stimuli with incomprehensible words, has an intact airway, and has a respiratory rate of 32/minute. His breathing is very deep and full. His radial pulse is weak and rapid. His skin is warm, dry, and flushed. The SpO₂ reading is 99 percent on room air.

2. Are there any immediate life threats?

3. What emergency care should you provide based on the primary assessment findings?

4. Explain possible causes for the respiratory rate and tidal volume.

5. What do the skin signs indicate?

6. Have you ruled out any conditions? What conditions are you still considering?

As you perform the secondary assessment, you note no evidence of trauma to the head; the pupils are midsize, equal, and reactive to light; and the mouth and nose are clear of any blood, vomitus, or secretions. The oral mucosa is pink but excessively dry. The tongue is furrowed. You note a peculiar odor on the breath that smells like fruity gum. The jugular veins are flat with the patient in a supine position. There is no tracheal deviation or subcutaneous emphysema. The breath sounds are equal and clear bilaterally, and the chest rise and fall are symmetrical. The abdomen is soft; however, the patient makes a facial grimace when you palpate the right upper quadrant. The peripheral pulses are barely palpable, and the patient moves all four extremities to a painful stimulus. There is no evidence of trauma to the chest, abdomen, posterior thorax, or extremities. The blood pressure is 82/64 mmHg, heart rate is 136 bpm, and respirations are 34/minute with a deep and full tidal volume. The skin is warm and dry and appears flushed. The blood glucose is 482 mg/dL. The parents indicate that the patient has no known medical history and takes no medications. He has not been feeling good for the past week or so and has felt worse over the past few days.

7. Based on the assessment findings, what condition do you suspect?

8. Explain the reason for the following findings:
   a. Tachycardia
   b. Warm, flushed skin

c. Decrease in mental status
d. Blood glucose level
e. Rapid deep respirations
f. Hypotension
g. Dry oral mucosa and furrowed tongue
h. Right upper quadrant pain

9. Which cells are getting glucose, and which cells are being deprived of glucose?

10. What emergency care should you provide?

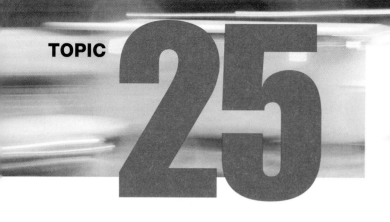

TOPIC

25

Standard Medicine

Competency Applies fundamental knowledge to provide basic and selected advanced emergency care and transportation based on assessment findings for an acutely ill patient.

PSYCHIATRIC DISORDERS

TRANSITION *highlights*

- *Overview of the frequency of psychiatric disorders in general, and the incidence of certain psychiatric conditions specifically.*

- *Basic pathophysiology of psychiatric disorders, as well as the changes seen in specific emergencies:*
  - Psychosis and schizophrenia.
  - Mood and anxiety disorders.
  - Somatoform disorders.
  - Factitious disorders.
  - Dissociative disorders.
  - Sexual and gender identity disorders.
  - Eating disorders.
  - Impulse control disorders.
  - Personality disorders.
  - Attention deficit hyperactivity disorders.
  - Autism spectrum disorders.
  - Substance related disorders.
  - Alzheimer disease.
  - Suicide.

- *Assessment and management of a patient with an acute psychiatric disorder.*

INTRODUCTION

Mental disorders are characterized by abnormalities in cognition, emotion, mood, or behavior. People with psychiatric disorders may display a wide variety of symptoms, which can influence how they behave and interact within society. By understanding the difference in various types of psychiatric conditions, the Advanced EMT can better assess and manage patients with these conditions. The patient with an apparent psychiatric complaint should always be screened for hidden medical conditions. The patient with a psychiatric condition will often require additional

communication skills, patience, and compassion from the AEMT (▶ Figure 25-1).

EPIDEMIOLOGY

Mental disorders affect an estimated one in every four adults in a given year. They are the leading cause of disability in the United States for those between the ages of 15 and 44. It is estimated that 48 percent of people with a mental disorder suffer from more than one diagnosable disorder. Many of these disorders co-occur with another psychiatric condition. Mental health–related chief complaints account for more than 6 percent of all emergency department visits, and this number is rising steadily. Among emergency mental health visits, substance-related disorders (30 percent), mood disorders (23 percent), anxiety disorders (21 percent), psychosis (10 percent), and suicide attempts (7 percent) are the most common.

PATHOPHYSIOLOGY

Unlike most medical conditions, many psychiatric conditions have no known cause. Many researchers believe that psychiatric conditions are caused by the interaction of a number of biological

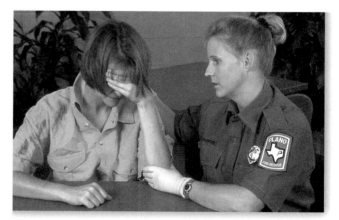

Figure 25-1 The patient with a mental disorder will require additional communication skills, patience, and compassion. Touch may be comforting to some patients, but do not touch a patient without the patient's consent.

and environmental factors. Some researchers believe that an individual's ability to cope with stress properly is also a factor in mental illness.

Physicians currently use the *Diagnostic and Statistical Manual of Mental Disorders, Fourth Edition, Text Revision* to diagnose psychiatric diseases. Psychiatric, medical, and psychosocial information is used during the evaluation. Medical disorders such as hypercalcemia, hypercarbia, hypoglycemia, hypoxia, hypothermia, lupus, organ failure, cerebrovascular disease, epilepsy, Huntington disease, multiple sclerosis, Parkinson disease, Addison disease, Cushing disease, and thyroid and parathyroid diseases, among others, must be ruled out as causes of the patient's condition before it is attributed to a mental illness.

Treatment for patients with psychiatric conditions often involves a combination of medications, therapies, counseling, and social support. Many patients with these conditions may not have access to proper medical treatment or may relapse. If left untreated, some disorders can result in dangerous behaviors or life-threatening complications.

Types of Psychiatric Disorders

PSYCHOSIS AND SCHIZOPHRENIA
Disturbances of perception and thought process fall into a broad category of symptoms referred to as *psychosis*. Schizophrenia is the most recognized psychotic disorder, affecting 1.1 percent of the population. It affects men and women equally; the onset usually occurs late in adolescence or in early adulthood. *Schizophrenia* is a complex illness or group of disorders characterized by bizarre hallucinations, delusions, behavioral disturbances, disrupted social functioning, lack of emotions, and other associated symptoms. *Schizo-affective disorder* is an illness that combines symptoms of schizophrenia with a major affective disorder such as major depression or bipolar disorder.

MOOD DISORDERS
Mood, or affective, disorders primarily reflect disturbances in one's mood, feelings, or tone. Approximately 9.5 percent of American adults in a given year have a mood disorder. Some of the main types include major depressive disorder, dysthymia, and bipolar disorder. *Major depressive disorder* is characterized by the deep and persistent presence of depressed mood

or loss of interest, changes in sleep or appetite, poor self-esteem, feelings of guilt, fatigue, poor concentration, hopelessness, despair, and thoughts of suicide. It affects women more than men. *Dysthymic disorder*, or dysthymia, is a chronic milder form of depression.

Bipolar disorder, also known as manic-depressive illness, is identified by shifts in a person's mood from periods of mania to depression. Manic episodes often include elated, euphoric, or grandiose thoughts and behaviors. During periods of depression, the patient may become withdrawn and show a lack of interest in life.

ANXIETY DISORDERS
Anxiety disorders include panic disorder, obsessive-compulsive disorder, posttraumatic stress disorder, generalized anxiety disorder, and phobias. They are the most common mental health problem in the United States, affecting about 18.1 percent of American adults. Most of these disorders appear during early adulthood. A *phobia* is an excessive and unreasonable degree of fear triggered either by exposure to or anticipation of a specific object or circumstance. People with specific phobias realize that their level of fear is excessive, but they still try to avoid any exposure to the feared object or circumstance.

Panic disorder is characterized by the presence of recurrent panic attacks. A panic attack is a sudden and intense burst of anxiety or fear that is accompanied by physical symptoms such as tachycardia, palpitations, dizziness, dyspnea, and diaphoresis. These attacks are often accompanied by a feeling of impending doom. A panic attack by itself is not considered to be a psychiatric disorder and can occur without being part of any syndrome.

Obsessive-compulsive disorder is characterized by recurrent, unwanted thoughts (obsessions) and/or repetitive behaviors (compulsions). The patient often performs repetitive behaviors such as hand washing, counting, checking, or cleaning in the hope of preventing or dismissing the obsessions.

Posttraumatic stress disorder involves the delayed response to an external traumatic event that produced extreme distress in an individual. This disorder occurs frequently after violent assaults, rapes, terrorism, natural or human disasters, and accidents. Patients with this condition often avoid remembering the event and can exhibit physiologic responses to any reminder of it.

Generalized anxiety disorder is characterized by persistent, excessive worry and tension events that can have an impact on one's daily life. Common worries concern financial matters, work or school, relationships, minor personal matters, health and safety issues, and community or world affairs.

Agoraphobia involves intense fear and anxiety of any place or situation from which escape might be difficult. This leads to the avoidance of situations such as being alone outside the home, traveling in a vehicle, or being in a crowded place.

Social phobia is characterized by the persistent fear and avoidance of a specific object or situation that involves performance, evaluation, or being judged by others. Almost 9 percent of adults have a social phobia, which typically began in childhood.

SOMATOFORM DISORDERS
Somatoform disorders are characterized by bodily symptoms that suggest a physical disorder but for which no underlying organic causes or known physiologic mechanisms can be found. The symptoms are presumed to be linked to psychological factors or conflict and are involuntarily produced by the patient. Some somatoform disorders include conversion disorder, somatoform pain disorder, somatization disorder, undifferentiated somatoform disorder, and hypochondriasis.

FACTITIOUS DISORDERS
Factitious disorders involve the conscious production of symptoms with the primary motivation of assuming the sick role and receiving treatment. Symptoms may be physical, psychological, or both. *Munchausen syndrome by proxy* involves a parent's projection of symptoms onto a child to indirectly assume the sick role. *Malingering* is characterized by intentionally producing symptoms for financial, legal, or personal gain.

DISSOCIATIVE DISORDERS
Dissociative disorders involve disturbances in memory, awareness, or sense of identity. Dissociation is a response, usually involving

> A panic attack is a sudden and intense burst of anxiety or fear that is accompanied by physical symptoms such as tachycardia, palpitations, dizziness, dyspnea, and diaphoresis.

stress or trauma, in which the mind attempts to distance or separate itself from the event or problem. Major dissociative conditions include dissociative identity disorder (formerly multiple personality disorder), dissociative amnesia, dissociative fugue, and depersonalization disorder.

SEXUAL AND GENDER IDENTITY DISORDERS
Sexual disorders are common in both men and women and are associated with significant distress or impairment. Sexual disorders include sexual dysfunction, paraphilias, and gender identity disorder. Gender identity disorders are conditions in which an individual feels a strong connection and desire to be the other sex.

EATING DISORDERS
An eating disorder is marked by extreme disturbances in eating behavior. Women are more likely than men to be diagnosed with an eating disorder. Anorexia nervosa, bulimia nervosa, and binge eating disorder are the three main types of eating disorders. *Anorexia nervosa* is characterized by a refusal to maintain, or attain, a minimally healthful body weight. *Bulimia nervosa* is characterized by recurrent episodes of binge eating followed by attempts to prevent weight gain or purging. *Binge eating disorder* is characterized by recurrent episodes of binge eating with no recurrent behaviors to purge calories or to prevent weight gain.

IMPULSE CONTROL DISORDERS
Impulsivity is the inability to resist an action that could be harmful to oneself or to others. Impulse control disorders are characterized by a building of tension around the desire to carry out any impulsive act that is relieved or gratified by engaging in the activity. There may be guilt, remorse, or self-reproach after the act. The six impulse-control disorders are *intermittent explosive disorder, kleptomania, pyromania, pathological gambling, trichotillomania,* and *impulse control disorders not otherwise specified.*

PERSONALITY DISORDERS
Personality disorders affect between 10 percent and 15 percent of the general population. Personality disorders are marked by patterns of maladaptive behaviors that deviate from the norms of society. Many patients display traits of more than one personality disorder. *Cluster A personality disorders* share the common features of being odd and eccentric. *Cluster B personality disorders* share features of being dramatic, emotional, and erratic. *Cluster C personality disorders* involve being anxious and fearful.

ATTENTION DEFICIT HYPERACTIVITY DISORDER
Attention deficit hyperactivity disorder (ADHD) is one of the most common mental disorders that develop in children. Children with ADHD have impaired functioning in relationships with peers and in multiple settings, including home and school. Although primarily seen in childhood, this disorder affects 4.1 percent of adults. ADHD is characterized by impulsiveness, hyperactivity, inattention, or a combination of the three.

AUTISM SPECTRUM DISORDERS
Autism spectrum disorders, or pervasive developmental disorders, cause severe impairments in thinking, feeling, language, and the ability to relate to others. These disorders are usually identified in early childhood and range in severity. *Autism* is the most severe form; *Asperger syndrome* is a milder form. Autism spectrum disorders are four times more prevalent in males than in females.

SUBSTANCE-RELATED DISORDERS
Substance-related disorders affect a large number of adults, half of whom have other underlying mental health conditions. The overindulgence in or dependence on the chemicals can negatively affect the physical and psychological well-being of the patient. Withdrawal from some substances, such as alcohol, benzodiazepines, or barbiturates, may also cause life-threatening conditions. Impaired judgment, altered mood, and inappropriate behaviors are commonly portrayed by these patients, who may pose a threat to themselves or others.

ALZHEIMER DISEASE
Alzheimer disease is a degenerative disease that affects 4.5 million Americans. It is the most common cause of dementia for people over age 65. The disease is gradual and progressive and produces a loss of mental and physical functioning. Memory, reasoning, personality, speech, movement, and functioning deteriorate over a period of years and lead to a dependency on others for survival.

Remember that not all dementia in the elderly is related to Alzheimer disease; in many cases, a medical condition (such as urinary tract infection, myocardial infarction, or stroke) is implicated. Furthermore, although Alzheimer disease is a condition that can cause symptoms similar to a psychiatric emergency, it is not truly a psychiatric condition.

SUICIDE
Suicide is a major preventable health problem that claims the lives of 33,000 people a year. More than 90 percent of suicide victims have diagnosable mental health disorders. Men are four times more likely than women to commit suicide; however, women are two to three times more likely to attempt it. Those who survive suicide attempts are often left with serious injuries that require medical attention.

ASSESSMENT FINDINGS
It is imperative for the AEMT to properly assess the patient to ensure that no underlying traumatic or medical condition is responsible for the presenting signs and symptoms. When in doubt, it is best to err on the side of the patient and treat him as if an underlying medical or traumatic cause (if suspected) is responsible for his behavior. During the assessment, the AEMT should focus on identifying, ensuring, maintaining, and supporting the vital functions of the patient's airway, breathing, and circulation (▶ Figure 25-2).

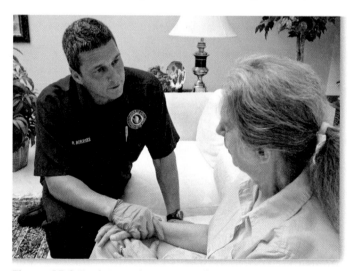

Figure 25-2 Explain to the patient who you are and maintain a nonjudgmental attitude. Assess the patient for trauma or a medical condition. Err on the side of the patient. (© *Craig Jackson/In the Dark Photography*)

The signs and symptoms seen in patients with mental health problems will vary with each individual. Overall, the signs and symptoms can impair the personal, social, and occupational functioning of the patient. The AEMT should remain respectful, empathic, and nonjudgmental. When performing your assessment, pay particular attention to the following:

- **Gaining consent for treatment.** A greater in-depth analysis of your patient's decisional capacity may be needed before appropriate informed consent or informed refusal of care can be obtained.

- **Assessing the mental status of the patient.** In addition to your normal assessment, note the patient's mood, posture, eye contact, dress, grooming, and facial expression. Be sure to note abnormal speech or movements (▶ Figure 25-3).

- **Conducting the verbal interview.** Significant information that will be used throughout the patient's care can be obtained from the interview. Unusual thoughts, suicidal or homicidal ideations, hallucinations, delusions, and phobias may be disclosed by the patient. Document all findings objectively. It may be necessary to obtain some information from family or bystanders about the patient's history, medications, behaviors, or norms. Take into consideration what information is disclosed and from whom the information is received.

RESTRAINT AND PATIENT SAFETY

Although techniques for de-escalation and calming often prevent the need for restraint, there are situations in which restraint becomes necessary.

The core principle behind restraint is that it is done safely and without harm to the patient or those providing the restraint. In many systems, the police are responsible for providing the restraint. EMS should not be directly involved with violent patients or those with weapons of any kind. As an experienced provider, though, you are likely also aware that EMS often does assist police and health professionals in restraint. When doing so, remember the following additional principles:

- Restraint should use only the force and techniques necessary to achieve the restraint effectively.
- Communicate with the patient during the process. Reassure the patient.
- Develop a plan before beginning restraint. Communicate with other personnel on scene to ensure efficient use of responders. Make sure that there is a safe escape if the violence escalates.
- Restrain patients face up.
- Do not bind the patient in a way that will restrict breathing. Do not hog-tie the patient.
- Use soft restraints (not handcuffs or flex cuffs).
- Monitor the restrained patient continuously. Patients who are agitated and then suddenly calm down may actually be experiencing a medical emergency and be near death (as discussed later).
- Restraint should never be punitive.

Agitated delirium is a term used to describe a condition that ultimately leads to the death of a patient with an apparent psychiatric emergency. It is often seen with those who have used drugs such as cocaine and has also been casually related to patients who have had sudden and

significant physical exertion (e.g., foot pursuit by police).

The patient will have the appearance of a psychiatric patient with psychotic behavior or hallucinations. Feats of "superhuman strength" have also been reported. An elevated body temperature is often present. This behavior usually ceases rapidly when the patient experiences respiratory arrest and death. These deaths in custody may be preventable and are a significant cause of liability for EMS providers and agencies.

In EMS, a common scenario occurs when an ambulance responds to assist police with a person in custody, due to an initial report of a psychiatric patient or an arrest. The patient is agitated and restrained by police (often handcuffed behind the back). The patient remains agitated and is transferred to the stretcher. Because the patient is agitated, police are hesitant to remove the handcuffs. When the patient "calms down," it is often because of respiratory arrest. Cardiac arrest quickly follows.

Even though there are many theories—and, likely, multiple causes—of death during restraint, AEMTs must follow the steps described here and monitor the patients closely for the entire time they are in their care.

EMERGENCY MEDICAL CARE

The treatment for a patient with a psychiatric condition will depend on the presenting signs and symptoms. If life threats exist, they should be managed immediately. The AEMT should identify any illnesses or injuries and treat them appropriately. Psychiatric conditions should be a secondary consideration to any underlying cause presented by the patient. If there is no illness or injury, the prehospital management of the patient with a psychiatric condition will be primarily supportive. Emergency care may include the following:

- **Safety of the provider and the patient is paramount.** Look for hazards within the scene that may indicate suicidal or homicidal intentions. Enlist the aid of trained public safety personnel if needed. This is particularly true if the patient verbalizes suicidal or homicidal thoughts.

- **Assess the patient for trauma or a medical condition.** Treat suspected

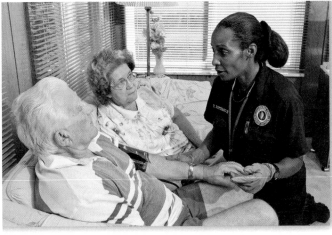

Figure 25-3 Be sure to note the patient's mood, posture, eye contact, dress, grooming, and facial expression.

traumatic or medical conditions appropriately.

- **If necessary, use restraints based on protocol.** Always use restraints appropriately and respect your patient. Never use restraints as a substitute for observation.

- **Provide a supportive environment for the patient to receive care.**

- **Transport the patient to a facility where he can get the necessary physical and psychological treatment.**

TRANSITIONING

REVIEW ITEMS

1. A patient states that he has lost interest in his normal activities, has withdrawn from family and friends, has lost his job, and has felt worthless for months. He states he has no desire to live. Based on his statements, you should suspect the patient may have _____.
   - a. major depressive disorder
   - b. agoraphobia
   - c. dissociative identity disorder
   - d. attention deficit hyperactivity disorder

2. A 64-year-old female patient presents with tachycardia, dyspnea, palpitations, diaphoresis, and anxiety. She tells you that her chest feels heavy and hurts. While obtaining her history, she discloses that she has a history of panic attacks. You should first suspect that the patient _____.
   - a. may have a somatoform disorder
   - b. may be having a heart attack
   - c. needs a psychiatrist
   - d. may be having a panic attack

3. Which of the following is *not* a physiologic response one might have to anxiety?
   - a. diaphoresis
   - b. bradycardia
   - c. palpitations
   - d. vertigo

4. Your patient has odd and bizarre behavior, delusions, hallucinations, and a flat affect. Which of the following psychological conditions might you suspect your patient could have?
   - a. social phobia
   - b. dysthymia
   - c. schizophrenia
   - d. gender identity disorder

5. Your patient's mother states that her teenage daughter has been hiding food and vomiting after meals. The mother states that she has found empty bottles of laxatives throughout the house. She states she has not noticed a change in her daughter's weight over the past month but is concerned because her daughter has been complaining of stomachaches and a bad sore throat. In addition to physical complications, you suspect the patient may have which of the following?
   - a. bulimia nervosa
   - b. binge eating disorder
   - c. anorexia nervosa
   - d. a factitious disorder

APPLIED PATHOPHYSIOLOGY

1. Discuss how a patient's impulsivity may negatively affect an emergency call.

2. Explain the difference between schizophrenia and dissociative identity disorder.

3. What information should be documented when assessing a patient's mental status?

4. Explain why it is important to ensure that no underlying traumatic or medical condition is responsible for the patient's signs and symptoms.

5. Differentiate between a mood disorder and an anxiety disorder.

CLINICAL DECISION MAKING

You are dispatched on a hot summer day to a local street corner for a patient behaving inappropriately. The call was placed by a passerby. As you and your partner approach the area, from a distance you notice a male in the middle of the road pacing back and forth.

1. Based on the scene size-up characteristics, list the possible conditions you suspect the patient is experiencing.

After securing a safe scene, you cautiously approach the patient. He appears to be about 25 years old and is dressed in several long layers,

with his buttons improperly fastened. The patient appears anxious and confused and keeps mumbling a phrase that makes no sense as he continues to pace back and forth in the road.

2. What are the life threats to this patient?

3. What immediate emergency care should you provide based on the primary assessment?

A bystander says that the patient lives on the next block in a local group home. He then states that he saw the patient walk to the corner and was on the phone to the facility when you arrived. The bystander denies witnessing any traumatic mechanisms that could cause injuries while he was watching the patient. You introduce yourself and your partner to the patient, who in turn says his name is Daniel. You do not observe any immediate life threats to his airway, breathing, or circulation. The patient informs you that voices in his head told him to come here. He denies any trauma and can tell you the date, time, and president's name. He also denies any substance or alcohol use. He verbally gives you consent to help him.

4. What conditions are you still considering as the possible cause?

5. Would you add any conditions as a possible cause? How could you rule them out?

During the secondary assessment, you note nothing physical out of the ordinary. He denies any physical complaints. His respirations are 12 *and adequate, pulse is strong at 72 beats per minute, and his blood pressure is 114/72. You obtain a blood glucose reading of 140 mg/dL. The woman at the group facility states on the phone that he has been off his medication for the past three days, is not allergic to anything, and has a history of schizophrenia and asthma. As you continue to interview your patient, he states that the voices have stopped, but he confides to you that they told him that he should let a car hit him. He says he is relieved that they are gone now because he doesn't really want to die.*

6. What conditions are you considering as a probable cause? Why?

7. What additional concerns do you have for this patient?

8. Based on your differential diagnosis, what are the next steps in emergency care?

9. Why?

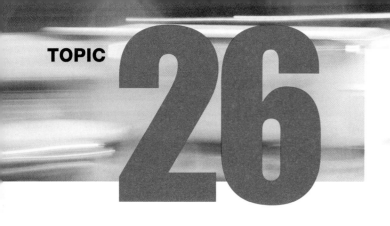

26

Medicine

Competency Applies fundamental knowledge to provide basic and selected advanced emergency care and transportation based on assessment findings for an acutely ill patient.

CARDIOVASCULAR EMERGENCIES: CHEST PAIN AND ACUTE CORONARY SYNDROME

TRANSITION *highlights*

- *Inclusion of the term acute coronary syndrome as an umbrella term for ischemic cardiac events.*

- *Pathophysiology of acute coronary syndrome.*

- *Increased emphasis on recognition of myocardial infarction and on emergency department door-to-intervention time.*

- *Changes in philosophy of oxygen administration to patients with acute coronary syndrome.*

- *Inclusion of aspirin and nitroglycerin administration for the acute care of acute coronary syndrome.*

- *Assessment findings indicative of cardiac arrest, as well as findings suggestive of a patient who may go into cardiac arrest.*

- *Importance of prehospital interventions and why they are successful in reversing cardiac arrest.*

INTRODUCTION

Cardiovascular emergencies are a common cause of EMS transports. The situation may be that the cardiovascular emergency was the precipitating cause for the ambulance (as in a heart attack) or that failure of another body system (such as the pulmonary system during an acute asthma attack) taxes the heart to a point that the patient is now suffering from cardiac compromise as well. These cardiac diseases and diagnosis are covered generically by a syndrome known as *acute coronary syndrome (ACS)*.

ACS is an umbrella term used to cover any cluster of clinical signs and symptoms related to diminished blood flow to the heart and the subsequent deterioration that comes from it. The spectrum of ACS can range widely from simple chest pain with exertion (angina) to a full heart attack (myocardial infarction) with resultant muscle death and the precipitation of pulmonary edema from left

heart failure. These life-threatening and often fatal disorders are a major cause of emergency medical care and hospitalization in the United States—as one would expect, as coronary heart disease is the leading cause of death in the United States today.

In any situation, a patient suffering from ACS requires diligent assessment and interview, specific and efficient treatment, and appropriate transport without delay to an appropriate emergency department to facilitate the best chance in patient survival.

EPIDEMIOLOGY

It has been estimated that more than 62 million Americans have some form of cardiovascular disease that commonly leads to coronary artery disease. Through previous research, the American Heart Association has found that approximately 7 to 8 million people each year will seek treatment in an emergency department in the United States for chest discomfort. Of those patients, approximately 2 million will actually suffer from a cardiac-related condition that involves the coronary arteries. About 1.5 million will suffer an actual heart attack, in which the coronary artery is occluded and a portion of the heart muscle begins to die. Of those patients, 500,000 will die from this heart attack, 250,000 of whom will die within one hour following the onset of the signs and symptoms.

In a more sobering light, about every 25 seconds an American will suffer a coronary event, every 34 seconds a heart attack will occur, and about once every minute someone will die from sudden cardiac arrest. These statistics are definite indications of the significance of cardiac-related emergencies and underscore the importance of having a thorough knowledge base regarding cardiac emergencies.

PATHOPHYSIOLOGY

To better understand the signs and symptoms of ACS, one must first understand the basic disease processes related to the condition. *Arteriosclerosis* is a condition that causes the smallest of arterial structures to become stiff and inelastic. This is often referred to as "hardening of the arteries." A form of arteriosclerosis is *atherosclerosis*. Atherosclerosis is a systemic arterial disease that is derived from the Greek word *athere*, meaning "gruel" or "porridge," and *scleros*, which means "hard."

Atherosclerosis is an inflammatory disease that starts in the intimal (innermost) lining of the blood vessels, where endothelial cells become damaged. Common risk factors that are thought to cause this endothelial injury include smoking, diabetes, hypertension, high levels of low-density lipoproteins (LDL), and low levels of high-density lipoproteins (HDL). Once injury occurs, intimal dysfunction and inflammation progress through the following five basic pathophysiologic events (▶ Figure 26-1):

- Intimal damage allows the migration of blood platelets and other substances in the blood (serum lipoproteins) into the vascular wall. This irritates and inflames the vascular wall.
- As a result of the irritation and inflammation, different types of cells migrate to the location, as do smooth muscle cells of the tunica media layer (muscular middle layer of the blood vessel).
- As these cells proliferate, longitudinal fatty streaks develop in the lumen of the blood vessel. The blood vessel weakens as intima and media are deprived of nutrients from the expanding plaque.
- In an attempt to "close off" the fatty streaks, smooth muscle cells produce collagen and migrate over the fatty streak to form a fibrous cap.
- Fibrous caps, however, are not stable and may rupture, which causes the body's clotting mechanism to activate with development of a thrombus (clot), which may occlude the blood vessel.

When a patient has a buildup of fatty deposits on the inside of the coronary arteries (atherosclerosis), the condition is called *coronary artery disease* (CAD). The narrowing of a coronary blood vessel increases the resistance to blood flow through the artery and decreases the amount of blood flow to the distal heart muscle. Also, the fatty deposits will reduce the coronary arteries' ability to dilate (become larger) and deliver additional blood flow to the heart when needed, such as during an increase in heart rate or more forceful pumping action, as needed during stress or exercise.

Although coronary artery disease is a vascular problem in and of itself, it sets up the body for an increased risk of additional emergencies, which is the real focus of this topic: acute coronary syndrome.

Acute Coronary Syndrome

As previously discussed, ACS results from any of a variety of conditions in which the coronary arteries are narrowed or occluded by fat deposits (plaque), clots, or spasm, all of which can affect the heart. The word *acute* refers to a sudden onset, *coronary* refers to a condition affecting the coronary arteries, and *syndrome* indicates a group of signs and symptoms produced by the condition.

Two conditions that are part of any acute coronary syndrome are *angina* (stable and unstable) and *myocardial infarction* (heart attack). A heart muscle that is not receiving an adequate amount of oxygenated blood because of narrowing of the coronary arteries by plaque or spasms, clot formation inside the coronary artery blocking the blood flow, an increase in the work of the heart that demands more blood flow than can be supplied through the coronary arteries, or any combination of these results in *cardiac cell hypoxia*, also known as myocardial ischemia. *Myocardial ischemia* is a state in which inadequate oxygen is delivered to the heart muscle.

Angina Pectoris

Angina pectoris (literally, "pain in the chest") is a condition and a symptom commonly associated with coronary artery disease and can manifest itself as one of the acute coronary syndromes (▶ Figure 26-2). Angina typically occurs when an increased workload is placed on the heart from an increase in the heart rate or the contractile function of the heart or when an increase in systemic vascular resistance causes the ventricles to work harder to keep blood moving.

In any instance, angina pectoris is a symptom of inadequate oxygen supply to the heart muscle, which is often caused by partial blockage of the coronary arteries that, in turn, produces cellular ischemia (reduced delivery of oxygenated blood) and tissue hypoxia (oxygen deficiency in the tissues).

Generally, angina pectoris occurs during periods of stress, either physical or emotional, at a time when the oxygen requirements of heart muscle are not met by oxygen delivery. Once the stress is relieved or the patient rests, oxygen requirements are reduced, and the pain will usually go away. Although more uncommon, angina may also occur in patients with valvular heart disease,

> About every 25 seconds an American will suffer a coronary event, every 34 seconds a heart attack will occur, and about once every minute someone will die from sudden cardiac arrest.

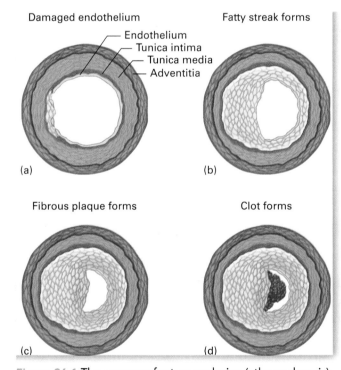

Figure 26-1 The process of artery occlusion (atherosclerosis): (a) The endothelium (inner wall) of the artery is damaged. (b) Fatty streaks begin to form in the damaged vessel walls. (c) Fibrous plaques form, causing further vessel damage and progressive resistance to blood flow. (d) The plaque deposits begin to ulcerate or rupture; platelets aggregate and adhere to the surface of the ruptured plaque, forming clots that may block the artery.

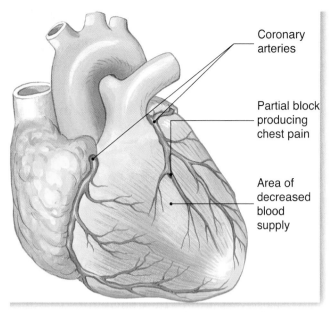

Figure 26-2 Angina pectoris, or chest pain, results when a coronary artery is blocked, depriving an area of the myocardium of oxygen.

Coronary arteries

Partial block producing chest pain

Area of decreased blood supply

enlarged hearts (cardiac hypertrophy), and hypertension. The pain is commonly felt under the sternum and may radiate to the jaw or down either arm, to the back, or to the epigastrium. The pain usually lasts for about 2 to 15 minutes.

Many patients will be able to tell you that they have had angina as part of their past medical history and will have nitroglycerin prescribed for this condition. Prompt relief of the symptoms after rest and administered nitroglycerin is a key finding typical of angina.

Angina pectoris has two subcategories, *stable angina* and *unstable angina*. Stable angina patients will experience episodes of chest pain of a more or less predictable nature. Commonly, the patient will know that certain levels of physical exertion (e.g., running versus walking) or extreme emotional or mental distress will precipitate the pain. Just as stable angina has a predictable onset, its resolution with rest and/or nitroglycerin is also predictable.

Unstable angina, conversely, is a subcategory of angina pectoris in which the onset of pain cannot be predicted. Unstable angina commonly occurs unexpectedly, in patterns that are not reliable. Although the underlying pathophysiology for unstable angina is still a diminishing of blood flow to distal capillary beds of the myocardium, it may occur during sleep, in the absence of physical exertion, or concurrently with other medical conditions such as infections or inflammations of the body. In addition, a change in the usual pattern of anginal episodes suggests unstable angina.

Variant angina (Prinzmetal angina) is a type of unstable angina in which a coronary artery spasm is the cause for diminished blood flow, but like unstable angina in general, the onset cannot be predicted.

Variant angina is highly correlated with secondary lethal dysrhythmias, myocardial infarction, and sudden cardiac death.

Myocardial Infarction

Pathophysiologically, a myocardial infarction (MI) is said to occur secondary to a coronary artery that becomes occluded following the rupture of an atherosclerotic plaque, which in turn leads to the formation of a clot (coronary thrombosis) that occludes distal blood flow. If a vessel becomes completely occluded, the myocardium tissue supplied by that vessel distally will become ischemic and hypoxic, resulting in tissue death after about 20 to 30 minutes without adequate reperfusion (▶ Figure 26-3).

The infarcted tissue consists of a necrotic core surrounded by marginal zones that can either recover normal function or become irreversibly damaged. One of the greatest determinants of MI size is the presence of any collateral blood flow. Collateral blood flow refers to an area of the heart that is also receiving blood from a blood vessel that is not occluded. This collateral blood flow is an important determinant of infarct size and of whether the marginal zones become irreversibly damaged.

Infarcted tissue does not contribute to tension generation during systole; therefore, it can alter ventricular systolic and diastolic functions, which in turn changes stroke volume and cardiac output, often detrimentally. Infarcted tissue can also interrupt normal electrical activity within the heart, leading to potentially fatal dysrhythmias.

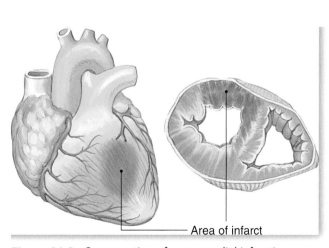

Area of infarct

Figure 26-3a Cross section of a myocardial infarction.

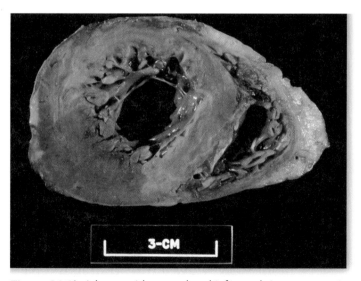

3-CM

Figure 26-3b A heart with normal and infarcted tissue.

If the MI affects the left ventricle, which is most common, the drop in cardiac function can lead to pulmonary vascular congestion and pulmonary edema. Infarcted tissue can also precipitate abnormal cardiac rhythms and conduction blocks that further impair global cardiac functioning and may become life threatening in some cases.

Reduced cardiac output and arterial pressure can activate baroreceptor reflexes that attempt to compensate for the drop in pressure by activation of numerous neurohumoral compensatory mechanisms, such as the sympathetic nervous system, as well as fluid retention systems, such as the renin–angiotensin and aldosterone systems. Renal hypoperfusion and sympathetic nervous system stimulation promote renin release—renin is converted into angiotensin II—and also aldosterone release, which enhance renal retention of sodium and water and promote vasoconstriction.

These negative feedback mechanisms cause the heart to work harder, thus increasing cardiac output. The retention of fluid by the kidneys drives up pressure by placing more fluid into the vascular system (explaining the elevated blood pressure and tachycardia seen in many MI patients). The pain and/or anxiety associated with a myocardial infarction further stimulates the sympathetic nervous system and results in ongoing peripheral systemic vasoconstriction and cardiac stimulation as catecholamines (such as adrenaline, norepinephrine, and dopamine) are released from the adrenal medulla.

Although the increased sympathetic tone and fluid retention help to maintain arterial pressure, they also lead to a large increase in myocardial workload and necessitate a greater myocardial oxygen need in an environment of diminished supply. This supply–demand mismatch can lead to more myocardial hypoxia, enlargement of the infarcted region, precipitation of cardiac dysrhythmias, and potentially a worsening in cardiac output. In addition, the sympathetic nervous system activation is responsible for the diaphoresis, anxiety, and nausea/vomiting commonly experienced by the patient.

After several weeks, if the patient survives the heart attack, the body remodels the infarcted tissue with a noncontractile fibrotic scar that does not contribute to ventricular strength. Long-term adaptation to the muscle loss includes development of compensatory hypertrophy or dilation, congestive heart failure, chronic dysrhythmias, and increased risk of sudden death. Table 26-1 provides an overview of the important body system changes secondary to an acute MI.

ASSESSMENT FINDINGS

Gathering a thorough history and physical exam is the foundation of assessment in patients with suspected myocardial ischemia or infarction. It is also important for the Advanced EMT to note that in some patients, in the absence of diagnostic tests performed by ALS providers or in the emergency department, the clinical picture of ischemia versus infarction may be nearly identical. As such, always assume the worst and treat the patient as if the acute coronary event with chest pain is actually an infarction.

The most classic features of MI include chest discomfort that is dull in nature and typically radiates into the left arm or jaw. Often the patient complains of dyspnea and nausea/vomiting and has tachycardia, changes in blood pressure, and diaphoresis. The presence of risk factors for coronary artery disease also increases the likelihood of the symptoms being related to ischemia or infarction. Such risk factors, as discussed earlier, include a past history of coronary or vascular disease, family history of coronary or vascular disease, smoking, hypertension, hypercholesterolemia, and diabetes mellitus.

Patients with classic angina will have a history of substernal chest pain or discomfort. The pain is usually described as a pressure or heaviness on the center of the chest; it usually occurs with activity and is relieved by rest. It may radiate to the left arm or jaw. The pain is frequently associated with dyspnea, nausea and vomiting, and diaphoresis. Depending on the significance of the myocardial ischemia, the patient may also display tachycardia and changes in blood pressure, inspiratory rales, or "cardiac asthma." ▶ Figure 26-4 lists common findings in patients with ischemic/infarction episodes.

Of special concern is the presentation of myocardial ischemia or infarction in women. Almost all common descriptions of the way ACS presents clinically have been taken from male cases. This is in part because medical literature at one time described only males with ACS, as they were primarily the ones who suffered cardiac events. However, as women have gained a more prominent presence in the workforce, higher rates of smoking, poor nutrition habits, higher stress levels, and so forth, they are now suffering from heart attacks at rates approaching those among men. In fact, because the incidence of MI in women is greater at older ages than in men, women are almost twice as likely to die from MI or its complications within the first few weeks following the event.

A woman may present with different signs and symptoms from a man when she is experiencing a cardiac event; however, the event is just as dangerous and can be as deadly. Therefore, the AEMT must be sure to recognize some of the more subtle signs and symptoms that women suffering from ACS experience.

TABLE 26-1	Effects of Myocardial Infarction on Body Systems
Neurohumoral effects	Enhanced sympathetic tone Increased circulating catecholamines Higher levels of angiotensin II and aldosterone Increased arginine vasopressin
Cardiopulmonary effects	Tachycardia Dysrhythmias Diminished stroke volume Increased oxygen requirements Pulmonary vascular congestion
Peripheral vascular effects	Increased vascular resistance (vasoconstriction) Elevations in blood volume Possible systemic edema

The most classic features of MI include chest discomfort that is dull in nature and typically radiates into the left arm or jaw.

	Angina Pectoris	Myocardial Infarction
Location of Discomfort	Substernal or across chest	Same
Radiation of Discomfort	Neck, jaw, arms, back, shoulders	Same
Nature of Discomfort	Dull or heavy discomfort with a pressure or squeezing sensation	Same, but maybe more intense
Duration	Usually 2 to 15 minutes, subsides after activity stops	Lasts longer than 10 minutes
Other symptoms	Usually none	Perspiration, pale gray color, nausea, weakness, dizziness, lightheadedness
Precipitating Factors	Extremes in weather, exertion, stress, meals	Often none
Factors Giving Relief	Stopping physical activity, reducing stress, nitroglycerin	Nitroglycerin may give incomplete or no relief

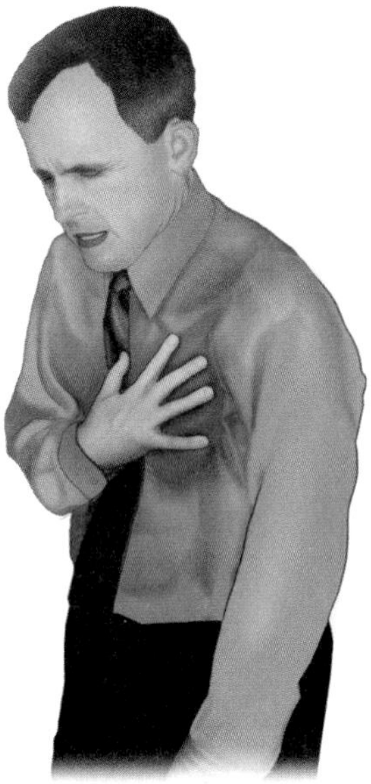

Figure 26-4 Both myocardial infarction and less serious angina can present symptoms of severe chest pain. Treat all cases of chest pain as cardiac emergencies.

The list of symptoms in Table 26-2 is common for women suffering from cardiac ischemia or infarction. Although you will see that some descriptions are the same as for men, many others are not.

Because when heart attack occurs the death rate for women is higher than that for men, the AEMT should have a high index of suspicion of ischemia/infarction when gathering a history from the female patient. Err on the side of the patient and provide emergency care for a potential myocardial infarction, despite a presentation of "atypical" signs of ischemia or infarction. Finally, note that diabetics and the elderly (Table 26-3) are also high-risk groups who may present with atypical findings.

EMERGENCY MEDICAL CARE

The treatment for the patient with angina pectoris or MI is geared toward ensuring patient comfort, improving oxygenation to the myocardium, diminishing enlargement of the injured area, and preserving normotension. Remember also that ischemia and infarction may at times be impossible for the AEMT to delineate in the field.

When the signs and symptoms of a myocardial ischemia or infarction are present, you should proceed rapidly with your assessment and management of the patient. This patient has the potential to go into cardiac arrest; therefore, assess the patient frequently and maintain a vigilant watch over the patient's condition. If at all possible, the patient should never be left alone while you are returning equipment to the EMS unit or retrieving and preparing the cot. The automated external defibrillator (AED) must always be available and close to the patient. The following is a summary of management considerations:

1. **Establish and maintain an open airway.**

2. **Provide oxygen** if the patient is dyspneic, hypoxemic, has obvious signs of heart failure, or has an SpO_2 reading of less than 94 percent. Initiate oxygen therapy via nasal cannula at 4 lpm and titrate oxygen therapy to maintain an SpO_2 reading of 94 percent or greater. If the breathing is inadequate, provide positive pressure ventilation at 10 to 12/min with high-flow supplemental oxygen.

3. **Administer 160 to 325 mg non-enteric coated aspirin.** Instruct the patient to chew the aspirin to promote a more rapid absorption.

4. **Initiate an intravenous line** of normal saline at a to-keep-open rate.

5. **Administer nitroglycerin** if the systolic blood pressure is greater than 90 mmHg or is less than 30 mmHg from the patient's baseline systolic

TABLE 26-2 Symptoms in Women with Cardiac Ischemia or Infarction

- "Classical" findings (not necessarily *common* findings)
  - Dull substernal chest pain or discomfort
  - Dyspnea or respiratory distress
  - Nausea, vomiting
  - Diaphoresis

- "Nonclassical" or "atypical" findings (not necessarily *uncommon* findings)
  - Neck ache
  - Pressure in the chest
  - Pains in the back, breast, or upper abdomen
  - Tingling of the fingers
  - Unexplained fatigue or weight gain (water weight gain)
  - Insomnia

| TABLE 26-3 | Special Considerations in Geriatric Cardiac Events |

History of diabetes mellitus	A geriatric patient with diabetes has long-term damage to the nerve endings in the body. This causes the typical pain from an MI to be perceived poorly, if at all, by the diabetic patient. Therefore, the diabetic patient experiencing an MI may complain only of respiratory distress or dizziness when standing, or even excessive weakness and dyspnea on exertion. It is important for the EMT to identify the patient with diabetes as potentially having an acute coronary event and to treat him appropriately. Contact ALS early, follow your local protocol, and ascertain whether additional or alternative therapies are desired by medical direction.
History of trauma	If the geriatric patient is a trauma patient, there must be a high index of suspicion for cardiac involvement as well. Geriatric patients who are traumatized can slip quickly into cardiac arrest and do not respond well to typical interventions. Geriatric patients with head trauma, chest trauma, abdominal trauma, or extremity trauma with severe bleeding are especially susceptible to cardiac arrest.
History of asthma	If a patient with a history of asthma goes into cardiac arrest, the cause may be acute bronchoconstriction that led to hypoxemia, acidosis, and cardiac arrest. Until the bronchoconstriction is reversed, the patient will not regain a pulse or start to breathe again. Early intercept or backup by an ALS unit will allow the administration of medications that may help reverse this condition.
History of COPD	Elderly patients commonly have some form of COPD (emphysema or chronic bronchitis). The arrest may have been caused by an exacerbation of the COPD, which led to hypoxemia, acidosis, and then arrest. ALS backup is needed during the resuscitation of this patient. Remember also that COPD disorders can weaken the lung tissue and cause the development of a pneumothorax and collapse of the lung. (This too may precipitate a cardiac arrest.) Be alert for the presence or the development of a pneumothorax during positive pressure ventilation, which may cause a bleb on the lung tissue to rupture.

blood pressure. Administer one nitroglycerin tablet every 3 to 5 minutes, up to a total of three tablets. Be sure the systolic blood pressure remains above 90 mmHg following the administration. Do not administer nitroglycerin if any of the following are present:

- A systolic blood pressure <90 mmHg, or 30 mmHg or greater below the patient's baseline systolic blood pressure
- Extreme bradycardia (<50 bpm)
- Tachycardia in the absence of heart failure (>100 bpm)
- Right ventricular failure

6. **Position the patient.** Semi- or high Fowler positioning will assist the patient in breathing and minimize the negative effects of fluid accumulating in the lungs. If positive pressure ventilation is being provided or frank hypotension is present, the patient will need to be placed supine for ongoing management.

7. **Ensure rapid transport to the emergency department.** Notify the receiving emergency department as early as possible. If the patient becomes pulseless and apneic (no pulse, no respirations), immediately apply the AED.

With the availability of mechanical measures, such as balloon angioplasty and stent placement, or medications, such as fibrinolytics and antiplatelet agents (new medications commonly referred to as "clot busters"), it may be possible to dissolve the clot, reopen the coronary artery, and restore perfusion to the ischemic heart muscle on arrival at the hospital. Prompt recognition and transport are necessary because the window of time to administer the fibrinolytic drugs is limited. In some jurisdictions, the AEMT may be capable of transmitting an ECG, which will reduce the time to mechanical (percutaneous cardiac) intervention or medical (fibrinolytic agent) intervention.

TRANSITIONING

REVIEW ITEMS

1. You are assessing a patient with chest pain characteristic of a myocardial infarction. Which of the following patient descriptions of the pain most accurately reflects an MI?
   a. "The pain is dull and radiates into my back from the center of my chest."
   b. "The pain is sharp and intermittent but gets easier when I burp."
   c. "It hurts real bad right beneath my shoulder blade, a burning type pain."
   d. "Right behind my breastbone it hurts, real sharp, and gets worse when I breathe."

2. Which of the following best describes the difference between myocardial ischemia and myocardial infarction?
   a. In ischemia, the heart muscle dies.
   b. In infarction, the heart muscle dies.
   c. Ischemia is from total occlusion of a coronary artery.
   d. Infarction occurs when myocardial oxygen needs are not being met adequately.

3. Which of the following is a modifiable risk factor for coronary artery disease?
   a. tobacco use
   b. age and gender
   c. family history of cardiovascular disease
   d. confirmed diagnosis of diabetes mellitus

4. Your 86-year-old female patient is complaining of dyspnea, weakness, swollen ankles, and diffuse chest discomfort. She has a history of coronary bypass and hypertension. She is allergic to penicillin. Currently her mental status is normal. Her vital signs are blood pressure 180/100, heart rate 108 beats per minute and irregular, respiratory rate of 18/minute. Given this scenario, what should your *first* action be?

a. Administer 365 mg baby aspirin orally.

b. Administer oxygen via a nasal cannula at 4 lpm.

c. Assist with the administration of her prescribed nitroglycerin.

d. Assist with the administration of her oral antihypertensive medication.

5. You arrive on scene to find a 45-year-old male patient with a chief complaint of chest pain. The patient states that the pain began while he was mowing the lawn but subsided after he sat on the couch for a few minutes. The patient has a cardiac history, and he states, "This just happened last week while mowing the lawn." Based on this information, from what do you think the patient is most likely suffering?

a. acute myocardial infarction

b. Prinzmetal angina

c. stable angina

d. congestive heart failure

APPLIED PATHOPHYSIOLOGY

A 48-year-old male patient is complaining of chest pain that he describes as dull and located substernally, with radiation to his neck. He rates the pain a 6 on a scale of 1 to 10 and complains of nausea and lightheadedness. His skin is cool and diaphoretic. His heart rate is 96 beats per minute, blood pressure is 124/82, respiratory rate is 14, and SpO_2 is 92 percent. He has taken two of his own nitroglycerin tablets prior to your arrival, without any relief.

1. Should you suspect that this patient is suffering from an ischemic or an infarction episode? Support your answer with the appropriate clinical findings provided.

2. Why might the administration of nitroglycerin to this patient be beneficial?

3. Describe the anticipated physiologic benefit(s) for each of the interventions that may be administered to a patient suffering

from a myocardial infarction. Also list the appropriate dosage for each medication:

a. Oxygen

b. Aspirin

c. Nitroglycerin

4. Discuss the differences in pathophysiology and presentation of the following acute coronary syndrome manifestations:

a. Stable angina pectoris

b. Unstable angina pectoris

c. Myocardial infarction

5. Describe the pathophysiologic changes that occur to the lumen of the blood vessel resulting in atherosclerosis and occlusion of coronary blood vessels.

CLINICAL DECISION MAKING

You are summoned to a retirement community for an unknown medical emergency. On your arrival you meet a 68-year-old man sitting beside a ladder he was attempting to climb so he could clean out his gutters. On further questioning, you learn that he experienced a sensation of vertigo nd nausea while climbing the ladder. A nearby family member stated that the patient was caught as he stumbled off the ladder and that no trauma occurred. The patient has also been experiencing "heartburn" for two days without relief. He last ate two hours earlier. His medical history includes hypertension, diabetes mellitus, a previous MI, and a "mini stroke" two years ago.

1. Based on the scene size-up characteristics, identify the clues that point to the field impression of either an ischemic or an infarction episode.

2. What medical condition does this patient have that could mask the common finding of an acute coronary syndrome?

The primary assessment reveals the patient to be alert and well oriented. His airway is clear; his breathing is rapid at 22/minute, respirations are slightly shallow, vesicular sounds are present, and slight inspiratory rales are noted. Peripheral pulses are also present and noted to be rapid and slightly irregular. His blood pressure is 132/92.

The neck veins are obviously engorged, and the SpO_2 reading on room air is 87 percent. His blood sugar is currently 142 mg/dL.

3. What are the life threats, if any, to the patient that you are currently aware of?

Further assessment reveals the patient's pupils to be equal and reactive, and the SpO_2 has increased to 94 percent with supplemental oxygen. Breath sounds are unchanged, and jugular venous distention is still present. His blood pressure is now 140/98, heart rate is 112 and irregular, and respirations have increased to 28/minute. The patient is starting to complain of chest "pressure" as well. During the ongoing management of the patient, you elect to administer the therapies listed below.

4. For each one, discuss in specific detail (1) the reason the intervention is warranted, (2) the expected outcome of that intervention, and (3) how you would assess to determine if the desired effect is occurring (i.e., the treatment worked).

a. Position patient in high Fowler position.

b. Administer oxygen.

c. Administer aspirin.

d. Administer nitroglycerin.

Standard Medicine

Competency Applies fundamental knowledge to provide basic and selected advanced emergency care and transportation based on assessment findings for an acutely ill patient.

TOPIC

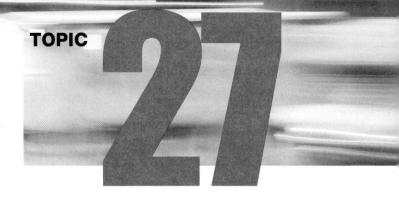

CARDIOVASCULAR EMERGENCIES: CONGESTIVE HEART FAILURE

INTRODUCTION

Not only is a patient with a cardiovascular emergency one of the most common patient scenarios the Advanced EMT will encounter prehospitally, but it may also be one of the most challenging, as the clinical presentation may vary widely, given the complexity of the underlying cardiovascular pathology. One such example of this is a patient with congestive heart failure (CHF).

Although CHF is a diagnosis given to a certain type of cardiac dysfunction, the patient with CHF may present with a wide variety of symptoms. The presentation of CHF could be as insidious as a patient complaining of weakness during normal daily activities to as severe as chest pain with acute pulmonary edema and systemic hypotension. In every situation, the AEMT must remain vigilant in assessing and managing these types of patients because although not all CHF patients will deteriorate acutely, when they do, the deterioration is commonly rapid and often fatal.

EPIDEMIOLOGY

In the United States, CHF is a disease state of significant concern. It has been estimated that the prevalence rate for CHF is about 1 to 2 percent in the adult population. In more specific numbers, more than 400,000 patients are diagnosed yearly with CHF, and currently about 3 million Americans have this disease state. In fact, this pathology is a common reason for hospital admittance, as up to 40 percent of CHF patients are hospitalized every year. CHF has been found to be the cause of death in blacks more often than in whites (blacks are 1.5 times more likely to die from CHF) and has a higher prevalence in men than in women (although in the population over 75 years of age, CHF shows no gender preferences).

As to be expected, the prevalence of CHF increases with age, affecting about 10 percent of the population older than 75 years. Finally, as a comorbid factor, patients with insulin-dependent diabetes have a significantly higher mortality rate.

PATHOPHYSIOLOGY

Congestive heart failure is a medical diagnosis, but—more important—it is a pathophysiologic state in which the heart

TRANSITION *highlights*

- *Frequency, ethnic and gender predisposition, and morbidity rates for patients with congestive heart failure.*

- *Pathophysiologic changes that accompany this disease process:*
  - Heart failure.
  - Left heart failure.
  - Right heart failure.

- *Common signs and symptoms of heart failure with specific findings that will best delineate between these emergencies.*

- *Assessment phases for a patient suffering from congestive heart failure and the specific etiologies that accompany this disease process.*

- *Treatment interventions:*
  - Oxygen.
  - Pulse oximetry.
  - Body positioning.
  - CPAP.
  - Intravenous therapy.

muscle is unable to pump the blood needed to meet the venous return of the body. The resultant drop in cardiac output most typically results in a condition in which a buildup of fluid (congestion) in the body occurs as a result of pump failure. In essence, it represents the condition in which the left, right, or both ventricles fail to meet the body's needs. It may be a chronic condition that develops over a period of time (perhaps years), or it may be more acute in nature should it be associated with a large myocardial infarction (MI) that affects the ventricle(s).

The many causes of CHF include coronary artery disease, valvular dysfunction, and myocardial disease. Other factors that may contribute to CHF include excessive salt or water intake, hypertension, thyrotoxicosis, pulmonary embolism, alcohol/drug abuse, and anemia.

> **The causes of CHF include coronary artery disease, valvular dysfunction, and myocardial disease.**

Heart failure, as discussed, results in the reduction of cardiac output and may be caused by a decrease in stroke volume or a change in heart rate. By definition, cardiac output is the amount of blood pumped by the heart for 60 seconds. The relationship of cardiac output (CO), stroke volume (SV), and heart rate (HR) is found in the following formula:

$$CO = SV \times HR$$

A reduction in cardiac output leads to compensatory mechanisms that act to restore cardiac output. For instance, when a patient sustains an MI, the dead heart muscle prevents the heart from pumping normally, thus leading to decreased cardiac output. The body senses the decrease in cardiac output by way of baroreceptors in the aortic arch and carotid bodies and tries to compensate by increasing sympathetic tone.

Because the myocardium cannot increase stroke volume because of the damaged pump, it must compensate by increasing the heart rate. If, however, a patient has a dysrhythmia that affects only the heart rate (i.e., bradycardia), the decreased heart rate leads to a decreased cardiac output. In that case, the body tries to compensate by increasing the stroke volume and systemic vascular resistance.

The body has several other mechanisms it can use to compensate for decreased cardiac output. These include vasoconstriction of peripheral vessels and activation of the hormonal systems of the body designed to increase intravascular volume. An example of the hormonal response is brain-type natriuretic peptide (BNP). This substance is released in response to distention of the ventricles seen in congestive heart failure. The substance, tested for as an indicator of CHF, promotes natriuresis and tends to lower blood volume. Unfortunately, these compensatory mechanisms actually increase myocardial oxygen demand and thus are potentially detrimental to myocardial function.

Heart failure is generally divided into left ventricular failure and/or right ventricular failure, although this is somewhat arbitrary in nature because the right and left ventricles perfuse different portions of the circulation. It can also be described as "backward failure" (leading to congestion) and "forward failure" (leading to diminished end-organ perfusion).

Left-Sided Failure

Left ventricular (LV) failure occurs when the left ventricle is unable to pump adequately; the heart pumps inadequately for multiple reasons. Dysfunction of the heart muscle itself, as is seen with MI, is one of the main causes of left ventricular pump failure. Dysrhythmias also inhibit the heart's ability to pump normally.

With *backward* failure of the left ventricle, pulmonary congestion (pulmonary edema) results, leading to signs and symptoms that are primarily respiratory in nature. With *forward* failure of the left ventricle, diminished peripheral perfusion and systemic circulation result. Conditions that may be responsible for this include obstruction of outflow from the heart, as is seen in valvular disease or chronic systemic hypertension.

Right-Sided Failure

In this type of heart failure, the right side of the heart fails to function as an adequate pump to the lungs, which commonly leads to back pressure of blood into the venous and systemic circulation with *backward* failure of the right ventricle. Backward failure of the right ventricle results in excess fluid that accumulates in the body, often in dependent extremities (▶ Figure 27-1), and may cause jugular venous distention (▶ Figure 27-2), enlargement of the liver, and possible abdominal distention in severe cases.

Right ventricular (RV) failure is most commonly caused by backward failure of the left heart muscle, which then causes an eventual backlogging of blood into the right heart circuit. Similar to the causes of left ventricular failure, other disorders that can cause the right side to fail include dysfunction of the heart muscle itself from chronic pulmonary hypertension or, in acute cases, right ventricular MI. Right ventricular MI is less common than left ventricular infarctions, but it is seen. Pulmonary hypertension and stenotic pulmonary valvular disease can also result in *forward* failure of the right heart and may result in lungs being underperfused, leading to subjective respiratory distress and diminished preload to the left heart circuit.

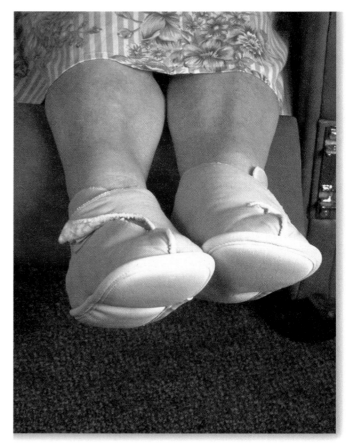

Figure 27-1 Edema to the lower extremities is a classic sign of congestive heart failure.

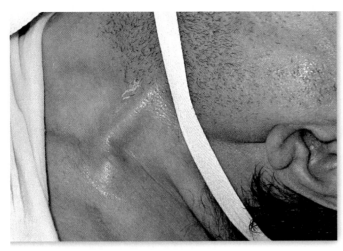

Figure 27-2 Jugular venous distention is a sign of right-sided ventricular heart failure. (© David Effron, M.D.)

Table 27-1 summarizes these pathophysiologic changes in right and left heart failure leading to the diagnosis of congestive heart failure. Remember, though, CHF is the underlying problem; when the medical condition exacerbates, the presentation is often centered around dyspnea, weakness, changes in breath sounds, possible chest pain, weakness, and fluid retention.

ASSESSMENT FINDINGS

The signs and symptoms of congestive heart failure will depend on the severity of the condition and whether it is an acute-onset or a long-term problem. During the AEMT assessment, recall that several exceptions apply to a simple left-versus-right division of heart failure symptoms. Left-sided *forward* failure overlaps with right-sided *backward* failure. Because the most common cause of right heart failure is left heart failure, patients may present with symptoms of both types (a condition known as *biventricular failure*). Regardless, the signs and symptoms of congestive heart failure include the following (▸ Figure 27-3):

- Marked or severe dyspnea (shortness of breath)
- Tachycardia (rapid heart rate, greater than 100 bpm)
- Difficulty breathing when supine (orthopnea)
- Suddenly waking at night with dyspnea (paroxysmal nocturnal dyspnea)
- Fatigue on any type of exertion
- Anxiety
- Tachypnea (rapid respiratory rate)
- Diaphoresis (sweating)
- Upright position with legs, feet, arms, and hands dangling
- Cool, clammy, pale skin
- Chest discomfort
- Cyanosis

- Agitation and restlessness from the hypoxia
- Edema (swelling) to the hands, ankles, and feet
- Crackles and possibly wheezes on auscultation
- Decreased SpO_2 reading
- Signs and symptoms of pulmonary edema
- Blood pressure normal, elevated, or low
- Distended neck veins—jugular venous distention (JVD)
- Distended and soft, spongy abdomen

Commonly, these patients will tell you that they are taking a "water pill." This is a diuretic that is used to reduce the amount of fluid in the body. They may also be on other drugs to strengthen the force of contraction of the heart and reduce the response of the sympathetic nervous system. They may also be on medications designed to control the rate and rhythm of the heart, as bradycardia and tachycardia can drop cardiac output and exacerbate the findings of CHF. Table 27-2 summarizes common findings of CHF and discusses the pathophysiologic change that underlies them.

EMERGENCY MEDICAL CARE

The treatment for the patient with CHF is geared toward improving oxygenation, diminishing fluid accumulation in the lungs, treating the patient for angina or MI should it concurrently be present, and maintaining normotension. Remember that exacerbation of CHF may be very scary to the patient, so good communication skills and verbal reassurance will also go a long way.

1. **Establish and maintain an open airway.**
2. **Provide oxygen** if the patient is dyspneic, hypoxemic, has obvious signs of heart failure, or has an SpO_2 reading of less than 94 percent. Initiate oxygen therapy via nasal cannula at 4 lpm and titrate oxygen therapy to maintain an SpO_2 reading of 94 percent or greater. If the breathing is inadequate, provide positive pressure ventilation at 10 to 12/min with high-flow supplemental oxygen.
3. **Use CPAP if protocol allows.** Continuous positive airway pressure (CPAP) will help shift fluid from the

TABLE 27-1	Pathophysiologic Changes in Right and Left Heart Failure
	Pathophysiologic Findings
Right heart failure	Right heart fails because of infarction, increased workload, valvular dysfunction, or a combination of these. It results in the congestion of blood in the vena cava, resulting in jugular venous distention, peripheral edema, enlarged liver, clear breath sounds, and probably hypotension.
Left heart failure	Left heart fails also because of infarction, increased workload (systemic hypertension), valvular dysfunction, or a combination of these. It results in the congestion of blood in the lungs, which increases pressure to a point at which fluid escapes into the alveoli, causing respiratory distress and pulmonary edema. Lung sounds often reveal crackles or "cardiac asthma," blood pressure is commonly normal to high, and peripheral congestion is absent.

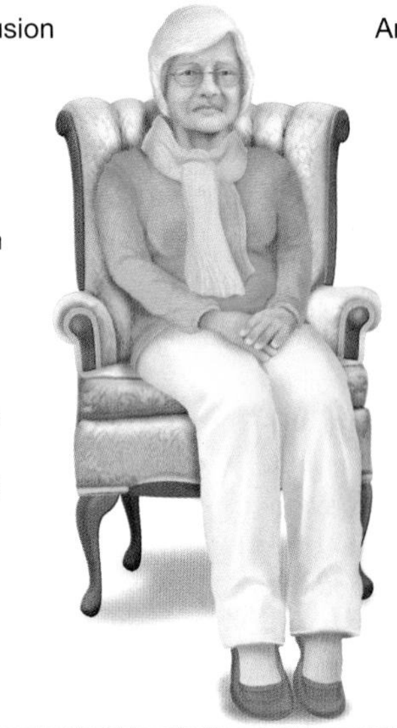

Mild to severe confusion

Cyanosis

Tachypnea

May cough up pink sputum

Low, normal, or high blood pressure

Rapid heart rate

A desire to sit upright

Anxiety

Distended neck veins (Late)

Crackles

Shortness of breath (dyspnea)

Pale, cool, clammy skin

Abdominal distention

Pedal and lower extremity edema

Figure 27-3 Signs and symptoms of congestive heart failure.

alveoli back into the vasculature. Usually CPAP is set at between 5 and 10 cmH$_2$O; follow local protocol (▶ Figure 27-4).

4. **Initiate an intravenous line of normal saline at a to-keep-open rate.**

5. **Administer nitroglycerin (follow your local protocol).** If the patient is concurrently presenting with a possible angina or infarction, the nitroglycerin will help relieve pain, and the peripheral vasodilation will make it easier for the failing heart to pump blood. Your local protocol may instruct you to administer nitroglycerin in LV failure even in the absence of chest discomfort. Follow your local protocol.

6. **Position the patient.** Semi- or high Fowler positioning will assist the patient in breathing and minimize the negative effects of fluid accumulating

TABLE 27-2 — Clinical Findings and Pathophysiologic Etiology of CHF

Clinical Finding	Pathophysiologic Etiology
Rapid breathing (tachypnea)	Multiple reasons, such as hypoxia, carbon dioxide retention, sympathetic discharge.
Shortness of breath (dyspnea)	Changes in O$_2$/CO$_2$ diffusion across alveoli; chemoreceptors in body detect changes in gas levels and cause the perception of dyspnea.
Shortness of breath while lying down (orthopnea)	On lying down, fluid accumulation in lungs from CHF tends to increase, which diminishes gas exchange across alveoli.
Constant waking at night (paroxysmal nocturnal dyspnea)	While lying down, fluid accumulates in the lungs and causes the person to wake up. Patient may state that the dyspnea eases after sitting or standing up from sleep.
Anxiety, tremors, nausea, vomiting	Sympathetic discharge caused by the changes in blood gases and/or cardiac output.
Low pulse oximetry readings	Poor oxygenation from fluid accumulation in lungs diminishes oxygen diffusion into the bloodstream.
Cool, pale, clammy skin	Sympathetic discharge from changes in cardiac output and oxygen/carbon dioxide levels.
Sitting upright and/or tripod positioning	Sitting upright eases dyspnea because of better diaphragmatic function; it also helps to ease fluid accumulation in lungs.
Chest discomfort	Possible angina, infarction in an acute setting.
Inspiratory crackles	Fluid accumulation in the alveoli from backward failure of left ventricle.
Wheezing (cardiac asthma)	Fluid accumulation in alveoli may migrate into bronchioles from breathing, causing stimulation of "irritant receptors" in lung tissue causing bronchoconstriction.
Distended neck veins, enlarged liver, distended abdomen	Increased venous pressure from backward failure of right ventricle.
Changes in blood pressure	Hypotension often caused by failing right ventricle (thereby diminishing left-sided preload). Hypertension often caused by left-sided failure in conjunction with heightened sympathetic tone.
Objective dyspnea findings: nasal flaring, retractions, tachypnea, tripod positioning, mouth breathing, etc.	Most commonly caused by combination of right and left ventricular failure.

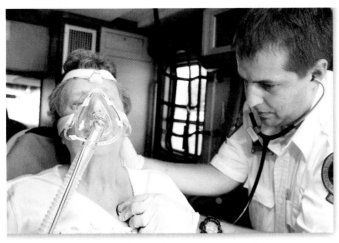

Figure 27-4 CPAP is a form of noninvasive positive pressure ventilation used in the awake and spontaneously breathing patient who needs ventilatory support. (© *Ken Kerr*)

in the lungs. If positive pressure ventilation is being provided or frank hypotension is present, the patient will need to be placed supine for ongoing management.

7. **Ensure rapid transport to the emergency department.** Notify the receiving ED as early as possible.

Continuously assess the patient and be prepared for respiratory failure and cardiac arrest. Should either of these occur, follow appropriate treatment and local protocol for supporting this lost function.

Patients suffering from exacerbation of congestive heart failure can be among the most challenging patients encountered by the AEMT. They may present anywhere on the continuum from being alert and oriented with only minimal symptoms to being unresponsive and just moments from complete cardiopulmonary arrest. Compounding this picture is that the CHF patient may go from one extreme to the other very quickly, without much warning for the AEMT. Therefore, the AEMT must always maintain a high degree of suspicion that these patients may deteriorate into arrest very suddenly.

TRANSITIONING

REVIEW ITEMS

1. During your interview, your patient tells you that she has "water on the lungs." This statement most closely reflects what pathophysiologic change in CHF?
   a. backward failure of the left ventricle
   b. frontward failure of the right ventricle
   c. biventricular failure
   d. elevation in central venous pressure

2. Of the choices here, which is most likely a determining factor causing the development of right-sided heart failure?
   a. high diastolic pressure
   b. preexisting left heart failure
   c. stenosis of the tricuspid valve
   d. history of diabetes mellitus

3. A patient presents with JVD, hypotension, clear breath sounds, and peripheral edema. These findings would be most representative of what type of heart failure?
   a. acute right ventricular failure
   b. acute left ventricular failure
   c. gradual right ventricular failure
   d. gradual left ventricular failure

4. Pulmonary edema would be a manifestation of what type of ventricular failure?
   a. acute right ventricular failure
   b. acute left ventricular failure
   c. gradual right ventricular failure
   d. gradual left ventricular failure

5. Diffusion of excessive alveolar fluid back into the perialveolar capillary bed would be best accomplished by what treatment intervention for the CHF patient?
   a. placing the patient supine
   b. providing high-flow oxygen
   c. administration of sublingual nitroglycerin
   d. continuous positive airway pressure (CPAP)

APPLIED PATHOPHYSIOLOGY

A 76-year-old female patient has a history of hypertension, insulin-dependent diabetes, and CHF. She summoned an ambulance because of weakness, mild chest pressure, and progressively worsening dyspnea over the past two days. The patient states that her trouble breathing got worse with physical exertion and when lying down at night to go to bed. Currently her vital signs are blood pressure 180/100, heart rate 102 beats per minute, respiratory rate 24, SpO2 92 percent on room air. During your assessment of the breath sounds, you note bilateral wheezing.

1. Identify if you believe this patient has right or left ventricular failure. Support your answer with the appropriate clinical findings.

2. Why might the administration of nitroglycerin to this patient be beneficial to the dyspnea?

3. Identify and discuss why the patient's wheezing should *not* be treated as it would be in an asthmatic or allergic-reaction patient.

4. Discuss the differences in pathophysiology and presentation of right versus left heart failure according to the following three assessment findings:

   a. Breath sounds:

   b. Systolic blood pressure:

   c. Vital sign changes:

5. Differentiate the pathophysiologic changes between *backward* and *forward* ventricular failure.

CLINICAL DECISION MAKING

Late one hot summer night, you are called for a patient suffering from acute respiratory distress. On arrival at the patient's home, you are escorted to an elderly female patient's bedroom on the second floor. As soon as you walk in, you see the patient lying on her back in bed with four or five pillows behind her head and shoulders, helping her to "sit up." The patient is alert and oriented; displays nasal flaring, retractions, and tachypnea; and is speaking in full sentences. On the nightstand beside the bed, you see four or five prescription bottles of medication.

1. Based on the scene size-up characteristics, identify the clues that point to the field impression of either CHF or acute pulmonary edema.

2. What common medications might you find on the patient's nightstand to support the field impression of CHF?

The primary assessment reveals the patient to be alert and well oriented. Her airway is clear, her breathing is rapid at 30/minute, respirations are slightly shallow, vesicular sounds are present and diminished, and slight inspiratory crackles are noted. Peripheral pulses are also present and noted to be rapid and slightly irregular. The neck veins are obviously engorged, and the SpO_2 reading on room air is 87 percent.

3. What are the life threats, if any, to the patient of which you are currently aware?

After managing and supporting the situation described, further assessment reveals the pupils to be equal and reactive, blood glucose level is 193 mg/dL, and the SpO_2 has increased to 94 percent with high-flow oxygen. Breath sounds are unchanged; the JVD is still present. The patient's blood pressure is 100/79, heart rate is 112 and irregular, and respirations are fast at 30/minute. The patient is now starting to complain of "chest pressure" as well.*

4. From what etiology of congestive heart failure is this patient likely suffering?

5. Explain the pathophysiologic cause for the following:

   a. Breath sounds

   b. Low pulse oximeter reading

   c. Jugular venous distention

6. During the management of the patient, you elect to administer the following therapies. For each one, discuss in specific detail (1) the reason the intervention is warranted, (2) the expected outcome of that intervention, and (3) how you would assess to determine whether the desired effect is occurring (i.e., the treatment worked).

   a. Positioning patient in high Fowler position

   b. Administration of oxygen

   c. Administration of nitroglycerin

   d. Application of CPAP at 10 cmH$_2$O pressure

Standard Medicine

Competency Applies fundamental knowledge to provide basic and selected advanced emergency care and transportation based on assessment findings for an acutely ill patient.

TOPIC

28

CARDIOVASCULAR EMERGENCIES: HYPERTENSIVE AND VASCULAR EMERGENCIES

INTRODUCTION

As has been discussed, cardiovascular disease is the leading cause of chronic morbidity and mortality in the United States today for both men and women. Because of the pathologic changes to the body's heart, blood vessels, and organs over time, a plethora of medical emergencies can arise in a patient that will require summoning EMS. Unfortunately, by the time cardiovascular disease is diagnosed, the disease process is usually very advanced, having progressed in the patient for decades; this typically results in a patient who becomes reliant on medications and lifestyle changes in an attempt to limit further bodywide deterioration.

The American Heart Association has identified the four most common manifestations of cardiovascular disease. The first is the precursor for angina and infarction: coronary heart disease. The next most common manifestations include stroke, high blood pressure, and heart failure.

Unfortunately, the list does not stop there; other forms of cardiovascular disease include cardiac dysrhythmias, rheumatic heart disease, congenital cardiovascular defects, diseases of the blood vessels, bacterial endocarditis, diseases of the pulmonary circulation, cardiomyopathies, valvular heart disease, diseases of the lymphatics, renal dysfunction, and other diseases of the circulatory system. Although this list is not all-inclusive, it does demonstrate the systemic tolls cardiovascular disease takes on the body.

In this topic, the focus is on three different emergencies that are caused by cardiovascular disease specifically as it affects the vascular system. These diseases are hypertensive emergency, aortic dissection, and aortic aneurysms. Any of these three conditions, if left untreated, can lead to rapid deterioration and death of the patient. This underscores the importance of the Advanced EMT understanding the pathophysiology, presentation, and management of these specific medical conditions.

EPIDEMIOLOGY

Current data suggest that more than 40 million people living in the United States today have hypertension, be it diagnosed or not. The National Center for Health Statistics has collected data

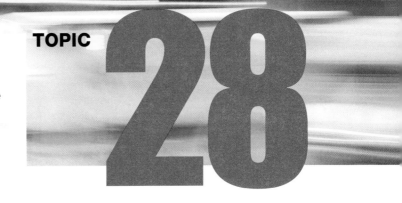

TRANSITION *highlights*

- *Frequency of hypertensive and other vascular disease emergencies.*
- *Pathophysiologic changes that accompany the vascular disease progression of arteriosclerosis and arthrosclerosis:*
  - Hypertension.
  - Aortic aneurysm.
  - Aortic dissection.
- *Common symptoms of hypertensive emergencies.*
- *Comparison of clinical findings found in aortic aneurysms versus aortic dissections.*
- *Assessment phases for a patient suffering from a hypertensive, aneurysm, or dissection disease process with integration of treatment considerations.*

on hypertension and has estimated the overall prevalence to be greater than 28 percent in the general population. Of these, more than 68 percent were aware of their medical condition, and roughly 58 percent were receiving medical care for the condition. There is a disproportionate distribution of hypertension in ethnic minorities, mainly African Americans, and also in underprivileged populations that commonly do not receive proper medical screening or care.

Regarding aortic aneurysms, there has been an increase in incidence rates as individuals and the population ages. Diagnosis is commonly made after the fifth decade of life. A gender disparity characterizes the development of aortic aneurysms, as they are five times more common in men than in women, and they are more common in white men than in African-American men. With diagnosis, ongoing care includes lifestyle changes, pharmacologic therapy, and in more extreme cases, surgical remedies. Ruptured aortic aneurysms have become the 13th leading cause of death in the United States. Although this may not seem common, this translates into roughly 15,000 people in the United States dying every year from a ruptured aortic aneurysm.

Aortic dissection is a true medical emergency. It is the most common catastrophic and fatal disease of the aorta, occurring more than twice as often as a rupture of an aortic aneurysm. When left untreated, one-third of all patients will die within 24 hours, and another 50 percent will die within the following 48 hours.

> **An aortic aneurysm is a weakening of all three layers of the aortic wall.**

True incidence rates for dissection are difficult to estimate, as most are based on autopsy studies. However, in population-based studies it has been estimated that roughly 6 to 10 new aneurysms occur per 100,000 person-years. Another study estimated roughly 2,000 new cases each year. Men are predominantly affected—typically, men older than the age of 50—and patients with connective tissue disorders, such as Marfan syndrome and Ehlers-Danlos syndrome, have higher risks as well.

PATHOPHYSIOLOGY

The genesis for almost all diseases of the arteries starts with cardiovascular risk factors. Because of lifestyle choices (such as diet, smoking, inactivity), genetics (gender, ethnicity, concurrent disease states), and age (risk increases with age), cardiovascular disease and damage to the intimal layers of the large blood vessels develop slowly, often insidiously, without clinical presentation until a catastrophic event, such as a ruptured aneurysm or hypertensive crisis, occurs. Some differences do exist, however, in the specific pathogenesis for these three emergencies.

> **Aortic dissection is the most common catastrophic and fatal disease of the aorta.**

Hypertensive Emergencies

Hypertension usually does not produce any clinical findings until vascular changes occur to organs such as the heart, brain, lungs, or kidneys.

Although hypertension is a very common finding in the United States, episodes of hypertensive emergencies are, fortunately, rare. A hypertensive emergency is defined as a severe hypertensive episode with a systolic pressure greater than 160 mmHg and/or a diastolic blood pressure greater than 100 mmHg and evidence of end-organ dysfunction. Typically, extremely high blood pressures are noted during the acute episode.

The constellation of findings may include acute left ventricular failure (congestive heart failure [CHF]), myocardial ischemia or infarction, acute renal failure, hypertensive encephalopathy, cerebrovascular accident (stroke), eclampsia, aortic dissection, or acute pulmonary edema. With hypertensive patients it is not so much the actual blood pressure that is detrimental; it is the speed at which the blood pressure rises that causes the patient's deterioration.

For example, a patient with chronic hypertension may be experiencing a stroke, and you are summoned to care for the stroke, not the elevation in blood pressure. It is just coincidental that the patient's blood pressure is up (which in that situation is "normal" for the patient). Conversely, if a rapid increase in blood pressure occurs in a patient who does not have chronic elevations, the patient may present with signs and symptoms related directly to the hypertensive crisis (such as a seizure). It is key to ascertain a thorough patient history in hypertensive emergency patients.

The two types of hypertensive patients are those with "primary" hypertension and those with "secondary" hypertension. *Primary hypertension* is most common and is characterized by a hypertensive state in which no specific etiology has been determined (idiopathic), although theories do exist as to the cause. The patient with primary hypertension most likely will be taking medications designed to keep the blood pressure low and will be on a diet that limits certain substances, such as sodium.

Secondary hypertension is said to occur when a patient is hypertensive from some other underlying disease process. For example, patients with renal disease are usually chronically hypertensive, as are patients with certain endocrine (thyroid, adrenal, etc.) disorders. Regardless of etiology, though, it is important for the AEMT to ascertain from the patient

whether he has chronic elevations in blood pressure. If he does, chances are that he has his blood pressure tracked and documented on a card that he carries with him. The AEMT should evaluate only what the patient's current blood pressure is in light of what a "normal" blood pressure is for him.

As another example, a patient may be experiencing a seizure but may coincidently have a diagnosis of high blood pressure for which he takes medication. A normal blood pressure for him might be 168/90 mmHg. If the patient's actual blood pressure during this emergency is near his average blood pressure, then the AEMT should focus on the seizure and not on the blood pressure directly. However, if a patient is found to be experiencing a seizure, but his normal blood pressure is 108/60 and his current blood pressure is 172/96 mmHg, the blood pressure may be considered during the concurrent management of the seizure because a sudden spike in the blood pressure is one etiology for seizures.

Aortic Aneurysm (Thoracic and Abdominal)

An aortic aneurysm is a weakening of all three layers of the aortic wall: the tunica intima (smooth inner layer), tunica media (muscular middle layer), and adventitia (fibrous outer layer). Within these walls of the aorta are concentric layers of smooth muscle, elastin fibers, and collagen fibers, which are designed to withstand the arterial pressure common to the aorta. As the aorta extends from its proximal thoracic origination to the distal termination point of the aorta in the abdominal cavity, a decrease in the number of medial elastin layers, a thinning of the medial layer, and a thickening of the intimal layer occur. This translates into an aorta that has increased strength to withstand arterial pressure closer to the heart and decreased strength as it descends distally into the abdominal cavity.

The development of an aneurysm leads to a change in elastin fibers (the principal load-bearing element of the aorta) in which elastin fibers start to degenerate and become fragmented. This also contributes to the weakening of the wall, which initially presents with ballooning of the aorta and may lead to rupture of the aneurysm. Because fewer elastin fibers are already present in the

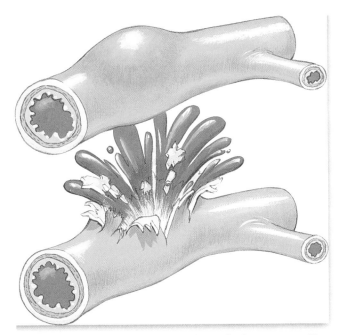

Figure 28-1 A weakened area in the wall of an artery will tend to balloon out, forming a saclike aneurysm, which may eventually burst.

abdominal aorta and smaller muscular layers of the tunica media, the abdominal aorta is pathophysiologically at a higher risk to develop an aneurysm. Again, aneurysms can develop in any portion of the aorta, but they most commonly involve the aorta below the renal arteries (abdominal aortic aneurysm [AAA]).

A generally accepted definition of an aortic aneurysm is a focal spot that dilates greater than 50 percent of normal arterial diameter. Clinically speaking, however, given the size of the aorta, a focal dilation of 3 cm or greater is also a commonly accepted definition of an aortic aneurysm.

The most disastrous clinical manifestation of an aortic aneurysm is a rupture. When this event occurs, it allows arterial blood to spill into the mediastinum, retroperitoneum, or abdominal cavity (depending on the aneurysm site), rapidly leading to an internal hemorrhage that results in hypovolemia, poor systemic perfusion, organ failure, and death (▶ Figure 28-1).

Aortic Dissection

An aortic dissection involves the dissection of the layers of the aorta, which is initiated by an intimal layer tear. Blood, under the force of arterial pressure, passes through the intimal tear and enters the media of the aorta and splits (dissects) the aortic wall. Dissection of the layers results in a false lumen, which then disrupts

normal blood flow patterns and can result in deranged organ perfusion and organ dysfunction. The aortic dissection typically begins as a tear in the tunica intima, usually in the ascending thoracic portion of the aorta about 10 cm above the aortic semilunar valve, although it can occur in the descending aorta as well.

Because the systolic pressure in the aorta is consistently high, over time a tear occurs to the tunica intima; the driving force of arterial blood flooding into this tear starts to dissect (or "split") the intimal and medial layers of the aortic wall from each other. The developing dissection may progress in either a forward (distal) or backward (proximal) direction, or both. Should the dissection progress proximally, it may involve the aortic valve and render it incompetent because of structural damage. It can also dissect into the peritoneal cavity, leading to acute tamponade. Conversely, should the dissection progress distally, it can disrupt the arteries that branch off the aortic arch and proximal descending aorta.

Aortic dissections are commonly confused with aortic aneurysms, but the ALS management of an aneurysm is drastically different from that of a dissection. The

AEMT may also hear about an aortic dissection being referred to as a "dissecting aortic aneurysm," but this is inappropriate, as an aneurysm does not have a "false passage" of blood flow, nor does a dissection result from a diffuse weakening of the vascular walls.

Pathophysiologically, the dissection results in altered blood flow through the aorta (typically the ascending aorta and aortic arch), and the aneurysm results in the hemorrhaging of blood into the abdominal or thoracic cavity because of a breach in all three vascular layers of the aorta. Table 28-1 summarizes the differences between aortic aneurysms and aortic dissections.

ASSESSMENT FINDINGS

Often, during the physical assessment and interview of a patient with a cardiovascular emergency, typical clues within the assessment findings and medical history can cue the AEMT into the underlying pathology causing the patient's clinical signs and symptoms. For example, patients with known hypertension or abdominal aneurysms are commonly on medications to help regulate blood pressure, and although aortic dissection is commonly an emergency that presents acutely, the AEMT may find a history of family members with this medical problem or may find that the patient has one of the connective tissue disorders that predisposes him to a dissection.

In any instance, the AEMT should always approach these patients with an open mind and perform a thorough assessment to prevent a pigeonhole approach to treatment. Just because a patient with one of these emergencies

TABLE 28-1	Differences Between Aortic Aneurysm and Aortic Dissection	
	Aortic Aneurysm	**Aortic Dissection**
Etiology	Primarily arteriosclerotic	Arterial hypertension
Pathophysiology	Weakening and dilation of all three aortic walls	Intimal tear leading to blood flow that dissects media from intima Creates false passage
Location	Primarily abdominal aorta	Primarily thoracic aorta
Incidence/Prevalence	Men > women Whites > blacks	Males > 50 Connective disease disorder

may be complaining of chest discomfort, the liberal use of nitroglycerin and other treatment modalities may prove harmful to the patient's hemodynamic status.

With patients who have a history of hypertension, a high blood pressure reading may well be normal for them—therefore, always attempt to find out the patient's normal blood pressure before interpreting the significance of the current blood pressure. If the patient has a blood pressure that is significantly higher than his normal pressure, however, consider the findings to be related to the hypertension. The following are the signs and symptoms of a hypertensive emergency:

- Strong, often bounding pulse (from increased peripheral perfusion)
- Skin possibly warm, dry, or moist (depends on degree of sympathetic discharge)
- Severe headache (from the high blood pressure increasing intracranial pressure)
- Ringing in the ears (auditory manifestation of neurological irritation)
- Nausea and/or vomiting (sympathetic discharge and/or neurological finding)
- Elevated blood pressure (typically higher than the patient's normal blood pressure)
- Respiratory distress (from poor pulmonary perfusion and/or fluid backing up into the lungs)
- Chest pain (increased workload on heart to overcome systemic resistance)
- Seizures (manifestation of neurologic irritation) or other mental status changes
- Focal neural deficits (manifestation of neurologic irritation)
- Possible nosebleed (elevated systolic pressure within the fragile nasal mucosa)
- Indications of organ dysfunction (stroke, heart attack, pulmonary edema)

Aortic aneurysms may remain asymptomatic indefinitely, meaning that they are clinically silent until they rupture. Once an aneurysm reaches about 5 cm in size, there is a high risk of rupturing; however, some aneurysms may reach more than 15 cm in diameter before rupturing.

The patient with a large aneurysm (which most commonly occurs within the abdominal cavity) may have a pulsatile mass superior to the umbilicus; however, in some patients with a large body habitus, this may be difficult to appreciate. The patient may also have foot pain, discoloration, or even sores on the toes arising from vascular occlusion because of material shed from the aneurysm. Other clinical findings include back pain, flank pain, throbbing or colicky abdominal pain, a sensation of abdominal fullness, and decreased femoral pulses. It is important for the AEMT to note that abdominal pain often indicates rupture and that the classic triad of "pain–hypotension–mass" may be noted.

The clinical presentation of aortic dissections can vary, depending on the type of dissection occurring to the patient. The management during the acute phase, however, is very similar. More than 95 percent of patients with an aortic dissection complain of a severe, sharp "tearing" type of chest pain radiating to the upper back or scapula. Anterior pain is associated with dissections that involve the ascending aorta, whereas posterior pain between the shoulder blades is more commonly associated with dissections involving the descending aorta. Depending on the vascular structures involved that originate off the aortic arch and descending aorta, neck or arm pain may also be present. Strokelike symptoms have been reported as a result of compromise of the carotid arteries.

Hypertension is another associated finding, seen in more than 60 percent of all patients. Depending on the location of the dissection, the patient may exhibit varied pulse pressures between the left and right sides of the body (that being if the dissection has progressed along the aortic arch and involved the arterial origins of the vessels located there). In addition, decreased carotid pulses may be present on one or both sides of the neck. Further or prolonged dissection may result in altered mental status or neurologic compromise from the vascular disruption. Additional signs or symptoms include any of the following:

- Loss of speech
- Dyspnea
- Paraplegia
- Myocardial infarction
- Abdominal pain (mesenteric infarction)
- Extremity weakness
- Hematuria (blood in urine)
- Decreased bowel sounds

Occasionally the pain from a dissection may be confused with the pain of either myocardial ischemia or infarction. Dissections, however, are not commonly associated with the other clinical findings consistent with an acute coronary syndrome, such as congestive heart failure, diaphoresis, and changes to the electrocardiogram, except that in some cases the dissection may dissect proximally and occlude the coronary arteries, leading to an ST-elevation myocardial infarction (STEMI). Table 28-2 compares the findings of abdominal aneurysms with aortic dissections.

EMERGENCY MEDICAL CARE

In the prehospital setting, the delineation between patients with a vascular emergency versus some other pathology caused by cardiovascular disease may be difficult to make without additional diagnostic tests available only in the emergency department. As such, the AEMT may find himself treating multiple abnormal pathologies. Regardless, always remember to support

TABLE 28-2	Assessment Findings of Aortic Aneurysm and Aortic Dissection	
	Aortic Aneurysm	**Aortic Dissection**
Pain location	Primarily abdominal	Primarily thoracic
Vital signs	Tachycardia and hypotension with rupture	Tachycardia or bradycardia, hypertension, pulse deficits
Important clinical symptoms	Clinically silent until rupture, abdominal fullness, abdominal pulsations, back pain	Sharp, "tearing" chest pain, pulse deficits, neurologic dysfunctions

lost functions to the airway, breathing, and circulatory components in these patients.

Remember also that the patient's hypertensive emergency or vascular emergency (aneurysm or dissection) can rapidly decompensate into cardiac arrest; as such, never leave the patient alone while retrieving equipment or preparing the cot, never allow the patient to walk down stairs or to the cot, and always keep the automated external defibrillator (AED) readily available. The following is a summary of management considerations:

1. **Establish and maintain an open airway.**

2. **Provide oxygen** if the patient is dyspneic, hypoxemic, has obvious signs of heart failure, or has an SpO_2 reading of less than 94 percent. Initiate oxygen therapy via nasal cannula at 4 lpm and titrate oxygen therapy to maintain an SpO_2 reading of 94 percent or greater. If the breathing is inadequate, provide positive pressure ventilation at 10 to 12/min with high-flow supplemental oxygen.

3. **Position the patient.** Semi- or high Fowler positioning will assist the patient in breathing. If positive pressure ventilation is being provided or frank hypotension is present, the patient will need to be placed supine for ongoing management.

4. **Initiate an intravenous line of normal saline.** In the case of a leaking or ruptured aortic aneurysm or aortic dissection, fluid administration may be necessary if the patient is hypotensive or exhibiting signs and symptoms of shock. Follow your local protocol and do not delay transport to initiate an intravenous line.

5. **Ensure rapid transport to the emergency department.** Notify the receiving ED as early as possible.

TRANSITIONING

REVIEW ITEMS

1. Which of the following statements best reflects the differences between chest pain from an acute coronary syndrome and that of an aortic dissection?
   a. Chest pain from a myocardial infarction is more intense than chest pain from a dissection.
   b. Dissection pain is commonly dull in characteristic, unlike that of a heart attack.
   c. Angina typically results in midsternal pain, whereas dissection pain radiates into the left and right arms.
   d. Dissection pain is typically "sharp and tearing," whereas ischemic pain is typically "dull" or "heavy."

2. Which of the following best describes why aneurysms are more likely to occur in the abdominal region rather than the thoracic region?
   a. The systolic blood pressure is higher in the abdominal aorta.
   b. The thoracic aorta is stronger than the abdominal aorta.
   c. The abdominal aorta has more arteries originating from it, allowing more locations for an aneurysm to develop.
   d. The venous pressure is lower in the thoracic aorta than in the abdominal aorta.

3. The most important determining factor for a hypertensive emergency is _____.
   a. the speed in which the pressure increases
   b. the age of the patient when diagnosed with hypertension

   c. whether the patient has primary versus secondary hypertension
   d. whether the systolic blood pressure is greater than 160 mmHg for two consecutive assessments

4. Your 72-year-old male patient is complaining of diffuse pain to the abdomen. Assessment reveals the abdomen to be globally distended with a palpable mass just above the umbilicus. Furthermore, you note a diminishment in the pedal pulses. The most likely cause for these findings is _____.
   a. hypertensive crisis
   b. descending abdominal aortic aneurysm
   c. descending thoracic aortic dissection
   d. myocardial infarction with mesenteric infarction

5. You suspect that a patient you are caring for is experiencing an aortic dissection. Other than the type and location of pain, what else would be a consistent finding that would help delineate a dissection from either a hypertensive crisis or abdominal aneurysm?
   a. systolic pressure over 140 mmHg
   b. presence of a severe headache associated with dizziness
   c. unequal pulse amplitudes or blood pressure in the upper extremities
   d. onset of a grand mal seizure in the absence of a diagnosed seizure problem

APPLIED PATHOPHYSIOLOGY

A 72-year-old white male patient is complaining of severe abdominal pain. You note that the patient has abdominal distension, low blood pressure, absent pedal pulses, and cyanotic legs and feet. His mental status is rapidly deteriorating, and the breathing and pulse rates continue to climb. Given this presentation, respond to the following questions:

1. From what medical emergency is this patient most likely suffering?

2. List the clinical findings that support your answer.

3. Explain the pathophysiology behind the findings you indicated as they relate to your field impression.

4. Discuss the differences in pathophysiology of the following vascular emergencies discussed in this topic:

a. Hypertensive emergency

b. Aortic aneurysm

c. Aortic dissection

Fill in the following chart with the appropriate information regarding the clinical findings of the vascular emergencies discussed previously:

	Heart rate	Respiration rate	Blood pressure	Type of pain	Location of pain	Mental status	Peripheral pulses
Hypertensive crisis							
Aortic aneurysm							
Aortic dissection							

CLINICAL DECISION MAKING

While returning from a long distant transport out of town, you and your partner have just reentered your EMS jurisdiction. Just before exiting the freeway, you are waved down by a police officer who has a car pulled over alongside the freeway. After you notify dispatch, activate your emergency lights, and safely position the ambulance, the police officer approaches and states that he happened on this car pulled off the road, so he decided to stop and investigate. He states that he found the driver slumped forward in the driver's seat, mumbling incomprehensible sounds. He adds that he did not detect any odor of alcohol, nor did he see any active bleeding or signs of injury.

1. Based on the scene size-up characteristics, identify at least five different medical emergencies caused by cardiovascular diseases that could result in this presentation.

The primary assessment reveals the patient to be an elderly black male who responds to verbal stimuli with garbled speech but moves his extremities symmetrically to noxious stimuli. His airway is clear, his breathing is rapid at 24/minute, respirations are slightly shallow, but alveolar breath sounds are present, and slight inspiratory crackles are noted. Peripheral pulses are present and noted to be rapid. The pulse oximeter reads 96 percent on ambient air, and blood pressure is measured at 168/102 mmHg. As you prepare to extricate the patient from the auto, he has a brief seizure and then vomits.

2. What are the life threats, if any, to the patient that you are currently aware of?

3. What treatment modalities should be employed to correct these life threats?

Secondary assessment reveals the pupils to be equal and reactive, breath sounds are unchanged, and the blood glucose level is noted to be 121 mg/dL. The skin is found to be warm and dry, and no unusual rashes or hives are noted on the skin. The patient is still moving his extremities symmetrically when noxious stimuli are applied. Peripheral pulses are present, equal, and bounding. The blood pressure is now 176/110 mmHg. The abdomen is soft to palpation, and you cannot find any signs of trauma to the body.

4. What medical emergency is the patient most likely experiencing?

5. What clinical signs and/or symptoms support your field impression?

Standard Medicine

Competency Applies fundamental knowledge to provide basic and selected advanced emergency care and transportation based on assessment findings for an acutely ill patient.

TOPIC

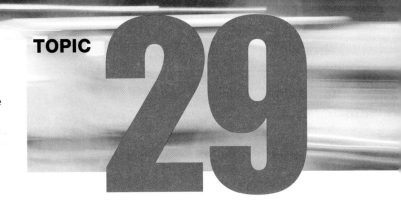

29

TOXICOLOGY: STREET DRUGS

INTRODUCTION

At one time, illicit drug use (sometimes referred to as "recreational drug use") was found almost exclusively in larger metropolitan areas, with the persons abusing drugs being typically on the lower socioeconomic status (SES) scale. In this scenario, it was easier in that time to identify the drug abuser, and because only a limited number of illicit drugs were abused, the assessment and management typically followed only one of a few pathways.

Over the past several years, however, the use of street drugs has migrated to more rural communities as well, and the number of abused agents has increased almost exponentially (▶ Figure 29-1). In addition, new varieties, through the mixing of one or more illicit drugs, have led to multiple combinations of new drugs that can have varied effects on the human mind and body. Further complicating the matter is that younger children and adults positioned higher on the SES scale are also using illicit drugs. Even the abuse of prescription medications and over-the-counter (OTC) medications continues to rise.

Although the approach to any patient with a toxicologic emergency from illicit drug use follows the same assessment process, the EMT needs to be cognizant of special problems regarding the effects of the toxic agent on the patient. This

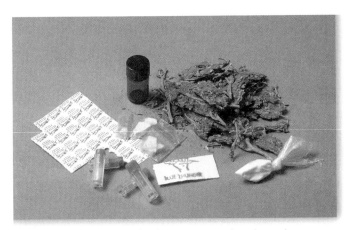

Figure 29-1 A variety of substances may be abused.

TRANSITION highlights

- Frequency with which certain drugs are abused in the United States.

- Many street drugs can be classified into clusters to help the AEMT recognize assessment patterns that indicate the category of drug abused:
  – Stimulants.
  – Depressants.
  – Cannabis.
  – Hallucinogens.
  – Inhalants.
  – Alcohol.

- Core assessment findings for each drug cluster discussed.

- Integration of the AEMT's assessment format and clinical findings with the appropriate medical care for a patient suffering from a street drug overdose.

segment of the text emphasizes the use of illicit or "street drugs" and discusses how Advanced EMTs should approach their assessment and management of the patient to ensure their own safety as well as provide appropriate care.

EPIDEMIOLOGY

The National Survey on Drug Use and Health (NSDUH) gathers information across multiple categories of illicit drug use. In 2007 a report was published estimating that more than 19.9 million Americans 12 years of age and older—8 percent of the population over age 12—had used illicit drugs within the 30 days prior to data collection (adding to the significance of these data is that the survey did not include the use of tobacco or alcohol).

The data also showed that the highest rates were in the 18-to-20-year-old age bracket, and overall, more than 77 percent of

In many situations, the person abusing drugs also has psychological problems.

the illicit drug use was by individuals between the ages of 14 and 29. Men were twice as likely to use illicit drugs. The most commonly abused illicit drugs (in descending order of frequency) were marijuana, psychotropic agents, cocaine, hallucinogens, inhalant agents, and heroin.

Alcohol abuse is also most common to the 15-to-24-year-old age bracket and has an incidence rate that includes more than 15.1 million people annually in the United States. The clarity of these statistics is sobering, and the chance that the AEMT will encounter one of these patients is very strong. Adding to the effect of illicit drug use is the fact that, in many situations, the person abusing the drugs also has psychological problems, he may be aggressive or combative, or he may also be suffering from concurrent trauma sustained while under the effects of the drug (e.g., motor vehicle collisions, fighting, and falls).

PATHOPHYSIOLOGY

Many times, the AEMT may not know the specific agent on which patient overdosed; even if a drug's name is available, there are so many different names (generic and "street" names) that there is a possibility the AEMT may not be familiar with it. In this situation, the AEMT may want to approach patient management based on the assessment findings of the patient.

Often, a pattern of findings (called a toxidrome) will indicate how the drug is affecting the body. For example, the AEMT may find either stimulatory or depressive effects on the central nervous system (CNS). As such, the best way to familiarize oneself with all these drugs is to appreciate the pathophysiologic effects by clusters—in other words, many drugs can be categorized into a cluster in which drugs share common findings. Table 29-1 lists the drug cluster name with the common drugs that fit that cluster (both generic and street names). The following section identifies these drug clusters and discusses the pathophysiologic changes that occur in the body as a result of abuse.

Stimulants

Stimulant overdoses typically have profound effects on the CNS that mimic a sympathetic discharge. As such, the resultant increase in heart rate and blood pressure may lead to profound hypertension. The respiratory rate often increases, and the pupils dilate. Core body temperature elevates, the body may start to tremble, and diaphoresis is often present. The blood pressure may rise to dangerously high levels, causing seizures, and the patient may experience a myocardial infarction and dysrhythmias due to coronary artery vasoconstriction. Psychologically, the patient may be aggressive, combative, or delirious.

Depressants (Narcotics and Sedatives)

Basically the opposite of stimulants, depressants will lead to a lowering of bodily activities, as the CNS is depressed as a result of the drug ingestion. Often the activity of the brainstem is depressed, which causes a lowering of the respiratory rate with concurrent shallow breathing and possible apnea. Cardiac output drops as the heart rate slows, and blood pressure commonly decreases. Because of CNS

TABLE 29-1	Commonly Abused Drugs			
Uppers	**Downers**	**Narcotics**	**Mind-Altering Drugs**	**Volatile Chemicals**
Amphetamine (Benzedrine, bennies, pep pills, ups, uppers, cartwheels) *Biphetamine* (bam) *Cocaine* (coke, snow, crack) *Desoxyn* (black beauties *Dextroamphetamine* (dexies, Dexedrine) *Methamphetamine* (speed, crank, meth, crystal, diet pills, Methedrine) *Methylphenidate* (Ritalin) *Phenmetrazine* (Preludin)	*Amobarbital* (blue devils, downers barbs, Amytal) *Barbiturates* (downers, dolls, barbs, rainbows) *Chloral hydrate* (knockout drops, Noctec) *Methaqualone* (Quaalude, ludes, Sopor, sopors) *Nonbarbiturate sedatives* (various tranquilizers and sleeping pills: Valium or diazepam, Miltown, Equanil, meprobamate, Thorazine, Compazine, Librium or chlordiazepoxide, reserpine, Tranxene or chlorazepate and other benzodiazepines) *Paraldehyde, pentobarbital* (yellow jackets, barbs, Nembutal) *Phenobarbital* (goofballs, phennies, barbs) *Secobarbital* (red devils, barbs, Seconal)	*Codeine* (often in cough syrup) *Demerol, dilaudid, fentanyl* (Sublimaze) *Heroin* ("H," horse, junk, smack, stuff) *Methadone* (dolly) *Morphine, opium* (op, poppy) *Meperidine* (Demerol) *Paregoric* (contains opium) *Tylenol with codeine* (1, 2, 3, 4)	**Hallucinogenic:** DMT, LSD (acid, sunshine) *Mescaline* (peyote, mesc) *Morning glory seeds,* *PCP* (angel dust, hog, peace pills) *Psilocybin* (magic mushrooms) *STP* (serenity, tranquility, peace) **Nonhallucinogenic:** *Hash, marijuana* (grass, pot, tea, wood, dope) *THC* **Mixed effects:** *Ecstasy* [stimulant, hallucinogen] *Gamma hydroxybutyric acid* (GHB) [depressant, visual disturbances, date rape] *Rohypnol* (roofies) [depressant, amnestic, date rape]	*Amyl nitrate* (snappers, poppers) *Butyl nitrate* (Locker Room, Rush) *Cleaning fluid* (carbon tetrachloride) *Furniture polish, gasoline, glue, hair spray, nail polish remover, paint thinner, typewriting correction fluids*

depression, the patient's orientation will diminish, and the patient may be comatose. Pupillary constriction is common, and visual disturbances can occur as well. Some depressant drugs may cause seizures, or seizures may occur due to the drop in cerebral perfusion or hypoxemia and acidosis.

Cannabis Products

Cannabis (marijuana) causes both psychological and physiologic effects on the body. Psychologically, the patient will display changes in perception (misinterpreting social situations), the mood may be elevated or depressed, euphoria may occur, and some patients may become paranoid. The patient will also have disturbances in short-term memory. Physiologically, the heart rate becomes elevated, but the systolic pressure usually drops as a result of peripheral vasodilation. The eyes may become reddened because of congestion of ocular blood vessels, and muscle groups may become ataxic, so the patient may be prone to accidental trauma from falls or motor vehicle collisions when driving or engaging in similarly demanding activities.

Hallucinogens

Hallucinogens are agents that largely affect the abuser's perception of reality. With hallucinogens, the patient's psychological stability is of greater concern than his physiologic stability. As a result of the cerebral effects, the patient will often state that he "hears" colors or "sees" sounds (known as *crossover sensations*). Often there is a distortion of shapes, sizes, and colors (either enhanced or diminished). Minimal changes occur to the patient's hemodynamic status, although sympathetic stimulation and even death can occur from extreme overdoses. With hallucinogens, the real danger is not so much the toxicity of the drug but, rather, the unpredictability of the psychological reaction.

Inhalants

Inhalants constitute a drug cluster that includes organic compounds that are very volatile in nature, and because they are sniffed or inhaled, absorption into the bloodstream and rapid distribution to the tissues of the body are nearly immediate. Often the inhaled substances are readily available in the household or are easily purchased. Sometimes inhalants are also referred to as "deliriants," as they can easily cause a state of delirium, as evidenced by the patient displaying excitement, confusion, depression, slurred speaking, and possible hallucinations.

Depending on the nature of the inhalant, damage to mucous membranes or the lungs (causing hypoxia, acidosis, or even pulmonary edema) can occur. Other pathologic changes can include changes in heart rate, confusion, possible coma, seizures, heart failure, and death. Because users typically inhale these compounds repeatedly, they put themselves at risk for fatal overdoses.

Alcohol

Otherwise known as ethanol, drinking alcohol is rapidly absorbed by the intestines and reaches the bloodstream, where it is circulated throughout the body with a multitude of effects. The first organ to be affected is the brain. The areas of the brain most susceptible to alcohol intoxication are those that control memory, attention, coordination, and sleep.

Initially, drinking alcohol will create a feeling of euphoria. With higher blood levels, alcohol causes an impairment of normal cerebral functioning, usually impairing cognitive abilities that control conduct and behavior. With moderate doses, the heart rate increases with slight peripheral vasodilation, which creates reddened skin (usually to the face and neck).

With even higher blood levels, alcohol becomes a depressant that depresses mental status to a point at which the patient becomes extremely ataxic, lethargic, comatose, and eventually unresponsive. At this point the patient is at great risk for aspiration and death from vomiting with loss of airway protection mechanisms. Compounding this effect is the type of patient: People who weigh less become intoxicated more quickly, and women feel the effects faster than men.

ASSESSMENT FINDINGS

Dispatch information may provide information prior to your arrival at the scene that will lead you to suspect a drug overdose. Clues at the scene may point to a potential illicit drug overdose, such as needles, drug paraphernalia, pills, alcohol, strong odors, family/bystander reports of the patient abusing drugs, or statements by the patient that he was abusing drugs.

> Cannabis (marijuana) causes both psychological and physiologic effects on the body.

It is of utmost importance that EMTs take every precaution to protect themselves from harm should the patient become aggressive or violent, or if the patient's environment is harmful to the EMS crew (e.g., if the patient was inhaling a chemical that is still concentrated in the air, it may afflict the EMS crew as well). The patient may also have remnants of the drug on his person, staining on the face from inhaling (▶ Figure 29-2),

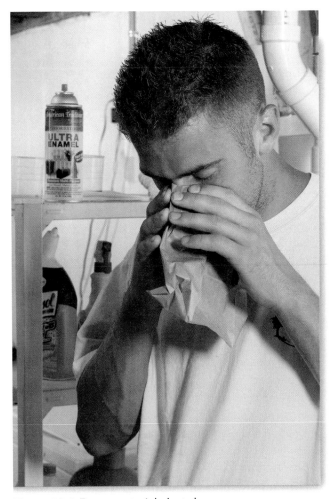

Figure 29-2 Exposure to inhalant drug.

partially chewed pills or vomitus in his mouth, and needle tracks on his arms from repeated drug abuse by injection (▶ **Figure 29-3**).

The following is a list of symptoms common to the drug clusters discussed earlier. The EMT is reminded to consider the changes in physiology from the abused drug as the patient illustrates the following signs and symptoms:

Stimulants (moderate doses)

- Increased alertness
- Mood elevation
- Excitation
- Euphoria
- Tachycardia
- Elevated blood pressure
- Insomnia
- Loss of appetite

Stimulants (higher doses)

- Dysrhythmias
- Angina
- Infarction
- Agitation and violence
- Increased body temperature
- Hallucinations
- Seizures
- Hypertension
- Altered mental status

Depressants (narcotics and opioids)

- Euphoria
- Drowsiness
- Lethargy
- Respiratory depression or apnea
- Constricted pupils
- Constipation
- Nausea
- Clammy skin
- Needle tracks with repeated injections

Depressants (sedatives and tranquilizers)

- Slurred speech
- Drowsiness
- Impaired thinking
- Incoordination
- Drunken behavior without smell of alcohol (EtOH)
- Shallow respirations
- Hypotension
- Seizures

Cannabis

- Euphoria
- Relaxed inhibition
- Increased appetite
- Dry mouth
- Disoriented behavior
- Fatigue
- Tremors
- Paranoia

Hallucinogens

- Motor disturbances
- Anxiety
- Paranoia
- Illusions and hallucinations
- Poor time/space perception
- Psychosis ("bad trip")
- Exacerbation of psychiatric problems
- Flashbacks

Inhalants

- Excitement
- Euphoria
- Feelings of drunkenness
- Giddiness
- Loss of inhibitions
- Aggressiveness
- Delusions
- Headache
- Nausea
- Drowsiness
- Staining to face
- Possible sudden cardiac arrest

Alcohol

- Euphoria
- Confusion
- Slurred speech
- Impaired balance
- Ataxia
- Erratic behavior
- Reddened eyes
- Dilated pupils
- Lethargy or coma
- Nausea and vomiting
- Death with acute severe intoxication

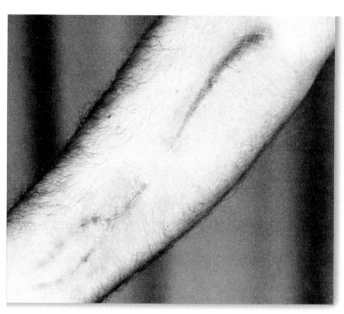

Figure 29-3 Needle track marks on the extremities are a sign of injected drug use.

EMERGENCY MEDICAL CARE

The assessment and management of a patient suffering from a toxicologic emergency related to illicit drug use can be a challenge for the AEMT. First, scene hazards may be present and can include threats of violence by the patient or bystanders, or toxic substances may still be present in the air or on the ground. Second, trying to gather information about the nature of the overdose is hampered by variables such as the clinical status of the patient, the patient's (or bystanders') unwillingness to provide information about the situation for fear of legal ramifications, or simply the patient being found unresponsive with no witnesses present.

If the illicit drug is identified by name, the AEMT should reference the name with a pocket guide to determine what cluster it belongs so he can best anticipate and recognize the presenting signs and symptoms. Regional poison centers are also a valuable resource. This information is also necessary for the hospital to provide definitive treatment. Although more specific medical interventions are identified here, the crux of the management will center around three specific areas, which can be solidified into "supporting lost function."

Of special note is the use of activated charcoal for ingested poisons. Activated charcoal (▶ **Figure 29-4**) is a medication carried on the ambulance that may be administered in certain ingested overdoses if it can be administered safely for the

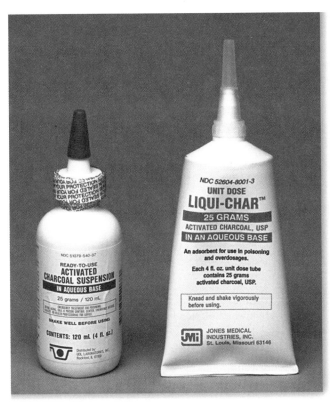

Figure 29-4 Activated charcoal.

patient, within a certain time frame of ingestion, and with permission of local medical direction. ▶ Figure 29-5 shows the way in which activated charcoal is administered.

The following are more specific guidelines to use when treating a patient with a known or suspected illicit drug overdose:

1. **Ensure an open airway.** Advanced airways may be used in respiratory or cardiac arrest if allowed by protocol. Many overdose patients with depressed respiratory drive still have an intact gag reflex. Common manual airway techniques are often sufficient and have less likelihood of causing vomiting. Be especially attentive to episodes of vomiting, which are common with illicit drug use in general and ingested drugs in particular.

2. **Provide oxygen.** If the patient is breathing adequately, consider a nonrebreather at 15 lpm. If the patient is breathing inadequately as evidenced by an extremely tachypneic or bradypneic rate, provide positive pressure ventilation (PPV) at 10 to 12/min with high-flow supplemental oxygen. Use pulse oximetry, and try to keep the reading greater than 95 percent.

3. **Position the patient as appropriate.** If the patient has an altered mental status, a lateral recumbent position will help maintain the airway should the patient regurgitate. And should the patient regurgitate, save the vomitus, as it may provide clues to the ED staff about the type of poisoning from which the patient is suffering. Suction the patient when necessary.

4. **Determine the blood glucose level.** If you identify a hypoglycemic component to the patient's status, the administration of IV D_{50} or oral glucose may be warranted, depending on airway status, if local protocol allows.

5. **For the patient who ingested an illicit substance, administer 1 gram/kilogram of activated charcoal** (if protocol allows or if advised by your poison control center or medical direction). Be sure that the patient is conscious and can follow directions and that there is minimal risk of aspiration.

6. **If a narcotic (opioid) overdose is suspected, administer naloxone** 0.4 to 2.0 mg titrated to adequate respiratory effort (▶ Figure 29-6). Naloxone may be administered IV, IM, SQ, or intranasally. If using a nasal atomizer, be sure to push the plunger of the syringe briskly to ensure that the medication sprays to the nasal mucosa (rather than dripping out).

7. **Provide rapid transport to the emergency department.** Notify the receiving emergency department as early as possible, and consider calling your local poison control center.

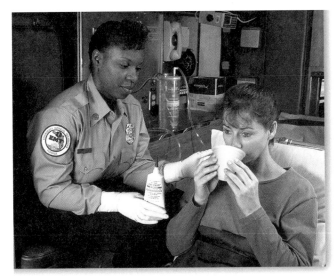

Figure 29-5 Administering activated charcoal. You may want to administer the medication in an opaque cup that has a lid with a hole for a straw.

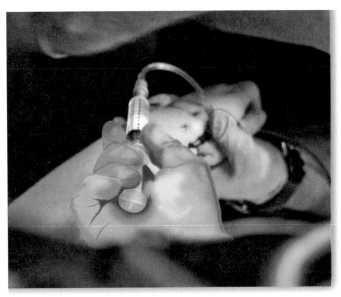

Figure 29-6 AEMT administering a medication (naloxone).

8. **If the patient becomes pulseless and apneic (no pulse, no respirations), immediately apply the automated external defibrillator and follow your protocol for arrest management.**

Providing care for a patient who has abused drugs often presents a number of challenges to AEMTs. As stated throughout this topic, the optimal treatment of an overdosing patient comes from rapid and accurate identification of the illicit substances. Because every patient situation is unique, a discussion with your regional poison center or medical command may help to establish the best treatment approach.

The treatment rendered by the AEMT is still largely supportive of lost function because of the toxic exposure. These interventions include airway skills, ventilatory support, circulatory support, and any other interventions needed should the situation be complicated by other conditions (such as seizures or stroke) or trauma (such as falls or motor vehicle crashes).

TRANSITIONING

REVIEW ITEMS

1. A patient who presents with anxiousness, tachycardia, hypertension, and dilated pupils was most likely abusing what type of illicit drug?
   a. stimulant
   b. depressant
   c. hallucinogen
   d. alcohol (EtOH)

2. What type of overdose is characterized by distortions of reality and delirium states but no real changes in vital signs?
   a. stimulant
   b. depressant
   c. hallucinogen
   d. alcohol (EtOH)

3. A patient is found unresponsive in a car that is parked on a deserted road. The patient presents with slow breathing, constricted pupils, and hypotension. This is most characteristic of what type of illicit drug use?
   a. stimulant
   b. depressant
   c. hallucinogen
   d. alcohol (EtOH)

4. Which of the following findings would be most consistent with a patient who has been inhaling a volatile chemical?
   a. altered mental status
   b. slow onset of signs
   c. nausea and vomiting
   d. staining of the face

5. What category of illicit drugs would be most responsive to administration of activated charcoal?
   a. injected
   b. ingested
   c. inhalant
   d. absorbed

APPLIED PATHOPHYSIOLOGY

A known drug abuser in a small community ingested a large amount of diet pills four hours prior to EMS notification. Upon EMS arrival, the patient is lethargic but becomes combative whenever the providers attempt to perform a physical assessment. After safely restraining the patient and completing a primary and secondary assessment, they note the following: The patient's airway is intact, mucous membranes are dry, he is breathing at 32 times a minute, but each breath is very shallow. The heart rate is 136 beats per minute and irregular, and the blood pressure is 232/114 mmHg. Pulse oximetry reads 93 percent on room air, and the patient's skin is very warm to the touch. Pupils are fully dilated, and the patient mutters something that sounds like, "My chest is on fire." Given this clinical presentation, discuss the following questions:

1. To what category (drug cluster) would this drug belong?

2. Why are there marked elevations in the patient's heart rate, blood pressure, and respiratory rate?

3. What would be three medical emergencies the patient may suffer as a result of this drug ingestion?

4. With what life threats, if any, is this patient presenting?

5. Because the patient ingested this medication, would the administration of activated charcoal be appropriate? Why or why not?

6. Describe the anticipated pathophysiologic changes in normal homeostasis for a patient who as abused the following illicit drugs:

   a. Stimulant

   b. Depressant

   c. Hallucinogen

7. What three clinical findings are most reliable for determining whether the patient has abused an inhalant drug?

8. In the following table, identify whether the given parameters would be elevated, depressed, or unremarkable for the given illicit drug abuse.

Type of Substance	Heart Rate	Respiratory Rate	Blood Pressure	Pupil Response	Mental Status	Muscle Tone
Stimulant						
Depressant						
Hallucinogen						
Cannabis						
Alcohol						

CLINICAL DECISION MAKING

You are dispatched for an "unknown medical" emergency for a 16-year-old male patient. On arrival at the residence, you are greeted by the patient's parents, who tell you that they had a recent argument with their son regarding their disapproval of his girlfriend, during which they demanded that he quit seeing her. Reportedly, hours after the fight, the patient again arrived at the girlfriend's house in a "confused state." His girlfriend decided to call his parents, who in turn called EMS when the patient stated he also took "all my mom's psycho pills." The patient became unresponsive shortly thereafter. The patient presents unresponsive to noxious stimuli, vomitus is in the airway, and the heart rate is 40 beats per minute with cool skin and no peripheral pulses.

1. Given this limited information, into which drug cluster would the type of drug taken most likely fit?

2. With what life threats, if any, is this patient presenting?

3. List your treatment, in order of priority, that you would administer for this patient, assuming his condition does not improve.

4. For each of your listed treatment interventions, briefly discuss how each would help restore the patient's hemodynamic status back toward normal.

5. How would you integrate any advanced modalities (e.g., advanced airways, medications) into your patient care?

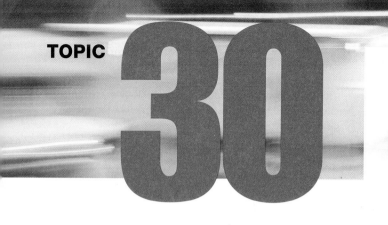
Standard Medicine

Competency Applies fundamental knowledge to provide basic and selected advanced emergency care and transportation based on assessment findings for an acutely ill patient.

RESPIRATORY EMERGENCIES: AIRWAY RESISTANCE DISORDERS

TRANSITION *highlights*

- *Frequency of airway resistance disorders in the United States.*

- *Pathophysiologic changes that occur with airway resistance disorders:*
  - Asthma (intrinsic and extrinsic).
  - Bronchitis (acute and chronic).
  - Bronchiolitis.

- *Relation of the assessment findings of respiratory distress to the pathophysiologic changes that occur due to the disease.*

- *Description of abnormal breath sounds commonly heard.*

- *Organized presentation of assessment findings to help the Advanced EMT delineate between different restrictive airway disorders.*

- *Treatment interventions and their relationship to improving the patient's respiratory status:*
  - Oxygen administration.
  - Positive pressure ventilation.
  - Administration of a beta-2 agonist via a metered-dose inhaler or nebulizer.
  - Patient positioning.

INTRODUCTION

Breathing, like the beating of your heart, is one of the most fundamental functions that your body does to stay alive. Fortunately, under normal conditions, breathing is essentially effortless and is under autonomic nervous system control, so we do not even have to think about it. This changes, though, when the respiratory system starts to fail because of disease or injury. Then the simple act of breathing becomes very difficult for the patient and serves as a common reason that EMS is

summoned to a patient's home. Few things are more frightening to the patient than the inability to breathe easily, and one of the most common symptoms of a respiratory emergency is shortness of breath.

For purposes of clarity, if the patient is complaining of *shortness of breath* (medically known as *dyspnea*), that refers to the patient's perception or sensation of respiratory distress. If, on assessment, the Advanced EMT finds physical signs of respiratory distress, this is known as *labored breathing*. It is important to remember that pulmonary conditions may present very similarly because many such findings arise from the body's attempt to improve breathing adequacy, not necessarily from the specific pulmonary condition.

Diseases discussed in this topic involve pathophysiologic changes that result in detrimental changes in the lung's resistance to airflow. Put another way, as these disease processes exacerbate, an increase in resistance to airflow results in labored breathing and dyspnea. The patient's presentation may be anywhere on a continuum of mild dyspnea to significantly labored breathing—so bad that the AEMT may have to intervene immediately with airway management, oxygenation, and ventilation.

In any instance, the AEMT should constantly assess the respiratory rate and tidal volume to ensure that the patient is breathing adequately. If at any time the respiratory rate or tidal volume becomes inadequate, the AEMT must be prepared to establish an airway and provide positive pressure ventilation and supplemental oxygen.

> One of the most common symptoms of a respiratory emergency is shortness of breath.

EPIDEMIOLOGY

One of the most common types of airway resistance disorders, which accounts for more than 2 million emergency department visits per year, is *asthma*. It is estimated that between 20 and 25 million people in the United States have asthma. Asthma typically presents in childhood; when patients have symptoms that persist into the second decade of life, they are likely to suffer from asthma through adulthood. Given these statistics, it is only a matter of time until the AEMT is confronted with a dyspneic patient with an asthmatic history.

Bronchitis, conversely, has been found to affect roughly 44 out of every 1,000 adults annually. More than 80 percent of these cases occur in the fall and winter months and are often associated with an upper respiratory infection (URI). Chronic bronchitis, a more severe form, has been diagnosed in more than 9.5 million people living in the United States.

Bronchiolitis is a highly contagious respiratory infection, primarily viral in etiology, which is contracted by infants during the first year or two of life. Respiratory syncytial virus (RSV) has been implicated in the majority of cases. Research has shown the incidence to peak during the fall and winter months, with the average age of those afflicted to be 2 to 6 months. Because of the maturing of the tracheobronchial tree, bronchiolitis is uncommon in children over 5 years of age. Thus, although this may not be seen as commonly by the AEMT as are adult airway resistance disorders, it is certainly common to the pediatric patient with respiratory distress.

PATHOPHYSIOLOGY
Asthma

Asthma is a common respiratory condition for which you will be called to the scene to manage. The most common complaint of the asthma patient is severe shortness of breath. Many asthma patients are aware of their condition and use medication to manage the disease and its signs and symptoms. You may be called to the scene for a patient who is suffering an early-onset asthma attack or for a patient whose medication is not reversing the attack.

In asthma, a paroxysmal narrowing of the bronchial airways results from mucus production and edema, which thicken the walls and decrease lumen size. In addition, smooth muscle constriction mediated by a trigger to which the patient is sensitive further constricts the airways, making it even harder for airflow to occur (▶ Figure 30-1).

Although the pathophysiology is similar, generally two different etiologies of asthma can be identified. *Extrinsic* asthma, or "allergic" asthma, usually results from a reaction to dust, pollen, smoke, or other irritants in the air. It is typically seasonal, occurs most often in children, and may subside after adolescence. *Intrinsic*, or "nonallergic," asthma is most common in adults and usually results from infection, emotional stress, or strenuous exercise. In either instance, the AEMT should recognize an asthma attack from its presentation, not exclusively from the patient's history.

Asthma is characterized by an increased sensitivity of the lower airways to irritants and allergens, causing bronchospasm and inflammation to the lining of the bronchioles. The following conditions in the asthma patient contribute to the increasing resistance to airflow and difficulty in breathing:

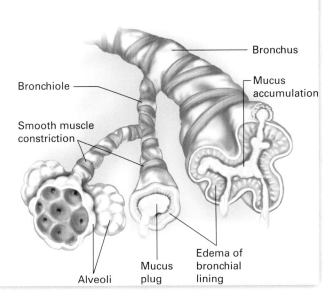

Figure 30-1 Pathophysiologic changes in the bronchioles in asthma contribute to higher airway resistance.

- **Bronchospasm.** Because of an antigen/antibody reaction, chemical mediators are released locally that promote smooth muscle constriction and restrict normal airflow.
- **Edema.** A thickening of the bronchial walls results from inflammation mediated by the asthmatic reaction. This also diminishes bronchial lumen size and inhibits normal airflow.
- **Mucus production.** Receptors located in the walls of the lung tissue detect any internal state abnormality. When this process is disrupted in asthma, an oversecretion of mucus can worsen airflow and cause smaller airways to plug.

With progression of this pathology, airflow and ventilation to the alveoli are diminished. Early in the progression, when mild bronchoconstriction is prevailing, the patient is able to inhale normally due to the active muscular contraction needed to do so. During exhalation, however, when airflow from the lungs is more passive, exhaled gases have a tendency to become trapped in the alveoli as the attack progresses. As this develops, the alveoli become distended with air; they have a tendency to collapse smaller nearby bronchioles when the lungs recoil, thereby contributing to more air trapping and making exhalation more prolonged.

Bronchoconstriction also is the underlying cause of wheezing that is heard with lung auscultation; it may be noted to be of differing qualities depending on the phase of the patient's ventilation. Because inhalation is active and airflow enters the lungs with a higher velocity, any mild bronchoconstriction may be countered by the rush of air coming in, and no wheezing may be evident. However, on passive exhalation, the airflow out of the lungs does not have the same velocity and, because it may not overcome early bronchoconstriction, expiratory wheezing will become evident. Because of this, wheezing is heard much earlier on exhalation during a mild (or early) asthma attack.

With worsening of the bronchoconstriction, edema, and mucus production, the patient is forced to use energy not only to breathe in, but also to eliminate the air from the lungs during exhalation. Thus, wheezing may be present during the entire ventilation cycle, and exhalation becomes an active process, requiring energy to push the air out of the lungs. This increased workload, coupled with diminished alveolar ventilation, leads to eventual exhaustion. Respiratory depression or arrest may follow shortly thereafter in severe cases. As such, the cessation of wheezing, which may suggest loss of air movement, may be an ominous sign of severe bronchoconstriction and deterioration.

Cessation of wheezing may be an ominous sign of severe bronchoconstriction and deterioration.

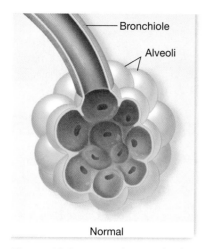
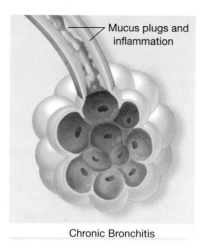

Figure 30-2 Mucus plugs and inflammation cause airway restriction in chronic bronchitis.

Unlike other chronic pulmonary diseases that result in permanent changes in the body's ability to ventilate and oxygenate and with which the patient is always experiencing some degree of respiratory distress, it takes a trigger to start an asthmatic attack. In addition, there is no structural damage, and the attacks are potentially "reversible." If the patient avoids the trigger, asthma attacks may be episodic, irregular, or even nonexistent for years. Between attacks, the patient usually has either no or very few signs or symptoms.

On the opposite end of the continuum, though, is a severe, prolonged, and life-threatening asthma attack that produces inadequate breathing and severe signs and symptoms—this is called *status asthmaticus*. Status asthmaticus is a severe asthmatic attack that does not respond to either oxygen or medication. Patients in status asthmaticus require immediate and rapid transport to the hospital.

The death rate from asthma has been rising in the past several years.

Acute Bronchitis and Chronic Bronchitis

As discussed elsewhere in this text, the conducting airways of the tracheobronchial tree are lined with mucous membranes that contribute to the humidification, filtration, and warming of inspired air. At times, however, this mucous lining can become inflamed from inhalation of an irritant, resulting in thickening of the mucosal wall and airway restriction from swelling and mucus production. These changes, when severe enough or when present in a patient who is susceptible to pulmonary dysfunction, can lead to respiratory distress and labored breathing. This condition is known as bronchitis, of which there are two categories, acute bronchitis and chronic bronchitis.

Acute bronchitis, as the name implies, is a respiratory dysfunction that has a short duration, typically no more than three weeks. During an episode of bronchitis, the bronchial tubes become inflamed, and occasionally sputum production will increase to the point at which the patient also has a productive cough. Acute bronchitis can be triggered by infectious agents (viruses and bacteria) or noninfectious agents (such as dust, smoking, or other inhaled pollutants). As a result of the narrowed lumen of the bronchi and bronchial structures from inflammation and an increase in sputum production and collection, the bronchitis patient may seek EMS care for respiratory distress and excessive coughing.

Chronic bronchitis is a disease process in the spectrum of chronic obstructive pulmonary disease (COPD) that involves inflammation, swelling, and thickening of the lining of the bronchi and bronchioles. This in turn leads to a narrowing of the lumen that the airflow must pass through. In addition, there is excessive mucus production from enlargement and multiplication of the mucus-secreting glands of the tracheobronchial tree, which leads to plugging of the smaller airways and further derangements in airflow.

The distal alveoli remain unaffected by the disease; however, the inflamed and swollen bronchioles and thick mucus restrict airflow to the alveoli so they do not expand fully, causing respiratory distress and possible hypoxia. The heavy mucus that resides in the conducting airway is difficult to expel; it traps inhaled particles that, if not eliminated from the body, can manifest into recurrent respiratory infections that leave scar tissue and further narrow the airways (▶ Figure 30-2).

In summary, the major pathophysiology associated with chronic bronchitis is the swelling and thickening of the inner lining of the lower respiratory tract and an increase in mucus production. The airways become very narrow, causing a high resistance to air movement and chronic difficulty in breathing. By definition, chronic bronchitis is characterized by a productive cough that persists for at least three consecutive months a year for at least two consecutive years.

Bronchiolitis

Bronchiolitis is the diagnosis given to young patients who have an acute onset of upper and lower airway inflammation that results in submucosal edema, damage to the ciliated cells that transport mucus out of the lower airway, and eventual occlusion of the smaller bronchioles. Interestingly, with bronchiolitis, bronchial smooth muscle constriction is rare. The pathophysiologic effect of bronchiolitis is disturbance in the ventilation/perfusion (V/Q) ratio and eventual presentation of subjective and objective findings consistent with labored breathing. As mentioned previously, this problem is generally confined to young infants. Older patients have larger and better developed bronchial structures that can handle this additional mucus accumulation and inflamed bronchial walls.

ASSESSMENT FINDINGS

Shortness of breath, abnormal upper airway sounds, faster or slower than normal breathing rates, poor chest rise and fall—these and other signs and symptoms of respiratory distress may be indications that the cells in the body are not getting an adequate supply of oxygen, which is the condition known as *hypoxia*. These signs and symptoms may also be directly related to obstructions of airflow occurring in either the upper or lower portions of the respiratory tract or from fluid or collapse in the alveoli of the lungs, causing poor gas exchange.

If adequate breathing and gas exchange are not present, the lack of oxygen will cause the body cells to begin to die. Some cells become irritable when they are hypoxic, causing the cells to function abnormally. The following is a listing of common findings that the patient with respiratory distress from a respiratory resistance disorder may display:

- Subjective complaint of shortness of breath
- Restlessness
- Tachycardia (early finding) or bradycardia (late and ominous sign)
- Changes to the rate of depth of breathing
- Pale cool skin (early) and cyanosis (late)
- Abnormal breathing, lung, or airway sounds
- Difficulty speaking or inability to speak
- Retractions (suprasternal, supraclavicular, subclavicular, intercostal)
- Altered mental status
- Abdominal breathing (excessive abdominal muscle utilization)
- Excessive coughing (with or without expectorating material)
- Tripod positioning
- Changes in pulse oximetry

Many patients who complain of breathing difficulty, especially those with a pulmonary resistance disorder, experience a condition in which the bronchioles of the lower airway are significantly narrowed from inflammation, swelling, and bronchoconstriction. This causes a drastic increase in resistance to airflow in the bronchioles, making inhalation and, particularly, exhalation extremely difficult and producing wheezing and breathing difficulty.

The patient may be prescribed a beta-2 specific agonist that is administered by metered-dose inhaler or home nebulizer. This medication, known as a *bronchodilator*, is designed to directly relax and open (dilate) the bronchioles, which results in an increase in the effectiveness of breathing and relief of the signs and symptoms. Some inhaled medications are steroids or parasympatholytics used for maintenance of a lower airway resistance and are not used as rescue drugs. The AEMT will learn of this medication while gathering the history.

Another common finding with patients who have an airway resistance disorder is the presence of abnormal breath sounds.

The AEMT should be aware of common abnormal breath sounds so the correct impression of the patient's underlying pathology can be determined and appropriate treatment rendered. Abnormal breath sounds the AEMT may encounter in a patient with respiratory distress include the following:

- *Wheezing* is a high-pitched, musical whistling sound best heard initially on exhalation. It may also be heard during inhalation in more severe cases. It is an indication of swelling and constriction of the inner lining of the bronchioles. Wheezing that is diffuse, heard over all the lung fields, is a primary indication for the administration of a beta-agonist medication by metered-dose inhaler (MDI) or small-volume nebulizer. Wheezing is usually heard in asthma, emphysema, and chronic bronchitis. It may also be heard in pneumonia, congestive heart failure, and other conditions that may cause bronchoconstriction.

- *Rhonchi* are snoring or rattling noises heard on auscultation. They indicate obstruction of the larger, conducting airways of the respiratory tract by thick secretions of mucus. Rhonchi are very often heard in chronic bronchitis, emphysema, aspiration, and pneumonia. One characteristic of rhonchi is that the quality of sound changes if the person coughs, or sometimes even changes position.

- *Crackles* (formerly known as *rales*) are bubbly or crackling sounds heard during inhalation. These sounds are associated with fluid that has surrounded or filled the alveoli or very small bronchioles. The crackling sound heard is commonly associated with the alveoli and terminal bronchioles "popping" open with each inhalation. The bases of the lungs posteriorly will reveal crackles first, due to the natural tendency of fluid to be pulled downward by gravity. Crackles may indicate pulmonary edema or pneumonia. This type of breath sound typically does not change with coughing.

Additional Assessment Findings

The following may also be found on assessment of a patient with asthma:

- Dyspnea (shortness of breath); may progressively worsen

- Nonproductive cough
- Wheezing on auscultation (typically expiratory)
- Tachypnea and tachycardia
- Anxiety and apprehension
- Possible fever
- Typical upper respiratory allergic signs and symptoms
- Chest tightness
- $SpO_2 < 95$ percent before oxygen administration

Patients with acute bronchitis may present with the following:

- Cough, most common finding, possibly productive
- Findings of mild to severe respiratory distress
- Sore throat, usually worse with coughing or swallowing
- Edematous nasal mucosa causing runny or stuffy nose
- General malaise, fatigue, muscle aches
- Infrequently: fever, nausea, vomiting, diarrhea

The following signs are often found in patients with chronic bronchitis:

- Typically overweight
- Chronic cyanotic complexion (often called "blue bloaters")
- Difficulty in breathing, but less prominent than with emphysema
- Vigorous productive chronic cough with sputum
- Coarse rhonchi usually heard on auscultation of the lungs
- Wheezes and, possibly, crackles at the bases of the lungs

Infants with bronchiolitis often present with the following findings:

- Increasingly "fussy" during feeding (early finding)
- History of a concurrent or recent URI; findings consistent with URI
- Progressive onset of dyspnea, usually over 2 to 5 days
- Tachypnea and tachycardia
- Cough, usually nonproductive
- Possible fever
- Fine inspiratory crackles and possible diffuse wheezing
- In severe cases: tachypnea (> 50/min) and low SpO_2

TABLE 30-1

TABLE 30-1   Findings for Respiratory Airway Disorders

Respiratory Airway Disorder	History Findings	Assessment Findings	Breath Sounds
Asthma	Commonly quick onset of distress. Often has a history of a known trigger.	Subjective and objective dyspnea. Respiratory distress findings may be severe.	Expiratory wheezing progressing with wheezing on inhalation and exhalation with more severe attacks. "Silent" chest is ominous.
Acute bronchitis	More gradual onset. May happen in patient with a recent URI.	Progressive but usually not debilitating dyspnea. Patient may have nonproductive cough.	Patient may display wheezing (with ronchi in more severe cases).
Chronic bronchitis	Patient may be chronically short of breath (more typically, CO_2 retainers), may experience acute exacerbations.	Chronic respiratory distress and tachypnea, overweight, low SpO_2. Acute exacerbations may lead to inadequate breathing.	Ronchi, diminished airflow, and wheezing should condition exacerbate.
Bronchiolitis	Gradual onset of respiratory distress, may follow URI. Common to pediatric patients under 2 years of age.	Progressively worsening cough, sore throat, stuffy nose, general malaise, muscle and joint aches.	Breath sounds may reveal crackles and diffuse wheezing.

Table 30-1 provides a summary of history, assessment findings, and breath sounds consistent for each of the emergencies discussed in this topic.

EMERGENCY MEDICAL CARE

Regardless of the specific respiratory etiology causing the breathing difficulty, salient interventions must always be performed in the respiratory emergency patient. Time is critical because of the detrimental effects of hypoxia on all cells and organs. Emergency medical care may include the following:

Establish and maintain an adequate airway.

- **Establish and maintain adequate ventilation and oxygenation.** A patient who is having difficulty breathing but has an adequate tidal volume (as evidenced by good speech patterns, adequate chest rise, and diffuse vesicular breath sounds) and an adequate respiratory rate is in respiratory distress. Because the minute and alveolar ventilations are still adequate, the patient is compensating and is in need of supplemental oxygen. Titrate the oxygen administration to achieve a SpO_2 reading of greater than 95 percent, reduce the complaint of dyspnea, and eliminate the signs and symptoms of hypoxia.

  If either the tidal volume or the respiratory rate becomes (or is) inadequate, the patient's minute and alveolar ventilation will be inadequate; the patient is then said to be in *respiratory failure*, as the respiratory tidal volume or rate is no longer able to provide an adequate ventilatory effort. This requires you to immediately begin ventilation with a bag-valve-mask device or other ventilation device. Supplemental oxygen must be delivered through the ventilation device. If a patient with inadequate breathing is not treated promptly, it is likely that he will deteriorate to respiratory arrest and probable cardiac arrest.

- **Place the patient in a position of comfort.** Position the patient in a semi- or high Fowler position to aid with breathing.

- **Administer a beta-2 specific agonist medication via a metered-dose inhaler or small-volume nebulizer** (▶ Figure 30-3). A common intervention in the patient with respiratory distress who has evidence of bronchoconstriction (primarily diffuse bilateral wheezing) is the administration of an inhaled beta-2 specific agonist medication, such as albuterol sulfate or levalbuterol. These bronchodilators are considered beta-2 specific agonists, which mimic the effects of the sympathetic nervous system in lung tissue. Specifically, these drugs relax the bronchiole smooth muscle, which dilates the airways. This decreases the resistance in the airways and improves the movement of air into the alveoli. Refer to ▶ Skill 30-1 for the procedure for administering a beta-2 specific agonist via a small-volume nebulizer.

- **Provide rapid transport to the medical facility.**

- **En route, establish an intravenous line of normal saline** at a to-keep-open rate if your protocol permits you to do so.

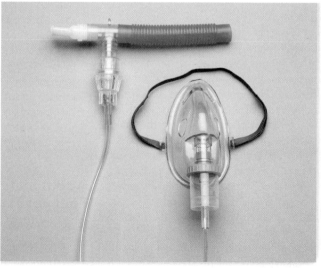

Figure 30-3 Small-volume nebulizer.

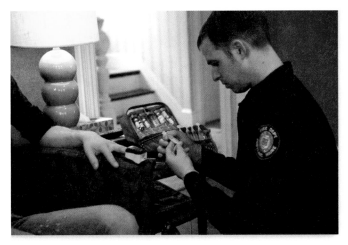

Assess the patient for need, follow your local protocol for the medication order, ensure adequate oxygenation of the patient, explain the procedure to the patient, and check for the right medication and expiration date.

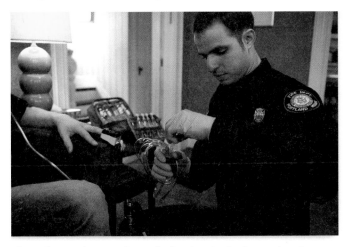

Place the medication for nebulization in the base chamber of the nebulizer. A total volume of 4 mL or greater must be used. If the drug is not already premixed, it may be necessary to dilute the medication with normal saline to a total volume of 4 mL or greater.

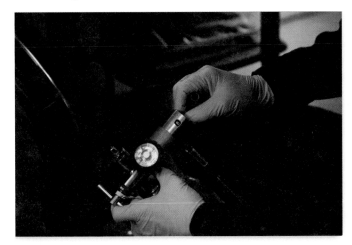

Attach the nebulizer oxygen supply tubing to the oxygen regulator. Set the flow rate at 6 to 8 L/minute to generate a fine mist.

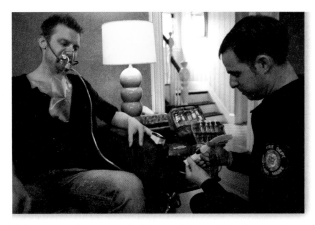

Select a mask or mouthpiece and assemble the equipment.

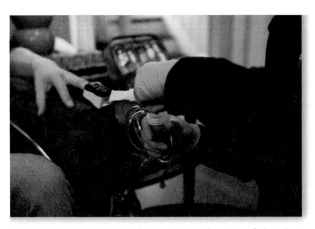

Continue with assembly by screwing the top of the device onto the medication holding chamber. Gently shake the nebulizer side to side to mix the medication.

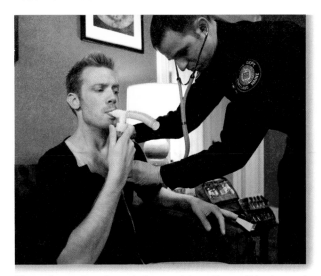

Place the patient in a sitting position. If possible, have the patient hold the nebulizer. Be careful that the patient does not invert the nebulizer and spill the medication out. Have the patient place the mouthpiece in his mouth and inhale slowly at a normal tidal volume for approximately 2 to 3 seconds, and then slowly exhale against pursed lips. Have the patient repeat this procedure until all the medication is gone, at which time the nebulizer typically begins to spurt. Reassess the patient and document the procedure.

REVIEW ITEMS

1. A patient with asthma is complaining of respiratory distress. He states that his chest feels "tight." This perception of feeling "tight" is likely caused by what physiologic change?
   a. hypotension
   b. bronchoconstriction
   c. heightened ventilatory effort
   d. increased fluid accumulation in the alveoli

2. A change in "airway resistance" refers to what?
   a. impaired diaphragm excursion
   b. difficulty with achieving alveolar ventilation
   c. increased opposition to airflow secondary to bronchoconstriction
   d. inability for the lung tissue to ventilate because of a loss of elasticity

3. Which of the following is a commonly cited contributor to bronchitis and emphysema?
   a. tobacco use
   b. age and gender
   c. family history of pulmonary disease
   d. confirmed diagnosis of lung cancer or asthma

4. Loss of adequate respiratory system function in the emphysemic patient is caused by what pathophysiologic change?
   a. destruction of the bronchi
   b. deterioration of the alveoli
   c. increased bronchoconstriction
   d. acute sputum production and bronchiole plugging

5. You arrive on the scene to find a 65-year-old male with a chief complaint of respiratory distress. The patient states that the dyspnea began about three days ago and is progressively worsening. The patient says he is not a smoker, has no known medical problems, and does not take any medications. Vitals are stable, and the SpO_2 is 96 percent on room air. The patient further adds that he has developed a nagging cough over the last day and that his granddaughter has a "bad cold" right now. Based on this information, from what do you think the patient is most likely suffering?
   a. asthma
   b. emphysema
   c. acute bronchitis
   d. chronic bronchitis

APPLIED PATHOPHYSIOLOGY

You are called to a local extended care facility for a male patient with respiratory distress. On entering the room, you hear the "hum" of the oxygen concentrator running beside his bed, and you note that the patient has a nasal cannula applied. His eyes are shut, he is overweight, and he keeps coughing. He does not respond to your verbal stimuli.

1. Identify the most likely chronic pulmonary conditions this patient may have.

2. What would be three assessment findings that could confirm your suspicion?

3. Describe the anticipated physiologic benefit(s) for each of the interventions that may be administered to a patient suffering from an acute asthma attack:

   a. Oxygen therapy
   b. Metered-dose inhaler
   c. Semi-Fowler positioning

4. Discuss the differences in pathophysiology and presentation of the following airway resistance disorders:
   a. Asthma
   b. Chronic bronchitis
   c. Bronchiolitis

5. Describe the pathophysiologic changes that occur to the lumen of the respiratory system that contribute to the respiratory distress and altered V/Q functioning in the bronchiolitis patient.

CLINICAL DECISION MAKING

You are called to a baseball field, where an 18-year-old boy has collapsed in the outfield. His teammates state that he was complaining of trouble breathing earlier in the game and that he said he forgot to bring his "inhaler" with him. As you approach the patient, you find him to be responsive to painful stimuli with purposeful motion. His breathing looks very labored.

1. Based on the scene size-up characteristics, identify the clues that point to a medical history of asthma.

The primary assessment reveals the patient to be alert to painful stimuli. His airway is clear, and his breathing is rapid at 28/minute, respirations are slightly shallow, vesicular sounds are markedly diminished, and coarse wheezing is present throughout the lungs. Peripheral pulses are also present and noted to be rapid and weak. The blood pressure is 110/68, the neck veins are obviously engorged, and the SpO₂ reading on room air is 87 percent.

2. What are the life threats, if any, to the patient that you are aware of currently?

3. Does this patient need oxygen by nonrebreather mask or by positive pressure ventilation? Why?

Further assessment reveals the pupils to be equal and reactive, and the pulse oximeter has increased to 94 percent with oxygen. Breath sounds are unchanged, and jugular venous distention is still present. The blood pressure is unchanged, heart rate is 118 and irregular, respirations have decreased to 24/minute. The patient is starting to become more responsive and mumbles something about his "inhaler." A family member, who has since arrived on the scene, says that she has the inhaler with her.

4. During the ongoing management of the patient, you elect to administer the following therapies. For each one, discuss in specific detail (1) the reason the intervention is warranted, (2) the expected outcome of that intervention, and (3) how you would assess to determine whether the desired effect is occurring (i.e., the treatment worked).

   a. Positioning patient in high Fowler position

   b. Administration of high-flow oxygen

   c. Administration of metered-dose inhaler

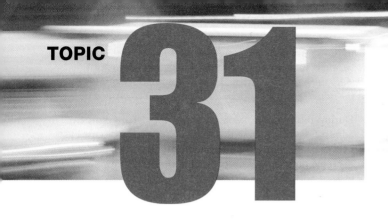

Standard Medicine

Competency Applies fundamental knowledge to provide basic and selected advanced emergency care and transportation based on assessment findings for an acutely ill patient.

RESPIRATORY EMERGENCIES: LUNG AND GAS EXCHANGE DISORDERS

TRANSITION *highlights*

- *Frequency with which various lung and gas exchange disorders occur in the United States.*

- *Pathophysiologic changes that occur with pulmonary diseases that hamper either gas exchange or lung compliance:*
  - Emphysema.
  - Pulmonary edema.
  - Pulmonary embolism.
  - Spontaneous (and tension) pneumothorax.
  - Cystic fibrosis.

- *Relation of the general assessment findings of respiratory distress to the pathophysiologic changes that occur due to the various diseases.*

- *Explanation of adequate and inadequate breathing as it is affected by lung and gas exchange disorders.*

- *Differential assessment findings that relate the pathophysiology to disease onset and clinical findings to help delineate each respiratory dysfunction.*

- *Various treatment interventions and their relationship on improving the patient's pulmonary function:*
  - Oxygen administration.
  - Positive pressure ventilation.
  - Medication administration via small-volume nebulizer or metered-dose inhaler (MDI).
  - Continuous positive airway pressure (CPAP).
  - Patient positioning.

INTRODUCTION

In the preceding topic, the focus of discussion was on respiratory disorders of a restrictive nature—that is, disorders that shared a pathophysiologic change of increased bronchoconstriction that contributed to a change in pulmonary function, resulting in labored breathing. In this topic, the focus will still be on respiratory disorders, but now we will look at disorders that alter either lung compliance or the ability of gases to exchange across the alveolar surface.

Lung compliance refers to the ability of the actual lung tissue to expand when air flows in. If the lungs are "stiff," then it becomes difficult for the patient to inhale sufficiently to ventilate the alveoli and respiratory distress results. Conversely, if the oxygen in the inhaled gases cannot diffuse across the alveoli because of some disturbance, the body will not be able to adequately oxygenate the tissues—and, again, respiratory distress results. These two pathologies are the focus of this topic.

EPIDEMIOLOGY

From a frequency standpoint, respiratory disorders, in young as well as in old patients, are one of the most common prehospital emergencies the Advanced EMT will encounter. Multiple conditions affect pulmonary function or the ability to circulate oxygenated blood, and almost all of these will lead to some degree of respiratory distress.

For example, the National Health Interview Survey has reported that emphysema occurs at an estimated rate of about 18 cases per 1,000 people in the United States. Another source estimates that 1.5 million people have been diagnosed with emphysema, and it is ranked 15th among chronic conditions that limit activities of daily living. Almost 18,000 people die annually of this disease.

Pulmonary edema, another gas exchange disorder, occurs in about 1 percent to 2 percent of the general population, most commonly those between the ages of 40 and 75 years. In patients over the age of 75 years, this emergency increases to about 10 percent of the population. Although pulmonary edema has a variety of causes, this disorder is commonly encountered by the AEMT.

Pulmonary embolism is another gas exchange etiology that causes respiratory distress. It occurs at an estimated rate of 1 per 1,000 persons in the United States, with about a quarter of a million cases occurring annually. An equal number of people are diagnosed at autopsy with a massive pulmonary embolism as are diagnosed clinically; this leads to revised estimates of 650,000 to 900,000 fatal and nonfatal events of this nature in the United States annually.

A pneumothorax, as discussed in Topic 40, "Chest Trauma," causes respiratory distress due to diminishing lung compliance. Illustrating a clear picture of the frequency of pneumothoraces is difficult because of the multiple etiologies that can cause this condition to occur. Generally, though, an adjusted rate of pneumothoraces in the United States of 6 to 7 cases per 100,000 individuals is cited. Pneumothorax occurs more often in men than in women. The incidence peaks in the early 20s for "primary" pneumothoraces (usually less clinically severe) and peaks again in patients over age 60 for "secondary" pneumothoraces (usually more clinically severe).

Cystic fibrosis (CF) is the most common lethal hereditary disease in Caucasians. Although it can occur in other ethnicities, it does so with a much lower frequency. CF has a prevalence rate of 1 case per 3,200 persons in the United States, which may seem uncommon, but those afflicted usually die of pulmonary complications in the second or third decade of life. Although CF causes derangements in many of the body's systems, the most common pathologies leading to death revolve around pulmonary disorders.

In conclusion, all the aforementioned conditions affect either lung compliance or the lung's ability to diffuse gases across the alveoli. Although the pathologies may not seem to occur that much individually, when one looks at the larger picture of lung compliance and gas exchange disorders, they become a common reason that a patient summons EMS.

PATHOPHYSIOLOGY

If lung compliance changes, this generally means that the ability of the lung tissue to expand and accommodate incoming airflow is hampered. If the disturbance is one that diminishes the ease by which gases diffuse across the alveolar wall and into and out of the bloodstream, then the patient will not be able to oxygenate appropriately. Recall that the key physiologic role of the lungs is to allow gas exchange, or the swapping of oxygen for carbon dioxide across the alveolar surface, thereby ensuring that adequate levels of oxygen are in the bloodstream as carbon dioxide is simultaneously removed. *External respiration*, as this is called, must occur in a sufficient manner; otherwise, the person will die.

Internal respiration is the process in which the body offloads oxygen in the

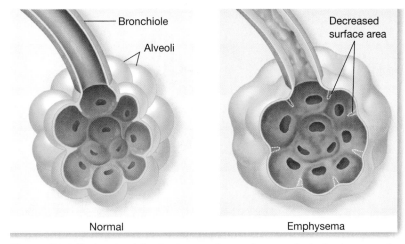

Figure 31-1 Pathophysiologic changes in emphysema include decreased surface area of the alveoli.

capillary beds for cellular utilization, while simultaneously picking up waste carbon dioxide and returning it to the lungs for the process to repeat. Any disorder or disease that inhibits the external respiration process by way of changing lung compliance or diminishing gas exchange across the alveoli affects an individual's overall health by decreasing the oxygen saturation in the blood while carbon dioxide levels rise.

Emphysema

Emphysema is a permanent disease process that is characterized by destruction of the alveolar walls and distention of the alveolar sacs. The primary causal factor is cigarette smoking, but people who are exposed continuously to environmental toxins are also predisposed to developing emphysema.

In healthy lung tissue, certain cells (macrophages and leukocytes) use toxic enzymes to eliminate inhaled irritants. Normally, the lung produces an inhibitor substance that prevents these toxic enzymes from actually attacking the lung tissue they are trying to protect. In patients with emphysema, however, this inhibition is lacking, and the enzymes start to attack the body's normal lung tissue as well. Progressively, the lung tissue loses its elasticity, the alveoli become distended with trapped air, and the walls of the alveoli are destroyed. Loss of the alveolar wall reduces the surface area in contact with pulmonary capillaries. This results in a drastic disruption in the body's ability to adequately facilitate gas exchange, and the patient becomes hypoxic and begins to retain carbon dioxide.

The distal airways also are involved and have greatly diminished lung compliance, making the very act of breathing problematic (▶ Figure 31-1).

Breathing becomes extremely difficult for the emphysema patient, and exhaling progresses to an active rather than passive process, requiring muscular contraction; therefore, the patient with emphysema uses significant amounts of muscular energy to breathe. Eventually the patient will usually complain of extreme shortness of breath on exertion, which may be simply walking across a room. In addition, the loss of lung elasticity, air trapping, and exaggerated use of respiratory muscles to breathe cause the chest to increase in diameter, producing the "barrel-chest" appearance typical with this disease.

> Cystic fibrosis is the most common lethal hereditary disease in Caucasians.

Pulmonary Edema

Acute pulmonary edema occurs when an excessive amount of fluid collects in the spaces between the alveoli and capillaries. This increase in fluid disturbs normal gas exchange and leads to hypoxia and hypercapnia, as oxygen diffusing into the bloodstream from the alveoli and carbon dioxide from the blood to the alveoli are both hampered (▶ Figure 31-2). The most significant problem associated with pulmonary edema is hypoxia, this being the primary reason underlying the respiratory distress complaint.

The two kinds of pulmonary edema are cardiogenic and noncardiogenic.

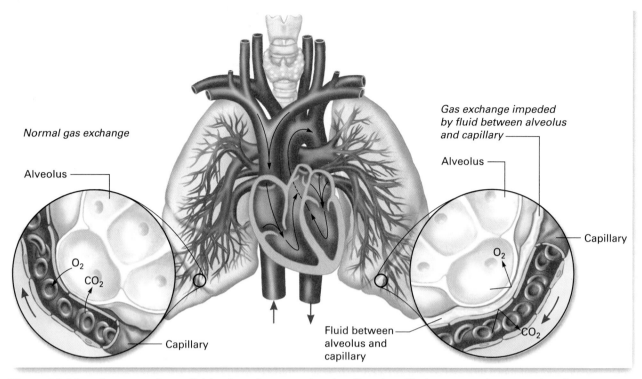

Figure 31-2 In pulmonary edema, fluid collects between the alveoli and capillaries, preventing normal exchange of oxygen and carbon dioxide. Fluid may also invade the alveolar sacs.

Cardiogenic pulmonary edema is typically related to an inadequate pumping function of the heart that drastically increases the pressure in the pulmonary capillaries, which forces fluid to leak into the space between the alveoli and capillaries and, eventually, into the alveoli themselves.

Noncardiogenic pulmonary edema, also known as *acute respiratory distress syndrome* (ARDS), results from direct destruction of the capillary bed that increases capillary permeability and allows fluid to leak out and into the interstitial spaces. Common causes of noncardiogenic pulmonary edema are severe pneumonia, aspiration of vomitus, near-drowning, narcotic overdose, inhalation of smoke or other toxic gases, ascent to a high altitude, and chest and lung trauma. Pulmonary edema is a life-threatening condition that presents with the same signs and symptoms, regardless of the etiology, and in some cases it is a dire emergency that requires immediate emergency care.

> **Pulmonary edema is a dire emergency that requires immediate emergency care.**

Pulmonary Embolism

A pulmonary embolism is not a disease state; rather, a pulmonary embolism is an emergency that arises from a complication of venous thromboembolism, more specifically and frequently from a deep venous thromboembolism (DVT) of the lower extremities (on rare occasions, they may originate from elsewhere in the venous system or the right side of the heart). Regardless, after the embolus breaks off, it travels through the venous system in increasingly larger blood vessels until it arrives at and is pumped through the right side of the heart.

After leaving the right ventricle, blood vessels continually get smaller and smaller as blood flows through the pulmonary system to the capillary beds of the lungs. As such, venous emboli can become trapped in one of these pulmonary blood vessels. Large emboli may lodge at the bifurcation of the main pulmonary artery (saddle embolism) or one of the smaller lobar branches. In this situation, the emboli may also cause significant hemodynamic compromise because the right ventricle will be unable to pump a sufficient amount of blood to the left side of the heart. Smaller emboli will travel more distally to smaller vessels in the lung. Occlusion here will likely cause respiratory distress in association with pleuritic (sharp, localized) chest

pain by initiating an inflammatory response in the parietal pleura.

The embolism prevents blood from flowing to the lung. As a result, some areas of the lung have oxygen in the alveoli but are not receiving any blood flow. This leads to a decrease in gas exchange and subsequent hypoxia, the severity of which depends on the size of the embolism or the number of alveoli affected. The hypoxia in this case is the result of the shunting of blood away from the oxygenated alveoli, creating a mismatch between ventilation and perfusion (▶ Figure 31-3).

Patients at risk for suffering a pulmonary embolism include the following:

- Patients who experience long periods of immobility (such as bedridden individuals)
- Patients who travel for a long period confined in one position
- Patients with long bone fractures or splints on extremities
- Patients with heart disease or a history of deep vein thrombosis
- Patients who have recently experienced surgery, venous pooling associated with pregnancy, cancer, or estrogen therapy
- Patients with underlying coagulation disorders
- Patients who smoke

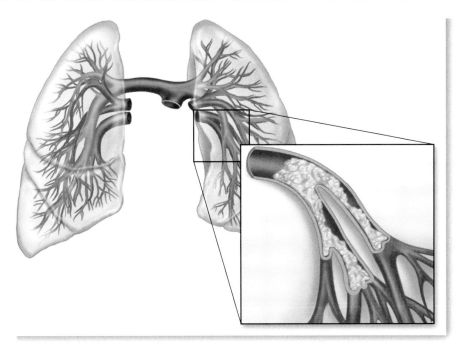

Figure 31-3 A blood clot, air bubble, fat particle, foreign body, or amniotic fluid can cause an embolism, blocking blood flow through a pulmonary artery.

Spontaneous Pneumothorax

As you are aware, during inspiration air is drawn into the lungs as the diaphragm and intercostal muscles contract, thereby enlarging the size of the thoracic cavity. As the chest wall moves out and the diaphragm drops, the parietal pleura moves, and because of the negative pleural space pressure, the visceral pleura gets drawn out as well, which enlarges the lungs. The mechanical process of breathing cannot be damaged or deranged without some compromise on breathing adequacy, which is what happens with a pneumothorax.

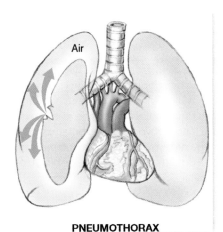

PNEUMOTHORAX

Figure 31-4 In pneumothorax, the lung collapse decreases lung tissue compliance and causes a disturbance in gas exchange that leads to hypoxia.

If air enters the pleural cavity, either from the outside (open pneumothorax) or from air escaping through a hole in the lung and into the pleural space (closed pneumothorax), the lung may collapse; with larger pneumothoraces, it becomes mechanically impossible for the patient to breathe. The lung collapse decreases lung tissue compliance and causes a disturbance in gas exchange that leads to hypoxia (▶ Figure 31-4).

With a particular type of significant pneumothorax known as a *tension pneumothorax*, air entering the pleural cavity has nowhere to escape, so it starts to depress lung tissue; eventually it will shift the mediastinal structures toward the uninjured lung. This may lead to severe shortness of breath as well as circulatory collapse. Tension pneumothorax is a life-threatening condition that requires urgent intervention.

Men are five times more likely to suffer a spontaneous pneumothorax than are women. Most of these male patients are tall, thin, and lanky and between the ages of 20 and 40. Many also have a history of cigarette smoking or a connective tissue disorder such as Marfan syndrome or Ehlers-Danlos syndrome.

Patients with a history of chronic obstructive pulmonary disease (COPD) are more prone to spontaneous pneumothorax because of areas of weakened lung tissue called *blebs*. It is thought that the reason tall, thin, lanky men are more likely to suffer a spontaneous pneumothorax is that the visceral pleura is stretched within the chest cavity beyond its normal limit. Often the stretched and weakened area ruptures when the patient experiences an increase in intrathoracic pressure from an activity such as coughing, lifting a heavy object, or straining.

Cystic Fibrosis

Cystic fibrosis (also known as CF, mucoviscidosis, or mucovoidosis) is a hereditary disease. Although it commonly causes pulmonary dysfunction because of changes in the mucus-secreting glands of the lungs, it also affects the sweat glands, the pancreas, the liver, and the intestines.

Lining almost the entire respiratory tree in the body is a layer of tissue that is coated with a mucus lining. This mucus lining is normally watery and helps to warm and humidify inspired air, and it also serves to trap any inhaled particles. In CF, however, an abnormal gene alters the functioning of the mucus glands lining the respiratory system, and there is an over-abundance of mucus, which is very thick and sticky. As this thick mucus layer develops, blockage of the airways occurs along with an increase in the incidence of lung infections, as bacteria can readily grow in the thick mucus.

Repeated lung infections, in turn, cause scarring of the lung tissue, reduce the ability of the lungs to clear the thick mucus, and promote ongoing pulmonary damage. As a result, there is progressive diminution in the efficiency of respiratory function, which leads to eventual pulmonary failure and death.

Pulmonary complications are the most common cause for a patient with this affliction to summon EMS. There is not yet a cure for CF, and many individuals with this disease die at a young age (20s–30s) because of pulmonary failure. In fact, CF is cited as one of the most common life-shortening genetic diseases. Because it is possible to detect CF in a patient at a very young age, it is common for the patient experiencing a crisis to already know of this diagnosis. Fortunately, medical research and treatment are lengthening the life span of some people to as high as 50 years. In terminal states of the disease, the final medical recourse, when all other interventions have failed, is lung transplantation.

ASSESSMENT FINDINGS

A patient suffering from a lung compliance issue or gas exchange deficit, as discussed in this topic, will almost certainly present with respiratory distress. The degree of respiratory distress can vary from very minimal, subjective dyspnea to severe dyspnea with objective findings of inadequate breathing present. The most important assessment the AEMT must do when dealing with a dyspneic patient is to determine whether the patient is breathing adequately.

> **The most important assessment the AEMT must do when dealing with a dyspneic patient is to determine whether the patient is breathing adequately.**

Recall that the patient's minute ventilation is a function of the respiratory rate and tidal volume. In almost all situations of illness or injury, the response of the respiratory rate is to increase, so identifying tachypnea is not all that uncommon or specific a finding. The tidal volume is more important to assess, however, as most all pulmonary diseases or injuries end up affecting the tidal volume (or the amount of air a patient takes with each breath).

Recall also that the body must ventilate through physiologic dead space prior to the air reaching the alveoli (physiologic dead space is about 150 mL of each tidal volume). As such, if a patient's tidal volume drops from 500 mL per breath to 200 mL per breath, the body will still fill 150 mL of dead space, which means only 50 mL of air available for gas exchange in the alveoli, as compared with the normal 350 mL in a patient who is breathing adequately. The point is, however, that you cannot look at a patient and determine how many milliliters of air he is moving with each breath unless you have diagnostic pulmonary equipment. What you can do, though, is assess the clinical adequacy of the tidal volume.

Although a long list of findings may be present if the patient is breathing adequately (a different list will apply if the patient is breathing inadequately), you really need to pay close attention to two assessment findings that will illustrate the quality of the patient's breathing.

First, listen to the patient's speech patterns. A patient speaking in full sentences without discomfort is still breathing adequately.

Second, assess vesicular breath sounds over the lung's periphery. Absent vesicular (alveolar) breath sounds indicates that the patient is not breathing adequately. If the patient's mental status precludes communication with you, determine breathing adequacy by assessing the rise and fall of the chest (chest wall excursion) along with vesicular breath sounds. It is not that the actual respiratory rate is unimportant; it is just that tachypnea is commonly seen with almost all medical/traumatic emergencies (other than late brainstem/head injury or depressant drug overdose), so except in cases of *extreme* tachypnea or *extreme* bradypnea, the rate is not that all clinically relevant.

Beyond the findings of general respiratory distress and/or labored breathing, the next sections give more specific findings for conditions addressed in this topic.

Additional Assessment Findings

Patients with emphysema may present with the following:

- On home oxygen
- Thin, barrel-chest appearance
- Coughing, but with little sputum
- Prolonged exhalation with pursed-lip breathing
- Diminished breath sounds
- Wheezing and rhonchi (rattles) on auscultation with exacerbation
- Extreme difficulty of breathing with minimal exertion
- Pink complexion (Emphysema patients are often called "pink puffers.")
- Tachypnea—breathing rate usually greater than 20 per minute at rest
- Tachycardia and diaphoresis
- Tripod position

The following may be found in patients with pulmonary edema:

- Dyspnea, especially on exertion
- Difficulty in breathing when lying flat (orthopnea)
- Cough (possibly productive), frothy sputum
- Tachycardia and tachypnea
- Anxiety, apprehension, combativeness, confusion
- Tripod position with legs dangling
- Crackles and possibly wheezing on auscultation
- Cyanosis or dusky-color skin
- Pale, moist skin
- Distended neck veins
- Swollen lower extremities
- Symptoms of cardiac compromise

Crackles (also called rales) are a sign of pulmonary edema. Be sure to auscultate the posterior lower lobes of the lungs to pick up early indications of crackles and pulmonary edema. If you are auscultating only the upper lobes, you may easily miss the condition because gravity is pulling the fluid downward into the lower portions of the lungs.

Patients with pulmonary embolism may present with the following:

- Sudden onset of unexplained dyspnea
- Signs of difficulty in breathing or respiratory distress; rapid breathing
- Sudden onset of sharp, stabbing chest pain
- Cough (may cough up blood)
- Tachypnea and tachycardia
- Syncope (fainting)
- Cool, moist skin
- Restlessness, anxiety, or sense of doom
- Decrease in blood pressure (late sign)
- Cyanosis (may be severe)
- Distended neck veins (late sign)
- Inspiratory crackles
- Swollen lower extremity
- Possible fever
- $SpO_2 < 95$ percent

It is important to note that not all the signs and symptoms of pulmonary embolism will always be present. Common signs and symptoms are chest pain, dyspnea, and tachypnea (rapid breathing) with tachycardia being the most common.

Additional assessment findings for spontaneous pneumothorax include the following:

- Sudden onset of shortness of breath
- Sudden onset of sharp chest pain or shoulder pain; may be pleuritic
- Decreased breath sounds to one side of the chest (most often apical)

TABLE 31-1   Differential Assessment Findings for Lung and Gas Exchange Disorders

Pulmonary Emergency	General Pathology	Onset of Dyspnea	Specific Differential Findings
Emphysema	Destruction of alveoli, air trapping, CO_2 retention (which is less common in emphysema)	Persistent dyspnea, acute deterioration with exacerbation	Diminished breath sounds, barrel chest, clubbing of fingers
Pulmonary edema	Fluid accumulation in alveoli from heart failure	Usually rapid onset with heart failure	Inspiratory crackles, jugular venous distention (JVD), frothy sputum
Pulmonary emboli	Occlusion of pulmonary blood vessel blocking blood flow to lung(s)	Sudden, unexplained; usually no precipitation event	Pleuritic chest pain, breath sounds possibly clear, unexplained tachycardia
Spontaneous pneumothorax	Collapse of lung tissue from air in pleural space	Sudden, may be related to straining	Pleuritic chest pain, unilateral diminishment of breath sounds
Cystic fibrosis	Excessive mucus plugging; final common pathway: respiratory failure	More gradual development, may progress to severe dyspnea	Coughing, ronchi, history of recurrent upper respiratory infection (URI), GI distress, general malaise

- Subcutaneous emphysema may be found
- Tachypnea and tachycardia
- Diaphoresis and pallor
- Cyanosis may be seen late and in a large pneumothorax
- $SpO_2 < 95$ percent

A patient who presents with a sudden onset of shortness of breath with decreased breath sounds on one side of the chest and no evidence of trauma should be suspected of having a possible spontaneous pneumothorax.

The following may be present in patients with cystic fibrosis:

- Commonly, a known history of the disease
- Recurrent coughing; rhonchi may be noted with auscultation
- General malaise (weakness, fatigue, not feeling well)
- Expectoration of thick mucus during coughing
- Recurrent episodes or history of pneumonia, bronchitis, and sinusitis
- GI complaints, possibly including constipation or other changes in bowel movements
- Abdominal pain from intestinal gas
- Malnutrition or low weight despite a healthy appetite
- Dehydration
- Clubbing of the digits
- Trouble speaking and breathing (dyspnea) with mucus buildup

Although the most common complaint the patient with CF will have is difficulty breathing, many of the other findings are due to dysfunction of other organ systems. The abdominal findings, such as dehydration, bowel changes, and poor weight gain, are from the damage the disease inflicts on the gastrointestinal (GI) tract. Pancreatitis can also cause abdominal pain, as can liver damage from the disease.

Table 31-1 summarizes the differential assessment findings for lung and gas exchange disorders.

EMERGENCY MEDICAL CARE

Treatment for lung compliance and gas exchange disorders share the same goals as treatment for other respiratory distress patients: Ensure that the patient's airway is clear and maintained, provide positive pressure ventilation should the patient be breathing inadequately or have fatigue of respiratory muscles, reverse hypoxemia and hypercapnia, and ensure that peripheral perfusion remains intact. The following is a summary of management considerations:

1. **Establish and maintain an open airway.**
2. **Establish and maintain adequate ventilation and oxygenation.** A patient who is having difficulty breathing but has an adequate tidal volume (as evidenced by good speech patterns, adequate chest rise, and diffuse vesicular breath sounds) and an adequate respiratory rate is in respiratory distress. Because the patient's minute and alveolar ventilation are still adequate, the patient is compensating and is in need of supplemental oxygen. Titrate the oxygen administration to achieve an SpO_2 reading of greater than 95 percent, reduce the complaint of dyspnea, and eliminate the signs and symptoms of hypoxia.

   If either the tidal volume or the respiratory rate becomes (or is) inadequate, the patient's minute and alveolar ventilation will be inadequate; the patient is then said to be in *respiratory failure*, as the respiratory tidal volume or rate is no longer able to support an adequate ventilatory effort. This requires you to immediately begin ventilation with a bag-valve-mask device or other ventilation device. Supplemental oxygen must be delivered through the ventilation device. If a patient with inadequate breathing is not treated promptly, it is likely that he will deteriorate to respiratory arrest and, potentially, cardiac arrest.
3. **Assist with administration of a beta-2 specific agonist medication** delivered via a small-volume nebulizer or metered-dose inhaler per your local protocol if bronchoconstriction is present.
4. **Initiate CPAP at 5 to 10 cmH2O, per protocol.** Patients with pulmonary edema, as well as many other pulmonary conditions, may benefit

from the "back pressure" delivered by a CPAP machine. Follow local protocol for when to and when not to administer CPAP.

5. **Position the patient.** Semi- or high Fowler positioning will assist the patient in breathing and minimize the negative effects of fluid accumulating in the lungs, especially for the patient with pulmonary edema. If positive pressure ventilation is being provided or frank hypotension is present, the patient will need to be placed supine for ongoing management.

6. **Provide rapid transport to the emergency department.** Notify the receiving ED as early as possible.

7. **En route, initiate an intravenous line of normal saline** at a to-keep-open rate if your protocol permits you to do so.

TRANSITIONING ● ● ● ● ● ● ●

REVIEW ITEMS

1. Which pulmonary gas exchange disorder typically has a rapid onset of dyspnea, commonly associated with pleuritic chest pain?
   a. pulmonary emboli
   b. pulmonary edema
   c. cystic fibrosis
   d. emphysema

2. Which of the following disorders would most likely have unilaterally diminished breath sounds?
   a. emphysema
   b. pneumothorax
   c. pulmonary edema
   d. pulmonary emboli

3. You are assessing a patient with dyspnea who you suspect has emphysema. Although he says he has not been to a doctor for years, what part of his history/presentation described here would best support your field impression?
   a. frequent use of antacids
   b. chronic use of antacids
   c. sudden onset of dyspnea
   d. inspiratory crackles with breathing

4. Your 86-year-old female patient is complaining of dyspnea and weakness. You note that she has jugular venous distention, inspiratory crackles, and diffuse expiratory wheezing. She has a history of coronary bypass and hypertension. Her current mental status is normal. Her vital signs are blood pressure 180/100 mmHg, heart rate 108 and irregular, respiratory rate 26/minute. Given this scenario, what should your *first* drug of choice be?
   a. Administer 365 mg baby aspirin orally.
   b. Administer oxygen 15 lpm via full face mask.
   c. Assist with the administration of her prescribed metered-dose inhaler.
   d. Assist with the administration of her oral antihypertensive medication.

5. Which of these body system/organ failures results in early death of cystic fibrosis patients?
   a. cardiac failure
   b. pancreatic failure
   c. pulmonary failure
   d. gastrointestinal failure

APPLIED PATHOPHYSIOLOGY

You are caring for a patient with respiratory distress. The patient presents with an intact airway, breathing is regular at 26/minute, and vesicular breath sounds are present bilaterally but markedly diminished. The patient states that he is normally slightly dyspneic, but over the past few days his dyspnea has progressively worsened. You note a low pulse oximeter reading, tachycardia, slightly erythemic skin, and a prolonged expiratory phase. He is on home oxygen, 2 lpm via cannula, per physician's orders.

1. Should you suspect this patient is suffering from a restrictive disorder or a compliance disorder? Support your answer based on your field impression. Why might the administration of higher concentrations of oxygen be beneficial for this patient?

2. Patients with cystic fibrosis may be recipients of bilateral lung transplants to sustain life; however, patients with emphysema are commonly not considered for this surgery. Basing your answer on progressive disease pathophysiology, briefly explain why this might be.

3. Discuss the differences in pathophysiology and presentation of the following gas exchange disorders of the pulmonary system:
   a. Pulmonary embolism
   b. Pulmonary edema

CLINICAL DECISION MAKING

You are summoned to a high school basketball game. There you find an elderly male patient who came to the game to see his grandson play. Shortly after sitting down near the top of the bleachers, he started to experience chest pressure that progressed into significant respiratory distress. He states he normally takes a nitroglycerin pill when his chest feels like this, but he forgot his nitro at home. You note that his jugular veins are engorged, he is using accessory muscles to breathe, and his speech is becoming more and more choppy. His medical history includes hypertension and "a bad heart."

1. Identify clues from the narrative that point to the field impression of pulmonary edema.

2. What medical condition does this patient have that could explain the onset of the pulmonary edema emergency?

The primary assessment reveals that the patient's airway is clear, his breathing is rapid at 28/minute, respirations are shallow, vesicular sounds are present, and inspiratory crackles are noted. Peripheral pulses are also present but are weak, rapid, and slightly irregular. His blood pressure is 182/104 mmHg. The neck veins are obviously engorged, and the SpO$_2$ reading on room air is 87 percent. The patient's mental status is rapidly deteriorating, and he mumbles something like, "Just let me lie down to rest a bit."

3. What are the life threats, if any, to the patient that you are currently aware of?

Further assessment reveals the pupils to be equal and reactive, and the pulse oximeter has increased to 94 percent with high-flow oxygen. Breath sounds are unchanged, and JVD is still present. The blood pressure is now 180/100 mmHg, heart rate is 112 and irregular, respirations have increased to 32/minute.

4. During the ongoing management of the patient en route, you elect to administer the following therapies. For each one, discuss in specific detail (1) the reason the intervention is warranted; (2) the expected outcome of that intervention; and (3) how you would assess to determine whether that desired effect is occurring (i.e., the treatment worked).

   a. Positioning patient in high Fowler position

   b. Administration of high-flow oxygen

   c. Application of CPAP

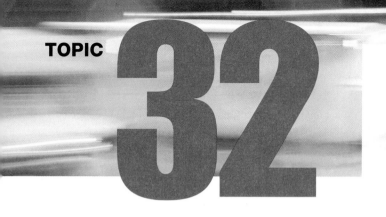
Standard Medicine

Competency Applies fundamental knowledge to provide basic and selected advanced emergency care and transportation based on assessment findings for an acutely ill patient.

RESPIRATORY EMERGENCIES: INFECTIOUS DISORDERS

TRANSITION highlights

- *Review of the frequency of which various infectious respiratory disorders occur in the United States and worldwide.*

- *Expanded discussion of common infectious disorders and how the pathophysiology is related to presenting signs and symptoms:*
  - *– Pneumonia.*
  - *– Pertussis.*
  - *– Viral respiratory infections.*

- *Common assessment findings as they relate to normal breathing, labored breathing, and inadequate breathing.*

- *Specific assessment findings as they relate to the aforementioned infectious disorders (beyond the general findings of respiratory distress).*

- *General emergency care for a dyspneic patient, as well as specific treatment considerations for infectious respiratory disorders.*

INTRODUCTION

As discussed in the previous two topics, respiratory distress or labored breathing is a common prehospital complaint with either medical or traumatic etiologies. Onset may be acute or gradual and can present mildly with minimal discomfort to the patient or severe enough that the patient may fear he will die if the cause is not rapidly identified and correct—and, to a large extent, that fear can be real. Breathing is an automatic process that is regulated in the brainstem and depends on functioning musculoskeletal, cardiovascular, and pulmonary systems; should one of these body systems fail, it can result in a serious condition requiring immediate intervention.

Because many findings of respiratory distress actually result from the body's attempt to improve breathing adequacy, not necessarily from the specific pulmonary condition, it is important to remember that pulmonary conditions may present very similarly. As such, many of the Advanced EMT's treatment modalities are similar for these varied conditions. In this topic, the focus will be on infectious disorders that afflict the pulmonary system and lead to respiratory distress. In any instance, however, it is important for the AEMT to recognize the signs and symptoms of respiratory emergencies, complete a thorough patient history and physical exam to determine the cause, and provide immediate intervention.

EPIDEMIOLOGY

Although cardiovascular disease is the leading cause of death in the United States and most developed nations, lower respiratory tract infections are the leading cause of death worldwide. Patients with immunosuppressive disorders or age extremes (very young and very old) are the ones most likely to succumb to a pulmonary infection that eventually robs them of the ability to ventilate and oxygenate adequately. With the ensuing increase in the work of breathing in an attempt to compensate for the pulmonary disturbance, the added workload to the respiratory muscles and cardiovascular system eventually leads to fatigue, acidosis, hypoxia, hypercapnia (high CO_2 levels), and death.

Pneumonia occurs more than 4.8 million times a year in the U.S. population, which can be extrapolated into more than 13,000 cases a day and 9 cases per minute. The vast majority of cases are found in nursing home and convalescent patients; pneumonia is a common cause of death in these populations. Patients infected with the human immunodeficiency virus (HIV) and others who are on immunosuppressive drugs, such as transplant patients, are also very prone to pneumonia. Additional risk factors include cigarette smoking, alcoholism, and exposure to cold temperatures.

Pertussis is a highly contagious childhood bacterial illness that is, fortunately, preventable with a vaccine. In the United States, most hospitalizations and nearly all deaths from pertussis are reported in infants aged less than 6 months (although morbidity does occur in other age groups). The Centers for Disease Control and Prevention (CDC) tracks documented cases of pertussis and have found in past years that the annual incidence is about 3.3 cases per 100,000 people; however, there has been a recent outbreak in the United States. When focusing on the age of the patient, the average annual incidence rate is highest (55.2 per 100,000) in infants less than 1 year of age. In older populations, only marginal increases in pertussis have been seen.

A third common infectious respiratory condition is viral respiratory tract infections (VRIs). VRIs are the most common cause of symptomatic disease among children and adults. Each year, approximately 2 to 4 respiratory tract illnesses occur in adults, compared with 6 to 12 respiratory tract illnesses in children. These infections may cause a wide variety of diseases, from the common cold to severe pneumonia, and may result in significant morbidity and mortality within age-extreme patients and those who are already immunocompromised. Because VRIs afflict the pulmonary system, the patient often presents with some degree of respiratory distress.

PATHOPHYSIOLOGY

Pneumonia

Pneumonia is primarily an acute infectious disease—caused by bacteria, a virus, or other pathogens—that affects the lower respiratory tract and causes lung inflammation and fluid- or pus-filled alveoli (▶ Figure 32-1). This leads to poor gas exchange across the alveoli and eventual hypoxia and hypercapnia. As oxygen and carbon dioxide diffusion across the alveoli becomes impaired, the patient will progress from subjective respiratory distress findings to objective findings. The progression may be slow and take days to weeks to develop, or, in the instance of bacterial pneumonia, the presentation of respiratory distress may occur more rapidly.

Often the virus or bacteria responsible for the condition initially resides in one of the lung's lobes; as it replicates itself it migrates up the respiratory tree and can settle in other lobes or even in the opposite lung. It is possible, early in the syndrome progression, that changes in breath sounds are present in only one lung or one lobe of a lung, a condition known as *lobar pneumonia*. Although viral pneumonia does occur, respiratory viruses commonly weaken the lung tissue, which then creates an environment conducive for the development of secondary pneumonia caused by opportunistic bacteria.

Finally, a type of pneumonia called *pneumonitis* can be caused by inhalation of toxic irritants or aspiration of vomitus or other toxic substances.

Pertussis

Pertussis (also known as "whooping cough") is a respiratory disease that is characterized by uncontrolled paroxysms of coughing. It is a highly contagious disease that affects the respiratory system and is caused by bacteria residing in the upper airway of an infected person. It is spread by respiratory droplets that are discharged from the nose and mouth during coughing. Pertussis has been found to occur in patients of all ages, but it is reported most often in children. Generally speaking, the younger the patient, the more severe the clinical condition.

Pertussis typically starts out very similar to a cold or a mild upper respiratory infection. Because of this, the parents of the infant or child (or in the situation of an older patient) may try "waiting it out" before seeking medical care; thus, by the time the patient presents to EMS, the condition may be severe. Within two weeks or so of onset, the patient will develop episodes of numerous rapid coughs (15–24 episodes) as the body attempts to expel thick mucus from the airway, followed by a "crowing" or "whooping" sound made during inhalation as the patient breathes in deeply and rapidly.

> **VRIs are the most common cause of symptomatic disease among children and adults.**

Complications of pertussis include pneumonia, dehydration, seizures, brain injuries, ear infections, and even death. Most deaths occur to younger patients who have not been immunized for this disease or to patients who are exposed before finishing the vaccination series. In younger patients, the ongoing and uncontrolled coughing can severely disrupt normal breathing, diminish gas exchange in the alveoli, and promote bacterial pneumonia.

Viral Respiratory Infections

A viral respiratory infection refers to a condition in the respiratory system caused by a virus. Common VRIs include bronchiolitis, colds, and influenza ("the flu"). In most situations for adults, VRIs are fairly mild, self-limiting, and confined to the upper respiratory system. In children, however, the infection has a greater propensity to spread

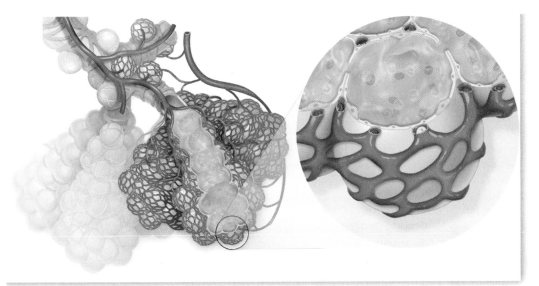

Figure 32-1 Pneumonia causes inflammation of the lungs and causes the alveoli to fill with fluid or pus, leading to poor gas exchange.

into the lower airways, where more significant infections can occur, resulting in patient deterioration.

Viral respiratory infections are commonly referred to by the medical community as *upper respiratory infections* (URIs) because the majority of symptoms are found in the nose and throat. In small children, however, VRIs can also cause infections of the lower airway structures, such as the trachea, bronchi or bronchioles, or lungs. When an infection involves these lower airway structures, depending on the site, the patient may be diagnosed with croup, bronchiolitis, or pneumonia. Known viruses that can cause VRIs include rhinoviruses, parainfluenza and influenza viruses, enteroviruses, respiratory syncytial virus (RSV), and some strains of the adenovirus.

> **Assess the patient's mental status and pay attention to speech patterns.**

The major pathophysiologic changes caused by these viruses on gaining entry into the body by way of patient-to-patient contact (and, to a lesser extent, through inhalation of respiratory droplets) is a triggering of the inflammatory process with increased mucus production to the upper respiratory structures. A fever, coughing, runny nose, and findings of mild respiratory distress may also be associated with the infection in the majority of cases. VRIs typically run a course of about 14 days, and unless extenuating circumstances are present (i.e., a secondary respiratory infection of the lower airways or severe respiratory distress), they rarely necessitate medical attention.

In any situation, however, it is nearly impossible (nor is it practical) for the AEMT to determine whether the associated findings of respiratory distress from a VRI etiology are in fact viral in nature or not, as there is no specific treatment for viral infections that the AEMT can administer. The mainstay of treatment for respiratory distress secondary to a VRI is supportive in nature and includes patient positioning, airway and breathing maintenance, oxygen administration, and transport to the hospital for ongoing diagnosis and management.

ASSESSMENT FINDINGS

Normal breathing (a normal respiratory effort) requires a minimal amount of energy expenditure and is almost effortless for the patient. Normal breathing is also quiet; it does not produce abnormal sounds or noises. When assessing the patient for normal respiratory effort, first start with the respiratory (breathing) rate, which is assessed by observing the patient's chest rise and fall. The normal respiratory rate range for an adult patient at rest is typically 8 to 24 breaths per minute.

Second, assess the patient's mental status and pay attention to speech patterns. A patient who is struggling to breathe can rarely speak in normal sentences, as his need to take another breath precludes this. However, for example, if you encounter a patient with a respiratory rate of 8 breaths per minute who is alert, oriented, and able to answer your questions without gasping for a breath or showing a struggle to breathe, 8 may be his normal respiratory rate, and no intervention is necessary.

As an additional confirmation of breathing quality, auscultate breath sounds. You should be able to hear air exchange in the bases of the lungs bilaterally (which indicates that the alveoli are being ventilated as well).

Also assess the respiratory (or breathing) rhythm—the regularity or irregularity of respirations. Normal breathing will have a normal respiratory rhythm, but remember that the respiratory rhythm can be easily affected by speech, activity, emotions, and other factors in the conscious and alert patient.

An abnormal respiratory rhythm, however—that is, an irregular pattern of respiration—in the patient with an altered mental status is a serious concern. It may indicate a respiratory medical illness or even a chemical imbalance or brain abnormality or injury. In situations of an irregular breathing rhythm (either from conscious control in an awake patient or during periods of altered mental status or unresponsiveness), it becomes more important to assess for breathing adequacy by assessing the respiratory rate and tidal volume.

In summary, the following findings are consistent with a patient who is breathing adequately:

- A patent (open) airway
- Adequate respiratory rate
- Adequate rise and fall of the chest
- Normal respiratory rhythm
- Breath sounds present bilaterally
- Chest expansion and relaxation occurring normally

- Minimal to absent accessory muscle use to aid in breathing

The following should also occur in a patient who is breathing adequately, providing there is no disturbance to other bodily systems:

- Alert and oriented
- Normal muscle tone
- Normal pulse oximeter reading
- Normal skin condition findings

As stated, the majority of patients the AEMT will encounter will display an adequate respiratory effort (normal breathing). This does not mean, however, that the AEMT will never encounter a patient with inadequate breathing or will never find that a patient who was initially breathing adequately has deteriorated to a point at which breathing is inadequate and insufficient to sustain life. In fact, failing to breathe adequately, even for short periods of time, not only will result in hypoxia and cellular death, but all the other bodily systems will start to falter as well.

The majority of findings seen in patients with respiratory distress are caused by the body's attempt to increase ventilator exchange. As such, many respiratory conditions may have remarkably similar findings; the following sections, however, list the characteristic findings common to the infectious respiratory conditions discussed in this topic.

Assessment of the Patient with Pneumonia

The signs and symptoms of pneumonia vary with the cause and the patient's age. The patient generally appears ill and may complain of fever and severe chills. Look for the following signs and symptoms:

- Malaise and decreased appetite
- Fever (may not occur in the elderly or infants)
- Cough—may be productive or nonproductive
- Dyspnea (less frequent in the elderly)
- Tachypnea and tachycardia
- Chest pain—sharp and localized and usually made worse when breathing deeply or coughing
- Decreased chest wall movement and shallow respirations
- Possibly, patient splinting his thorax with his arm

- Possibly, crackles and rhonchi heard on auscultation
- Altered mental status, especially in the elderly
- Diaphoresis
- Cyanosis
- SpO$_2$ < 95 percent

Assessment of the Patient with Pertussis

Pertussis actually has three stages. Stage 1 is characterized by findings consistent with a common cold or upper respiratory infection. Stage 2 is characterized by coughing that continues to worsen to the point that medical care is sought (EMS is summoned), and thus the suspicion for pertussis (whooping cough) is made. Stage 3 is the recovery stage; recovery is usually gradual, taking several weeks until resolution is reached. More specific findings for pertussis include the following:

- History of upper respiratory infection
- Sneezing, runny nose, low-grade fever
- General malaise (weakness, fatigue, "not feeling well")
- Increase in frequency and severity of coughing
- Coughing fits usually more common at night
- Vomiting from coughing hard
- Inspiratory "whoop" heard at the end of coughing burst
- Possibly, cyanosis developing during coughing burst
- Diminishing pulse oximetry finding
- Exhaustion from expending energy during coughing burst
- Trouble speaking and breathing (dyspnea) during coughing burst

Assessment of the Patient with a Viral Respiratory Infection

As stated, most people do not seek medical attention or summon EMS for a typical VRI due to the minimal clinical findings that are easily treated with over-the-counter cold medications for symptomatic relief. However, if the patient's condition and findings of respiratory distress are severe enough to call EMS, chances are that the infection has spread into the lower airways and is starting to impinge on normal oxygenation by the lungs. Signs and symptoms of viral respiratory infections include the following:

- Nasal congestion
- Sore or scratchy throat
- Mild respiratory distress, coughing
- Fever (usually around 101°F–102°F)
- Malaise
- Headaches and body aches
- In infants, irritability and poor feeding habits
- Tachypnea
- Exacerbation of asthma if patient is asthmatic and contracts a VRI

Regardless of the mechanism of respiratory distress, remember the discussion in Topic 31 regarding the determination of respiratory distress. If the conscious patient is unable to speak in normal sentences *or* does not have vesicular breath sounds, his breathing is inadequate, even though other classic findings of dyspnea may not yet be present. If the patient is unresponsive, the absence of vesicular breath sounds *or* minimal chest wall movement is indicative of inadequate breathing. In both these situations, positive pressure ventilation and oxygen therapy are the most important intervention the AEMT can provide.

EMERGENCY MEDICAL CARE

For all the topics that have focused on different respiratory conditions, the AEMT will notice a stark similarity in the management of these symptomatically related (but pathophysiologically diverse) respiratory conditions. This is because the primary goal for any patient with difficulty breathing is to calm his apprehension with verbal reassurance, place him in a position of comfort that facilitates breathing (normally a semi- or high Fowler position), provide oxygen therapy, and in cases of respiratory failure, provide airway support and positive pressure ventilation. En route to the medical facility, consider establishing an intravenous line of normal saline at a to-keep-open rate (follow your local protocol). The following sections offer more condition-specific interventions the AEMT may consider.

Emergency Medical Care for Pneumonia

The pneumonia patient is managed no differently from any other patient having difficulty breathing. Ensure adequate oxygenation and breathing. Pneumonia is an acute infectious disease process that is not usually associated with severe bronchoconstriction, unless it occurs as a complication of asthma or COPD. Therefore, you would not expect the patient to have a metered-dose inhaler (MDI) or home nebulizer for this condition, nor would you necessarily consider its use unless indications of bronchoconstriction are present. Follow your local protocol regarding the administration of a beta-2 agonist medication via a metered-dose inhaler or nebulizer (see Topic 30 for more detailed information).

Emergency Medical Care for Pertussis

Treatment of pertussis is similar to that for many other respiratory problems. It is focused on ensuring oxygenation, reversing hypoxia, and preventing airway obstruction. The patient should remain in a comfortable position, and the AEMT should administer high-flow oxygen at 15 lpm via a nonrebreather mask. The AEMT should also encourage the patient to expectorate any mucus that is brought up with the coughing. The administration of humidified oxygen may help the mucus become less viscous and be expelled more easily. The patient will probably be anxious and/or frightened, so the AEMT should also try to ensure a quiet and calm environment. Expedite transport, and consider an ALS intercept.

In addition, remember that pertussis is a very contagious disease. The AEMT should take all precautions necessary to prevent cross-contamination (including putting a simple mask on the patient to catch expelled airway droplets), as long as doing so does not impinge on the patient's breathing. Following transport of a known patient with pertussis, consider totally disinfecting the patient compartment of the ambulance.

> **Remember that pertussis is a very contagious disease.**

Emergency Medical Care for VRIs

The majority of VRI cases do not present to EMS because the clinical presentation is confined to nasal and pharyngeal discomfort. In the susceptible patient, however, the presence of concurrent lower-tract infections can cause some degree of respiratory distress. In all but the most severe (and uncommon) of cases, supportive treatment of positioning, oxygen therapy, emotional support, and gentle transport to the hospital are all that are necessary. If the infection is allowed to persist without medical attention, however, and it develops into a more serious viral infection (especially for the very young or very old), high-flow oxygen and, occasionally, positive pressure ventilation may become warranted.

Despite the often minimal presentation, the AEMT should always maintain a high index of suspicion for deterioration in a patient who does not respond favorably to the aforementioned supportive measures.

TRANSITIONING

REVIEW ITEMS

1. A patient presents with respiratory distress with a gradual onset, has a slight fever, and has diminished breath sounds in the lower right lobe. This presentation is most consistent with what infectious disease process?
   - a. pertussis
   - b. pneumonia
   - c. chronic bronchitis
   - d. upper viral respiratory infection

2. Which of the following patients is most likely to develop pneumonia?
   - a. a recent lung transplant patient
   - b. a patient with a history of long bone fractures
   - c. a pediatric patient with a history of Down syndrome
   - d. an elderly patient with diagnosed Parkinson disease

3. What type of secondary lung infection is a patient with a recent diagnosis of VRI most likely to acquire?
   - a. tuberculosis
   - b. pneumonia
   - c. pertussis
   - d. asthma

4. What type of infectious lung disease would most readily spread through a day care center or kindergarten classroom?
   - a. bronchiolitis
   - b. bronchitis
   - c. pertussis
   - d. asthma

5. EMS is rarely summoned for patients with viral respiratory infections because _____.
   - a. early respiratory distress is often mild
   - b. findings are often self-limiting with use of over-the-counter medications
   - c. most insurance companies will not reimburse the EMS bill for VRI patients
   - d. the actual incidence of VRI in the United States is very rare in all age groups

6. At what stage of pertussis would EMS most likely be summoned for a patient with shortness of breath?
   - a. stage 1
   - b. stage 2
   - c. stage 3
   - d. stage 4

7. A patient with severe pneumonia is found to be tachypneic and warm to the touch, has an altered mental status, and displays absent vesicular breath sounds on auscultation. The single most important treatment for this patient is _____.
   - a. oxygen
   - b. aspirin for the fever
   - c. placement in a position of comfort
   - d. provision of positive pressure ventilation

APPLIED PATHOPHYSIOLOGY

1. Discuss the pathologic process by which a viral respiratory infection could result in the patient developing bacterial pneumonia.

2. Why would an elderly patient have a less severe (or more atypical) presentation of pneumonia than patients in younger age groups?

3. Identify the pathogenic etiology for the following signs and symptoms given the listed infectious disease state:
   a. Diminished breath sounds in the patient with pneumonia
   b. Tachypnea and low pulse oximetry readings in the patient with pertussis
   c. Increased mucus production and coughing in the patient with a VRI
   d. Tripod positioning, nasal flaring, shallow breathing, and altered mental status in all three of the discussed infectious respiratory conditions

CLINICAL DECISION MAKING

Family members call you to the home of a bedridden patient with a known neuromuscular disease. The family states that the patient seems to be "very uncomfortable" while trying to breathe. As you approach the patient, you see an oxygen concentrator beside his bed. The patient looks at you as you approach but cannot speak due to stoma placement. You note that the stoma's inner cannula is properly placed. The skin appears "dusky," the patient has weak coughing spells that are bringing up some white phlegm through the stoma, and the conjunctiva of the eyes appear somewhat dehydrated.

1. Based on the scene size-up characteristics, identify the infectious respiratory diseases from which the patient is most likely suffering. Defend your answer.

Further assessment reveals that the 58-year-old male patient is alert and will blink his eyes as directed. The family states that he gets these "attacks" once or twice a year, and the hospital diagnoses a respiratory infection. Pulse oximetry is 97 percent on room air. Auscultation of the chest during breathing reveals clear upper lobe sounds, with diminished lower right and left breath sounds with mild inspiratory crackles.

The heart rate is 102/minute, respirations are 24, and the blood pressure is 142/82 mmHg. The patient's core is warm to the touch.

2. Does this additional information support or contradict your initial field impression? Why?

3. What immediate emergency care should you provide based on the provided assessment findings?

4. What conditions are you still considering as the possible cause? Would you add any conditions as a possible cause, and if so, which ones?

5. What are one or two possible differential diagnoses for this patient?

6. Following your treatment, what would be key indications that the patient's pulmonary function and general status are improving? What would be important indications of continued deterioration?

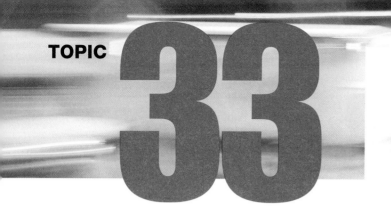

Standard Medicine

Competency Applies fundamental knowledge to provide basic and selected advanced emergency care and transportation based on assessment findings for an acutely ill patient.

HEMATOLOGY: BLOOD DISORDERS

TRANSITION *highlights*

- *The ethnic predisposition and frequency in which blood disorders occur in the United States.*

- *Types of cells found in the blood (red and white), and the role of platelets.*

- *Disorders and disease processes that can afflict the blood:*
  - Red blood cell diseases:
    - Anemia.
    - Sickle cell disease.
    - Polycythemia.
    - Thalassemia.
  - White blood cell diseases:
    - Leukopenia/neutropenia.
    - Leukocytosis.
    - Leukemia.
    - Lymphoma.
  - Platelet diseases/clotting disorders:
    - Thrombocytopenia.
    - Thrombocytosis.
    - Hemophilia.
    - Von Willebrand disease.
    - Disseminated intravascular coagulation.
    - Multiple myelomas.

- *Brief overview of basic assessment findings.*

- *General treatment interventions for a patient suffering from a hematologic disorder.*

INTRODUCTION

Hematology is the study of the blood and blood products. Blood consists of plasma, red blood cells, white blood cells, and platelets. Various medical conditions result from changes associated with these components. Lab tests, combined with history and physical exams by physicians, are needed to accurately diagnose hematologic conditions.

EPIDEMIOLOGY

Hematologic conditions are common but do not often present as the primary complaint of patients in the prehospital environment. Some conditions are not very common in the overall population but are more prevalent in a specific population. For example, one of the more common hematologic conditions encountered by the Advanced EMT in the prehospital environment is sickle cell disease, also known as sickle cell anemia. Sickle cell anemia occurs in about 1 in every 400 African Americans in the United States. The sickle cell trait is found in 8 percent to 10 percent of African Americans in the United States.

PATHOPHYSIOLOGY

The composition of the blood is a primary factor associated with hematologic conditions. It is necessary to understand the basic functions of each of the blood components to gain a better understanding of hematologic disorders.

Blood is composed primarily of plasma, red blood cells, white blood cells, and platelets. *Plasma* is the pale yellow liquid portion of blood; it is composed primarily of water but also contains proteins, chemical messengers, gases, salts, and other nutrients. Plasma transports the cellular components throughout the body and conveys the cellular waste products to the kidneys, lungs, and liver to be removed.

Red blood cells, or *erythrocytes*, are disk-shaped cells responsible for the transport of oxygen from the lungs to the tissues and carbon dioxide transport in the reverse direction. Red blood cells contain *hemoglobin*, a protein chemical that contains iron, which is bright red in color. Oxygen transport is influenced by the amount of hemoglobin, its oxygen affinity, and blood flow (▶ Figure 33-1).

White blood cells, or *leukocytes*, are the body's primary defense against infections. They are capable of moving outside the bloodstream to reach tissues being invaded by microbes.

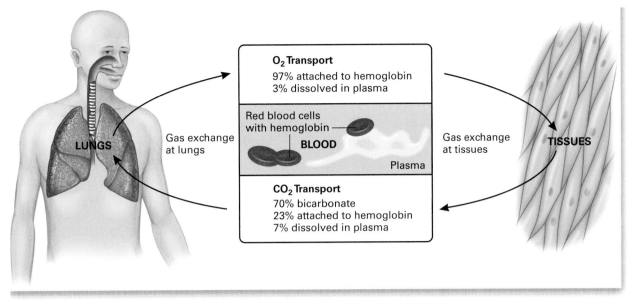

Figure 33-1 Oxygen is transported in the blood in two ways: attached to hemoglobin and dissolved in plasma. Carbon dioxide is transported in the blood in three ways: as bicarbonate, attached to hemoglobin, and dissolved in plasma.

The five major types of white blood cells are basophils, eosinophils, lymphocytes, monocytes, and neutrophils. When an infection occurs, the number of white blood cells within the body will significantly increase.

Platelets, or *thrombocytes,* are cell-like particles that help in the clotting process. They gather at a bleeding site and clump together to form a hemostatic plug. They also release substances that help promote further clotting.

Red Blood Cell Diseases

ANEMIA *Anemia* is a condition defined by a reduced number of red blood cells that results in a decreased ability to carry oxygen effectively in the blood. The types of anemia are listed in Table 33-1. Blood loss, lack of red blood cell production, or high rates of red blood cell destruction are the three main causes of anemia. These causes may stem from a number of disorders, such as vitamin deficiencies, or other factors.

Mechanisms that help maintain tissue oxygenation in patients with gradual onset of anemia include peripheral vasodilation, increased cardiac output, change in the oxygen–hemoglobin dissociation curve, and the shunting of blood away from circulation-rich organs to critical organs. With severe or long-lasting anemia, the lack of oxygen in the blood

can damage the heart, brain, and other organs of the body.

SICKLE CELL DISEASE *Sickle cell disease* is an inherited blood disorder that results in the production of abnormal hemoglobin. The hemoglobin deoxygen-

ates and clumps together, causing the red blood cells to become stiff and develop a crescent or C shape or sickle form. These sickle-shaped cells can block blood vessels and can prevent adequate oxygenation of the tissues, contributing to severe pain and organ damage.

TABLE 33-1	Types of Anemia	
Cause	**Type**	**Pathophysiology**
Inadequate production of red blood cells	Aplastic	Failure to produce red blood cells.
	Iron deficiency	Iron is the primary component of hemoglobin.
	Pernicious	Vitamin B_{12} is necessary for correct blood cell division during its development.
	Sickle cell	A genetic alteration, in low oxygen states, causes production of a hemoglobin that changes the shape of red blood cells to a C, or sickle shape.
Increased red blood cell destruction	Hemolytic	Body destroys red blood cells at a rate greater than production; red blood cell parts interfere with blood flow.
Blood cell loss or dilution	Chronic disease	Hemorrhage leads to cell loss; excessive fluid leads to a dilution of red blood cell concentration.

Sickle cell crises, or *vaso-occlusive crises*, are episodes of pain resulting from the blockages that are usually followed by periods of remission. Illness, physical stress, cold temperature, or being at high altitudes may increase the risk of a crisis. The most serious dangers associated with a sickle cell crisis are acute chest syndrome, long-term damage to major organs, stroke, and complications during pregnancy, such as high blood pressure in the mother and low birth weight in the infant. The mean life expectancy for people diagnosed with sickle cell anemia is 48 years for women and 42 years for men.

POLYCYTHEMIA *Polycythemia*, or *erythrocytosis*, is a condition resulting from an abnormally high level of red blood cells in the blood. The increase is usually due to an excess production of red blood cells. Pseudoerythrocytosis may appear secondary to dehydration. The higher the red blood cell levels, the greater is the risk of thrombosis in the individual.

THALASSEMIA *Thalassemia* is an inherited blood disorder that results in the decreased production of hemoglobin and red blood cells. It usually affects people of Mediterranean or Asian ancestry. Severe thalassemia is normally identified by the age of 2 years. Signs and symptoms include pallor, anorexia, listlessness, and jaundice.

White Blood Cell Diseases

LEUKOPENIA/NEUTROPENIA *Leukopenia* is the condition involving too few white blood cells. This indicates a problem with either production of white blood cells in the marrow or the destruction of white blood cells. *Neutropenia* is said to exist when a patient's peripheral neutrophil count is lower than usual. Yemenite Jews and black individuals have an increased risk of developing neutropenia. Neutropenia is most commonly induced by chemotherapeutic agents.

> **Most of the symptoms of blood disorders are vague and nonspecific.**

LEUKOCYTOSIS *Leukocytosis* is the condition involving too many white blood cells. Leukocytosis is usually caused by a bacterial infection or arises when the body is particularly stressed—for example, because of rheumatoid arthritis, diabetic ketoacidosis, pain, or exercise.

LEUKEMIA *Leukemia* is a cancer of the bone marrow and blood that results from the rapid production of abnormal white blood cells. These cells are unable to fight infection and impair the production of red blood cells and platelets in the bone marrow. The two main types of leukemia are called *lymphocytic leukemia* and *myelogenous leukemia* based on the predominant blood cell type. Leukemia can be acute or chronic.

LYMPHOMA *Lymphoma* is a cancer of the lymphatic system. Abnormal white blood cells called *lymphocytes* form cancerous lymphoma cells, which multiply and collect in the lymph nodes. These cells can impair the immune system and the body's ability to fight infection. The two main types of lymphoma are Hodgkin lymphoma and non-Hodgkin lymphoma. About half the blood cancers that occur each year are lymphomas.

Platelet Diseases/Clotting Disorders

THROMBOCYTOPENIA *Thrombocytopenia* is an abnormal decrease in the number of platelets. It can be caused by a decrease in the number of platelets produced in the blood marrow, sequestration of platelets in the spleen, or destruction of the platelets. Some medications, including heparin, contribute to thrombocytopenia.

THROMBOCYTOSIS *Thrombocytosis* is an increase in the number of platelets. This is usually caused by an increase in the production of platelets. This condition is often seen with leukemias, autoimmune disorders, and acute hemorrhage.

HEMOPHILIA *Hemophilia* is a blood disorder in which one of the proteins necessary for blood clotting is missing or defective. This results in the blood not clotting properly and increases the risk of severe hemorrhage from what would appear to be a minor injury. Males are affected more than females. Patients with hemophilia may suffer from damage to their joints, tissues, and organs caused by internal bleeding and typically present with acute painful swelling in the joint (hemarthrosis).

VON WILLEBRAND DISEASE *Von Willebrand disease* is an inherited disease that results from a deficiency or defect in the body's ability to make von Willebrand factor, a protein that helps blood clot. Von Willebrand disease is usually milder than hemophilia and can affect both males and females.

DISSEMINATED INTRAVASCULAR COAGULATION *Disseminated intravascular coagulation* (DIC) is a condition in which blood clots form throughout the body's small blood vessels. These blood clots can reduce or block blood flow through the blood vessels, which can damage the body's organs. This reduces the number of platelets and clotting factors in the blood needed to control bleeding, and excessive bleeding occurs. DIC is typically seen late in severe infections.

MULTIPLE MYELOMA *Myeloma* is a cancer of white blood cells called plasma cells. In myeloma, the cells overgrow, forming a mass or tumor that is located in the bone marrow. These cells may spread to other bones in the body. These abnormal cells interfere with the production of normal blood cells and the body's ability to fight infection. Kidney damage, bone destruction, and fractures can result from myelomas.

ASSESSMENT FINDINGS

Patients who have hematologic problems often present with various signs and symptoms. Most of the symptoms of blood disorders are vague and nonspecific. Symptoms that may suggest an underlying blood disorder include fatigue, weakness, shortness of breath, bleeding or bruising easily, headache, dizziness, confusion, jaundice, and many others. Obtaining a good history and anticipating complications from a hematologic condition is very important.

EMERGENCY MEDICAL CARE

Emergency medical care for patients with hematological emergencies is primarily supportive. Patients may present with a wide variety of signs and symptoms, based on their underlying condition, that require emergency medical care. The emergency care may include the following:

- **Establishing and maintaining a patent airway.** This may require the insertion of a mechanical airway device or suction if necessary.

- **Administration of oxygen based on the patient's presentation.** Maximize oxygenation in a patient suspected of having a vaso-occlusive crisis. If the patient is breathing adequately, use a nasal cannula or nonrebreather mask. Use a ventilation device in the patient who requires ventilation.

- **Provide positive pressure ventilation** if the tidal volume or respiratory rate is inadequate.

- **Control external hemorrhage.** Anticipate complications from these disorders, and treat the patient for shock if indicated.

- **Consider contacting paramedics** based on the patient's presentation, especially if pain control is needed.

- **Initiate transport** and provide comfort measures.

TRANSITIONING

REVIEW ITEMS

1. A patient presents with excessive bleeding from a small laceration on the forearm, which has not been easily controlled by direct pressure. Based on that initial finding, you should suspect _____.
   - a. anemia
   - b. hemophilia
   - c. leukemia
   - d. lymphoma

2. Which of the following blood components contains hemoglobin?
   - a. plasma
   - b. red blood cells
   - c. white blood cells
   - d. platelets

3. Leukocytes respond to infection by _____.
   - a. increasing hemoglobin production
   - b. decreasing clotting factors
   - c. decreasing in number
   - d. increasing in number

4. Which of the following conditions results when excessive clotting is followed by excessive hemorrhage?
   - a. disseminated intravascular coagulation
   - b. von Willebrand disease
   - c. non-Hodgkin lymphoma
   - d. myelogenous leukemia

5. Clotting is primarily a function of which blood component?
   - a. erythyrocytes
   - b. thrombocytes
   - c. leukocytes
   - d. plasma

APPLIED PATHOPHYSIOLOGY

1. List four compensatory mechanisms used to help maintain tissue oxygenation in patients with gradual anemia.

2. What are the two major classifications of lymphoma?

3. Explain the difference between thrombocytopenia and thrombocytosis.

4. Explain how a vaso-occlusive crisis occurs in a patient with sickle cell anemia.

CLINICAL DECISION MAKING

You are dispatched to a residence for a patient complaining of severe pain in his legs. After determining the scene to be safe, you approach the patient, a 19-year-old African-American male, who is sitting in bed and appears to be in significant pain. No apparent mechanisms of injury are present, and the patient denies any trauma.

The primary assessment reveals that the patient is anxious, alert, and oriented. He has a respiratory rate of 24/minute with adequate chest rise and fall. The patient has a strong radial pulse of 120 beats per minute. The skin is pale, very warm, and dry. The SpO$_2$ reading is 90 percent.

1. What are the life threats to this patient?

2. What immediate emergency care should you provide based on the initial assessment?

The patient states he is having severe pain in his legs. He says that the pain began two days ago and has continued to get worse. He reluctantly admits that he called now because he has had a painful erection for the past four hours that has not gone away.

3. List the possible conditions you suspect the patient may be experiencing.

4. What cultural considerations might influence your care for this patient? Why?

During the secondary assessment, the patient also complains of dizziness, fatigue, and weakness. You note jaundice in the sclera of his eyes. The abdomen is soft and nontender, pelvis is stable, and there are ulcers on the lower extremities. No deformities are noted to the extremities. The patient does have a priapism. His peripheral pulses are present. The patient has no known allergies, has a history of sickle cell disease, and states he used to take prescribed medication for the pain but has not been able to afford it for the past couple of months. He has been drinking a lot of water and ate some cereal for breakfast about five hours ago. He admits to taking 800 mg of Motrin for the pain after breakfast. His blood pressure is 160/92 mmHg, heart rate is now 112 beats per minute, and his respirations are 20 per minute.

5. What conditions are you considering as a probable cause? Why?

6. Based on your differential diagnosis, what are the next steps in emergency care? Why?

Standard Medicine

Competency Applies fundamental knowledge to provide basic and selected advanced emergency care and transportation based on assessment findings for an acutely ill patient.

TOPIC

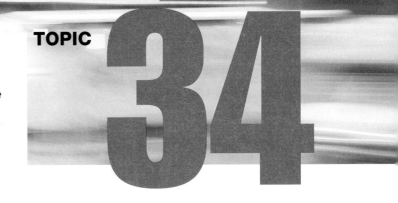

RENAL DISORDERS

INTRODUCTION

Renal emergencies primarily affect the kidneys' ability to function properly. Renal conditions can result in life-threatening complications if they are left untreated. These conditions require the Advanced EMT to perform an accurate patient assessment and to provide prompt emergency care.

EPIDEMIOLOGY

Kidney disease affects about 20 million people in the United States. An estimated 11.5 percent of adults over the age of 20 have physiologic evidence of chronic kidney disease. Approximately 350,000 Americans receive dialysis for end-stage renal disease every year. More than 33 billion dollars in public and private spending has been used in the treatment of kidney failure. More than 50,000 Americans die each year from kidney disease.

PATHOPHYSIOLOGY

The major functions of the kidneys include the production and elimination of urine from the body. The kidneys also play a role in homeostasis by regulating the body's pH (acid/base levels) and electrolytes, controlling the blood volume, eliminating waste products, and regulating the blood pressure.

Traumatic and nontraumatic causes can damage the kidneys and affect their ability to function properly. Inflammation, infection, physical obstruction, and hemorrhage are factors that can cause renal emergencies. Initially, many patients who experience renal emergencies will complain of abdominal or flank pain (▶ Figure 34-1). It is not necessary to try to pinpoint the exact cause of the pain, but it is necessary to properly assess and manage the patient based on the presentation.

Renal Conditions

Three of the most common renal emergencies that will be seen in the prehospital environment involve kidney stones, renal (kidney) failure, and dialysis-related emergencies. Dialysis and kidney transplantation may be necessary for patients who have kidney failure.

TRANSITION *highlights*

- Frequency and mortality rates for renal diseases in the United States.
- Overview of normal renal function and its role on homeostasis.
- Pathophysiologic changes that can occur with renal disease and overview of common renal conditions:
  – Kidney stones.
  – Renal failure (acute and chronic).
- Role of dialysis as therapy for renal patients:
  – Hemodialysis (done in a medical facility).
  – Peritoneal dialysis (done in the home).
- Important SAMPLE and OPQRST considerations/findings when caring for a patient with kidney stones or renal disease.
- Treatment strategies the Advanced EMT can employ when caring for a patient with a renal emergency.

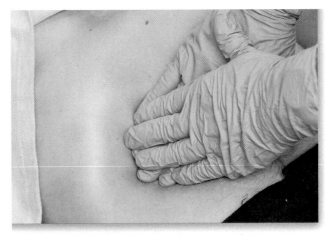

Figure 34-1 Patients who experience a renal emergency may complain of abdominal, flank, or lower back pain, or tenderness on palpation.

KIDNEY STONES *Kidney stones*, or *renal calculi*, are crystals of substances such as calcium, uric acid, struvite, and cystine that are formed from metabolic abnormalities (▶ Figure 34-2). Renal calculi are believed to originate in the kidneys and must pass through the rest of the urinary system to be eliminated from the body.

Visceral pain noted unilaterally in the flank is normally followed by severe pain as the stone is dislodged and passes through the ureter into the bladder. Hematuria is a common finding when the stone is being passed, although this is commonly seen only by testing the urine.

Lithotripsy or other surgical interventions may be necessary if the patient is unable to pass the stones on his own. If left untreated, renal calculi can lead to loss of kidney function, obstruction of the urinary tract, or kidney damage.

RENAL (KIDNEY) FAILURE *Renal failure*, or *kidney failure*, occurs when the kidneys fail to function adequately. The two main types of kidney failure are acute renal failure and chronic renal failure.

- *Acute renal failure* (ARF) normally occurs over a period of days and often results from a significant decrease in urine elimination. Some causes of ARF include decreased blood flow to the kidneys, trauma, cardiac failure, surgery, shock, sepsis, and urinary tract obstruction. It is imperative that this condition be identified as soon as possible because, depending on the cause and extent of the damage, it is sometimes reversible. Some patients with ARF will require dialysis. If left untreated, ARF can lead to life-threatening metabolic derangements.

- *Chronic renal failure* (CRF) normally occurs over a period of years and results from a permanent loss of nephrons (the functional units of the kidneys). The causes of chronic renal failure are numerous; however, diabetes and hypertension are linked to a majority of the cases. Chronic renal failure leads to an accumulation of waste products and fluids that cannot be removed from the body properly. These uremic changes can affect every organ system in the body. CRF is a permanent and life-threatening condition. Symptoms of CRF range from mild at first to severe when end-stage renal failure develops. Patients ultimately will require dialysis or a kidney transplant for survival.

Dialysis

Dialysis is an artificial process used to remove water and waste substances from the blood when the kidneys fail to function properly. It generally works through osmosis and filtration of fluid across a semipermeable membrane. In general, the blood containing waste products passes on one side of the membrane while a dialysate (special fluid used for dialysis) passes on the other side. When this occurs, the water and waste products travel from the blood across the membrane and into the dialysate, thus removing the waste from the patient.

The two major types of dialysis are hemodialysis and peritoneal dialysis.

- **Hemodialysis.** In hemodialysis, a machine containing the dialysate is connected to an access site on the patient. The access site may be a shunt, fistula, port, or graft. The patient's heparinized blood is then pumped through the access site and into the machine, where the waste is removed. The EMT should *not* take the blood pressure of a dialysis patient on the side of the patient's access site. In general, care must be taken not to occlude the access site.

- **Peritoneal dialysis.** In peritoneal dialysis, the dialysate is run through a tube into the patient's abdomen. The peritoneal membrane functions as the semipermeable membrane. The fluid remains in the abdomen for several hours so it can absorb the wastes, and then it is drained out of the body through a different tube.

Although dialysis provides a necessary treatment for patients with kidney failure, it has risks that can result in life-threatening complications such as hypotension, muscle cramps, peritonitis, hemorrhage, infection, or cardiac arrest. If they miss their dialysis treatments, patients who require dialysis also may experience life-threatening problems, such as life-threatening elevations in potassium or pulmonary edema.

ASSESSMENT FINDINGS

After ensuring a safe scene, it is important to determine whether the patient has been injured or is suffering from a medical illness. Some patients may become dizzy or weak and may fall as a result of their medical condition. Remember that dialysis patients may be on heparin, a blood thinner.

Form a general impression of your patient and determine whether the patient is alert and oriented. An altered mental status may reflect changes occurring as a result of the disease process. Pay attention to the airway, ventilation, oxygenation, and circulation.

Kidney failure and metabolic derangements can affect every organ system in the body and may precipitate shock or other life threats. Because of this, aggressive management of any potential life threats is necessary. Priority transport should be provided if the patient has a poor general appearance, has an altered mental status, shows signs of shock, or is in severe pain.

When gathering a history, in addition to the standard information collected, be sure to inquire about the following:

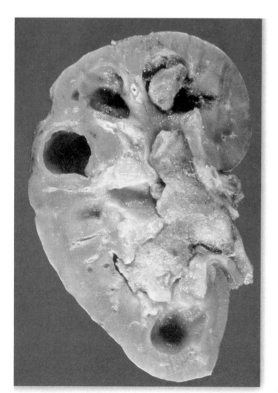

Figure 34-2 Sectioned kidney with kidney stones. (© *SIU/Photo Researchers, Inc.*)

- How long has the patient been sick or suffering from these signs and symptoms?
- What is the patient's medical history? When was the last time he saw a doctor for his medical condition? Has he had any surgeries?
- Is there any genital pain or discharge? If so, what are the color, consistency, and odor like?
- Is there a change in urine? If so, what are the color and odor like?
- Does the patient receive dialysis? If so, when was the last treatment received? When is the next treatment due?
- Does the patient have any abdominal, pelvic, or flank pain?
- Has the patient had any nausea or vomiting? If so, when and how much?
- Does the patient have any pain associated with urination, defecation, or sexual intercourse?

The physical exam will focus primarily on the renal complaint and will normally involve the abdominal and pelvic area. Because renal conditions can affect other body systems, you must assess them all. Perform the physical examination of the abdomen carefully and gently. Begin by inspecting and palpating the abdomen. Determine whether there is any bleeding, pain, or tenderness. You should also note whether a urinary catheter is in place.

Obtain and document the patient's vital signs. Hypertension or hypotension may exist based on the underlying cause. Make sure that you do not obtain a blood pressure in the arm with the fistula or shunt. Decreased blood pressure, tachycardia, and pale, cool, moist skin are indicators of shock.

When performing your physical exam, you may find a variety of signs and symptoms, depending on the cause of the emergency. Some common signs and symptoms of renal emergencies include the following:

- Urine with an abnormal color, consistency, or odor
- Abdominal, pelvic, or flank pain or tenderness
- Malaise, nausea, and vomiting
- Fever or chills
- Syncope or altered mental status
- Pain or burning during sexual intercourse, urination, or bowel movement
- Frequent or urgent need to urinate or decreased urine output
- Blood in the urine (hematuria)
- Edema of the feet, ankles, and/or legs
- Hypertension or hypotension
- Anorexia
- Tachycardia

EMERGENCY MEDICAL CARE

Do not try to isolate the exact cause of abdominal or pelvic pain or a renal condition. Correctly assess and identify the signs and symptoms and provide the proper emergency medical care.

1. **Maintain manual spinal stabilization** if trauma is suspected.
2. **Keep the airway patent.** Always be alert for vomiting and the potential for aspiration. It may be necessary to place the patient in the left lateral recumbent position to protect the airway if the patient has an altered mental status. Be prepared to suction.
3. **If breathing is adequate, administer oxygen based on the SpO$_2$** reading and patient signs and symptoms. If the SpO$_2$ reading is greater than 95 percent and no signs or symptoms of hypoxia or respiratory distress are present, oxygen may not be necessary. In this case, you may choose to apply nasal cannula at 2 to 4 lpm. If signs of hypoxia or respiratory distress are present, or the SpO$_2$ reading is less than 95 percent, place the patient on a nonrebreather mask at 15 lpm.

> **Make sure that you do not obtain a blood pressure in the arm with the fistula or shunt.**

4. **Control any major bleeding if present;** recheck the access site for bleeding in a dialysis patient.
5. **Place the patient in the position of comfort if no trauma is suspected.** If spinal stabilization is required, fully immobilize the patient on a backboard. If signs or symptoms of shock are present, then place the patient in a supine position. If pulmonary edema is suspected, place the patient in an upright position.
6. **Calm and reassure the patient.** Be supportive and nonjudgmental.
7. **Initiate a quick and efficient transport.**
8. **If an IV is initiated, do so en route to the hospital.** Do not use an arm that has a shunt for IV access. Use caution with IV fluid administration. Administer fluid boluses cautiously to patients with renal failure and those on dialysis.
9. **Continuously monitor and reassess your patient.**

TRANSITIONING

REVIEW ITEMS

1. A patient presents with severe unilateral flank pain. Based on that initial finding, you should suspect the patient most likely will also present with _____.
   a. warm and dry skin
   b. tachycardia
   c. bradycardia
   d. hypotension

2. Which of the following is commonly associated with chronic renal failure?
   a. hypotension
   b. Graves disease
   c. diabetes mellitus
   d. Crohn disease

3. About how many Americans are affected by kidney disease?

    a. 5 million   b. 10 million

    c. 15 million   d. 20 million

4. Kidney stones can usually be composed of all of the following *except* _____.

    a. calcium   b. potassium

    c. uric acid   d. cystine

5. Severe pain from renal calculi is most commonly experienced as the stone passes through the _____.

    a. kidney

    b. ureter

    c. urinary bladder

    d. urethra

APPLIED PATHOPHYSIOLOGY

1. List the primary functions of the kidney.

2. Explain the difference between acute renal failure and chronic renal failure.

3. Differentiate between hemodialysis and peritoneal dialysis.

4. What complications could occur if chronic renal failure is left untreated?

5. Explain why dialysis or kidney transplantation is necessary if a patient has end-stage renal failure.

CLINICAL DECISION MAKING

You are called to a residence for a 28-year-old male patient with abdominal pain. On arrival, you encounter the patient pacing on the front porch of his residence with his hands on his back. You note that he appears to be in significant distress and there is no sign of trauma. As you determine the scene is safe, you approach the patient, who states that he is in severe pain.

1. Based on the scene size-up characteristics, list the possible conditions you suspect the patient is experiencing.

The primary assessment reveals that the patient is anxious, restless, alert, and oriented. He has adequate respirations at a rate of 22/minute with good chest rise and fall. His radial pulses are strong and regular at a rate of 112 beats per minute. His skin is pale, cool, and clammy. The SpO$_2$ reading is 95 percent.

2. What are the life threats to this patient?

3. What immediate emergency care should you provide based on the primary assessment?

4. What conditions are you still considering as the possible cause? Would you add any conditions as a possible cause?

During the secondary assessment, you note no signs of any traumatic injuries. The patient states that he was playing basketball when he suddenly had a severe pain in his lower back. He said the pain started about 15 minutes earlier and that he has vomited because of the pain. He describes the pain as the worst in his life and says it feels like it is moving down into his groin. He denies any head, neck, or chest pain. His abdomen is soft and tender on palpation. He says that when he urinated it was bloody and painful. His pelvis is stable, and no deformities or trauma to the extremities are evident. The patient has no known allergies or past medical problems, and he takes no prescription medication. He states that he had eaten a sandwich and drank bottled water about an hour prior to your arrival. His blood pressure is 134/72 mmHg, heart rate is now 106 beats per minute, and his respirations are 16/minute.

5. What conditions have you ruled out in your differential field diagnosis? Why?

6. What conditions are you considering as a probable cause? Why?

7. Based on your differential diagnosis, what are the next steps in emergency care? Why?

Standard Medicine

Competency Applies fundamental knowledge to provide basic and selected advanced emergency care and transportation based on assessment findings for an acutely ill patient.

TOPIC

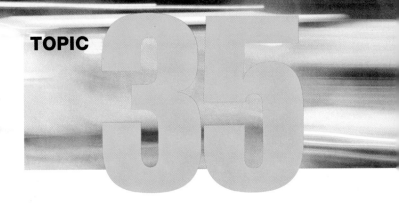

GYNECOLOGIC EMERGENCIES

INTRODUCTION

Gynecology refers to the study of female health and the female reproductive system. A variety of gynecologic emergencies may cause abdominal pain, vaginal bleeding, or discharge. These emergencies can be both medical and traumatic in nature. If left untreated, gynecologic conditions can deteriorate into life-threatening complications. Knowledge of the female reproductive system and its function is pertinent for accurate assessment, differential diagnosis, and treatment of these conditions. Take time to review the anatomy of the female reproductive system (▶ Figure 35-1).

EPIDEMIOLOGY

More women every year are taking steps to improve their overall health. Each year an estimated 19.4 million women receive a preventive gynecologic examination. But even with routine preventive screenings, gynecologic emergencies can arise. Pathophysiology specific to vaginal bleeding, traumatic vaginal bleeding, pelvic inflammatory disease, pregnancy, and sexual assault is discussed in the next section.

PATHOPHYSIOLOGY

Vaginal Bleeding

Vaginal bleeding is a common chief complaint among women requesting emergency medical care. Normal vaginal bleeding occurs cyclically in women who have achieved menarche. This typically starts at approximately 12 to 13 years of age until the onset of menopause, around the age of 51. The regularity of the menstrual cycle is dependent on a complex feedback mechanism involving the hypothalamus, pituitary gland, uterus, and ovaries. Duration of the normal menstrual cycle is an average of four days, with a blood loss of approximately 50 mL.

Abnormal vaginal bleeding occurs in women of all ages and can result from a variety of causes, such as anatomic abnormalities, complications of pregnancy, malignancies, infection, systemic diseases, and endocrine imbalances.

Approximately 5 percent of women 30 to 45 years of age will seek medical attention for abnormal non-pregnancy-related

vaginal bleeding, also known as dysfunctional uterine bleeding. Thirty percent of all women report having prolonged or excessive uterine bleeding occurring at regular intervals.

Dysfunctional uterine bleeding is more prevalent in extremes of age during the reproductive years. It also affects 50 percent of premenopausal women. There is no distinction among races; however, black women have a higher incidence of uterine fibroids, which inherently cause vaginal bleeding. (Vaginal bleeding in conjunction with pregnancy is discussed in Topic 49, "Obstetrics (Antepartum Complications).")

Obtain an accurate history of the chief complaint to establish the extent of the emergency at hand. Question the patient as to when the bleeding started. Ascertain whether the bleeding started at the scheduled onset of a menstrual period. Ask the patient about the volume and duration of the bleeding. Useful

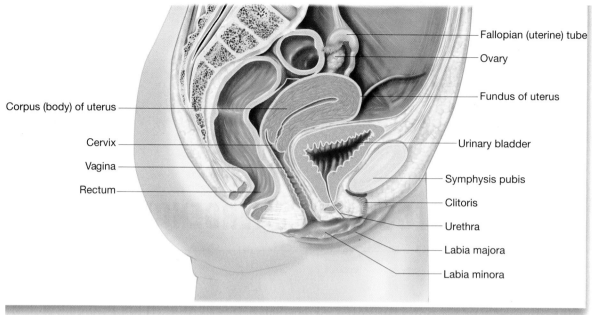

Figure 35-1 Anatomy of the female reproductive system.

information includes the number of tampons or pads changed over the preceding 12 to 24 hours.

A tampon or pad holds an average of 20 to 30 mL of vaginal effluent. Women with heavy bleeding typically change pads or tampons a minimum of every 3 hours. Determine whether the pads are saturated and whether blood clots are present. Clots with a diameter of greater than 1 cm are associated with menstrual blood loss of at least 80 mL.

Do not discount the possibility of the patient being pregnant. Has the patient missed a period? Some bleeding may actually occur during implantation of the embryo, making the patient believe that the bloody vaginal discharge is her normal period. Does she have unprotected sex? Has she had sexual intercourse since her last menstrual cycle? Obtain a menstrual history in the premenopausal patient to include the date of the last period, any change in the frequency of periods, whether the flow is usually heavy or prolonged, and whether

> **Do not discount the possibility of the patient being pregnant.**

> **Seventy-five percent of the vaginal lacerations reported by women who are requesting emergency medical care require repair.**

the patient has had similar episodes of bleeding. A gynecologic and obstetric history should include methods of contraception, the outcome of all prior pregnancies (miscarriages, abortions, and deliveries), pregnancy complications, and previous pelvic infections.

The physical exam is aimed at determining the amount of blood loss and attempting to identify the underlying etiology of the bleeding. Inspect the abdomen for a mass or distention and palpate to localize the area of abdominal tenderness. Baseline vital signs are obtained to assess hemodynamic stability. Postural changes in vital signs can be indicative of the patient's volume status. Hypotension and tachycardia, as well as pale skin and conjunctiva, are indicative of hypovolemic shock and require aggressive management.

Traumatic Vaginal Bleeding

Although obstetric-related trauma is the most common cause of injury to the female genital tract, nonobstetric trauma is not uncommon. Vaginal lacerations and traumatic vaginal bleeding occur more often than recognized. These lacerations can result in significant blood loss and life-threatening hypovolemic shock if not properly managed.

Vaginal lacerations not related to childbirth vary greatly in comparison to obstetric lacerations. Nonobstetric vaginal lacerations are generally classified

into two groups. The first group is associated with the first encounter of sexual intercourse or even with normal sexual intercourse. This results in a relatively minor laceration to the vagina and resolves with minimal or no treatment. The second group of vaginal lacerations is deeper, is more extensive, and causes copious vaginal bleeding. These lacerations can lead to significant blood loss and require rapid intervention.

Seventy-five percent of the vaginal lacerations reported by women who are requesting emergency medical care require repair. These patients present with marked vaginal bleeding. In addition, an average of 15 percent of these patients have perineal and/or lower abdominal pain. In addition, hemorrhagic shock manifests in 15 percent of these cases.

The most common mechanism of injury for nonobstetric vaginal lacerations is sexual intercourse. Predisposing factors that can account for this injury are virginity, disproportion of male and female genitalia, insertion of foreign bodies, previous surgery, stenosis or scarring of the vagina from congenital abnormalities, and atrophic vagina in postmenopausal women. Be certain not to discount the possibility of sexual assault in these patients. Many women with these injuries are embarrassed and do not seek help until self-treatment is unsuccessful. These patients then present late with significant blood loss and impending hypovolemic shock.

Noncoital reproductive tract injuries can include blunt and penetrating trauma. Traumatic vaginal bleeding can be the consequence of trauma to the abdomen, especially trauma involving pelvic fractures. In addition, straddle injuries are known to cause substantial vaginal laceration and bleeding. Although straddle injuries are more commonly seen in children with bicycle injuries, these injuries can be seen in adults involved with activities such as water or jet skiing.

Physical exam and emergency care of traumatic vaginal bleeding should focus on accurate assessment and treatment of clinical presentation. Swiftly determine the cause and amount of hemorrhage. Place a pad to help absorb the hemorrhage, but do not pack the vagina. Obtain baseline vital signs, and establish the effects of blood loss to the patient. Expeditiously transport the patient, and frequently reevaluate for signs and symptoms of shock.

Pelvic Inflammatory Disease

Pelvic inflammatory disease (PID) is a community-acquired infection of the upper female reproductive system. It includes the uterus, fallopian tubes, and neighboring pelvic structures. PID is a serious condition initiated by an infectious process that ascends from the vagina and cervix. The inflammatory response and infectious process can result in endometritis, salpingitis, oophoritis, peritonitis, or tubo-ovarian abscess. A delay in diagnosis and treatment of PID can lead to chronic pelvic pain, adhesions, and even infertility (▶ Figure 35-2).

PID is the most common serious infection reported among women 16 to 25 years of age. In the United States, 1 million women are estimated to experience an episode of PID per year. It has a higher incidence in white females of a lower socioeconomic status. An estimated 10 percent to 20 percent of untreated gonorrheal and chlamydial infections turn into PID. More than 100,000 women are estimated to become infertile each year because of this condition. However, only 0.29 in every 100,000 women 15 to 44 years of age succumb to PID. The most common cause of

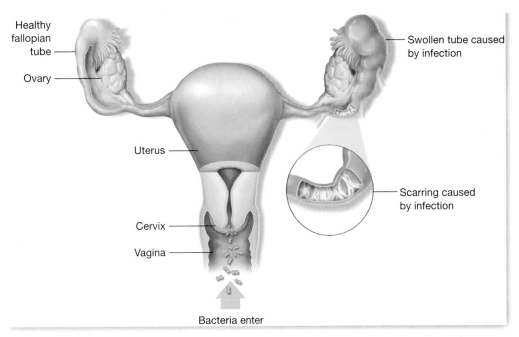

Healthy fallopian tube
Ovary
Uterus
Cervix
Vagina
Swollen tube caused by infection
Scarring caused by infection
Bacteria enter

Figure 35-2 Illustration of the way in which pelvic inflammatory disease (PID) affects the reproductive organs.

death in these cases is secondary to rupture of a tubo-ovarian abscess.

Evaluation of risk factors for sexually transmitted disease (STD) and risk factors that increase the probability for PID can be helpful in the diagnosis of this condition. Risk factors for STD include age less than 25 years, nonbarrier contraception or oral contraception, multiple or symptomatic sexual partners, and first intercourse at a young age. Factors that potentially facilitate PID include a history of the disease, sex during menses, vaginal douching, bacterial vaginosis, and the use of an intrauterine device.

This community-acquired infection is typically caused by a sexually transmitted disease. *Neisseria gonorrhoeae* and *Chlamydia trachomatis* are usually identified in women with PID. Gonococcal disease tends to have a rapid onset of symptoms, whereas chlamydial disease has a more insidious onset. Lower abdominal pain is the cardinal presenting symptom in patients with PID, experienced by 90 percent of patients. Pain that worsens with coitus and jarring movement or after menses is also suggestive of PID.

On exam, abdominal pain is usually diffuse in the lower quadrants and may or may not be symmetrical. Rebound tenderness and decreased bowel sounds are also common findings. In addition to abdominal pain, abnormal uterine bleeding occurs in one-third of patients with PID. Other associated signs and symptoms

that are not specific to PID but are typically present include purulent vaginal discharge, fever, and chills. Purulent vaginal drainage is seen in approximately 75 percent of patients.

Pregnancy

A woman's reproductive years start at the onset of menstruation and end at the cessation of menstruation, or menopause. When evaluating a female patient in her reproductive years, it is important to remember the possibility of her being pregnant. In some cases, the patient's current complaint is the first sign that she is pregnant. In the United States, each year more than 6 million women are clinically recognized as being pregnant.

Most women experience signs and symptoms of pregnancy as early as three weeks after conception. The cardinal sign of pregnancy is amenorrhea or absence of menstrual flow. Pregnancy should be suspected whenever a woman of childbearing age has a cessation of menstruation or delay of menstruation greater than one week. In addition to amenorrhea, sexual activity without contraception or misuse of contraception should also increase your suspicion of pregnancy.

Other signs and symptoms of early pregnancy include nausea, vomiting, breast tenderness, increased urinary frequency, and fatigue. The term *morning sickness* refers to the tendency for most pregnant women to develop nausea, and

> **As an AEMT, you are required to report sexual assault cases to law enforcement and the proper authorities.**

in some cases vomiting, between 6 and 12 weeks of gestation. The nausea is typically worse in the mornings and improves as the day progresses. If nausea and vomiting are accompanied by fever, dizziness, headache, or abdominal pain, however, then a cause other than pregnancy should be considered. Pregnant women often notice an enlargement in their breasts with a strong sensation of soreness. This is due to estrogen and progesterone fluctuations. Pregnancy causes an increased total urinary output, which leads to an increase in urinary frequency. Finally, profound fatigue is frequently seen in pregnancy. It is most common in the first trimester and becomes less prominent in the second and third trimesters.

You can ask specific questions to help verify your suspicion of pregnancy. Inquire about when the patient's last menstrual period occurred and whether it was normal. Ask whether the patient has been sexually active since her last menstrual cycle. If she has been sexually active, did she use a form of contraception, and did she use it properly? It is unlikely that you will be able to determine early pregnancy by physical exam. However, your assessment of the signs and symptoms, as well as the patient's history, can help you determine the likelihood of pregnancy. Maintain a high index of suspicion in women of childbearing age, even if the history is not consistent with the diagnosis.

Sexual Assault

Sexual assault refers to an act of violence in which sexual intercourse and/or sexual activities are performed without consent. Although anyone can be a victim of sexual assault, victims of such crimes are typically women and often know their assailant. It is not uncommon for victims who know their assailant not to report the crime to the proper authorities. However, as an Advanced EMT, you are required to report sexual assault

> **During your secondary assessment, continue to protect the patient's privacy and modesty.**

cases to law enforcement and the proper authorities. Make sure you follow your local protocol when caring for these patients.

On arrival at the scene of a sexual assault, ensure scene safety. Law enforcement is often dispatched to these calls for service; however, they are not always on scene at the time you arrive. Be cautious about the possibility that the assailant may still be present. Once the scene is secure for you to enter, address the safety needs of the patient and others at the scene.

Once the scene is safe, you can assess the patient for life-threatening injuries and provide the appropriate emergency care. Make certain that you provide emergency care that addresses both the physical and emotional needs of the patient. In addition, you want to emphasize the need for the patient to seek medical evaluation and collection of evidence at the hospital.

If the patient agrees to emergency care and evidence collection, explain how to preserve the evidence until it can be collected. Do not allow her to bathe, brush her teeth or hair, change her clothes, urinate or defecate, smoke, eat, or drink. If possible, do not cut or touch the patient's clothing unless it interferes with emergency care.

Let the patient know that most of her clothing will be taken for evidence. Offer to bring a clean change of clothes with her or have someone bring clothing to the hospital. If the patient has already changed her clothing, collect it in a separate bag and handle the evidence as little as necessary. Initiate transport to the hospital and, when applicable, transport the patient to a facility other than the one to which the suspect has been taken.

En route to the hospital, provide physical as well as emotional care as appropriate. Provide a safe environment for the patient. Remain nonjudgmental and protect confidentiality by asking only questions that are pertinent to the assessment and emergency care of the patient. Do not touch the patient unnecessarily, and ask for consent before performing procedures. Obtain a baseline set of vital signs and evaluate for any other associated injuries. Be certain to document all your findings objectively and accurately. Be familiar with the hospitals in your area that have specialized personnel and facilities for sexual assault victims; it is preferable to transport the patient to those facilities.

ASSESSMENT

As always, use your dispatch information to help you determine what is taking place at the scene. This information should trigger you to think of possible causes for the chief complaint. Dispatch information can also lead you toward whether the patient is suffering from a traumatic injury or a medical condition. If sexual assault is a possibility, ensure that law enforcement has been notified. Remember that it is always possible that the assailant may still be at the scene. Once you arrive, ensure that the scene is safe for you to enter and use Standard Precautions before you approach the patient.

As you approach the patient, look around the scene to obtain a general impression. Assess the situation to determine whether a traumatic injury is involved. If you suspect an injury, establish manual stabilization of the spine. Ensure that the patient's airway is open and clear of any potential obstruction. Evaluate the rate, rhythm, and quality of the patient's respirations. In addition to clinical assessment findings, use a pulse oximeter to determine whether the patient requires oxygen administration.

Pay particular attention to the patient's circulatory status. Bleeding can be both external and internal. Avoid missing internal bleeding by evaluating the patient's pulses, skin color, and temperature. A patient who presents in shock needs to be aggressively treated and rapidly transported to an appropriate medical facility. Patients who require expeditious transport include those presenting with poor general appearance, altered mental status, severe pain, uncontrolled bleeding, and shock.

Obtain a baseline set of vital signs, including blood pressure, and begin your physical exam. Typically, the physical exam focuses on the gynecologic complaint; however, be sure to examine the rest of the body for other associated signs and symptoms. Remember that it is not necessary to diagnosis the exact cause of the gynecologic complaint, but it is necessary to rule out the cause as stemming from another body system.

During your secondary assessment, continue to protect the patient's privacy and modesty. Be mindful that it is necessary to ask the patient personal questions and that she may be hesitant to answer, especially in the presence of many people. Be compassionate and professional when obtaining a history and physical exam from patients who have been sexually assaulted.

EMERGENCY MEDICAL CARE

As mentioned previously, it is not imperative that you diagnose the exact cause of the patient's abdominal pain and/or vaginal bleeding. However, it is imperative that you accurately assess and identify the patient's signs and symptoms. Then you can provide appropriate emergency care based on the patient's clinical presentation. Emergency care should include the following:

- **Maintain manual spinal stabilization.** If you suspect trauma, take precautions to maintain spinal immobilization.
- **Maintain a patent airway.** Be prepared for the possibility that the patient may vomit. If no trauma is suspected, transport the patient in a left lateral recumbent position to protect the airway.
- **Determine the patient's respiratory status.** Administer oxygen based on the patient's signs and symptoms and the SpO$_2$ reading. If the SpO$_2$ reading is greater than 95 percent and the patient is asymptomatic, oxygen administration may not be necessary. However, you can apply a nasal cannula with 2 to 4 lpm of oxygen if you feel it is appropriate. If the SpO$_2$ reading is less than 95 percent and the respirations are adequate, place the patient on a nonrebreather mask at 15 lpm. Inadequate respirations require positive pressure ventilation with a bag-valve mask and high-concentration oxygen.
- **Control any major bleeding.** If vaginal bleeding is present, place a pad to absorb the flow. Do not pack the vagina.
- **Initiate transport.**
- **IV access and fluid administration may be warranted en route.** Follow local protocol for guidelines on IV fluid boluses.
- **Calm and reassure the patient.** Be supportive and nonjudgmental, especially in cases of sexual assault.

TRANSITIONING

REVIEW ITEMS

1. What is the best indicator of blood loss in a patient presenting with vaginal bleeding?
    a. "This is more bleeding than normal for my period."
    b. "I noticed a small blood clot on my sanitary napkin."
    c. "My tampons are saturated, and I have changed them four times in the last hour."
    d. "I have had a period for the last seven days."

2. What is the most common nonobstetric cause for traumatic vaginal bleeding?
    a. vaginal delivery of a baby   b. straddle injuries
    c. sexual intercourse   d. none of the above

3. Which of the following is not a risk factor for PID?
    a. sexual intercourse during menstruation
    b. multiple sex partners

    c. age less than 25 years
    d. consistent condom use

4. Which is the most common sign of pregnancy?
    a. amenorrhea
    b. breast tenderness
    c. increased urinary frequency
    d. morning sickness

5. Who is most likely to be a victim of a sexual assault?
    a. 4-year-old girl
    b. 10-year-old boy
    c. 25-year-old woman
    d. 35-year-old man

CLINICAL DECISION MAKING

You are called to the scene of an 11-year-old girl suffering from what appears to be a straddle injury from a bicycle accident. The child is lying supine on the ground next to the bicycle, with blood saturating her pants. As you approach the child, her eyes are closed, and she is not crying.

1. Would you manually stabilize the spine in this patient? Why or why not?

2. What technique would you use to open the patient's airway? Why?

The SpO$_2$ reading is 90 percent with a respiratory rate of 16 and adequate respirations.

3. What oxygen therapy would you provide to this patient?

When assessing the circulation you observe pale skin, weak pulses and a heart rate of 180. After exposing the patient, you observe a heavy flow of blood from the vagina.

4. How would you treat the vaginal bleeding?

5. Why does the patient have weak pulses, tachycardia, and pale skin?

6. Would you expect the blood pressure to be normotensive, hypotensive, or hypertensive?

7. Would you begin an IV for fluid administration? If so, what would you use to determine the amount of intravenous fluids you should administer?

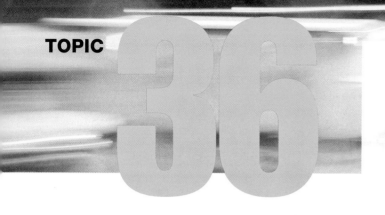

Standard Medicine

Competency Applies fundamental knowledge to provide basic and selected advanced emergency care and transportation based on assessment findings for an acutely ill patient.

EMERGENCIES INVOLVING THE EYES, EARS, NOSE, AND THROAT

TRANSITION *highlights*

- *Frequency, types, mortality, and morbidity of facial injuries.*

- *Overview of how kinetic energy produces the forces causing the various types of facial injuries.*

- *Pathophysiologic changes that occur with facial emergencies likely to be encountered in the prehospital environment:*
  - *– Eye injuries.*
  - *– Epistaxis.*

- *Specific questions to ask and assessment findings pertinent to these types of emergencies.*

- *How to use a Morgan Lens kit for eye irrigation.*

- *General treatment parameters the Advanced EMT can employ when caring for a patient an emergency involving the eyes, ears, nose, and throat.*

INTRODUCTION

Trauma to the eye, face, or neck can cause a patient not only significant injury, but emotional stress as well. Patients often experience fear and panic when they think of the possible outcomes from their injury. In some situations, these injuries can bring about loss of vision, scarring, and permanent disfigurement. As an Advanced EMT, you will have to care for not only physical trauma, but emotional trauma as well.

Moreover, an injury to the face or neck can pose significant airway and circulatory compromise. With eye, face, and neck injuries, the likelihood for airway compromise, severe bleeding, and shock is high. In addition, trauma to the face and neck has the potential to cause spinal column or cord injury. You must anticipate the complications that accompany these injuries. Always maintain a high level of awareness, and give priority to

caring for life-threatening airway, ventilatory, and circulatory compromise.

Knowledge of the anatomy of the eyes, face, and neck is imperative when treating these emergencies. Attentiveness to the location of structures and major blood vessels can allow you to predict the complications that often arise with these injuries (▶ Figure 36-1 and ▶ Figure 36-2).

EPIDEMIOLOGY

More than three million facial injuries occur in the United States each year. In urban communities, facial trauma is most commonly secondary to assaults, motor vehicle crashes, and industrial accidents. The number-one cause of facial injuries in the rural setting is motor vehicle crashes, followed by assaults and recreational activities. Injuries to the midface, such as LeFort fractures, occur most commonly in motor vehicle crashes with patients who were not wearing a seatbelt. In assaults, zygomatic and mandible fractures are commonly seen. Other important causes of facial injuries include penetrating trauma, domestic violence, and abuse in children and the elderly.

The incidence of major injury accompanying high-impact facial fractures is as high as 50 percent, as compared with 21 percent in low-impact fractures. Associated cervical spine injury varies between 0.2 percent and 6 percent. Mortality is as high as 12 percent in high-impact fractures; however, this is rarely due to the maxillofacial injury. Mortality typically arises from a secondary injury associated with impact, such as head injury. Maintain a high index of suspicion for other injuries when caring for these patients.

PATHOPHYSIOLOGY

The dispersion of kinetic energy during deceleration produces the force that results in injury. Kinetic energy, defined as the energy possessed by an object because of its motion, equals mass (weight in pounds), times the velocity (feet per second) squared, divided by two:

$$\frac{\text{Mass} \times \text{Velocity}^2}{2}$$

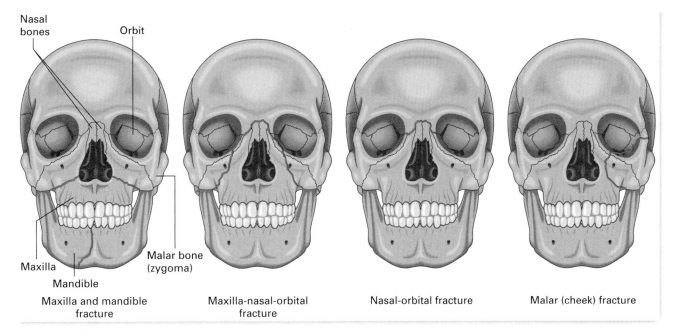

Figure 36-1 Types of facial fractures.

Maxilla and mandible fracture

Maxilla-nasal-orbital fracture

Nasal-orbital fracture

Malar (cheek) fracture

Nasal bones

Orbit

Maxilla

Mandible

Malar bone (zygoma)

High-impact force is defined as a force greater than 50 times the force of gravity. Low-impact force is less than 50 times the force of gravity. The zygoma (cheek) and nasal bone need only a low-impact force to cause damage. The supraorbital rim of the eye, mandible (jaw), and frontal bones require a high-impact force to cause injury.

Finally, the most common of all facial fractures are simple nasal fractures.

ASSESSMENT

Primary assessment in a patient with an injury to the eye, face, or neck should include inline manual stabilization of the spine as you approach the patient. These injuries are traumatic in nature and have the potential to cause injury to the cervical spine. Use a jaw-thrust maneuver to open the airway. Suction blood and any other secretions or potential obstruction from the airway.

If breathing is inadequate, provide positive pressure ventilation and high-concentration oxygen via the ventilation device at a rate of 10 to 12 ventilations per minute in the adult patient. Infants and children should be ventilated at a rate of 12 to 20 ventilations per minute. Should the respiratory function be adequate, provide oxygen.

Control any major bleeding with direct pressure. Consider early notification of ALS for the patient you suspect may need more advanced airway maneuvers, has continued respiratory distress, or has major bleeding you are unable to control.

Once life-threatening conditions are managed, obtain a history. Important questions to ask include the following:

- Did the patient lose consciousness? If so, for how long was the patient unconscious?
- Does the patient have any vision problems, such as blurred vision, diploplia, or photophobia?
- Does the patient have any hearing problems, such as muffled tones or ringing in the ear?
- Does the patient have any clear-fluid drainage from the nose or ears that may be indicative of cerebrospinal fluid?
- Does the patient have malocclusion or misalignment of the teeth?

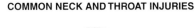

COMMON NECK AND THROAT INJURIES

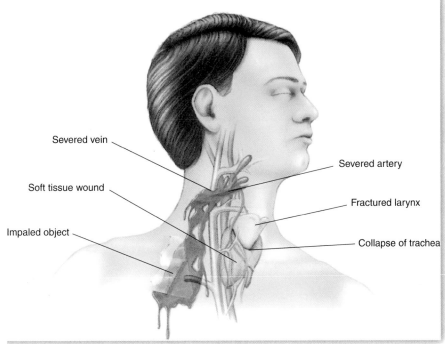

Severed vein

Soft tissue wound

Impaled object

Severed artery

Fractured larynx

Collapse of trachea

Figure 36-2 Common neck and throat injuries.

- Does the patient have numbness or tingling in the face?
- Is the mechanism of injury secondary to abuse or domestic violence?

EMERGENCY CARE

Whether you are treating an injury to the eye, face, or neck, emergency care focuses on airway, breathing, and circulation. Emergency care may include the following:

- Establish manual inline stabilization of the spine, followed by complete immobilization.
- Open the airway, using a jaw-thrust maneuver.
- Suction the airway.
- If there are signs of hypoxia, provide oxygen. Administer positive pressure ventilation and supplemental oxygen to the patient with inadequate respiratory function.
- Control major bleeding with direct pressure.
- Consider early notification of advanced life support and initiate rapid transport.
- Provide emotional support.

SPECIFIC EMERGENCIES AND MANAGEMENT

Eye Injuries

In some eye injuries, irrigation of the eye may be necessary. These instances include chemical burns and attempting to remove foreign particles from the eye such as dirt, sand, or other particles that tears may not wash away naturally.

Should it be determined that eye irrigation is necessary, you may flush the eye with clear, clean water. The water does not necessarily have to be sterile, but it should be clean. Hold the eyelids apart and flush the water from the inner canthus of the eye downward to the outer edge of the eye. Position the patient's head to facilitate drainage of the water as it passes over the eye into a basin and to not contaminate the uninjured eye.

In cases of chemical burns, flush the eye continuously for 20 minutes. If the chemical involves alkali, flush the eye for at least an hour or until arrival at the hospital.

MORGAN LENS Use of the Morgan Lens® is beneficial in flushing a patient's eye, especially during the prolonged irrigation of chemical burns. The Morgan Lens is a contact-lens type irrigation device that provides slow, continuous eye irrigation. The lens itself is attached to intravenous tubing primed with saline or Ringer's lactate. With a slow, steady flow, place the lens onto the patient's eye. Have the patient look downward and set the lens on the upper aspect of the eye and allow the lid to sit over the lens (▶ Figure 36-3A). Then have the patient look upward to facilitate the placement of the lens on the lower aspect of the eye. Allow the eyelid to cover the bottom aspect of the lens (▶ Figure 36-3B).

The steady flow of irrigant during placement prevents the Morgan Lens from sitting directly on the cornea. Secure the tubing to the patient's head and adjust the flow accordingly. Take caution to not allow the solution to run dry. Absorb the overflow of irrigant into a towel. To discontinue the use of the Morgan Lens, continue the flow. Retract the lower eyelid and hold it in position. Then remove the lens downward and terminate the flow of the solution. Pat the excess solution dry while instructing the patient not to rub the eyes.

Epistaxis

Epistaxis, or nosebleed, is a common problem, occurring in 60 percent of the general population. Epistaxis is more likely to affect children before the age of 10 and adults between 45 and 65 years of age. There is a male predominance for epistaxis prior to the age of 49, but the sex distribution equalizes thereafter. This can be attributed to the protective effects of estrogen in women through relief of capillary permeability. There is a higher proportion of epistaxis in the winter months, caused by the increased incidence of upper respiratory tract infections, allergic rhinitis, and mucosal changes associated with fluctuations in the temperature and humidity during the winter months.

Epistaxis is often self-limiting in nature. It is classified by the source of bleeding: anterior and posterior. Anterior epistaxis frequently originates from the nasal septum. It is the most common, accounting for 90 percent of all nosebleeds. Posterior epistaxis does not occur as regularly, but it can result in significant hemorrhage, and even hemorrhagic shock, if not controlled properly.

Epistaxis often results from mucosal trauma or irritation. Nose picking is the most common cause; however, there are numerous other causes, including low moisture content in the ambient air, mucosal hyperemia secondary to allergic or viral rhinitis, nasal steroid use for seasonal allergies, presence of a foreign body, chronic excoriation from intranasal drug use, and facial trauma. Epistaxis can also be secondary to several medical conditions, such as hemophilia, platelet disorders, conditions requiring the use of anticoagulants or blood thinners, and nasal neoplasms.

The primary assessment of epistaxis should focus on evaluation of airway

> Epistaxis is a common problem, occurring in 60 percent of the population.

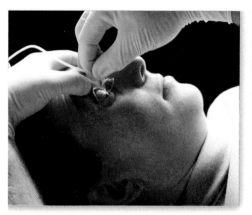 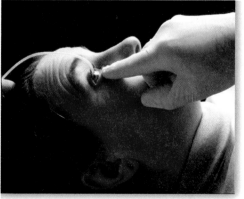

Figure 36-3 Inserting the Morgan Lens: (A) Have the patient look downward; set the lens on the upper aspect of the eye, and allow the lid to sit over the lens. (B) Have the patient look upward to facilitate placement of the lens on the lower aspect of the eye. Allow the eyelid to cover the bottom aspect of the lens.

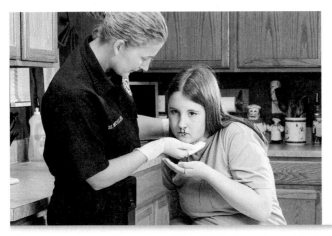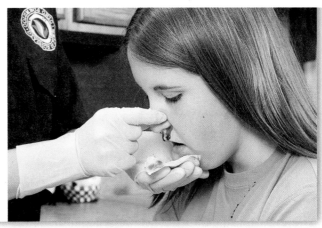

Figure 36-4 Controlling a nosebleed: (A) Have the patient sit and lean forward. (B) Pinch the fleshy part of the nostrils together.

management, respiratory function, and cardiovascular stability. Ensure that the patient's airway is clear of blood and secretions. If necessary, suction the airway so it is free of any potential obstruction. If your patient is awake and alert, you can provide him with a hard suction catheter so he may clear any secretions as often as he prefers.

Assess the patient's respiratory rate and adequacy of ventilation. Provide high-concentration oxygen as needed (although bleeding control has priority, which may prevent the use of a mask or nasal cannula). Evaluate the patient's circulatory status by palpating central and peripheral pulses for rate and quality. Also, use a skin assessment to help determine the patient's circulatory status. Cool,

clammy skin with a weak pulse could indicate hypovolemic shock.

Once it is determined that the patient's airway, breathing, and circulatory function are adequate, the next step is to achieve hemostasis (▶ Figure 36-4). Properly instructed patients may achieve this by holding direct pressure and pinching the fleshy portion of their nostrils together. Instruct the patient to exert pressure by grasping the nostrils distally and pinching them tightly against the septum.

The patient must maintain direct pressure for 10 consecutive minutes. Ensure that the patient does not check to see whether the bleeding has stopped prior to holding direct pressure for 10 minutes. In addition, you may have the patient sit

down and bend forward at the waist. This will help the patient expectorate blood accumulation in the pharynx and prevent him from swallowing excess blood. If possible, apply ice or a cold pack to the bridge of the nose to facilitate vasoconstriction.

Once hemostasis is achieved, the timing, frequency, and severity of the epistaxis should be determined. Is this an isolated episode or one of many? Are there any medical conditions that can be exacerbated by blood loss? Examples of these conditions include coronary artery disease and chronic obstructive pulmonary disease. Is the patient experiencing any signs or symptoms associated with these conditions, such as chest pain, dyspnea, weakness, or dizziness?

TRANSITIONING

REVIEW ITEMS

1. Which method is the simplest, most effective way of managing anterior epistaxis?
   a. direct pressure
   b. nasal packing
   c. cauterization
   d. ice application

2. In which situation would you consider irrigation of the eye with a Morgan Lens?
   a. chemical burn to the eye
   b. ruptured globe
   c. corneal abrasion
   d. impaled metal object into the cornea

3. Which solution should you use with a Morgan Lens?
   a. normal saline
   b. 5% dextrose in water
   c. 50% dextrose in water
   d. hypertonic saline

4. Which situation would make you consider ALS backup?
   a. inability to keep the airway clear of secretions and potential obstruction
   b. inability to provide adequate positive pressure ventilation to a patient with poor respiratory effort and severe facial trauma
   c. inability to control bleeding to the neck
   d. all of the above

APPLIED PATHOPHYSIOLOGY

1. List five causes of epistaxis.

2. Which epistaxis poses the biggest threat of significant hemorrhage—anterior or posterior?

3. Describe the process of inserting a Morgan Lens.

4. List five injuries you expect to see in a patient with high-impact trauma to the face.

CLINICAL DECISION MAKING

You are dispatched to the local bike trail for a male patient who crashed his bicycle. When you arrive on scene, you observe a man lying prone on the cement approximately five feet away from his bicycle. Bystanders state he struck an object in the roadway and flipped over the handlebars.

1. What is your first step in rendering care and positioning of this patient for adequate assessment?

Once the patient is supine, you observe multiple abrasions and contusions about his face. There is a large hematoma to the right eye, causing the eyelid to be swollen shut. There are bloody secretions flowing out of his mouth and a broken tooth on the ground near his head. There is auditory gurgling with the patient's respirations. His respirations are shallow and slow. Aside from the bleeding in the oral cavity, there does not appear to be any other major bleeding.

2. Summarize the steps you will take to care for the patient's ABCs.

3. Would you consider requesting ALS backup for this patient? Why or why not?

Standard Shock and Resuscitation

Competency Applies a fundamental knowledge to provide basic and selected advanced emergency care and transportation based on assessment findings for a patient in shock, respiratory failure or arrest, cardiac failure or arrest, and post-resuscitation management.

TOPIC

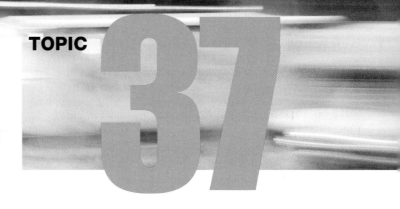

ISSUES IN CARDIAC ARREST AND RESUSCITATION

INTRODUCTION

Each patient the Advanced EMT encounters in the prehospital environment is, in some sense, unique and challenging. This requires the AEMT to remain ever vigilant during all steps of assessment and management to ensure optimal patient outcomes. However, few EMS responses can rival a cardiac arrest when it comes to the need for scene control and choreography, efficient and focused assessment, prioritization and integration of prehospital skills, and overall expenditure of provider energy and thought processing.

When faced with a patient either deteriorating into cardiac arrest or already in cardiac arrest, the skills the AEMT provides must be measured by both efficacy and time, as this patient may suffer irreversible cardiac and brain injuries in a matter of minutes if care is either delayed or inappropriate. If EMS can have a dramatic impact on both the patient and the patient's family in any one situation, it is here. Whether the patient ultimately lives or dies, this situation will leave a permanent emotional mark in the memories of all.

EPIDEMIOLOGY

Cardiovascular disease is the most prevalent chronic condition in the United States, as well as the leading contributor to death. It has been said that cardiovascular disease is actually a "young person's" disease process that results in "old age" complications. In other words, the way a younger person treats his body in the present time will have a direct impact on disease presence and progression by the time he reaches late adulthood. In fact, with many cardiovascular disease processes, the first clinical indication of its presence may well be the patient's first heart attack, stroke, or even sudden cardiac arrest.

The statistics representing cardiovascular disease are as alarming as the disease process itself. It has been estimated that more than 62 million Americans have some form of cardiovascular disease (this number does not include those yet to be diagnosed). As the result of cardiovascular disease, 1.5 million people will suffer a heart attack each year, which will result in cardiac arrest and the death of 500,000 of them.

TRANSITION *highlights*

- *Frequency of annual cardiac arrest rates and similar trends over the past several years.*

- *Pathophysiologic changes that occur in cardiac arrest, how quickly cells may become injured and die.*

- *Electrical changes to the heart that accompany cardiac arrest.*

- *Relationship between cardiac arrest and the metabolic changes that lead to cellular damage and death.*

- *Assessment findings indicative of cardiac arrest, and findings suggestive of a patient who may go into cardiac arrest.*

- *Importance of prehospital interventions and why they are successful in reversing cardiac arrest.*

- *The best way to integrate care interventions for a successful reversal of cardiac arrest:*
    - Difference in management of witnessed and unwitnessed cardiac arrests.
    - Provision of high-quality CPR.
    - Automated external defibrillator operation.
    - Proper airway and ventilation.
    - Importance of not interrupting compressions.

Studies from 2009 indicate that up to 350,000 of patients suffer cardiac arrest within one hour following the onset of the signs and symptoms, which means that the majority of cardiac arrests will occur in the prehospital environment—in fact, about 60 percent of all cardiac arrests are treated by EMS. In a more sobering light, about once every minute someone will collapse from sudden cardiac arrest.

Sudden cardiac arrest is not always caused by cardiovascular disease. Statistics described previously have shown that cardiovascular disease is the leading cause of arrest; however, some

30 percent to 35 percent of cardiac arrests occur because of other etiologies. These include traumatic injuries (head and chest), nontraumatic hemorrhage (GI bleeds, aortic rupture, intracranial bleeds), drug overdoses (accidental or purposeful), and pulmonary embolism.

Regardless of etiology, all cardiac arrest patients require the same assessment and treatment goals: rapid identification and assessment, airway maintenance, support of absent breathing, artificial circulatory support, provision of electrical therapy as warranted, and attempts at reversing or remediating the offending cause of the arrest situation.

PATHOPHYSIOLOGY

To better understand the signs and symptoms of cardiac arrest, the AEMT must first understand the basic pathophysiologic underpinnings related to the condition. *Cardiac arrest* (also known as *cardiopulmonary arrest* or *circulatory arrest*) is the cessation of normal circulation of the blood; if this is unexpected (as it often is), it can be termed a *sudden cardiac arrest* (SCA).

With cardiac arrest, ventricular contraction is absent or ineffective, resulting immediately in the cessation of blood flow and systemic circulatory failure—in fact, it is the final common pathway to human death. Although it is often difficult to determine the cause of cardiopulmonary arrest at the time of presentation, a working differential diagnosis of the causes can be formulated based on the patient's history, physical examination, and automated external defibrillator (AED) rhythm analysis.

With stoppage of the heart, blood flow ceases, and no oxygenated blood is being delivered to the capillary beds of the body. Lack of blood flow initially causes pulselessness and unresponsiveness in the patient, but the lack of oxygen supply to the body's cells results in irreversible tissue damage and death.

All organs have different susceptibilities to ischemic injury from cardiac arrest, with the brain being the most vulnerable. Literature suggests that brain damage occurs after 4 to 6 minutes of normothermic cardiac arrest, and the damage is irreversible. The heart is the second most susceptible organ to ischemic injury. The renal, gastrointestinal, musculoskeletal, and integumentary systems are much more resistant to ischemia than the heart and brain; these organs rarely sustain irreversible damage in patients who are successfully resuscitated. As such, for the best chance of survival and neurologic recovery, immediate and decisive treatment is imperative.

Cardiac arrest can also be caused by multiple etiologies, either medical or traumatic. As discussed, the primary risk factor for an acute coronary syndrome is coronary artery disease. Although cardiac arrest is commonly caused by an acute coronary syndrome, it can also be caused by myriad other conditions. For example, a traumatized patient may be in arrest following severe head trauma or significant blood loss.

A person who accidentally or intentionally overdoses on his medication may be in arrest due to the effects of the medication or asphyxia. Even stroke or seizure patients may go into cardiac arrest secondary to permanent brain damage from inadequate oxygenation of cerebral tissue.

It is also important to note the common changes that occur to the electrical conduction system of the heart when a person experiences cardiac arrest, as there are specific treatment modalities that may be necessary based on the heart rhythm. During cardiac arrest, the normal electrical impulses are usually absent or disrupted, or the mechanical response to the electrical impulse does not occur. In most situations of cardiac arrest caused by cardiovascular disease, instead of smooth, coordinated contractions the heart often shows a different type of electrical activity, most commonly the uncoordinated twitching known as *ventricular fibrillation*, which cannot produce any ventricular contraction.

Conversely, in some situations in which the cause of arrest was hemorrhagic or trauma related, the heart may show organized electrical activity without evidence of actual mechanical contraction or blood flow because of the loss of volume or direct damage to the heart muscle itself. The final common pathway in these and other arrest scenarios is that after cardiac arrest has existed for several minutes, the heart will eventually cease all electrical activity, and the patient will "flatline" (an ECG rhythm known as *asystole*). Asystole is the least viable rhythm, which most often leads to an unsuccessful resuscitation attempt.

Tissue metabolic concerns also must be taken into account when managing any patient in cardiac arrest. Research has indicated that, during cardiac arrest, the metabolic demands of the cells are no longer being met secondary to the lack of perfusion. Despite this, the cells still attempt to maintain functioning as long as possible with the residual oxygen and metabolic substrates remaining in the adjacent bloodstream. Eventually the normal cellular activity and ongoing creation of energy (adenosine triphosphate, ATP) becomes so deranged from a lack of perfusion that the cells cease aerobic metabolism in favor of anaerobic metabolism in an attempt to maintain ATP production.

The consequence of this metabolic shift is the creation of overwhelming acidosis that actually hastens ongoing cellular damage and death. This has a clinical consideration regarding the management of cardiac arrest (the provision of cardiopulmonary resuscitation, artificial ventilation, and AED operation), based on the estimated downtime of the patient and whether or not bystander CPR was started prior to EMS arrival. These considerations will be discussed more thoroughly in the Emergency Medical Care section of this topic.

The discussion thus far has centered on cardiac arrest in the adult patient. However, cardiac arrest can also occur in the pediatric patient—the most common etiologies are acute airway/breathing compromise or body system trauma. In children, the presenting cardiovascular change is typically caused by airway/breathing compromise with resulting bradycardia, which, left untreated, will eventually deteriorate into asystole. However, in about 15 percent to 20 percent of pediatric cardiac arrests, the patient may present with ventricular tachycardia or fibrillation, which is managed with the AED. Thus, the need for rapid defibrillation should be considered in children who meet AED utilization criteria with sudden cardiac arrest not preceded by respiratory symptoms.

ASSESSMENT FINDINGS

Dispatch may provide information that will lead you to suspect cardiac arrest. Reports that a patient has no pulse or that emergency medical responders are performing CPR clearly indicate cardiac arrest. But also be alert to the possibility of cardiac arrest in calls to patients with other complaints including chest pain or discomfort, difficulty in breathing, seizures, unresponsiveness, or serious motor vehicle accidents or other significant trauma.

Often the patient in cardiac arrest is not hard to identify. During the primary assessment, the AEMT will note the patient in cardiac arrest to be unresponsive, pulseless and apneic, and frequently cyanotic. The determination of pulselessness is commonly determined in a large core body artery, at either the carotid or femoral locations. Determining pulselessness can be difficult; therefore, a pulse check should be limited to 10 seconds or less. According to the 2010 American Heart Association (AHA) Guidelines for Cardiopulmonary Resuscitation and Emergency Cardiovascular Care, unresponsiveness and absence of breathing or absence of normal breathing should be the key assessment indicators of cardiac arrest. Health care providers perform pulse checks simultaneously with assessment for unresponsiveness and apnea or agonal respirations.

Usually following cessation of blood flow, the patient will lose consciousness within 15 seconds; this may be followed by brief seizure activity. A near-immediate loss of bowel/bladder control may also occur with the onset of arrest. Agonal or gasping respirations may last up to 60 seconds. Pupils also typically dilate within 60 seconds of arrest.

Dependent lividity and rigor mortis, which are also associated with cardiac arrest patients, will not develop for hours after cardiac arrest occurs. If those signs are present, they are indicative of a prolonged downtime; in these cases, the patient should not be resuscitated. The following are the most important clinical indications of cardiac arrest:

- Unresponsiveness (usually occurs about 10 to 15 seconds after the heart stops)
- Absence of breathing or normal breathing (breathing may last up to 60 seconds following arrest)
- No detectable pulse (central)

Historical information gathered from on-scene family or bystanders may provide key information regarding etiology and potential outcome. If the cardiopulmonary arrest is witnessed, there exists a potential for bystander/heath care provider CPR, which increases the likelihood of a successful resuscitation. If the cardiac arrest occurs prior to arrival of the EMS, then information obtained from family, bystanders, or other emergency personnel may provide key information that will assist in resuscitation of the patient. Important historical information includes the following questions:

- Was the arrest witnessed?
- How quickly was CPR started?
- Was an AED used?
- How much time passed since the arrest was first recognized (remembering that such estimates are often inaccurate)?
- What was the patient doing at the time of arrest and during the several hours just prior to the arrest?
- What are the patient's past medical history and current medications?

Not all patients with chest pain will experience cardiac arrest, nor will all unresponsive or traumatized patients. What is important to note is that these patients can rapidly deteriorate to cardiac arrest. In these situations, in which the patient is suspected to be in critical condition, it may be best to bring the AED from the ambulance to the patient on initial approach. If cardiac arrest is known or suspected, an ALS unit should also be sent immediately to the scene to provide backup support and additional therapies.

EMERGENCY MEDICAL CARE

Although medical direction and protocol will ultimately determine what interventional steps are recommended or taken, the AEMT should follow the current guidelines for cardiopulmonary resuscitation as written by the AHA. Remember also the importance of the "chain of survival," which underscores the importance of a systematic approach toward cardiac arrest management.

The 2010 American Heart Association Guidelines for Cardiopulmonary Resuscitation and Emergency Cardiovascular Care emphasize the need to begin chest compressions in the cardiac arrest patient immediately and minimize any interruptions once the chest compressions are begun.

> If cardiac arrest is known or suspected, an ALS unit should also be sent immediately to the scene.

The standard ABC sequence of initial assessment is altered to CAB in suspected cardiac arrest patients. In cardiac arrest, chest compressions (C) are initiated immediately, and after 30 compressions the airway is opened (A) and the first two ventilations (B) are delivered. This sequence reduces the delay to first compressions.

The following are some treatment considerations during the management of a patient in cardiac arrest:

1. Witnessed versus unwitnessed cardiac arrest. If the EMS personnel did not witness the cardiac arrest, immediately initiate CPR beginning with chest compressions and continue for 2 minutes (five cycles of 30 compressions and two ventilations). During the CPR, the AED should be prepared and applied to the patient. After 2 minutes of CPR, allow the AED to analyze the rhythm and defibrillate if indicated. Following defibrillation or rhythm assessment, immediately resume CPR beginning with chest compressions.

The reason for this change is because a heart that has not been beating for several minutes consumes the residual oxygen and metabolic substrates available in the adjacent bloodstream in an attempt to remain viable. Eventually these metabolic needs are no longer met, and acidosis overwhelms the cells. Should a defibrillation be delivered during this period of cellular hypoxia, hypercapnia, and acidosis—even in the presence of ventricular fibrillation—the all-too-common outcome is asystole and death. With high-quality CPR for approximately 2 minutes, it has been shown that the reperfusion of oxygenated blood into the coronary arteries for cellular consumption by myocardial tissue cells facilitates an environment that is more responsive to the electrical therapy, and conversion rates on defibrillation to a perfusing

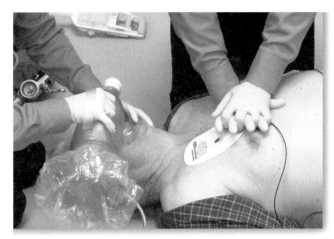

Figure 37-1 Direct ventilation with high-concentration oxygen.

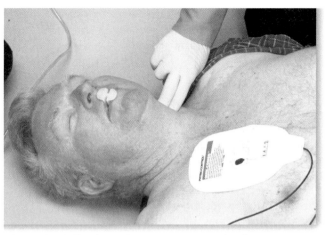

Figure 37-2 Checking the patient's carotid pulse (maximum 10 seconds).

rhythm improve. This, in turn, contributes to overall survival rates.

If the EMS personnel witnessed the cardiac arrest, immediately initiate CPR beginning with chest compressions, attach the AED as soon as it is available, and analyze the rhythm as quickly as possible. The goal is to defibrillate within 3 minutes from the onset of cardiac arrest; therefore, in the witnessed cardiac arrest patient, application of the AED and immediate rhythm analysis is performed as soon as possible. Do not wait until five cycles of CPR are completed.

2. Open the airway, insert an oro-pharyngeal airway, and ventilate the patient with a bag-valve mask and 100 percent oxygen (▶ Figure 37-1).
Ventilate the patient carefully, being sure not to exceed the recommended ventilation rate of one ventilation after every 30 compressions (8 to 10/minute). Research has indicated that overventila-tion (ventilations that are either too fast or deliver too large a tidal volume) is detrimental to cardiac output in arrested patients. Remember, in the cardiac arrest patient, chest compressions precede opening the airway and ventilation (CAB). Adequate resources are often available in the prehospital setting to perform airway management simultaneously with chest compressions. The key is to not interrupt or compromise the effectiveness of chest compressions at any time.

In nonarrest states, blood is returned to the heart via muscular contraction of the muscles that "milk" the veins in conjunc-tion with the one-way valves in the veins' lumina. Blood also returns to the heart

via gravity from the head and upper torso and because of the negative intrathoracic pressure created during spontaneous breathing (known as the cardiothoracic pump). In a cardiac arrest, obviously the patient will be motionless, which elimi-nates blood return facilitated by muscu-lar contraction. Furthermore, the arrested patient is typically in a supine position; therefore, gravity cannot facilitate blood return to the heart. Finally, if the patient is apneic and positive pressure ventilation (PPV) is being provided, there is minimal generation of negative intrathoracic pres-sure during the recoil of chest compres-sions to facilitate blood flow to the lungs.

Although the first two influences (supine position and lack of motion) cannot realistically be mediated by the AEMT, the third influence (provision of PPV) and its effect on the cardiothoracic pump can be at least minimized by pro-viding ventilations at a rate of 8 to 10 per minute, with a tidal volume just sufficient to achieve visible chest rise. Only after an advanced airway (such as the ETC or KingLT) is in place should ventilations be delivered asynchronously to chest com-pressions at a rate of 8 to 10 ventilations per minute. In support of this, it has been shown through recent research that, his-torically, the patient in cardiac arrest has been overventilated by care providers, which in turn diminishes cardiac output states during compressions by altering cardiac preload. Ultimately it was shown that overventilation is negatively corre-lated with cardiac arrest survival rates.

3. Assess the pulse and provide car-diac compressions. As noted previously,

assess a core pulse location for deter-mining whether cardiac compressions are warranted. Traditionally the carotid pulse is used for this determination, but some research has shown that lay provid-ers and health care providers alike may have trouble determining whether the pulse is present or absent in a hemo-dynamically unstable or critical patient. Therefore, quickly (maximum 10-second count) assess the pulse (▶ Figure 37-2). This is done correctly by being sure to assess the pulse on the same side as the AEMT, assessing with the fingertips of the first and second digit (do not use the thumb), and never assessing for carotid pulses simultaneously on each side of the neck. If the patient is unresponsive, with no breathing or agonal breathing, and a central pulse cannot be quickly located, immediately begin chest compressions. Do not waste precious compression time trying to ensure that the patient is pulse-less. Chest compressions delivered to patients who are not pulseless rarely lead to significant injury.

The second concern with assessing the pulse and providing compressions is the fashion in which the AEMT delivers external compressions. Since 2005, the AHA has been advocating "push hard, push fast" to underscore the importance of high-quality compressions in increas-ing survival rates of arrested patients. It has been well documented in previous research that even perfectly performed compressions can achieve only a small portion of normal cardiac output. It has been more recently documented in the literature that shallow compressions, slow compressions, or frequent interruptions

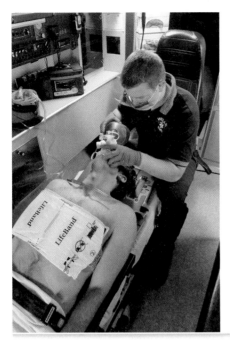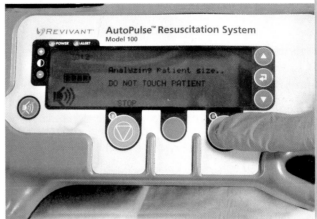

Figure 37-3 The AutoPulse™ Model 100: (A) applied to a patient; (B) close-up view.

of compressions result in reduced cardiac output, which ultimately translates into poor survival rates. Research has shown that compressions that are delivered at a rapid rate (100/min) and depress the sternum to a depth of at least 2 inches with complete recoil of the chest wall will optimize the effectiveness of compression.

The AEMT must also realize that any interruption of compressions, even for brief periods, causes the cardiac output and coronary perfusion to drop to nothing. On resumption of compressions it can take up to 45 seconds of constant compressions to return cardiac output to what it was prior to ceasing compressions. As such, always minimize the number of times you have to stop compressions and minimize the length of time compressions have to be stopped (this is also why the compression/ventilation ratio is now 30:2 and why the initial focus in cardiac arrest is on chest compressions).

Advocating and performing the "push hard, push fast" approach to compressions at a 30:2 ratio is correlated with increased cardiac output and is correlated with higher survival rates in arrested patients.

4. Examine other cardiac arrest considerations. Additional CPR adjuncts and interventions may become more commonplace during prehospital management of arrested patients. One device is a mechanical CPR adjunct that will alleviate one person from performing CPR. Because it is mechanical in nature, it may provide more consistent compressions; however, no adjunct to date has been proven to be superior to standard manual CPR (▶ Figure 37-3).

Another intervention is the use of "controlled hypothermia" during the postarrest resuscitation phase. It has been learned through controlled clinical trials that by carefully lowering the body core temperature, metabolic demands decrease, edema diminishes, and increased survival rates have been realized. This intervention is implemented into some EMS protocols, although there is no clinical evidence that early hypothermia improves outcomes, and there is actual danger if the process is not continued during the hospital phase of care.

Although specific chronological interventions for the management of a cardiac arrest patient in the prehospital environment were not discussed in their entirety, the previous discussion was intended to address the current research and physiology regarding cardiac arrest management and how to maximize the effects of the interventions to improve resuscitation rates. Treatment for the patient in cardiac arrest must be delivered in a timely manner, without error. Failure to do so will invariably lead to lower success rates in patient resuscitation.

When caring for a patient in cardiac arrest, always do your best in each of the interventions you are providing. Remember to "push hard, push fast" with compressions so that the brain and heart can still receive blood flow during arrest management. Ensure adequate ventilations and provide oxygen during the arrest as well. Minimize the amount of time that CPR is interrupted.

The automated external defibrillator should be used specifically as addressed earlier in this topic so that patients in ventricular fibrillation or pulseless ventricular tachycardia will have the greatest opportunity for survival. Patients in nonventricular fibrillation cardiac arrest (identified by a "no shock" message on the AED) should also receive this high level of care so that they too may have the greatest chance for survival.

The person with impending cardiac arrest, in cardiac arrest, or just coming out of cardiac arrest is probably one of the most challenging and dynamic patients the AEMT will ever encounter. The situation requires a thorough understanding of the body, application of multiple skills simultaneously, coordination of multiple EMS providers—all done in the shortest time possible so the patient can be transported to the hospital for definitive care.

REVIEW ITEMS

1. Of the following clinical findings, which is most reliable for determining whether the patient is in cardiac arrest or not?
   a. unresponsiveness
   b. brief seizure activity
   c. agonal breathing pattern
   d. absence of a core pulse

2. What is the most significant contributor to cardiac arrest in the prehospital environment?
   a. trauma
   b. cardiovascular disease
   c. gastrointestinal hemorrhage
   d. occlusion of a cerebral artery

3. A patient is found in cardiac arrest; no bystanders or family were present. All that is known is that it took EMS 8 minutes to arrive. Given this, the first intervention should be to _____.
   a. start CPR
   b. attach the AED

   c. contact medical control
   d. initiate ventilations at 12 per minute

4. In which of the following situations would the AED be applied prior to a full 2-minute cycle of CPR?
   a. 3-week-old infant in respiratory arrest with a pulse
   b. 69-year-old male who suffered a witnessed cardiac arrest
   c. 78-year-old female patient who suffered cardiac arrest 5 minutes prior to arrival
   d. 30-year-old male with traumatic cardiac arrest, with rescuers needing 20 minutes to gain access to the patient

5. Overventilation of the patient in cardiac arrest can have what detrimental effect?
   a. inability to properly compress the sternum
   b. failure of the AED to read the cardiac rhythm correctly
   c. decrease in cardiac output achieved through compressions
   d. hyperventilation causing hyperoxemia, which damages the central nervous system

APPLIED PATHOPHYSIOLOGY

While nearing the end of your 12-hour night shift, you are paged for a possible cardiac arrest in a 67-year-old man. On arrival at the scene 9 minutes later, the family member who found the patient states that he was "fine last night." Currently nothing is being done for the patient, who is in fact pulseless and apneic. The patient is still warm to the touch, there is cyanosis to the fingertips and hands, and no rigor or dependent lividity is present.

1. Should the AEMT initiate CPR or apply the AED first, assuming both could be done simultaneously?

2. Explain your rationale in support of your answer to the preceding question. What clinical condition or change in the circumstances would have to be present for you to change your answer?

3. Describe the anticipated physiologic benefit(s) for each of the interventions that may be administered to a patient suffering from a cardiac arrest.
   a. PPV delivered at a rate of 10–12/min:
   b. Providing compressions at a rate > 100/min:

   c. Use of AED after 2 minutes of CPR in an unwitnessed cardiac arrest:

4. What three clinical findings are most reliable for determining that an adult patient is in cardiac arrest?

5. Explain the pathophysiologic changes that occur at the cellular level as the body shifts from aerobic to anaerobic metabolism and what effect that has on defibrillation success rates.

6. What are four or five specific questions regarding the patient's history that the AEMT should try to ascertain as rapidly as possible when confronted with a patient in cardiac arrest?

7. What is the most common underlying etiology to pediatric cardiac arrest, and what is typically the presenting cardiac rhythm in these patients?

CLINICAL DECISION MAKING

You are transporting to the hospital a 59-year-old obese patient with a history of hypertension and diabetes secondary to chest pain. Thus far, you have placed the patient in a position of comfort, administered

oxygen via nonrebreather mask, and assisted in the administration of two doses of nitroglycerin. While reassessing the patient's vital signs, he moans loudly and then suddenly loses consciousness. You then witness him experiencing a mild full-body seizure that lasts about 10 seconds. You can visually see the patient is now apneic, and his skin is rapidly becoming ashen in color.

1. Based on the information provided, what assessment parameter should the AEMT determine first, before initiating any other patient care interventions?

2. What cardiac rhythm disturbance does this patient most likely have?

After confirming that the patient is unresponsive to external stimuli and is apneic and pulseless, as you reach for the AED, the ambulance stops and an AEMT from a backup unit from the same EMS company climbs into the back of the ambulance with you, and you are again en route to the hospital with lights and sirens.

3. What are your immediate interventions? Support your answer with an understanding of the metabolic changes seen in cardiac arrest.

After another 5 minutes of transport time toward the hospital, you now have an airway in place, compressions are ongoing, and the patient is receiving positive pressure ventilation via bag-valve mask attached to high-flow oxygen. You notice that your partner is ventilating the patient at a rate of about 18 per minute.

4. Is this an appropriate rate for an adult patient in cardiac arrest? If not, what is the appropriate rate?

5. What detrimental effects, if any, may occur secondary to the overventilation of a patient in cardiac arrest?

TOPIC

Standard Shock and Resuscitation

Competency Applies a fundamental knowledge to provide basic and selected advanced emergency care and transportation based on assessment findings for a patient in shock, respiratory failure or arrest, cardiac failure or arrest, and post-resuscitation management.

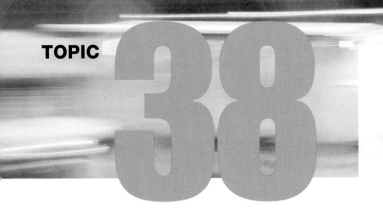

SHOCK

TRANSITION highlights

- Review of the speculative rates for hypoperfusion and shock, including mortality rates.

- Aerobic and anaerobic metabolism and its relation to hypoperfusion.

- The final common pathway of a hypoperfusive state leading to cellular death.

- Pathologic basis of the cellular stages of shock:
  - Initial stage.
  - Compensatory stage.
  - Progressive stage.
  - Refractive stage.

- Etiologies of shock and comparison with the aforementioned general pathophysiology.

- Comparison of common assessment parameters as they present according to the etiology of shock.

- Treatment strategies for managing a patient with hypoperfusion and shock, regardless of the etiology of the disturbance.

INTRODUCTION

Hypoper-fusion can be characterized as a global diminution of perfusion to the body's cells.

In 1743, while describing a state of poor tissue perfusion from battlefield injuries, a young French surgeon used the phrase "shock and agitation" in his written description of the clinical syndrome that a soldier experienced after being struck by a bullet, and the term *shock* was born. The term was quickly adopted by the Germans and the French and was initially used exclusively in connection with describing wounds and injuries. As time passed, however, the word became associated with other medical con-

ditions such as insulin shock, electrical shock, spinal shock, burn shock, psychiatric use, and, even in the effects of war, as shell shock.

Despite the medical community's attempt to remove this term due to its now varied meanings, it is still used widely today to describe myriad conditions causing patient instability.

In the traditional sense of the word, *shock* describes what occurs at the cellular level when the supplies of oxygenated blood and metabolic nutrients are insufficient to meet the body's needs, while removal of cellular waste products from this metabolic activity is simultaneously inadequate. Essentially, when cells become injured and die from shock, widespread tissue death results. With significant tissue death, the associated organ begins to dysfunction. Organ dysfunction will subsequently result in body system disturbances, and if the disturbance is grave enough, then death of the patient will ensue from this cellular "shock."

Although the term *shock* will probably never leave the lexicon of medical terms, more recently *hypoperfusion* has been introduced to better reflect what is actually happening at the cellular and tissue level and is gaining more widespread acceptance in the medical community.

EPIDEMIOLOGY

As discussed, hypoperfusion can be characterized as a global diminution of perfusion to the body's cells. Because adequate perfusion necessitates three components (adequate heart function, adequate blood supply, and adequate vascular tone) to exist properly, hypoperfusion can occur from the failure of one or more of these components—which would initially be caused by some emergency. For example, a myocardial infarction (MI) could weaken the heart muscle to a point at which it can no longer maintain an adequate cardiac output level, which in turn can cause hypoperfusion to cells, which enter into a shock state and die.

As such, it is difficult to get a precise reflection of the incidence or prevalence rates for hypoperfusion in general because of the varied etiologies and interpretations of the syndrome. It has been speculated that in the United States more than 1 million cases of hypoperfusion (from various etiologies) are seen annually in emergency departments. Mortality rates from hypoperfusion in general have been reported to consistently exceed 20 percent, with some specific etiologies of shock causing up to 90 percent mortality.

PATHOPHYSIOLOGY

Hypoperfusion from any etiology (cardiac, volume, or vascular) is a multifaceted clinical and physiologic syndrome that can disrupt normal homeostatic mechanisms along many dimensions. Despite the uniqueness of each etiology of hypoperfusion, they all share one final pathway: the deterioration in cellular oxygenation and buildup of cellular waste in the terminal tissue beds. Although this syndrome does have clinical markers, hypoperfusion is truly a cellular disturbance that results in a cascade of events that progress from cellular and tissue death, to organ breakdown, to system failure, and ultimately to global dysfunction and patient death.

Early medical literature characterized shock as "a momentary pause in the act of death." Because the cell and microcirculation are the first to suffer the insult from hypoperfusion and inadequate oxygenation, it is best to have a functional knowledge of how the cell and microcirculation normally operate before introducing the pathophysiologic changes from inadequate perfusion and inadequate oxygenation.

Cellular respiration follows two critical pathways for the creation of energy:

- **Aerobic metabolism.** Within the cellular mitochondria, in the utilization of oxygen, glucose, amino and fatty acids, 1 molecule of glucose converts into 34 to 36 total molecules of cellular-sustaining energy (ATP). The outcome of this process is energy, water, heat, and carbon dioxide. Energy is stored as ATP, and the carbon dioxide is eliminated from the body via the pulmonary system.

- **Anaerobic metabolism.** In the absence of oxygen, glucose refinement can progress only through the glycolysis phase, which liberates only two molecules of ATP. This process also results in pyruvate, which in the absence of oxygen is converted into lactic acid, which is released back into the cellular fluid and body fluids, creating a detrimental and often fatal drop

in blood pH. The end result of this process is insufficient energy production and harmful production of acids.

The benefit of understanding the preceding explanation is to appreciate how any disturbance in blood perfusion pressure, or the diminution of oxygen at the cellular level, results in the conversion of aerobic metabolism to anaerobic metabolism, with the consequences of inadequate energy supply and overwhelming acidosis. This in turn causes the failure of normal metabolic activities, and the cell dies. With cellular death, the walls of the cell deteriorate rapidly, and enzymes that are normally safely held within the cellular walls are liberated. These damaging enzymes start to exert their enzymatic activity on neighboring cells, causing their walls to collapse and the cells to die—leading to more enzyme release and more widespread cellular damage. In addition, capillary beds develop small permeations that allow fluid to exit the vascular system, causing more hypoperfusion.

As the blood becomes more acidic and cold, platelets start to clump together and form microemboli in the vascular system. The clotting systems of the body fail, and the cellular and vascular acidosis becomes overwhelming. The damage that started in just one capillary bed in one region of the body, given this progression of injury, now leads to tissue deterioration elsewhere in the body—it becomes a vicious circle of hypoperfusion, hypoxia, acidosis, and cellular death until the patient dies.

In summary, it is this widespread cellular death that causes tissue–organ failure, which in turn causes organ–system dysfunction, and when applied on an organism (or patient) level, death of the person results.

Stages of Shock

As stated, shock is a widespread response to inadequate perfusion and oxygenation. Cells are forced into anaerobic metabolism, which causes widespread cellular hypoxia and acidosis. Cells are injured first and die, which contributes to tissue death, organ dysfunction, system failure, and patient death. Shock has been found to be a progressive syndrome, progressing through four primary stages:

- **Initial stage.** Blood flow and oxygenation to distal capillary beds start

to drop, secondary to the underlying disturbance (trauma and/or medical emergency). During the initial stage the cells continue to extract oxygen from the adjacent bloodstream, but when this can no longer be done, the cells will enter into anaerobic metabolism. In the early stages of shock, very subtle clinical indications, if any at all, are noted. Despite the lack of clinical indications during this stage, serum lactate levels in the bloodstream start to rise and, thus, may be detected clinically at the hospital.

> **Widespread cellular death causes tissue–organ failure, which in turn causes organ–system dysfunction.**

- **Compensatory (nonprogressive) stage.** During this stage, the body will incorporate its own compensatory mechanisms (negative feedback mechanisms) to maintain cellular homeostasis. Be aware that during compensatory shock, however, oxygen delivery to the distal capillary beds is already markedly reduced, and lactic acid levels continue to rise.

Three compensatory mechanisms are largely initiated and regulated by the sympathetic nervous system during this stage: the chemical, neural, and hormonal mechanisms. As these compensatory mechanisms are used, they create many of the signs and symptoms seen early in the shock syndrome. The clinical problem with the use of compensatory mechanisms at this stage is that they can mask low blood volume, poor cardiac output, failing pulmonary efficiency, and other hemodynamic variances.

Keep a high index of suspicion regarding what is going on at the cellular level based on often vague clinical findings. Be aware that by the time the most obvious clinical findings of shock are present, significant, if not irreversible, damage has already occurred at the cellular level. Table 38-1 provides a summary of these compensatory mechanisms.

- **Progressive (decompensatory) stage.** The progressive stage of shock, also referred to as the decompensatory stage, is literally the beginning of the end of the shock syndrome. Until this point, the compensatory

TABLE 38-1	Compensatory Mechanisms in Hypoperfusion
Mechanism	Effects at the Cellular and System Levels of the Body
Neural	The body has several strategically placed sensors to monitor its internal state. Baroreceptors in the aortic arch and carotid sinuses detect the drop in pressure and trigger the sympathetic nervous system. This nervous system is also triggered by the chemoreceptors in the body that detect elevating CO_2 and acid levels and faltering O_2 levels. The result of these stimuli is enhanced sympathetic tone, which results in tachycardia, narrowing pulse pressure, tachypnea, pupillary dilation, CNS excitation, and diaphoresis.
Chemical	With ongoing shock and faltering blood chemistry (diminished oxygen levels and increased levels of hydrogen and carbon dioxide), the adrenal glands will release epinephrine and norepinephrine. These hormones work together to increase cardiac output by way of elevating the heart rate, strength of contraction, and electrical conduction speed (epinephrine), and by further promoting peripheral vasoconstriction (norepinephrine) in an attempt to maintain adequate perfusion pressure.
Hormonal	Low arterial pressure causes the release of renin–angiotensin–aldosterone hormones that collectively increase thirst perception, promote vasoconstriction, and prompt reabsorption of sodium by the kidneys to preserve body fluid levels. Antidiuretic hormone release from the posterior pituitary gland further promotes vasoconstriction to nonvital tissues while enhancing reabsorption of water by the kidneys.

mechanisms have been functioning at capacity to maintain adequate perfusion and oxygenation to the body's tissues. Many of the symptoms and signs seen at that stage were the result of the body trying to maintain perfusion to essential organs including the heart, lungs, brain, and kidneys at the expense of the rest of the body. However, if the etiology of the hypoperfusion syndrome was not treated, was treated improperly, or worsened despite treatment, the patient will enter the third phase of shock.

The progressive stage of shock is hallmarked by the body's inability to maintain perfusion. Autoregulation of small capillary beds is lost, and the vessels vasodilate, which results in blood pooling in the periphery and diminished venous return. Microcirculation begins to form microemboli as platelets start clumping together, resulting in obstructed blood flow through tissues and organs and ongoing necrosis. The formation of clots depletes the body's clotting factors, and a condition known as *disseminated intravascular coagulation* (DIC) can develop, which leaves the body subject to hemorrhage.

Anaerobic metabolism is still ongoing, with progressive cellular death and liberation of enzymes and other intracellular components. Along with increasing nearby cellular death, cardiac rhythm instability may be caused by electrolyte disorders from ruptured cells and the liberation of their contents. Digestive enzymes liberated

from necrotic cells can also travel to the lungs and start to deteriorate the alveolar surfaces, which further hampers the diffusion of gases. Although the patient has a chance for recovery with efficient and expedient treatment, the chances of recovery are rapidly diminishing. Table 38-2 summarizes the progressive effects of shock on certain body organs.

- **Refractory (irreversible) stage.** At this stage of shock, the compensatory mechanisms have failed despite treatment (or in the absence of treatment). The widespread shift from aerobic to anaerobic metabolism has now resulted in permanent cellular destruction and tissue death. Multiple organ failure occurs, and the primary body systems (cardiovascular, neurologic, and pulmonary) fail to maintain perfusion pressure and oxygenation to the body's most important organs (heart, brain, lungs, kidneys). Death will ensue regardless of the medical interventions applied at this time. A patient at this stage of shock is typically unresponsive.

The tachycardic pulse starts to become bradycardic due to ischemia and acidosis, the respiratory rate that was once tachypneic will now start to wane, blood pressure begins to decrease (although not yet to the point of hypotension), pulse pressure narrows, pulses become weak, urinary

TABLE 38-2	Effects of Shock on Body Organs and Systems
Organ or System Affected	Progressive Hypoperfusion
Brain	Ischemia, hypoxia, disrupted nerve transmission.
Heart	Tachydysrhythmias, poor coronary artery perfusion, decreased strength, low cardiac output.
Lungs	Breathing becomes rapid and shallow; diminished blood flow causes poor oxygenation, alveolar surface deterioration, pulmonary edema, and ARDS
Pancreas	Dysfunction from ischemia, release of myocardial toxin factor from hypoperfusion.
Kidneys	Drop in urine production, elevation in blood toxins, eventual renal failure.
Integumentary	Skin pales and cools from vasoconstriction; diaphoresis occurs; eventual mottling from cardiovascular system impairment.
Gastrointestinal	Ulcerations from stress; ischemic bowel releases more toxins into bloodstream.
Hematologic	Cold, acidic, severe hypoxemia; DIC from clotting substance depletion; widespread inflammatory response.

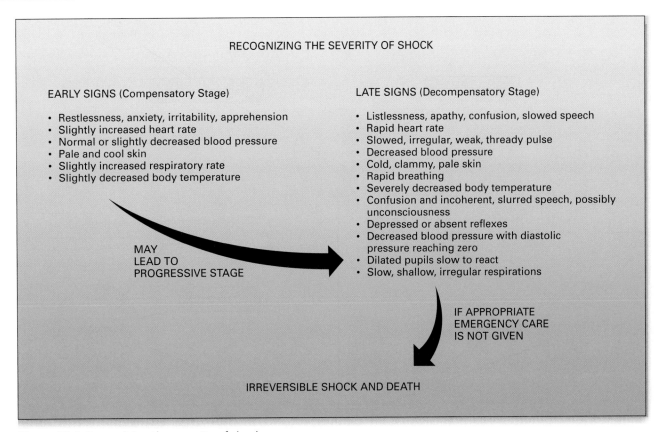

RECOGNIZING THE SEVERITY OF SHOCK

EARLY SIGNS (Compensatory Stage)

- Restlessness, anxiety, irritability, apprehension
- Slightly increased heart rate
- Normal or slightly decreased blood pressure
- Pale and cool skin
- Slightly increased respiratory rate
- Slightly decreased body temperature

MAY LEAD TO PROGRESSIVE STAGE

LATE SIGNS (Decompensatory Stage)

- Listlessness, apathy, confusion, slowed speech
- Rapid heart rate
- Slowed, irregular, weak, thready pulse
- Decreased blood pressure
- Cold, clammy, pale skin
- Rapid breathing
- Severely decreased body temperature
- Confusion and incoherent, slurred speech, possibly unconsciousness
- Depressed or absent reflexes
- Decreased blood pressure with diastolic pressure reaching zero
- Dilated pupils slow to react
- Slow, shallow, irregular respirations

IF APPROPRIATE EMERGENCY CARE IS NOT GIVEN

IRREVERSIBLE SHOCK AND DEATH

Figure 38-1 Recognizing the severity of shock.

output ceases, bowel sounds are absent, and the patient will slip into cardiopulmonary arrest. Resuscitation at this point is often futile.

This is the "rude unhinging of the machinery of life" described as shock by early medical researchers when observing the effects of trauma. In actuality, however, this progression will occur not only from trauma but also from any etiology of hypoperfusion or hypoxia, as discussed next. ▶ Figure 38-1 discusses common findings consistent with each stage of shock.

Etiologies of Shock

As mentioned repeatedly in this topic, shock starts as a cellular syndrome of hypoxia, ischemia, and eventual death secondary to hypoperfusion and inadequate oxygen supply. These effects will occur regardless of the etiology creating this poor perfusion state. Just as stated previously in this text, to have a sufficient supply of oxygen and other metabolic needs delivered to the cell, an adequate pump (heart), adequate blood supply (volume), and an intact vascular system (container) are necessary.

Not only must these three components exist, but they must also all operate in relation to each other. For example, the container (vasculature) may be intact, but if it becomes too large (massive vasodilation), the perfusion pressure within will drop and may be insufficient to meet the metabolic needs of the body.

▶ Figure 38-2 shows the relationship among the etiologies of shock. Other etiologies of shock are discussed in Table 38-3.

ASSESSMENT FINDINGS

Shock (hypoperfusion) can be characterized as a syndrome that requires both clinical and physiologic diagnoses. More simply put, the Advanced EMT must be able to recognize that the tissues of the body are not receiving an adequate amount of oxygen and other metabolic needs, and the dysfunction that results provides the clinical indication that shock is present.

It is also a physiologic diagnosis, as the AEMT must first recognize the clinical findings of shock and then couple this information with the patient's history to arrive at a conclusion of which physiologic

system is at fault (volume, pump, or container). Only with proper recognition of the clinical findings of shock in light of the physiologic disturbance will the EMT be able to provide the best care possible.

The symptoms seen in shock states are a function of the body's tissues and cells not receiving an adequate supply of oxygen and other metabolic substrates. The clinical findings are then a result of organs not receiving what they need to function. Poor kidney perfusion will result in a drop in urine production, hypoperfused muscles will become limp, poor perfusion to the brain will cause changes in mental status, and so on. Although varied by etiology, Table 38-4 identifies common characteristics of the major categories of shock.

Shock requires immediate interventions to save the patient's life. As such, early recognition of its presence is imperative, even if the exact etiology of shock is not as readily apparent. From an overall perspective, when a patient presents with alterations in major organ function, significant disturbances in vital signs, or a history consistent with a shock state, the EMT should initially presume that the patient is in shock or may soon go into

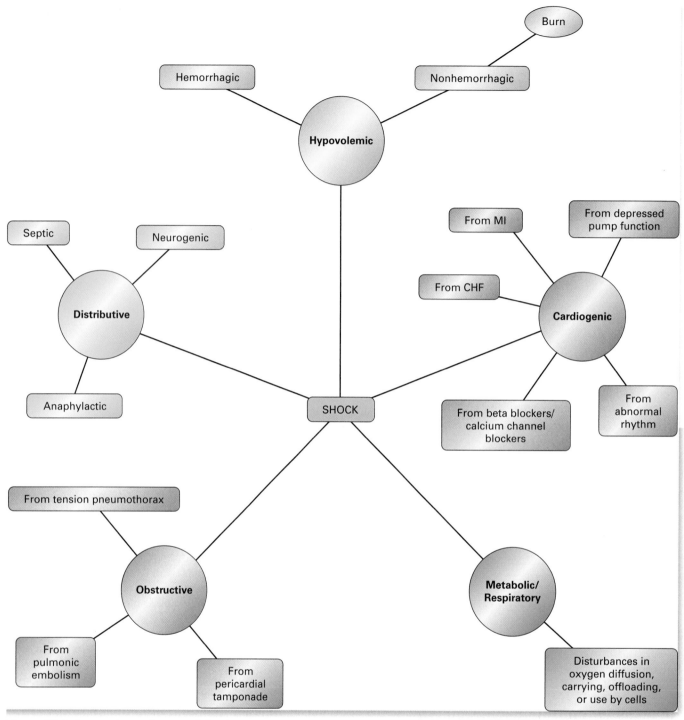

Figure 38-2 Categories and types of shock.

shock. Only through this high index of suspicion will the ill effects of the syndrome be adverted prehospitally.

EMERGENCY MEDICAL CARE

Medical direction and protocol will ultimately determine the recommended interventional steps that should be followed with the patient presenting with shock. The shock state occurs as the result of a failure of body systems (e.g., shock could happen with traumatic bleeding, an MI, or an anaphylactic reaction).

As such, providing a specific recommendation of care in this text is difficult without first identifying the type of shock the patient is experiencing. For this reason, the following recommendations are centered around global treatment considerations that should be undertaken for any patient displaying a shock syndrome.

Spinal Immobilization Considerations

In any patient with a known traumatic insult, especially one involving the head and neck, manual spinal stabilization

TABLE 38-3 Etiologies of Shock

Type of Shock	Basic Pathophysiology	Causes/Etiologies
Fluid loss (▶ Figure 38-3)	Fluid in the vascular system is insufficient to carry oxygen and nutrients to the capillary beds.	External hemorrhage, internal hemorrhage, significant vomiting and/or diarrhea, excessive diaphoresis, burns.
Pump failure (▶ Figure 38-4)	Heart muscle can no longer adequately maintain cardiac output needed to ensure perfusion.	Myocardial infarction, congestive heart failure, significant vasoconstriction, excessive tachycardia or bradycardia, AV valve damage, aortic valve stenosis.
Container failure (▶ Figure 38-5)	Vascular system is disproportionately too large or permeable ("leaky") for volume of blood—massive vasodilation is present.	Sepsis, anaphylaxis, neurogenic, certain types of drug overdoses, spinal cord injury.

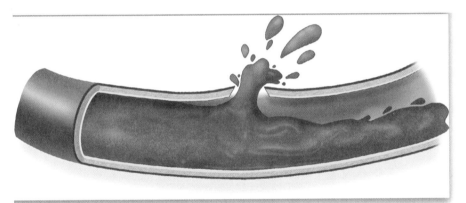

Figure 38-3 Etiology of shock: fluid loss.

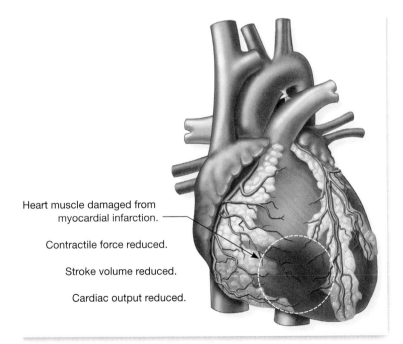

Heart muscle damaged from myocardial infarction.

Contractile force reduced.

Stroke volume reduced.

Cardiac output reduced.

Figure 38-4 Etiology of shock: pump failure.

should be provided. If the patient's history is unclear or the patient is unresponsive, it is best to provide manual stabilization and eventual spinal immobilization as a precautionary measure.

Airway Considerations

A patient in shock will eventually have alterations in mental status that will render him incapable of protecting his own airway. This is an important skill that must be performed correctly 100 percent of the time. Provide suctioning as necessary, and then progressively provide ongoing airway techniques starting with manual maneuvers (jaw thrust, head tilt-chin lift), then using simple mechanical adjuncts (oropharyngeal or nasopharyngeal airways), and eventually advanced mechanical adjuncts (such as the ETC or KingLT), until the airway is clear and secure. Failure to do so will doom any future interventions to defeat.

Breathing Considerations

If the patient is breathing adequately, provide high-flow oxygen via a nonrebreather mask to ensure that adequate levels of oxygen are present to meet cellular metabolic needs. If the patient is apneic or breathing inadequately, ventilate with a bag-valve mask and 100 percent oxygen at a rate of 10 to 12 ventilations per minute.

Ventilate the patient carefully, being sure not to exceed the recommended ventilation rates. Recall that blood is returned to the heart via contraction of the muscles that milk the veins in conjunction with the one-way valves in the vein's lumen. Blood also returns to the heart via gravity from the head and upper torso and, finally, from the negative thoracic pressure created during spontaneous breathing (known as the cardiothoracic pump).

Typically, a shock patient will be motionless, which eliminates venous blood flow facilitated by muscular contraction. In addition, the shock patient is commonly supine, so gravity cannot facilitate blood return to the heart. Finally, if positive pressure is being provided, there is never a moment of negative intrathoracic pressure to facilitate blood flow to the lungs.

Although the first two influences cannot realistically be mediated by the AEMT (supine position and motionless), the third influence (provision of positive pressure ventilation) and its effect on the

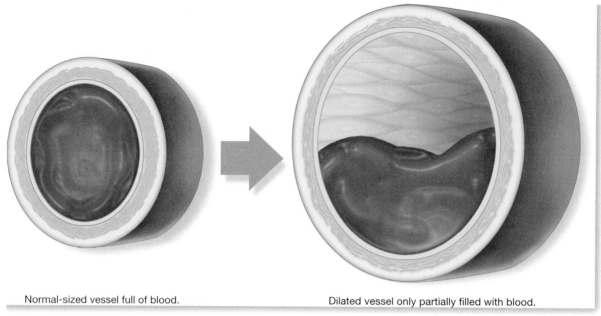

Normal-sized vessel full of blood.   Dilated vessel only partially filled with blood.

Figure 38-5 Etiology of shock: vasodilation.

cardiothoracic pump can be at least minimized by providing ventilations at a recommended rate, with a tidal volume just sufficient to achieve visible chest rise and produce alveolar breath sounds. It has been shown through recent research that overventilation is negatively correlated with almost all patient outcome measures and cardiac arrest survival rates.

Circulatory Considerations

Assess for a core pulse in any patient presenting with shock findings. Should compressions be warranted due to cardiac arrest, start compressions immediately, recalling the "push hard, push fast" recommendation by the American Heart Association. It has been well documented in the literature that shallow compressions, slow compressions, or frequent

TABLE 38-4	Characteristics of the Major Categories of Shock				
Type of Shock	Heart Rate	Respirations	Blood Pressure	Skin	General Findings
Fluid loss	Elevated initially; in final stages of shock heart rate will abruptly slow.	Elevated initially; in later stages respirations may become tachypneic and shallow.	Systolic maintains initially; pulse pressure narrows, eventual systolic hypotension.	Cool to the touch, diaphoretic, pallor; late stages result in mottling of the skin.	History of trauma or internal bleeding; patient may complain of thirst early. Early CNS stimulation with later confusion, disorientation, and unresponsiveness.
Pump failure	Rate most often elevated; extreme heart rates (fast or slow) may be seen. Rhythm disturbances (tachycardia or bradycardia) may be noted.	As shock ensues, respiratory rate typically increases.	Normal or elevated pressure initially; with MI, systolic pressure may drop suddenly.	Cool to the touch, diaphoretic, pallor; late stages result in mottling of the skin.	Patient may have history consistent with myocardial event (MI, ischemia). Pitting peripheral edema and inspiratory crackles may be present; jugular vein distention (JVD) may also be evident.
Container failure	Heart rate may be normal or slowed in neurogenic (spinal) shock; with other forms of massive vasodilation, heart rate is typically elevated.	Respirations may be fast and shallow with absent intercostal muscle use with spinal shock; other forms of vasodilation result in tachypnea.	Blood pressure is commonly found in the "low" range of normal, or frank systolic hypotension may be present.	In early shock from vasodilation, skin is often warm to the touch and reddened; with ensuing hypoperfusion, skin temperature cools with mottling.	May have history of trauma with spinal shock, may also display priapism. Other forms of vasodilatory shock (sepsis) may have history of general illness, and a rash may be present. Anaphylactic shock may reveal hives, redness, and itching.

interruptions of compressions result in reduced cardiac output, which ultimately translate into lower survival rates. Compressions that are delivered at a rapid rate (> 100/min) while using a 30:2 ratio and that depress the sternum to a depth of at least 2 inches with complete recoil of the chest wall optimize the effectiveness of compression.

Another circulatory consideration is external hemorrhage. Whereas it is known that arterial bleeding can be life threatening, so can venous bleeding. The safest approach to interpreting the significance of a bleed is that if it simply looks heavy enough to cause shock and/or death of the patient, it is a significant bleed. Apply direct pressure with a pressure dressing to stop the bleed; should this fail, apply a tourniquet.

INTRAVENOUS THERAPY Do not delay transport to initiate an intravenous line. En route to the medical facility, initiate an intravenous line of normal saline. If volume expansion is needed, use a large-bore catheter (14 or 16 gauge) and a large vein. Run the fluid at a rate based on the clinical findings for the patient. Always follow your local protocol.

VOLUME LOSS ETIOLOGY If the etiology of shock is associated with volume loss (hypovolemia), the patient may benefit from the administration of fluid. The most common type of hypovolemic shock is from hemorrhage. Use the following as a guide for fluid administration. Emergency care may vary; therefore, always follow your local protocol.

UNCONTROLLED HEMORRHAGE If internal bleeding is suspected or an exter-nal hemorrhage cannot be controlled, infuse fluid at a rate to maintain a systolic blood pressure of 80 to 90 mmHg or until radial pulses are able to be palpated. Once this is achieved, back off the fluid infusion. Continue to titrate fluid to a SBP of 80 to 90 mmHg or presence of radial pulses.

CONTROLLED HEMORRHAGE If an external hemorrhage is controlled by direct pressure or a tourniquet, continued bleeding is not present, and no internal bleeding is suspected, infuse fluid to maintain the systolic blood pressure above 90 to 100 mmHg.

In a brain-injured patient, infuse fluid to maintain the systolic blood pressure above 90 mmHg regardless of a controlled or uncontrolled hemorrhage or suspected internal injury.

VASODILATION ETIOLOGY If the etiology of shock is from massive vasodilation, two treatment recommendations to increase perfusion and blood pressure are (1) increase vascular resistance by decreasing the vessel size, and (2) fill the vessel with fluid. As an AEMT, you will not likely be able to administer vasopressor medications to constrict vessels; however, you can infuse fluids to fill the vascular space. Anaphylactic, septic, and vasogenic shock are all distributive types of shock that are typically associated with hypotension from systemic vasodilation.

CARDIOGENIC ETIOLOGY A cardiogenic etiology of shock is typically associated with left ventricular failure from a myocardial infarction, congestive heart failure, or some other cause of ventricular failure such as cardiac rhythm disturbance or cardiomyopathy. The patient is typically normovolemic and is experiencing difficulty in moving the existing volume of blood. Therefore, it is extremely important to restrict fluid administration to a keep-open rate once the intavenous line is initiated.

Other Considerations

Always attempt to maintain normothermia in the patient. In shock states the body will cool down, and this cooling worsens the effects of hypoxia and acidosis.

In the shock patient, maintaining or reestablishing perfusion to the body's capillary beds and cells to oxygenate and remove waste products should guide all treatment. Because the shock syndrome can rapidly cause irreversible tissue damage and death, focus on only the interventions that will have a direct and immediate impact on meeting this goal. This is perhaps best achieved by recognizing the shock state, providing high-flow oxygen, initiating ventilation as needed, and supporting the circulation while providing rapid transport to the hospital.

> **Should compressions be warranted, start them immediately, recalling the "push hard, push fast" recommendation by the American Heart Association.**

TRANSITIONING

REVIEW ITEMS

1. A patient is suspected of having suffered a spinal cord injury between C5 and C6. What impact will this injury have on the patient's ability to breathe?
   a. The patient will become apneic.
   b. The patient will be able to breathe normally.
   c. The patient will be able to breathe, but it will be labored.
   d. Spontaneous breathing will be present, but it will be slow (bradypneic).

2. During the terminal, prearrest stage of any hypoperfusion syndrome, what can be said regarding the efficiency of cellular production of ATP?
   a. Cellular efficiency increases as higher levels of ATP are created.
   b. Cellular production of ATP decreases as the cells change from aerobic to anaerobic metabolism.
   c. There is no change in cellular efficiency until all residual oxygen in the blood is used; then only nerve cells fail.

d. Tissue cells enter into a hypermetabolic state in which energy and glucose are released to overcome the physiologic disturbance.

3. In which of the following types of hypoperfusive shock states will the heart rate be unable to increase as a negative feedback mechanism for enhancing cardiac output?
   a. neurogenic shock
   b. cardiogenic shock
   c. anaphylactic shock
   d. hypovolemic shock

4. A patient who presents with confusion, tachypnea, a systolic pressure of 118 mmHg, and a narrow pulse pressure is probably in what stage of shock?
   a. early
   b. initial
   c. progressive
   d. irreversible

5. Your female patient is experiencing a heart attack. She is borderline hypotensive, pulses are weak and rapid, and you identify other early indications of hypoperfusion. Given her history and presentation, what etiology of shock would you suspect?
   a. neurogenic
   b. cardiogenic
   c. hypotensive
   d. hypovolemic

APPLIED PATHOPHYSIOLOGY

A 32-year-old male patient is hit by a car while riding his bike through the park. Although he was struck at a low rate of speed, bystanders state that the patient's torso was run over by the vehicle's tires. Upon your arrival, the patient presents as unresponsive.

1. Given this history and basic presentation, if the patient is in shock, what cause(s) is/are most likely?

Upon completion of your primary assessment, you find the patient's breathing to be very shallow and tachypneic at 38/minute, the heart rate is 64/minute, blood pressure is 98/60 mmHg, and the peripheral pulses are bounding. Mental status is yet unchanged.

2. With this additional information, what etiology of shock is most likely the cause of this patient's presentation?

3. What clinical findings support your field impression?

Describe the anticipated physiologic benefit(s) for each of the interventions that may be administered to the patient hit by the car.
   a. Oxygen
   b. Positive pressure ventilation
   c. Spinal immobilization
   d. Fluid administration

In the following chart, indicate if the requested assessment parameter is elevated (E), normal (N), or decreased (D) during the initial and compensated stages of shock:

Type of Shock	Heart Rate	Respiratory Rate	Blood Pressure
Hypovolemic			
Cardiogenic			
Anaphylactic			
Neurogenic			

CLINICAL DECISION MAKING

You are called to the scene of a collision between a compact car and an SUV. Upon your arrival, the fire department on scene directs you to the driver of the compact car, who is still trapped in the driver's seat.

As you approach the patient, he keeps screaming, "Get me out of here—my leg is bleeding bad!" His leg, however, is pinned under the dashboard, and there is no way to apply direct pressure to the heavy bleed. His pant leg is soaked, and blood is collecting on the floor of the car. His breathing is unlabored but rapid, distal radial pulse is very weak, and he is becoming agitated.

1. Based on your initial assessment findings, identify clues that indicate the likely cause of his early shock signs.

2. What other conditions may the patient have that could cause you to identify similar findings?

About 10 minutes later, the patient is finally extricated from the car. At this point you perform a quick reassessment and find that the patient arouses to verbal stimuli, his airway is still clear, and his breathing is rapid and shallow at 36/minute with no vesicular sounds present. Peripheral pulses are now absent, and the blood pressure is 82/palpation. The neck veins are flat when positioned supine.

3. Of what life threats, if any, to the patient are you currently aware?

4. Into what stage of shock would you categorize this patient?

5. During the ongoing management of the patient, you elect to administer the following therapies. For each one, discuss in specific detail (1) the reason the intervention is warranted, (2) the expected outcome of that intervention, and (3) how you would assess to determine if that desired effect is occurring (i.e., the treatment worked).

   a. Administration of high-flow oxygen

   b. Fluid administration

   c. Maintaining normothermia

TOPIC

39

Standard Trauma

Competency Applies fundamental knowledge to provide basic and selected advanced emergency care and transportation based on assessment findings for an acutely injured patient.

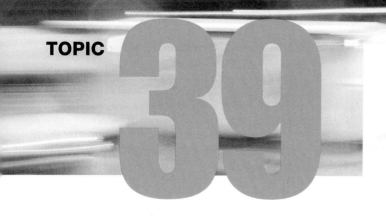

BLEEDING AND BLEEDING CONTROL

TRANSITION *highlights*

- **Rates of unintentional trauma and victim death from exsanguination (bleeding to death).**
- **Types of hemorrhage:**
  - External hemorrhage.
  - Internal hemorrhage.
  - Exsanguinating hemorrhage.
- **Types of assessment findings the Advanced EMT will identify in a patient with internal or external bleeding.**
- **The currently recommended procedure for progressively managing an external bleed.**

INTRODUCTION

Experience from recent military conflicts has consistently shown that bleeding from extremities is among the leading causes of preventable battlefield deaths. Although it is always difficult to compare military and civilian medicine, avoiding preventable death by controlling external hemorrhage is an important lesson EMS should learn from the experience of military medics. Although internal bleeding is an important subject, this topic focuses primarily on recognizing and treating external hemorrhage.

EPIDEMIOLOGY

According to the National Safety Council, unintentional injury is the fifth leading cause of death in the United States and the leading cause of death in patients 1 to 44 years of age. It is difficult to pinpoint how many of those deaths are related purely to bleeding, but some studies point to exsanguination (bleeding to death) as accounting for more than 40 percent of trauma-related deaths. Although the vast majority of these deaths are related to internal bleeding, external hemorrhage still accounts for a significant number of preventable trauma deaths each year.

PATHOPHYSIOLOGY

Blood is the supply system for the cells. Oxygen binds to red blood cells, dissolves in plasma, and is pumped to cells by the heart. Carbon dioxide and other waste products are removed and transported back to the alveoli for elimination. This perfusion of the cells is essential for life; when it fails, shock sets in. A leading cause of shock is hypovolemia, which occurs when perfusion fails because of a lack of blood. Although there are other causes of hypovolemia, actual blood loss is most common.

A patient may lose blood for a variety of reasons. Remember that bleeding can be external or internal. Massive hemorrhage can occur internally without any evidence on the outside.

External bleeding, however, depends greatly on the extent and location of the injury. Damage to large vessels will typically create larger volumes of blood loss. Furthermore, damage to the higher-pressure arteries will result in a more rapid loss of blood.

Bleeding may also be associated with fractured bones, gastrointestinal tract disorders, abdominal or chest trauma, and problems in the reproductive system.

Exsanguinating Hemorrhage

Exsanguinating hemorrhage is a very specific and very rare classification of bleeding. In this case, an artery or series of blood vessels has been damaged significantly enough to allow massive, life-threatening blood loss. This type of bleeding is typically associated with trauma to the large blood vessels, such as the femoral and brachial arteries, and the hemorrhage exceeds what we normally consider "severe bleeding." In this case, the patient may bleed to death in less than 1 minute. When this type of bleeding is identified, it must become the most important treatment priority.

ASSESSMENT FINDINGS

Your primary assessment will give you a rapid opportunity to identify blood loss. At this point, you will visually inspect the patient for bleeding. Remember to check void spaces and bulky clothing with your hands if you cannot see all areas of the patient. You will also assess for basic shock findings such as mental status, the presence (or lack) of a radial pulse, and skin condition. Pale skin, rapid pulse and respirations, and delayed capillary refill time can both indicate the presence of internal hemorrhage and shock.

Remember that not all bleeding can be seen externally. Often the most severe bleeding is occurring internally and must be assumed based on other signs and symptoms.

External hemorrhage must be evaluated rapidly. *If you identify exsanguinating hemorrhage, you must act immediately!* In cases of exsanguinating hemorrhage, the traditional ABC model of the primary assessment now becomes XABC, with the X standing for "exsanguinating hemorrhage." In these rare instances, treating the massive bleeding is more important than even addressing airway concerns (although it would be best if both could be addressed simultaneously).

Other, less severe, hemorrhage will need to be evaluated and treated using good clinical judgment. Typically, even serious external bleeding will be less of a priority than airway and breathing concerns. When identified in the primary assessment, take steps to control the external blood loss. Your immediate decision-making process will focus on how fast the patient is bleeding and how much volume he is losing. Keep in mind that exsanguinating hemorrhage is exceptionally rare.

EMERGENCY MEDICAL CARE

The urgency of bleeding control will vary depending on decisions you make during your primary assessment. Your assessment will help you define how severe the bleeding is and, in turn, how urgent is the need for bleeding control.

Your assessment will also help you identify the importance of bleeding control within the list of immediate priorities. For example, if you identify a moderate external hemorrhage on a trauma patient without a viable airway, you should open the airway before controlling the bleeding. In this case, the airway is certainly more important than the bleeding. On the other hand, if the bleeding were exsanguinating, then your priorities would have to change (unless you had enough resources to treat both issues simultaneously). With assessment questions answered, you will then select the most appropriate treatment options.

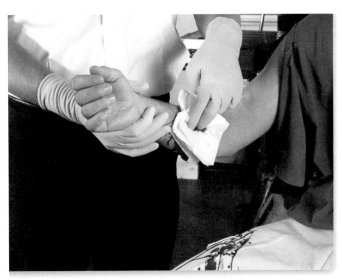

Figure 39-1 When treating external bleeding with direct pressure, apply gloved fingertip pressure over a dressing directly on the point of bleeding.

Bleeding Control Priority

If you identify an arterial (pulsating), high-volume hemorrhage (previously described as exsanguinating hemorrhage), you must address this injury before undertaking any other treatment steps. This level of bleeding is immediately life threatening and, if left untreated, will kill the patient in the next few minutes. Ideally, hemorrhage control can be multitasked, with other high-priority treatments, such as airway and breathing concerns, initiated simultaneously. However, if resources must be delegated, treatment of exsanguinating hemorrhage must come first.

Bleeding Control Progression

Unless the injury is known to be purely isolated (e.g., a limited extremity laceration), you should always assume that the worst bleeding is occurring internally. The true treatment for internal bleeding is rapid transport and delivery to an appropriate trauma facility. Remember the golden hour and focus most of your on-scene priorities on rapid evacuation.

DIRECT PRESSURE Most external bleeding control begins with direct pressure. Direct pressure forces blood from the small surface vessels and aids in clot formation. For an overwhelming number of external hemorrhage cases, direct pressure is the only necessary treatment. Direct pressure is accomplished by placing a clean—preferably sterile—dressing over the wound and applying force to the wound area and proximal surrounding tissue (▶ Figure 39-1). It is best if this pressure can be distributed over a wide area to avoid pinpoint "poking" force. The exception to this rule is when a wound is wide, or gaping, and a bleeding point can be identified. In this case it is appropriate to place pinpoint pressure directly on the bleeding vessel.

Direct pressure is best when applied over bone so that soft tissue is compressed between the force and a rigid surface. Consider the angle you are using to apply force to ideally compress the wound against a bony backstop.

Direct pressure must be a constant force. A common mistake in bleeding control is frequent checking of the wound. Direct pressure must be applied for a minimum of 5 minutes (longer in more severe bleeding) to be effective. Frequent checking often destroys newly formed clots and is counterproductive to stopping the bleeding. Direct pressure needs steady, firm pressure. For severe arterial bleeding, you may need to use heavy force, such as leaning onto the wound with body weight. Always use good clinical

> **Not all bleeding can be seen externally.**

> **If resources must be delegated, treatment of exsanguinating hemorrhage must come first.**

judgment to determine the appropriate amount of force.

DRESSINGS   A dressing is used to protect and cover a wound, not to hide bleeding. Beware of using too many absorbent dressings only to hide severe bleeding. Direct pressure is still necessary as long as bleeding continues. Pressure dressings—dressings combined with a tight (nonoccluding) bandage—are helpful in simple bleeding control. Consider using a bandage that allows for tight application of the dressing without cutting off blood flow to the distal extremity. Keep in mind that direct pressure may still be necessary for more severe bleeding.

HEMOSTATIC AGENTS   A number of commercially available hemostatic agents are designed to aid in the control of external hemorrhage. Be sure to check local protocol before using these products. Hemostatic agents come in powders, pouches, and impregnated dressings and are designed to be placed into and around wounds to aid the clotting process (▶ Figure 39-2). In general, they work as a drying agent to help remove the liquid portion of the blood and promote clot formation. They can be very effective, but some have specific side effects. Some agents produce heat, whereas others can

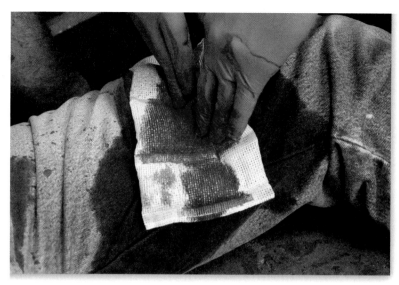

Figure 39-3 Application of a hemostatic dressing.

elicit allergic reactions. Always follow the manufacturer's recommendations for use.

Hemostatic agents are typically applied directly against or into the wound. When possible, avoid applying the agent into a puddle of blood. First wipe the wound clean, and then apply the agent (▶ Figure 39-3). Direct pressure should immediately follow application.

SPLINTING AND POSITION   The splinting of fractures can often assist in bleeding control. Proper positioning and the application of a splint often are effective methods of slowing and stopping bleeding. Elevation can sometimes aid in bleeding control. When possible, elevate the extremity above the heart. Keep in mind, however, that elevation of potentially fractured extremities may increase blood loss if done prior to appropriate splinting. Always follow local protocol.

Tourniquets

Tourniquets were once thought to be dangerous, "life or limb" treatments to be used only when we were willing to trade loss of a limb to keep our patient alive. Recent experiences in the operating room and anecdotal

evidence from battlefield prehospital medicine, however, have shown us that tourniquets may be safer than we once assumed. In many cases, early tourniquet application is an important element of treating severe bleeding.

It is important to remember that tourniquets are still a last resort. All other bleeding control options should be exhausted prior to their application. That said, it is important to move to this step rapidly when other treatments fail.

There are many commercially available tourniquets (▶ Figure 39-4). Tourniquets can also be created from improvised materials, such as the windlass method, or even using a blood pressure cuff. Regardless of where a tourniquet is obtained, there are common elements all tourniquets must have.

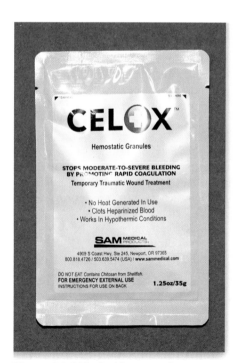

Figure 39-2 Topical hemostatic agents, such as Celox™, are a recent development in wound care.

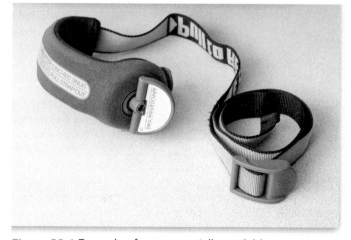

Figure 39-4 Example of a commercially available tourniquet.

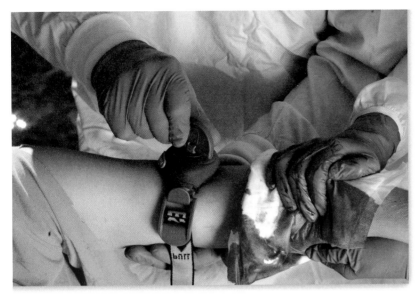

Figure 39-5 Proper placement of a tourniquet is proximal to the wound, between the wound and the heart.

Tourniquet application is a painful process. Many patients who need a tourniquet may be conscious. In these cases, you should anticipate a reaction to the pain. Take steps to address the emotional component and provide a clear understanding that although it is a painful treatment, it is absolutely necessary.

Putting It All Together

Bleeding control is a linear process. It starts simply and adds steps when initial treatments fail. Direct pressure is the most important element and forms the foundation for many other treatments. Concentrate on the proper application of direct pressure and escalate to more aggressive treatments when necessary.

Intravenous Fluid Replacement

As mentioned in Topic 38, "Shock," fluid replacement had been the mainstay of care for bleeding and shock. Many think of shock as a protective mechanism and not as much in need of correction as previously thought. Always follow local protocols in reference to IV fluid replacement.

Although intravenous therapy as a skill is believed to be foundational for the advanced provider, the need for proper assessment and recognition of developing shock and the ability to recognize the need for transport to a trauma center with surgical capabilities is perhaps an even more important skill for any EMS provider.

- Tourniquets must be a wide band (most references state at least 1 to 2 inches wide). More narrow bands must be avoided as they can cut into soft tissue as they tighten.

- Tourniquets must have a method of applying mechanical force to tighten. That is, there should be a way to twist or ratchet the tourniquet to tighten it, as opposed to simply pulling it tight. Hand tightening may not provide enough force to stop the bleeding of a major artery.

APPLYING A TOURNIQUET Tourniquets are used in extremity injuries only.

They should be applied proximal to the wound, between the wound itself and the heart (▶ Figure 39-5).

Remember that the idea of a tourniquet is to compress and occlude an artery. In lower extremities, such as the tibia/fibula and radius/ulna, the major arteries run between the bones. As a result, occlusion of these arteries by a tourniquet is difficult. For this reason, some experts recommend that tourniquets should never be used distal to the elbow or the knee. Always follow local protocol on tourniquet location. In general, tourniquets should be tightened until the bleeding stops and a distal pulse is lost in the extremity.

TRANSITIONING ● ● ● ● ● ● ●

REVIEW ITEMS

1. Which of the following signs of bleeding would you consider the most life threatening?
   a. delayed capillary refill time and pale skin
   b. oozing blood from an abrasion
   c. venous bleeding from a hand laceration
   d. vomiting with warm, pink skin

2. You are assessing a patient following a motor vehicle crash. He complains of abdominal pain, and you note that he has a rapid heart rate and is a bit pale. He has no obvious bleeding. You should suspect _____.
   a. internal hemorrhage
   b. external hemorrhage
   c. the patient has no injury
   d. the patient is simply upset

3. Massive, life-threatening bleeding from a major blood vessel can be otherwise defined as _____.
   a. exsanguinating hemorrhage
   b. venous hemorrhage
   c. capillary hemorrhage
   d. extracorporeal hemorrhage

4. Direct pressure should be applied for a minimum of _____.
   a. 5 minutes
   b. 5 seconds
   c. 30 minutes
   d. 30 seconds

5. Proper placement of a tourniquet includes which of the following elements?

    a. application proximal to the wound

    b. application distal to the wound

    c. application between the wound and the end of the extremity

    d. application directly over the wound

APPLIED PATHOPHYSIOLOGY

1. List three signs of exsanguinating hemorrhage.

2. Explain how exsanguinating hemorrhage might differ from another "severe" hemorrhage.

3. Discuss how exsanguinating hemorrhage might change the normal progression of the primary assessment.

4. Describe the components of proper direct pressure when used for bleeding control.

CLINICAL DECISION MAKING

An 18-year-old man has been shot in the upper thigh. On arrival, you find the patient lying on the ground. You note a massive, spurting hemorrhage coming from the leg wound and a large amount of blood already on the ground.

1. Assuming the scene is safe, and given your general impression, what immediate actions are necessary?

2. Would you classify this bleeding as exsanguinating hemorrhage? If so, why?

To control the bleeding you apply a bulky dressing and apply direct pressure. Bleeding immediately soaks through the dressing.

3. What is the next step in the progression of bleeding control?

4. At what point should you consider the use of a tourniquet?

5. Please describe the following components of proper tourniquet application:

    a. Location (where it should be placed)

    b. Width of band

    c. Tightness

You arrive by yourself to treat this gunshot wound patient. Bystanders note that they do not think he is breathing.

6. How might this fact affect your immediate treatment? Please discuss which primary assessment problem (bleeding or breathing) you would treat first, and why.

7. During which part of the call would you start an IV? At what rate would you run the IV?

Standard Trauma

Competency Applies fundamental knowledge to provide basic and selected advanced emergency care and transportation based on assessment findings for an acutely injured patient.

TOPIC

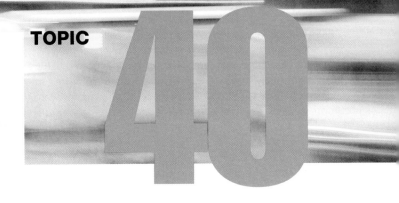

CHEST TRAUMA

INTRODUCTION

Thoracic injuries can be very dramatic and may present with obvious physical findings that lead to immediate identification and management during the primary assessment or, following exposure, in the secondary assessment. As an example, a large open wound to the anterior thorax can be easily found on inspection of the supine patient who is in a well-lit environment.

On the other hand, some patients with thoracic injuries may exhibit very subtle signs and symptoms that can be easily missed initially, partly because of the extremely uncontrolled environment in which EMS personnel function and partly because of limitations in physical diagnosis (e.g., small hemothorax). A small gunshot or stab wound to the thorax, for example, can be missed when assessing a patient in a poorly lit, chaotic setting.

Accurate assessment requiring differentiation of breath sounds can also be hampered by loud background noises produced by crowds, music, television, passing vehicles, or your own ambulance engine. A high index of suspicion, accurate assessment, and frequent reassessment are necessary to identify the apparent and less obvious thoracic injuries that could lead to lethal consequences. Also, remember that a thoracic injury may be considered minor or moderate in a relatively healthy adult patient, yet the same injury may be severe in an elderly patient or one with a history of pulmonary disease.

EPIDEMIOLOGY

Approximately 20 percent to 25 percent of trauma deaths each year in the United States are caused by thoracic trauma. The deaths are most often associated with motor vehicle crashes in which severe blunt trauma ruptures the myocardial wall or thoracic aorta. Those deaths are usually immediate and occur at the scene. Other early deaths from thoracic trauma are associated with a tension pneumothorax, pericardial tamponade, flail segment, open pneumothorax, and hemothorax.

MECHANISM OF INJURY

Thoracic injury may result from both penetrating and blunt trauma. Penetrating trauma has a tendency to be more obvious in the initial phases of assessment because of the presence of an open

TRANSITION *highlights*

- Annual injury and death rates for patients who are victims of chest trauma.

- Importance of mechanism of injury in determining presence of chest trauma.

- Pathophysiologic changes that occur with chest trauma and their effect on normal physiology:
  – Tension pneumothorax.
  – Open pneumothorax.
  – Flail chest.
  – Hemothorax.
  – Acute pericardial tamponade.

- Identification and differentiation of clinical findings of chest trauma with the altered physiology creating them.

wound to the thoracic wall. External bleeding may or may not be present. The amount of external bleeding is not an indicator of the potential or severity of internal bleeding associated with an underlying trauma.

High-velocity gunshot wounds and bullets that enter the thoracic cavity and ricochet can produce multiple organ, vascular, and structural damage. The physical location of the gunshot entrance or exit wound does increase one's index of suspicion of underlying internal organ and structural damage; however, it does not provide a precise prediction of the complete scope of the internal injury. Low-velocity wounds to the chest, such as those produced by a knife, produce more predictable underlying organ and structural damage because of the kinematics associated with the injury.

The amount of external bleeding is not an indicator of the potential or severity of internal bleeding associated with an underlying trauma.

Blunt trauma may produce gross physical findings such as large contusions, tenderness, fractured ribs, and flail segments, or relatively little external evidence of injury. The chest wall may be severely compressed during the application of the blunt force, causing the internal organs to be stretched, torn, or sheared. After the blunt force is removed, the chest may recoil, leaving significant, moderate, or minor evidence of the temporary cavitation that occurred during the impact.

If little external injury is evident, one may suspect minor or no internal thoracic damage, whereas the patient may be suffering from multiple and severe organ, vascular, and structural injury. In both cases, rely on patient complaints and physical exam findings to increase your index of suspicion of internal organ and structural injury.

Blunt and penetrating trauma may produce injury to several structures within the thoracic cavity. Some injuries have a much higher incidence when associated with a specific mechanism, such as acute pericardial tamponade related to penetrating injury to the chest and upper abdomen, and esophageal injury associated with penetrating trauma to the neck and upper chest. Anatomic structures that have the potential to be injured in thoracic trauma are the chest wall, lung tissue, pulmonary tract, myocardium, great vessels (inferior and superior vena cava, and aorta), esophagus, and diaphragm. Thus, the injury may involve muscles, bones, organs, and vessels.

PATHOPHYSIOLOGY

A compromise in ventilation, oxygenation, and circulation may occur because of the anatomic structures typically involved in thoracic trauma. Injuries such as rib fractures and flail segment may interfere with the "bellows" action of the chest and lead to inadequate mechanical ventilation. Oxygenation may be impaired by a large pulmonary contusion that is restricting gas exchange through the collection of blood within the alveoli and the alveolar–capillary interface, or from a large area of collapsed lung tissue resulting from a pneumothorax. Hypotension from blood loss from a hemothorax or a reduction in cardiac output from a mechanically compressed myocardium associated with an acute pericardial tamponade can produce significant circulation and tissue perfusion disturbances.

> Overventilation may lead to exacerbation of a pneumothorax and the conversion to a tension pneumothorax.

Some injuries, such as a tension pneumothorax, may lead to ventilatory, oxygenation, and circulation compromise, which can produce lethal results quickly if not rapidly identified and managed. Some injuries, such as simple rib fractures, may produce such excruciating pain that the patient intentionally hypoventilates to reduce chest wall movement and becomes secondarily hypoxic.

As with any patient, the focus in the treatment of thoracic trauma is to establish and maintain an adequate airway, ventilation, oxygenation, and circulation. This may involve emergency management aimed at preventing further organ or structural involvement, reducing the existing life threat, or minimizing the progression of the pathophysiologic compromise.

ASSESSMENT

The basic principles of assessment apply to thoracic trauma. A systematic approach is critical to ensure that all potential life-threatening injuries are identified and managed rapidly. Thoracic injury is also associated with a relatively high incidence of extrathoracic trauma, especially when a blunt mechanism of injury is involved.

A shotgun approach to assessment may lead to missed or late identification of life-threatening injuries, potentially resulting in a poor patient outcome as a result of lack of immediate emergency intervention, or failure to identify the severity of the patient's condition, producing unnecessarily long on-scene times, lack of proper notification of the receiving medical facility, or an improper destination decision. Developing tunnel vision in the assessment approach and focusing just on the thoracic injury may cause the EMS practitioner to miss injuries to other body systems and cavities. Similarly, continued reassessment is required, especially if the patient's condition deteriorates.

The primary assessment is designed to identify and manage life threats to the airway, ventilation, oxygenation, and circulation. As previously noted, these may all be compromised in thoracic trauma. Airway obstruction, hypoventilation, hypoxia, and severe hypotension are often the primary reasons for deterioration and death in the trauma patient.

Once the scene is secured, and as you approach the patient, get a general impression. Identify, through a quick body scan, any obvious life-threatening injuries or conditions that may require immediate management, such as an obvious open chest wound, especially if it is producing a sucking sound; blood, vomitus, or other substances in the oral cavity that may result in aspiration; major bleeding (arterial or venous); and a flail segment, although the early signs are often subtle.

Provide manual spinal stabilization if a spinal injury is suspected. Establish and maintain an open airway, inspect inside the oral cavity, and suction or remove any substance that can be aspirated or lead to an airway obstruction.

Assess the tidal volume and respiratory rate carefully. If the tidal volume and respiratory rate are both adequate, and the patient is suspected of having a significant thoracic injury or is exhibiting signs of hypoxia, maximize oxygenation by applying a nonrebreather mask at 15 lpm. If either the tidal volume or respiratory rate is inadequate, immediately begin positive pressure ventilation at a rate of 10 to 12 ventilations per minute (one ventilation every 5 to 6 seconds) in the adult and 12 to 20 ventilations per minute (one ventilation every 3 to 5 seconds) in the infant and child.

Be sure to provide very controlled ventilation rates and volumes. Do not overventilate the patient. Overventilation may lead to exacerbation of a pneumothorax and the conversion to a tension pneumothorax; reduction of preload, cardiac output, blood pressure and perfusion, especially in patients with significantly increased intrathoracic pressure; and other secondary barotrauma.

Assess the status of circulation by comparing the amplitude of peripheral and central pulses, obtaining a heart rate, and observing skin temperature, color, and condition. If the thoracic trauma patient presents with pale, cool, and clammy skin; tachycardia; and weak or absent peripheral pulses, you should suspect the possibility of bleeding in the thoracic cavity, mechanical compression of the heart and great vessels, or bleeding in another area of the body.

Following the primary assessment, a rapid secondary assessment will be conducted to identify all other potentially life-threatening injuries. Immediately life-threatening thoracic injuries include tension pneumothorax, open pneumothorax, pericardial tamponade, severe hemothorax, and a flail chest. These conditions are identified through inspection, palpation, auscultation, and percussion.

The vital signs, including a systolic and diastolic blood pressure, heart rate, respiratory rate, and skin findings, along with a pulse oximeter and end-tidal carbon dioxide reading, will provide valuable information in the recognition and differentiation of thoracic injuries. It is necessary to understand and link thoracic injury to possible findings in other areas of the body when conducting your rapid trauma assessment. For example, inspecting the pupils is not only necessary to assess for the possibility of a brain injury, but sluggish pupillary reaction may also indicate significant hypoxia related to a chest injury.

Likewise, jugular venous distention, especially if associated with the inspiratory phase of respiration (referred to as the Kussmaul sign) may be an indication of a thoracic injury that has resulted in a high intrathoracic pressure (i.e., tension pneumothorax) or interference with ventricular filling and cardiac output (i.e., pericardial tamponade). This may be a subtle finding; however, a patient with tension pneumothorax and pericardial tamponade may present with signs that mimic those of a hypovolemic patient. One would not suspect jugular venous distention in hypovolemia, however, because of the low venous pressure. Recognizing the jugular venous distention, even though it may be very subtle or late, may be one sign that gets the Advanced EMT thinking about a condition other than hypovolemia.

Also, do not rule out the possibility of pericardial tamponade or tension pneumothorax when jugular venous distention is not found, as a large percentage of patients with chest injury may also be hypovolemic, resulting in a low venous pressure that will preclude the jugular veins from engorging. It is necessary to think critically and process and consider all the assessment information during the exam.

Signs of other chest injuries that may be identified during the secondary assessment may include rib fractures, simple pneumothorax, simple hemothorax, pulmonary contusion, and cardiac contusion. The specific signs, symptoms, and emergency care of the most immediately life-threatening conditions will be discussed in the following section.

EMERGENCY MEDICAL CARE

The most immediately life-threatening thoracic injuries that require rapid recognition and intervention and expeditious transport are tension pneumothorax, open pneumothorax, flail chest, massive hemothorax, and acute pericardial tamponade. Focus on establishing and maintaining an airway and on adequate ventilation and oxygenation. As with any other trauma patient, an intravenous line of normal saline or lactated Ringer's should be initiated once the patient is en route to the medical facility.

Do not delay transport to start an IV line. Use a large-bore catheter (14 or 16 gauge) and run the fluids to maintain a systolic blood pressure of 80 to 90 mmHg or until radial pulses are regained. Once this is achieved, reduce the fluid infusion and titrate to maintain the systolic blood pressure at 80 to 90 mmHg or to maintain radial pulses. Some protocols require that the systolic blood pressure be maintained at 70 mmHg to reduce the incidence of hemodilution and increased bleeding associated with aggressive fluid administration in the trauma patient with uncontrolled bleeding. Follow your local protocol.

Tension Pneumothorax

A tension pneumothorax occurs from the disruption of the parietal pleura, visceral pleura, or tracheobronchial tree associated with blunt or penetrating trauma, or iatrogenically from certain medical procedures, such as the use of positive end-expiratory pressure (PEEP) with ventilation or central venous catheter insertion. Also, excessively aggressive ventilation with high pressure and excessive tidal volumes may convert a simple pneumothorax to a tension pneumothorax.

The disruption allows air to escape into the pleural space. Typically, the injury to the pleural lining creates a one-way valve that allows air to enter the pleural space during periods of negative intrathoracic pressure associated with inhalation; however, when air attempts to escape with the increase in intrathoracic pressure, the one-way valve is forced closed, trapping the air in the pleural space. With each inhalation, more air enters the pleural space and becomes trapped. The air begins to build rapidly, collapsing the involved lung.

Because of the nature of lung tissue, the lung has a natural tendency to recoil and collapse, similar to a rubber band when stretched and released. When the water seal is broken between the visceral and parietal pleura, the lung will continue to exert a pulling effect inward and recoil while continuing to create a relative negative pressure inside the pleural space that promotes air entry.

As the air collects in the pleural space on the injured side, the volume and pressure continue to build. This will eventually cause the mediastinum to shift away from the injured hemithorax and contralaterally toward the uninjured hemithorax, resulting in compression of the uninjured lung, right atrium, and vena cava (▶ Figure 40-1). Because the injured lung has already collapsed, compression of the uninjured lung will lead to severe ventilatory and oxygenation compromise. The patient will exhibit signs of severe respiratory distress and hypoxia.

Compression of the vena cava and right atrium will lead to reductions in preload, left ventricular end-diastolic filling volume, and cardiac output. Hypotension, tachycardia, and other signs of poor perfusion will become evident. A tension

> **Do not rule out the possibility of pericardial tamponade or tension pneumothorax when jugular venous distention is not found.**

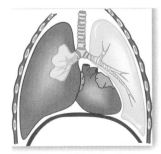

Figure 40-1 In a tension pneumothorax, air continuously fills the pleural space, the lung collapses, pressure rises, and the trapped air compresses the heart and the other lung.

pneumothorax causes both significant respiratory and circulation compromise, making it an immediate life-threatening condition that requires rapid identification and intervention.

The following are the early signs and symptoms associated with a tension pneumothorax:

- Dyspnea
- Tachypnea
- Tachycardia
- Chest pain
- Anxiety
- Fatigue
- Decreased breath sounds on the injured side

The following are the late findings in a tension pneumothorax:

- Altered mental status
- Hyperexpanded chest wall from hyperinflation of the pleura on the injured side (asymmetrical chest wall)
- Severe respiratory distress to respiratory failure
- Hypotension
- Severely decreased or absent breath sounds on the injured side
- Decreased breath sounds on the uninjured side
- Cyanosis
- Increased resistance to bag-valve ventilation
- Bradypnea (ominous sign of impending respiratory or cardiac arrest)
- Pulsus paradoxus (decrease in systolic blood pressure by > 10 mmHg during inhalation)
- A reduction in peripheral pulse amplitude during inspiration
- Jugular venous distention (may be seen early during inspiration, or not at all if the patient is hypovolemic)
- Displacement of the apical pulse
- Tracheal deviation away from the injured side (late, inconsistent, and very difficult to accurately assess and find)
- Hyperresonance on the injured side
- Subcutaneous emphysema

The first priority of management on identification of a tension pneumothorax is to reduce the pressure of the affected pleural space. If an occlusive dressing has been applied to an open pneumothorax, it is necessary to remove the dressing and allow any air that has been built up to

escape. Be sure to leave the dressing off for a few exhalations. If this is ineffective or if the patient does not have an open pneumothorax, needle decompression of the affected pleural space is necessary. This is an advanced life support skill that is necessary for an immediate life-threatening condition; thus, it would be prudent to seek assistance from an ALS provider as early as possible.

Ensure that you have established and are maintaining an adequate airway, ventilation, and oxygenation. If ventilating the patient, use minimal rates and tidal volumes. Rapidly transport the patient to an appropriate medical facility capable of managing thoracic trauma. If the tension pneumothorax was relieved in the field, continuously reassess the patient and be cognizant of the redevelopment of a tension pneumothorax.

Open (Communicating) Pneumothorax

When air enters the pleural space through an open wound in the chest wall and parietal pleura, it is termed an *open pneumothorax* or *communicating pneumothorax*. As the air enters the pleural space, it collapses the lung as in a simple pneumothorax. The difference between the two is that in an open pneumothorax the air enters the thoracic cavity from a wound to the chest wall and not from the trachea as in normal ventilation (▶ **Figure 40-2**). The wound creates an alternative conduit for air to enter the chest when the intrathoracic pressure becomes negative during inhalation.

If the opening in the chest is large enough, a majority of the air will follow the pathway of least resistance and enter the pleural space directly through the

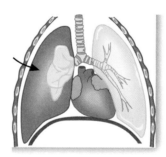

Figure 40-2 In an open pneumothorax, air enters the chest cavity through an open chest wound or leaks from a lacerated lung. The lung then cannot expand.

open wound, bypassing the respiratory tract and lungs. A large or significant wound is thought to be two-thirds of the internal diameter of the trachea. In an average-size adult, this means that the wound may need to be only the size of a nickel to be significant.

If a majority of the airflow is into the pleural space and not the lungs, the patient will develop hypoxia rapidly from lack of effective ventilation and oxygenation. The patient will appear to be breathing while the chest wall moves during inspiration and expiration; however, with each chest wall expansion, the negative pressure that is created inside the thorax will draw more air into the open wound, causing the lung to collapse further.

If not impeded by skin, muscle, bone, or other tissue, the open wound may allow air to escape during exhalation. One might think that this would then pose no real danger for the patient, as the air is escaping with each breath. However, remember that the significant wound will draw the majority of air into the pleural space and not the lung, drastically reducing lung ventilation and oxygenation. Even with the escape of air during exhalation, the patient will deteriorate rapidly from the loss of effective alveolar ventilation.

If the air is prevented from escaping during exhalation, the condition may quickly develop into a tension pneumothorax. If the patient is initially assessed in a quiet environment and the open wound is large enough, it may be possible to hear a sucking sound with inhalation and possibly with exhalation. This rare episode is referred to as a sucking chest wound.

The following are the signs and symptoms of an open pneumothorax:

- Open wound to the thorax
- Decreased breath sounds on the affected hemithorax
- Tachypnea
- Tachycardia
- Dyspnea
- Subcutaneous emphysema
- Deteriorating SpO$_2$ reading
- Frothy blood at open wound
- Other signs of respiratory distress

The priority in management of an open pneumothorax is to occlude the open wound to the thorax. This should be done immediately on its identification. You can initially occlude it with a gloved hand as soon as it is found and, as rapidly as

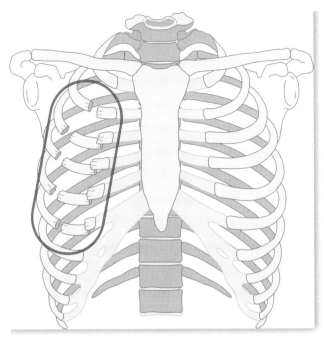

Figure 40-3 Flail chest occurs when blunt trauma causes the fracture of two or more ribs, each in two or more places.

possible, apply an occlusive dressing taped on three sides. Plastic wrap, Vaseline™ Gauze, plastic covering from an oxygen mask, or a commercial device such as an Asherman chest seal can be used.

Once the wound is sealed, proceed with the standard trauma care to include establishing and maintaining an airway and ventilation, maximizing oxygenation, maintaining circulation, and providing rapid transport to the medical facility. Carefully reassess the patient because the open pneumothorax can develop into a tension pneumothorax, especially if the visceral pleura is injured, allowing air to escape internally into the pleural space from the injured lung.

Flail Chest

Flail chest is defined differently by various sources. Most define it as two or three adjacent ribs fractured in two or more places, which creates a free-floating segment within the chest wall (▶ Figure 40-3). The flail could be anterior or posterior, or it could involve the sternum with ribs on both sides fractured. It typically takes a significant blunt force applied to the thorax to produce a flail segment. In patients with some type of pathology that causes the ribs to weaken, such as osteoporosis, less force may be required to create a flail chest. When such significant force is applied to the chest, the lung has a

tendency to become contused. Thus, pulmonary contusion is a second injury common to this type of injury, which may be more lethal than the flail chest.

When a true flail segment is present, it has the ability to move independent of the remainder of the chest wall. Thus, when the chest wall is expanding, the negative intrathoracic pressure will draw the free-floating flail segment inward as the remainder of the chest is moving outward. As the chest wall begins to reduce its size during exhalation, the positive intrathoracic pressure will cause the free-floating flail segment to move outward (▶ Figure 40-4). This abnormal chest wall movement may interfere with effective generation of intrathoracic pressure and lung inflation.

The pulmonary contusion allows blood to seep into the alveolar–capillary interface and within the alveoli. This interferes with the ability of oxygen and carbon dioxide to cross the alveolar membrane and alveolar–capillary interface and enter into the capillary, impeding effective gas exchange.

The flail segment and pulmonary contusion will cause respiratory compromise.

Both conditions may lead to severe hypoxia and hypercarbia.

Pain associated with the rib fractures is typically a predominant complaint, along with signs and symptoms of respiratory distress. The severe pain may cause the patient to intentionally hypoventilate, leading to hypoxia and hypercarbia. The respiratory distress, hypoxia, and hypercarbia may also be associated with a large pulmonary contusion. A poor SpO_2 reading; pale, cool, and clammy skin; and cyanosis may be present.

Paradoxical movement is often thought to be the predominant sign of a flail segment. When the ribs fracture, however, the intercostal muscles may spasm, and the patient may intentionally limit his breathing, causing the flail segment initially to be stabilized. Thus, the paradoxical movement may be missed on initial inspection of the chest; however, palpation will reveal the unstable segment. This is one reason that palpation of the chest is necessary during the secondary assessment. As the intercostal muscles fatigue, the flail segment becomes more apparent on inspection.

As for other chest injuries, emergency management is aimed at establishing and maintaining an airway, effective ventilation, oxygenation, and circulation. Remember, the patient may be intentionally hypoventilating because of the pain and not as a result of some other respiratory pathology. If the respiratory rate or tidal volume is ineffective, begin positive pressure ventilation with a bag-valve device. Maximize oxygenation by nonrebreather mask at 15 lpm in the adequately breathing patient or attached to the bag-valve

(a) 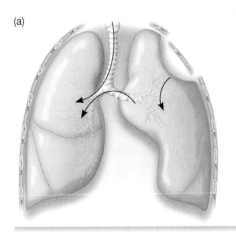 (b)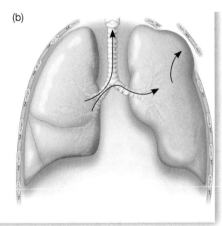

Figure 40-4 With a flail chest, (a) the flail segment is drawn inward as the rest of the lung expands with inhalation; (b) the flail segment is pushed outward as the rest of the lung contracts with exhalation.

device through a reservoir if providing assisted ventilation.

Stabilization of the flail segment with sandbags or other devices is no longer recommended. The patient may be able to self-splint using a pillow and his own arm. Rapidly transport the patient to a medical facility capable of managing the chest injury.

Hemothorax

A hemothorax is very similar to a pneumothorax; however, blood instead of air fills the pleural space and collapses the lung. The source of bleeding varies but is associated with laceration or rupture of the lung tissue itself or a vascular structure within the thoracic cavity as a result of blunt or penetrating trauma, causing the blood to collect in the pleural cavity.

As in a pneumothorax, as the blood continues to collect, it places inward pressure on the lung tissue, collapsing the lung (▶ Figure 40-5). Because of gravity, the blood is pulled downward and has a tendency to collect in the lower bases of the lung in the seated patient or posteriorly in the supine patient. This is important to consider when assessing the patient's breath sounds.

In a pneumothorax, the air moves upward and collects in the superior portion of the lungs in the seated patient and the anterior portion in the supine patient. Thus, the breath sounds would be decreased or absent in the upper lobes in the seated patient or anteriorly in the supine patient, whereas in a hemothorax the breath sounds would be decreased or

absent in the lower lobes in the seated patient or posterior in the supine patient. Because blood, and not air, is the source of lung collapse, the patient is not only prone to respiratory compromise, but he can also experience hypovolemia.

The patient with a hemothorax presents with signs and symptoms very similar to those of a patient with a pneumothorax; however, due to the blood loss, signs and symptoms of hypovolemia usually predominate. (It is common for a pneumothorax and hemothorax to occur together. This condition is referred to as a *hemopneumothorax*.)

The following are the signs and symptoms of a hemothorax:

- Dyspnea
- Tachypnea
- Decreased or absent breath sounds to the affected hemithorax
- Tachycardia
- Pale, cool, and clammy skin
- Decreasing systolic blood pressure
- Narrow pulse pressure
- Decreasing SpO$_2$ reading
- Evidence of blunt or penetrating trauma to the thorax

Emergency care focuses on management of the airway, ventilation, oxygenation, and circulation. The AEMT is limited in managing the hemothorax in the field and should focus on reversing life threats found in the primary assessment and on expeditious transport. Administration of fluids to expand the existing blood volume should be restricted, even in a hemothorax. Fluids will dilute the blood, making it less viscous, and will increase the blood pressure, allowing the wound to bleed faster and potentially dislodge a clot. Follow your local protocol when infusing fluids in the trauma patient.

Acute Pericardial Tamponade

Acute pericardial tamponade is seen in approximately 2 percent of patients with penetrating trauma to the chest and upper abdomen. It is rarely seen in patients with blunt thoracic trauma and is most often associated with stab wounds to the chest. This is a critical chest injury that can cause the patient's condition to deteriorate in minutes. Rapid recognition and subsequent expeditious

transport are imperative to patient survival.

Pericardial tamponade occurs when an injury to the heart causes blood to collect in the pericardial sac, a tough fibrous sac surrounding the heart. As the volume of blood in the pericardial sac increases, it compresses the atria and ventricles and does not allow them to fill adequately (▶ Figure 40-6). This reduces the stroke volume, the amount of blood being ejected with each ventricular contraction.

A decrease in stroke volume causes a decrease in cardiac output. A decrease in cardiac output decreases the blood pressure. This, in turn, affects perfusion of the vital organs. As the blood pressure decreases, the body attempts to compensate by increasing the heart rate and total peripheral vascular resistance (PVR) through vasoconstriction. Thus, tachycardia and pale, cool, clammy skin are signs of pericardial tamponade. Because the blood is not moving forward effectively through the heart, aorta, and arteries, the blood backs up in the venous system, causing the veins—especially the large veins close to the heart, such as the jugular veins—to become distended.

Signs and symptoms of acute pericardial tamponade are very similar to those of a tension pneumothorax, with the exception of significant dyspnea because there is no associated lung injury in pericardial tamponade. Therefore, the breath sounds will remain equal bilaterally, and there will

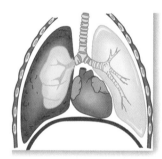

Figure 40-5 In a hemothorax, blood leaks into the chest cavity from lacerated vessels or the lung itself, and the lung compresses.

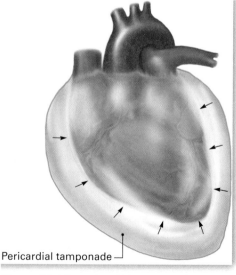

Pericardial tamponade

Figure 40-6 In pericardial tamponade, accumulating blood compresses the heart inward.

TABLE 40-1   Differential Field Diagnosis of Chest Injury

Sign or Symptom	Tension Pneumothorax	Open Pneumothorax	Flail Chest	Hemothorax	Pericardial Tamponade
Breath sounds	Severely decreased or absent unilaterally and possibly decreased on the uninjured side	Decreased on the injured side	Decreased on the injured side	Decreased on the injured side	Present, clear, and equal bilaterally
Blood pressure	Decreased with a narrow pulse pressure	Normal if not associated with other trauma	Normal if not associated with other trauma	Decreased with a narrow pulse pressure	Decreased with a narrow pulse pressure
Pulse	Weak and rapid peripheral pulses	Tachycardia possibly present due to hypoxia, but peripheral pulses normal unless with other associated trauma	Tachycardia possibly present due to hypoxia, but peripheral pulses normal unless with associated trauma	Weak and rapid peripheral pulses	Weak and rapid peripheral pulses
Jugular veins	Distended (late finding) if patient not hypovolemic	Normal	Normal	Flat	Distended (late finding) if patient not hypovolemic
Respiratory distress	Severe	Present	Present	Present	Possible
Pulsus paradoxus	Present	Absent	Absent	Absent	Present
Asymmetrical chest	Present	Absent	Absent	Absent	Absent
Paradoxical chest movement	Absent	Absent	Present	Absent	Absent
Decreased SpO$_2$	Severe	Present to severe	Present to severe	Present	Present

be no tracheal deviation. Signs and symptoms include the following:

- Tachycardia
- Anxiety or anxiousness
- Hypotension
- Cyanosis
- Pulsus paradoxus (decrease in systolic blood pressure by > 10 mmHg during inhalation)

- A reduction in peripheral pulse amplitude during inspiration
- Jugular venous distention

Emergency care focuses on management of the airway, ventilation, oxygenation, and circulation. The EMT is limited in managing a pericardial tamponade in the field; however, early recognition of the condition and expeditious transport could

be lifesaving. The emergency care should focus on reversing life threats found in the primary assessment.

Differentiating among these chest injuries could be difficult (see Table 40-1). Some of the injuries may present with more subtle signs and symptoms initially. Having a high index of suspicion is imperative to making a good clinical decision and differential field diagnosis.

TRANSITIONING

REVIEW ITEMS

1. A patient with a stab wound to the anterior chest presents with a decrease in mental status; circumoral cyanosis; very weak and rapid radial pulses; pale, cool, and clammy skin; blood pressure 72/56 mmHg; heart rate 132 beats per minute; and respirations 28/minute with adequate chest rise. You note jugular venous engorgement on inspiration. The patient has equal and clear breath sounds bilaterally. You should suspect _____.

   a. tension pneumothorax   b. hemothorax
   c. open pneumothorax   d. pericardial tamponade

2. A patient with a penetrating chest injury has jugular venous engorgement and a decrease in pulse amplitude on inspiration. You should suspect _____.

   a. an increase in intrathoracic pressure
   b. excessive blood loss into the pleural space
   c. a decrease in peripheral vascular resistance
   d. fluid collection in the alveolar–capillary interface

3. A patient was kicked in the anterior chest during a fight. He complains of severe pain to the chest on inhalation and difficulty breathing. His radial pulse is 128/minute, respiratory rate is 38/minute and shallow, and blood pressure is 148/92 mmHg. His breath sounds are clear and equal but decreased bilaterally. You should suspect _____.

   a. a hemothorax
   b. a tension pneumothorax
   c. a chest wall contusion
   d. a pericardial tamponade

4. A patient with an open chest injury is anxious and agitated. You should suspect that this response is most likely caused by_____.

   a. pain associated with the injury
   b. a normal reaction to trauma
   c. a narrowing pulse pressure
   d. a decrease in oxygenation

5. Which of the following would most likely differentiate a tension pneumothorax from a pericardial tamponade?

   a. unilateral decreased or absent breath sounds
   b. jugular vein distention and a narrow pulse pressure

   c. severe tachycardia and hypotension
   d. peripheral and core cyanosis

6. You are providing emergency care to a patient with a gunshot wound to the chest. He is responding to verbal stimuli with moaning. His SpO_2 is 86 percent; radial pulse is absent; skin is pale, cool and clammy; his carotid pulse reveals a heart rate of 123 bpm; his respirations are 22/minute with adequate chest rise; and his blood pressure is 66/48 mmHg. You should _____ .

   a. initiate two-large bore IVs and run both at a wide-open rate until the blood pressures reaches a normal range
   b. initiate one large-bore IV and run at a rate to achieve a systolic blood pressure of 80 to 90 mmHg or until radial pulses are regained
   c. initiate one large-bore IV line and keep it at a to-keep-open rate
   d. not initiate an IV line in the chest-injured patient

APPLIED PATHOPHYSIOLOGY

1. Explain the difference in the presentation between a patient suspected of having a tension pneumothorax and one having a pericardial tamponade.

2. Explain the difference in the presentation between a patient suspected of having a hemothorax and a patient in hypovolemic shock with no chest injury.

3. Explain the difference in the presentation between a patient suspected of having a tension pneumothorax and a patient in hypovolemic shock with no chest injury.

4. Explain the pathophysiology of hypotension and hypoperfusion in a pericardial tamponade.

5. Explain the pathophysiology of hypotension and hypoperfusion in a tension pneumothorax.

6. Explain why a patient with a flail segment can become severely hypoxic.

7. Explain why it is important to restrict fluid administration in the patient with a chest injury.

CLINICAL DECISION MAKING

You are called to treat a 19-year-old male patient who was involved in an altercation. He is sitting upright against the wall outside a club. He is very anxious and agitated and is complaining that he cannot breathe. You note a large bloodstain on the front of his shirt.

1. Based on the scene size-up and characteristics of the scene, list the possible conditions you should suspect.

The primary assessment reveals that the patient is alert, anxious, agitated, and confused; complains of severe shortness of breath; and has circumoral cyanosis. His respirations are 38/minute; radial pulse is barely palpable at 148 beats per minute; skin is pale, cool, and clammy; and SpO_2 is 72 percent. You expose the patient and find what appears to be a stab wound to the right chest.

2. What are the immediate life threats?

3. What immediate emergency care should you provide based on the life threats found in the primary assessment?

4. Explain the related pathophysiology of the anxiousness and agitation.

5. Explain the related pathophysiology of the confusion.

6. What conditions have you ruled out from the scene size-up? What conditions seem more plausible based on the primary assessment?

During the secondary assessment, you note that the patient is becoming less agitated; however, his mental status continues to decrease. His jugular veins appear to be engorged, and you note subcutaneous emphysema when palpating the neck. The breath sounds are absent on the right and decreased on the left. A small stab wound is noted to the right anterior chest at approximately the fourth intercostal space at the midclavicular line. No evidence of trauma is noted to the abdomen, pelvis, or extremities. The abdomen is soft and nontender and the pelvis is stable. The peripheral pulses are absent, and the skin is extremely pale, cool, and clammy. You note cyanosis to the distal extremities, face, and neck. The blood pressure is 72/60 mmHg, heart rate is 148 beats per minute, respirations are 42/minute and labored, and SpO$_2$ is 68 percent.

7. What condition should you suspect?

8. Explain the differential indicators as to why you suspect that condition.

9. What further emergency care should you provide?

10. Why is the patient's blood pressure only 72/60 mmHg? Explain the reason for the narrow pulse pressure.

11. Explain why the patient became less agitated. Why is this a critical finding in this patient?

TOPIC

Standard Trauma

Competency Applies fundamental knowledge to provide basic and selected advanced emergency care and transportation based on assessment findings for an acutely injured patient.

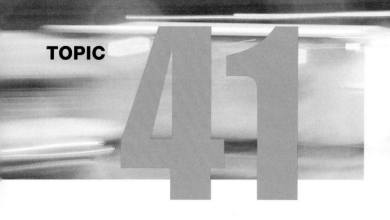

ABDOMINAL TRAUMA

INTRODUCTION

Children sometimes play a game called "mystery box," in which they take turns guessing about an unknown object contained within a closed box. In many ways, this game is similar to the assessment and treatment of a patient with an abdominal injury. You cannot see what is inside the abdomen, and indeed, it is full of surprises.

As an Advanced EMT, you have some clues, however. You have a working knowledge of anatomy, and you have an assessment that will allow you to gather information and help you form reasonable conclusions. In some cases, your assessment of the abdomen will point you to likely problems. In other cases, you may never know for sure what is wrong.

That said, it is important to remember that in our game of mystery box, the goal is not necessarily to pinpoint the exact problem but, rather, to identify when that problem is causing a critical life threat. With abdominal trauma, the focus must always be on the big picture.

EPIDEMIOLOGY

Trauma is the leading cause of death of patients between the ages of 1 and 44. The specific frequency of death associated with isolated abdominal trauma is difficult to pinpoint. However, when you consider internal bleeding and multisystem trauma

cases, blunt abdominal trauma is consistently among the leading causes of trauma-related death.

PATHOPHYSIOLOGY

The abdomen itself is a container. Housed within this container are a series of vital structures that can be generally classified among three categories: hollow organs, solid organs, and blood vessels. Although these structures are generally well protected, they are subject to damage associated with trauma.

Damage can come in the form of direct force, such as a blow to the abdomen; compression forces, such as organs being squeezed between a seatbelt and the spinal column; and shearing/deceleration injury, such as an organ being torn out of place as the body decelerates. How these organs will respond to these offending forces will depend largely on their specific makeup.

HOLLOW ORGANS Hollow organs in the abdomen include (among others) the stomach, intestines, urinary bladder, and gallbladder. Hollow organs generally respond well to trauma, as they tend to be flexible and possess the capability of stretching. However, when excessive force is exerted on these organs, the internal pressure changes will often cause the hollow structure to rupture.

Rupture of the structure and associated bleeding can be problematic in itself, but often the larger problem is the release of air and fluid contents into the abdominal vault. Depending on the organ, spilled contents can cause inflammation and life-threatening infection.

SOLID ORGANS Solid organs in the abdomen include the liver, spleen, pancreas, and kidneys. Solid organs are dense and are often very rich in blood supply. Because of their solid makeup, they do not respond well to trauma. External forces often cause direct damage to the organ, which can result in excessive bleeding.

BLOOD VESSELS Several large blood vessels make their way through the abdominal cavity. The abdominal aorta and the inferior vena cava are among the largest. Trauma to these vessels can lead to massive blood loss that is not visible, and this is the leading cause of death in abdominal injuries.

Trauma to the Abdomen

Abdominal structures can be damaged by a variety of forces. When considering abdominal injuries, it is important to understand the nature of the energy exerted on them.

DIRECT FORCE INJURY Direct force results from energy being applied specifically onto a point in the abdomen. This can come in the form of penetrating trauma, such as a gunshot wound, or in the form of blunt trauma, such as a poorly placed lap belt striking the lower abdominal quadrants. In direct force injuries, the energy of the offending object is transferred directly to whatever organ or structure happens to be in its path.

COMPRESSION INJURY With a mechanism similar to that of direct force, compression injuries exert forces directly onto organs and other structures. In this case, an organ is squeezed, or compressed, between other structures. For example, when an unbelted driver in a car crash is thrown forward into the steering wheel, the wheel will be driven into his abdomen. As it drives backward into the area of his liver, that organ will be compressed between the wheel and the spinal column, potentially resulting in organ damage.

SHEARING/DECELERATION INJURY Isaac Newton found that objects in motion tend to stay in motion. When a body is stopped abruptly, as in a motor vehicle crash, its organs continue moving forward until they are stopped. If the force is great enough, these organs may be torn from their tethering structures. Often this rapid deceleration can damage the organ. In some cases, the tethering ligaments may actually slice through the solid organs they normally hold in place. This shears the organ into pieces and results in massive hemorrhage. Shearing injuries are common in both the liver and aorta.

Abdominal trauma can penetrate the muscular walls and skin and cause an open injury. Occasionally internal organs can protrude through holes (this is called an *evisceration*). More commonly, however, injuries are caused by blunt forces that do not penetrate the abdominal walls. This type of injury is referred to as a *closed abdominal injury*.

ASSESSMENT FINDINGS

Abdominal injuries frequently result in severe internal bleeding. Therefore, the real focus of the assessment of abdominal trauma is the rapid identification of life threats. We will discuss techniques that may assist you in identifying a likely abdominal problem; however, you should never become so focused on the differential diagnosis that you neglect the larger priorities.

A thorough primary assessment is critical in a patient with abdominal trauma. Remember that although the abdominal wound may be dramatic, airway and breathing issues may still be the higher priority. It is assuredly true that the best way to keep a trauma patient alive is to manage the airway and ventilation. This is true regardless of the nature of his injuries.

Your primary assessment may also reveal signs of shock that would indicate internal bleeding long before you examine the abdomen. Keep in mind that if you identify shock, treatment must begin immediately, regardless of what part of the abdomen is causing the problem.

Once you have completed the primary assessment (and treated any necessary deficits), you can use your knowledge of abdominal anatomy to help you identify other potential problems that may be associated with trauma. Here you will consider both the mechanism and location of injury to better understand the potential for damage.

Recall that the abdomen is divided into four quadrants (▶ Figure 41-1). The umbilicus is the center and divides both upper and lower and left and right. Knowing the general location of key organs (Table 41-1) will help you predict the potential for damage.

When assessing the abdomen, consider the mechanism of injury. What forces impacted the abdomen? How much energy was transferred? High energy can be expected to cause more damage than low energy. Consider, for instance, the difference between being struck by a rock and being struck by a bullet. Consider also the path the energy took.

Certain areas of the abdomen are more vulnerable to damage caused by trauma. Recall the location of the solid organs. For example, when trauma impacts the right upper quadrant, the liver is vulnerable. Because the liver is a vascular, solid organ,

> **Although the abdominal wound may be dramatic, airway and breathing issues may still be the higher priority.**

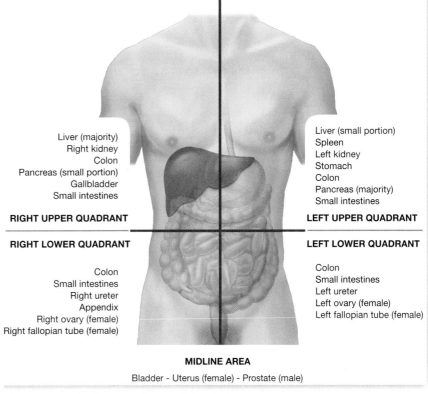

Liver (majority)
Right kidney
Colon
Pancreas (small portion)
Gallbladder
Small intestines

RIGHT UPPER QUADRANT

Liver (small portion)
Spleen
Left kidney
Stomach
Colon
Pancreas (majority)
Small intestines

LEFT UPPER QUADRANT

RIGHT LOWER QUADRANT

LEFT LOWER QUADRANT

Colon
Small intestines
Right ureter
Appendix
Right ovary (female)
Right fallopian tube (female)

Colon
Small intestines
Left ureter
Left ovary (female)
Left fallopian tube (female)

MIDLINE AREA

Bladder - Uterus (female) - Prostate (male)

Figure 41-1 The four quadrants of the abdomen.

TABLE 41-1 Contents of the Abdominal Quadrants

Right Upper Quadrant	Left Upper Quadrant
• Liver	• Liver
• Gallbladder	• Spleen
• Right kidney	• Stomach
• Colon/small intestine	• Left kidney
• Pancreas (head)	• Colon/small intestine
	• Pancreas (tail)

Right Lower Quadrant	Left Lower Quadrant
• Appendix	• Colon/small intestine
• Colon/small intestine	• Ovary/fallopian tube (women)
• Ovary/fallopian tube (women)	• Bladder
• Bladder	

damage to this area often results in severe bleeding. Use your knowledge of anatomy to predict which structures are most likely to be involved in the injury.

Penetrating Versus Blunt Trauma

PENETRATING TRAUMA Penetrating trauma disrupts the integrity of the abdominal wall. Some object, such as a knife, a bullet, or a handlebar, has physically been inserted into the abdominal cavity and displaced and destroyed the tissue and structures that happened to be in the way. In some cases, the path of damage is easy to predict. In a truly open wound, the path may actually be visible. However, you should always remember that penetrating trauma is not always easy to assess.

Small external holes can result in huge internal injuries. Consider a small bullet hole (▶ Figure 41-2). Although the offending object is small, the energy behind it is great. This impact can cause massive organ damage beneath the skin, despite leaving only a small entrance wound.

Occasionally, with penetrating trauma, an exit wound may be visible as well. This may help predict the path of destruction, but the process is inherently unreliable because of bullet fragmentation and ricochet.

Consider also a cone of damage with penetrating weapons such as a knife. By looking at the object we may be able to predict depth, but remember that the object may have been moved inside the body and therefore may have caused damage to a larger area than the immediate pathway.

When assessing penetrating trauma, be sure to fully expose patients. Small puncture wounds are often difficult to find. Be sure also to examine all four sides of the abdomen: anterior, posterior, and the two flanks or sides.

BLUNT TRAUMA Blunt trauma results from force spread out over a larger area such that the abdominal wall is not disrupted (a closed abdominal injury). Make no mistake, however; the energy behind the offending force can be immense. The difficulty in assessing a closed injury is that there is no clear pathway. In some cases, you can identify the likely point of impact, but even in these cases the damage beneath the skin is often unpredictable.

In blunt trauma, you will need to assume the worst and use other findings, such as vital signs, to indicate shock and other life threats. When assessing closed abdominal injuries, consider the patient's position at the time of impact. Is the patient guarding his abdomen (▶ Figure 41-3)?

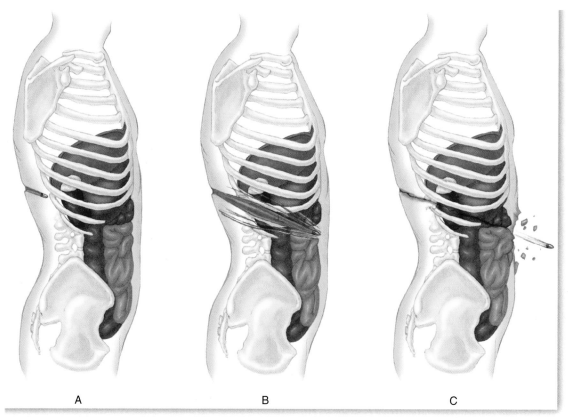

A   B   C

Figure 41-2 Bullets cause damage in two ways: from the bullet itself (A and C) and from cavitation, which is the temporary cavity caused by the pressure wave (B).

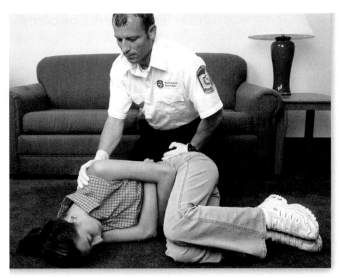

Figure 41-3 A typical "guarded" position for a patient with acute abdominal pain.

Look for pain, rigidity, and discoloration that may indicate an underlying injury (▶ Figure 41-4). Use palpation of all four quadrants to assess for tenderness, rigidity, and guarding. Remember also that abdominal injury is often missed when treating a patient with multisystem trauma. Often blunt trauma (a closed injury) is difficult to identify when the patient is unconscious or distracted by other injuries. When possible, complete a secondary survey that includes palpation of the abdomen to help better identify abdominal problems.

Abdominal Pain

Abdominal pain is a useful indicator of injury. Localizing abdominal pain can be helpful in identifying likely injured structures. Discuss pain with the patient. Palpate the abdomen to identify point tenderness.

Remember that abdominal pain can also be referred to other areas (called referred pain), such as a spleen injury causing shoulder pain. At the same time, keep in mind that damaged organs may be bleeding rapidly without causing significant pain. Other injuries, such as extremity trauma or spinal cord injury, can often distract the patient from abdominal pain. A lack of pain should never rule out a potential abdominal injury, especially in the presence of other physical findings.

Abdomen or Lung?

Injuries to the abdomen quite frequently involve lung tissue. Remember that on inspiration, the diaphragm can drop as low as the umbilicus and therefore expose lung tissue to what would otherwise be an abdominal injury. Always suspect a lung injury with abdominal trauma, and carefully assess breathing to identify possible lung and/or chest complications.

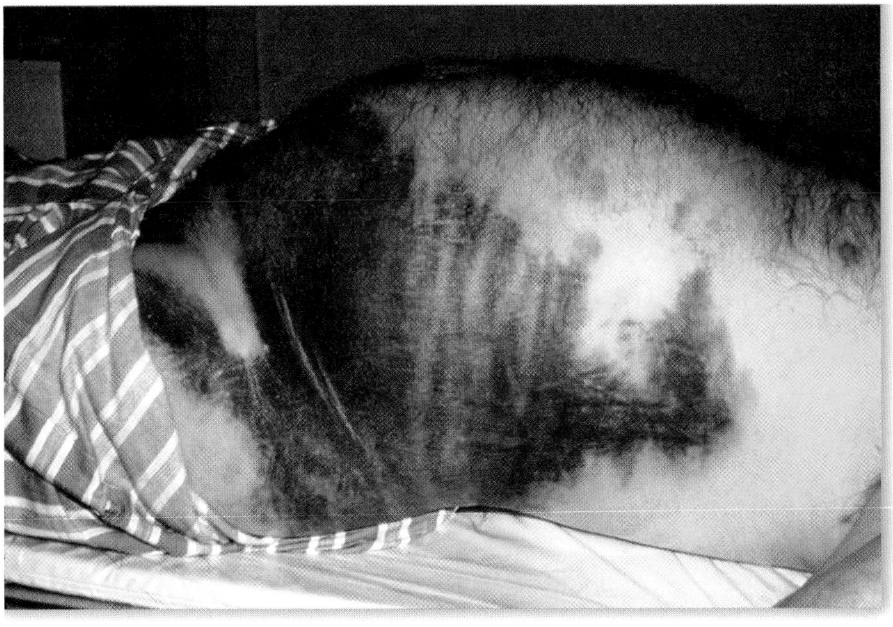

DECISION MAKING: SHOCK AND ABDOMINAL TRAUMA

Mechanism of Injury + Shock = Critical Patient

You should always keep this formula in mind when assessing a patient with abdominal trauma. In the presence of any abdominal injury (even a minor one), keep a keen eye out for the signs and symptoms of shock, including altered mental status, tachycardia, increased respiratory rate, and delayed capillary refill. Any of these signs can indicate an underlying critical injury.

Pediatric Considerations

The organs in a pediatric abdomen are more exposed, as they are covered less by the rib cage than those in an adult. The abdomen also makes up a larger portion of the overall torso and therefore is more exposed to trauma. Always consider abdominal injuries in blunt force trauma in children. Your index of suspicion should be especially high in car-versus-pedestrian injuries, as often the abdomen is directly in the line of the majority of the energy being transferred by the car.

EMERGENCY MEDICAL CARE

The most important elements of care for a patient with abdominal trauma are directed by findings in the primary assessment. Treat airway, breathing, and circulation with the highest priority.

Airway and Breathing

Regardless of how dramatic the abdominal injury, airway and breathing will always take precedence. Providing oxygenation and ventilation to the trauma patient is a crucial element in improving outcomes.

Open abdominal injuries may not only disrupt the abdominal cavity, but they also may also disrupt the chest cavity. If the penetration is high enough to involve lung tissue, the hole in the abdomen may be interfering with respiratory mechanics. Consider using a nonporous dressing with any question of lung involvement. These dressings seal abdominal wounds to prevent air entry and potentially preserve the integrity of the chest cavity as well.

Figure 41-4 Abdominal bruising is a sign of blunt trauma and probable internal bleeding.

Circulation

Recognize and treat shock. Apply high-concentration oxygen, maintain normal temperature, and initiate rapid transport to an appropriate facility. Manage external hemorrhage when possible, and always have a high index of suspicion for internal bleeding in abdominal trauma. Transport patients with suspected shock rapidly.

Initiate a large-bore IV with normal saline and administer as necessitated by the patient's clinical picture and per local protocol.

Other Treatment Concerns

Open abdominal injuries sometimes cause eviscerations. Be sure to cover exposed internal organs with a moistened saline dressing and then seal the wound with a nonporous dressing (▶ Figure 41-5). Never replace protruding internal organs.

First take Standard Precautions.

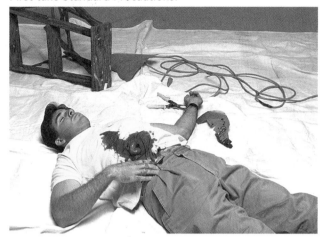

Open abdominal wound with evisceration.

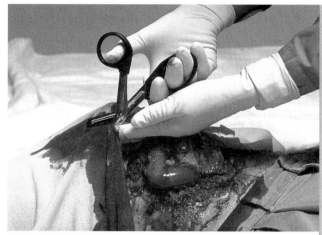

1. Cut away clothing from the wound.

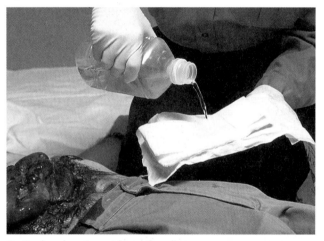

2. Soak a dressing with sterile saline.

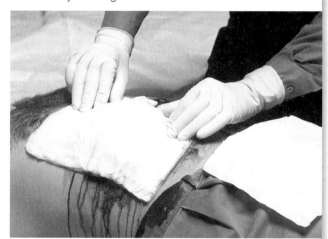

3. Place the moist dressing over the wound.

Cover the dressed wound to maintain warmth. Secure the covering with tape or cravats tied above and below the position of the exposed organ.

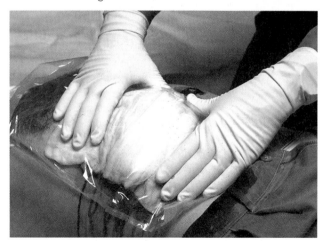

4. Apply an occlusive dressing over the moist dressing if local protocols recommend that you do so.

Figure 41-5 Steps in dressing an open abdominal wound.

When treating an impaled object, stabilize it in place. Never remove the object.

Constantly reassess patients with abdominal injuries, as their status can change rapidly. Internal bleeding can quickly lead to a decompensated patient, and it is your obligation to recognize such deterioration.

When appropriate, transport the patient with abdominal injuries in a position of comfort. Often a knee-flexed position will be preferred. Ensure that your destination choice has the capability to care for the injuries that may be present.

Always remember that identification of the specific abdominal injury is less important than treating immediate life threats. Refer back to the primary assessment and treat life threats first.

TRANSITIONING

REVIEW ITEMS

1. Which of the following would be considered a hollow organ?
   a. gallbladder
   b. liver
   c. spleen
   d. kidney

2. You are treating a patient who was struck in the abdomen by a hockey stick. He complains of left shoulder pain despite the fact he sustained no trauma to the shoulder. You should suspect _____.
   a. a spleen injury
   b. a prior shoulder injury that has been exacerbated
   c. a shoulder injury that is referring pain to the abdomen
   d. a gallbladder injury

3. You are treating a patient with a puncture wound to the upper right quadrant. The organ you should be most concerned about is the _____.
   a. liver
   b. spleen
   c. stomach
   d. appendix

4. You are assessing a patient who has been stabbed in the upper left quadrant. He complains of difficulty breathing and is coughing up blood. These findings are most likely caused by _____.
   a. lung tissue damage from the abdominal injury
   b. referred pain from the abdomen
   c. a chest injury you missed on your assessment
   d. a stomach injury

5. You are treating a patient with an abdominal evisceration. Your primary assessment reveals vomit in his airway, 6 respirations per minute, and a carotid pulse of 130. You should first _____.
   a. suction the airway
   b. ventilate with a bag-valve mask
   c. apply moist sterile dressings
   d. apply an occlusive dressing

APPLIED PATHOPHYSIOLOGY

1. For each of the following organs, indicate in which quadrant it is found and whether it is a hollow or solid organ.

4. Describe how a deceleration/shearing force would injure an abdominal organ.

Organ	Location	Hollow or Solid
Spleen		
Liver		
Stomach		
Gallbladder		

2. List three signs of a closed abdominal injury.

3. Describe why a solid organ might be more vulnerable to trauma compared with a hollow organ.

5. Discuss why penetrating trauma to the abdomen is often difficult to assess. Why is it unpredictable?

CLINICAL DECISION MAKING

You are called to respond to a 17-year-old male patient who has been struck by a car. On arrival, bystanders note that he was hit by the grille of a car traveling approximately 35 miles per hour and was thrown 10 feet onto the street. The scene is safe, and you approach. Your general impression finds the patient on the ground with an angulated femur fracture. He is moaning in pain. You note that he is pale and diaphoretic.

Your primary assessment reveals a patent airway, rapid breathing with bilateral lung sounds, and no radial pulse. He does, however, have a carotid pulse at a rate of 124.

1. Is this patient critical? Why or why not?

2. What immediate actions must you take?

The patient states, "My leg hurts!" He denies any further complaint. Your rapid trauma assessment finds tenderness and guarding in the upper left quadrant of his abdomen and the obviously fractured femur.

3. Is this patient in shock? If yes, what is the most likely cause of the shock?

4. Given the tenderness in the upper left quadrant, what organ(s) might you be concerned is/are affected?

5. Explain the pathophysiologic cause for the following:

    a. Absent radial pulse:

    b. Pale skin:

    c. No complaint of pain even though his belly is tender to palpation:

6. You begin a large-bore IV on the patient and run normal saline. What is the goal for your fluid resuscitation?

Standard Trauma

Competency Applies fundamental knowledge to provide basic and selected advanced emergency care and transportation based on assessment findings for an acutely injured patient.

TOPIC
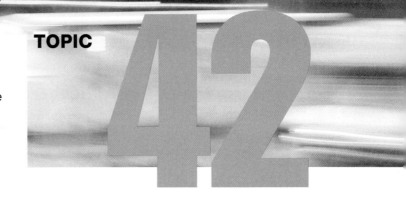

SOFT TISSUE INJURIES: CRUSH INJURY AND COMPARTMENT SYNDROME

INTRODUCTION

Crush injuries and compartment syndrome damage tissues in a very specific way. Crush injury is a form of blunt trauma, whereas compartment syndrome is a complication of blunt trauma. These particular types of injury present the Advanced EMT with very specific challenges to patient assessment and care. Compartment syndrome requires an AEMT to think long term and prevent ongoing injury, whereas crush injuries force the AEMT to consider some very different treatment modalities. In this topic we discuss both of these specific circumstances as they pertain to blunt trauma.

Even with these specific circumstances in mind, remember the basic principles of assessing and treating blunt force trauma. In particular, recall that when dealing with soft tissue injuries you must consider not just the outside of the skin, but also the potential for injury beneath the skin.

Blunt trauma damages by applying force and stretching tissues beyond their normal tolerances. A *crush injury*—a particular type of blunt trauma—damages tissues by compressive force

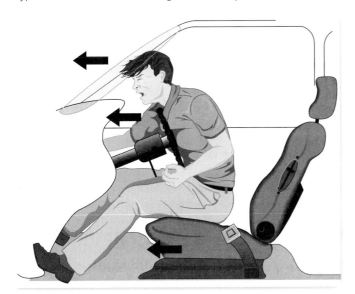

Figure 42-1 Direct force can cause crush injuries, some resulting in open wounds.

(▶ Figure 42-1). This force is generally applied over larger areas and damages more tissue, either through direct compression (direct, crushing force) or by compressing tissues and limiting blood flow (perfusion) to the cells in that area. Crush injuries can occur over a relatively small area, such as striking the thumb with a hammer, or over a large area, such as traumatic asphyxia of the chest. The mechanism of injury remains similar.

This type of injury can occur from either external or internal forces. An example of external direct compression might be a beam that has fallen and trapped a patient's leg. A different mechanism that might have a similar net effect would be *compartment syndrome*. In compartment syndrome, internal swelling causes high pressure to build up within the relatively closed muscular compartment of an extremity. This pressure can damage nerve, muscle, and vascular tissue and limit perfusion to that area. As compartment syndrome emerges, tissue is destroyed just as it would be by direct force.

EPIDEMIOLOGY

The broad definition of soft tissue injury (nonbony, non–organ injury) accounts for the vast majority of traumatic injuries. Crush injuries are only a small portion of this category, but they result from a wide range of mechanisms.

Direct Force

Direct force crush injuries are the most common types of crush injuries. In this case, an object (or objects) applies force and destroys tissue by direct compression. Examples of this include injuries caused by falling objects and blunt trauma distributed over larger areas.

Entrapment/Weight-Based Compression

In this situation, compression of tissue is caused by the patient's position. This damage typically manifests over hours—and sometimes days. The inability of a patient to shift position causes compression and restricts blood flow. Cells are deprived of oxygen, and waste products build up. Dramatic examples of this include victims trapped and pinned by earthquakes and bomb blasts, but more common examples occur in patients who fall and are unable to get up; their weight causes the crushing force on dependent structures.

> **Crush injuries can restrict and even stop blood flow to the areas that are being compressed.**

Consider a stroke patient who collapses and pins her own leg beneath her body weight (▶ Figure 42-2). Her stroke renders her unable to get up or even change her position. Her own body weight compresses her leg and causes a crush-type injury.

Internal Compression

Internal swelling causes compartment syndrome and damages tissue by direct, internal compression and by limiting perfusion.

PATHOPHYSIOLOGY

Direct compression destroys cells in the same manner as any other direct force trauma does. Energy is transferred from an offending object into the tissues. When tissues are stretched beyond their normal tolerances, damage occurs. With crush injuries, that damage can be spread over wide areas and extend deep into tissues below the skin.

Blood flow—for delivery of oxygen and nutrients and for the removal of waste products—is essential to cells. Crush injuries can restrict and even stop blood flow to the areas that are being compressed. These types of injuries are common when, for example, a patient's lower extremities are pinned under rubble after a building collapse. As the legs are compressed, cells are destroyed, not just by the direct force but also by the lack of perfusion.

If compression continues over an extended time (typically longer than four hours), the muscle tissue will actually begin to break down and may cause systemic problems by releasing toxins into the bloodstream. These toxins can cause cardiac problems, a drop in blood pressure, and even kidney failure.

Compartment Syndrome

Compartment syndrome is compression from the opposite direction. *Fascia* is a fibrous membrane that serves to separate areas of muscle. Because fascia does not stretch, these muscular compartments form relatively closed containers. When bleeding or swelling occurs inside these compartments, pressure can build up. If this pressure continues to rise, it can reduce perfusion and destroy cells; this buildup of pressure is compartment syndrome.

ASSESSMENT FINDINGS

Remember that all assessment begins with a thorough primary assessment. Although your attention may be immediately grabbed by pinned extremities, the airway and breathing still take precedence. Treat life-threatening emergencies first.

Crush injuries often cause massive internal hemorrhage. Be vigilant for the signs and symptoms of shock. Again, dramatic injuries may mask more serious underlying issues.

The actual crush injury will generally appear similar to any other blunt trauma wound. Typically, the chief complaint will be pain in the affected area. Discoloration—such as bruising, tenderness, and even deformity—can indicate such an injury. In prolonged or massive compression injuries, blood vessels and nervous tissue may be destroyed. As such, it is not uncommon to see diminished circulatory, sensory, and motor function in distal areas (▶ Figure 42-3).

Assessment may be extremely difficult if the patient is trapped under an object. Understand the limitations of your assessment at this point, and be prepared for further injuries and unexpected complications once the patient is disentangled.

Assessment of Compartment Syndrome

Compartment syndrome typically occurs in the extremities; however, it can also occur in the buttocks and even the abdomen. Compartment syndrome is generally not an acute problem and typically takes hours and even days to develop. As such, much of your assessment will be geared to preventing compartment syndrome rather than identifying it.

Signs and symptoms of compartment syndrome include the following:

- Pain, discomfort, and/or burning sensation in the affected extremity, especially pain that continues or increases after immobilization
- Tenderness (pain on palpation) in the affected extremity
- Unusual firmness or rigidity in the affected area
- Altered motor function, circulation, or sensation in the distal areas of the extremity (*Note:* Loss of a distal pulse is an unusual finding in compartment syndrome. Typically a pulse is present, even though circulation may be impaired. This pulse may feel weaker

Figure 42-2 A stroke patient who has fallen and trapped her right leg beneath her body weight.

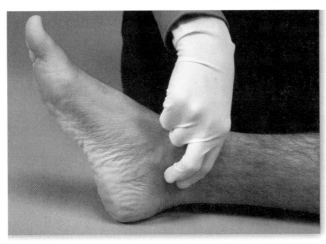

Figure 42-3 Assess circulation in an extremity following a crush injury.

than the same pulse in the unaffected extremity. Delayed capillary refill time may be a more important finding.)

- Weakness or paralysis of the muscles

Remember that assessment of soft tissue injuries will often be a lower priority than treating the ABCs. Always ensure that the primary assessment has been completed prior to evaluating such wounds.

EMERGENCY MEDICAL CARE

Scene safety will be an important element in treating crush injuries. Before initiating any patient contact, ensure that the mechanism of injury that injured the patient will not injure you. Treating patients in a collapse zone requires specialized training and rescue resources. Be sure to know what resources are available in your area and how to access those resources when necessary.

The most important care in crush injuries will be to treat immediate life threats first. Always address airway and breathing complications and life-threatening hemorrhage immediately. Only after treating these more important priorities should you be concerned with addressing soft tissue injuries. Beware of being distracted by a dramatic soft tissue injury while more subtle complications rapidly kill your patient.

Crush injuries can encompass virtually any area of the body. As a result, you will have to tailor your treatment to best treat the affected area. For example, crush injuries to the chest, such as

traumatic asphyxia, might require immediate ventilatory support. Massive crush injuries will also require immediate and rapid transport to an appropriate trauma facility.

Often, soft tissue injuries will mask more serious internal injuries, such as internal bleeding. Always think of the structures that lie beneath the outer injury and consider how damaging those structures might affect your patient's overall status.

In compression-related injuries (whether they are caused by an external force or by the patient's position), relieving the pressure is important. Restoring blood flow to the affected area will limit tissue damage.

Keep in mind that patients who have been trapped for prolonged periods may have systemic complications as a result of their compression-related injuries. When compression is released, waste products and toxins from the affected area may be released into the patient's system. These toxins can cause cardiac dysrhythmias, hypotension, and other systemic complications. With patients who have been trapped longer than four hours, consider starting a large-bore IV line and contacting medical control prior to removing large objects (when possible). Run IV fluids at a rate guided by medical direction or local protocol.

Remember also that large, entrapping objects may be limiting hemorrhage in the affected area and, when released, may allow massive bleeding to occur. Always be prepared for rapid patient deterioration after removal from entrapment.

In general, treat crush injuries as you would any other blunt force trauma. Immobilize potential fractures, elevate the involved extremity, and use ice to reduce swelling and for pain control. Consider spinal immobilization when appropriate.

Preventing and Treating Compartment Syndrome

As stated, compartment syndrome generally develops over long periods of time. As a result, it is typically not a major concern for the short contact times of most EMS systems. However, in many situations EMS may be in prolonged contact with patients, and in such circumstances preventive measures will help avoid compartment syndrome.

The following actions are necessary to prevent compartment syndrome:

- **Elevate extremities.** Although some experts disagree, it is generally accepted that keeping an extremity elevated above the level of the heart will help minimize swelling and maximize the work of the lymphatic system to remove accumulated fluid from the area.
- **Beware of constricting immobilization.** Although splinting material may be just right at the time of initial immobilization, remember that swelling can cause these same bands to become constricting. Monitor equipment frequently to ensure appropriate tightness. Remove any constrictive jewelry.
- **Apply cold.** Appropriately applied cold packs and ice can help limit edema and mitigate pain.
- **Monitor distal circulatory, sensory, and motor function.** Changes in these findings can indicate rising pressure and could identify a reason to modify response and/or transport modalities.

Crush injuries and compartment syndrome are infrequent circumstances that require critical decision making. Use good patient assessment to identify life threats and treat specific injuries appropriately.

> **Beware of being distracted by a dramatic soft tissue injury while more subtle complications rapidly kill your patient.**

REVIEW ITEMS

1. Which of the following would be considered a mechanism of injury leading to a crush injury?
   a. a stroke patient who falls and traps his leg under his body weight for eight hours
   b. a stab wound to the left thigh
   c. a syncope patient who falls and strikes his head against the dresser
   d. an angulated tibia/fibula fracture

2. Which of the following signs would potentially indicate compartment syndrome in an injured extremity?
   a. firmness or rigidity
   b. swelling at the site of the fracture
   c. red discoloration
   d. decreased capillary refill time in the distal areas

3. Which of the following is a step you might take to prevent compartment syndrome?
   a. Elevate the extremity.
   b. Use compression bandages to wrap the extremity.
   c. Place the extremity in a position below the heart.
   d. Apply heat packs.

4. Which of the following patients would have the potential for systemic effects of a crush injury?
   a. a patient recently freed after having his extremities pinned for four hours
   b. a patient recently freed after having his extremities pinned for four minutes
   c. a patient who has crushed his thumb with a hammer
   d. a patient who has broken his leg while inline skating

5. Which of the following would cause damage as the result of compartment syndrome?
   a. internal compression
   b. direct compression
   c. entrapment/weight-based compression
   d. organic/inorganic compression

APPLIED PATHOPHYSIOLOGY

1. List three signs of compartment syndrome.

2. Describe how the mechanism of entrapment/weight-based compression damages soft tissue.

3. Describe the relationship between fascia and compartment syndrome.

CLINICAL DECISION MAKING

You respond to a roof collapse with people trapped. On arrival, you stage and wait for rescue personnel to secure the scene. About four hours later, you are directed in. Rescue workers bring you to a patient whose legs are trapped beneath a collapsed beam. The workers state they are almost ready to lift the beam off the patient.

1. What types of injuries would you expect from this mechanism?

2. What immediate assessment steps should you take?

Your partner completes the assessment as you prepare the stretcher. Your partner tells you the patient is breathing only four times per minute. At that moment, the captain of the rescue team tells you to step back, as rescue workers are now ready to move the beam.

3. What should your next action be?

4. Is ventilating the patient worth delaying extrication?

The beam is moved, and you move the patient to the backboard for transport. Your partner tells you, "I don't think he has a pulse."

5. Explain why the patient may have gone into cardiac arrest now (there may be more than one reason).

6. Why might having advanced life support on scene prior to removal of the beam be important?

Standard Trauma

Competency Applies fundamental knowledge to provide basic and selected advanced emergency care and transportation based on assessment findings for an acutely injured patient.

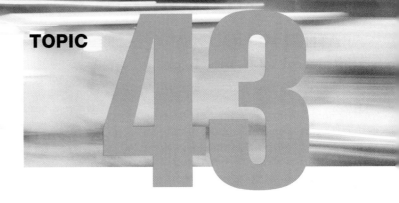

TOPIC

43

HEAD AND TRAUMATIC BRAIN INJURY

INTRODUCTION

As an Advanced EMT, on a regular basis you will be faced with caring for patients suffering from head injuries. In the United States, 1.5 million people per year incur a head injury. These injuries require a high level of suspicion, as signs and symptoms can manifest days and even weeks after the original injury, especially in the very young and the elderly. Assessment of these patients can be complicated because altered mentation is a common presentation in head injuries. In addition, drugs or alcohol may also compound the situation, making assessment even more difficult. You must overcome these challenges to promptly evaluate the condition and prevent further neurologic damage to your patient.

Understanding the anatomy of the skull and its contents is imperative for determining the specific type of head or traumatic brain injury (TBI) your patient is displaying. The skull is the part of the skeletal system that protects the brain and a portion of the spinal cord. It is formed by the fusion of several flat bones held together by cranial sutures. The brain occupies 80 percent to 90 percent of the space within the skull. Therefore, the space in which the brain can swell or bleed is grossly limited. The other 10 percent to 20 percent of the space is filled with cerebrospinal fluid (CSF), which cushions the brain within the skull.

Inside the skull, the meninges protect the surface of the brain. The three *meninges*, or layers of tissue, are the dura mater, the arachnoid meninge, and the pia mater. The *dura mater*, literally meaning "hard mother," is composed of a double layer of thick, fibrous tissue and is the outermost protective layer. Directly beneath the dura mater is the *arachnoid meninge*. The *pia mater* is the layer that is in direct contact with the brain.

The gap between the arachnoid and pia mater is called the *subarachnoid space*. It is composed of fibrous, spongy tissue and cerebrospinal fluid. The brain itself is divided into three parts: the cerebrum, cerebellum, and brainstem. (These parts are discussed at length in Topic 17, "Neurology: Altered Mental Status.")

EPIDEMIOLOGY

Head injuries are the leading cause of death among accident victims younger than 45 years of age. Each year 50,000 people

TRANSITION *highlights*

- *Incidence and death rates for traumatic brain injury along with age and gender predispositions for these injuries.*

- *Pathophysiology of brain injuries to include types of injuries, effects on cerebral tissue, and effects on normal brain functioning:*
  - Intracerebral hemorrhage.
  - Diffuse axonal injury.
  - Concussion.
  - Epidural hematoma.
  - Subdural hematoma.
  - Subarachnoid hemorrhage.

- *Assessment steps and considerations for victims of brain injury, with special emphasis on four topics:*
  - Brain herniation.
  - Importance of mental status.
  - Decorticate and decerebrate posturing.
  - Glasgow Coma Scale.

- *Current treatment parameters for patients with both herniating and nonherniating brain injuries.*

die from TBIs. About 50 percent of head injury patients requiring surgical intervention arrive to the emergency department with a Glasgow Coma Scale (GCS) score ranging from 9 to 15. These patients have improved results if surgical intervention takes place prior to their neurologic demise—which emphasizes the importance of transport to a trauma center.

Epidemiologies specific to intracerebral hemorrhage, diffuse axonal injury, epidural hematoma, subdural hematoma, and subarachnoid hematoma are discussed in the following section.

PATHOPHYSIOLOGY

Intracerebral Hemorrhage

Intracranial hemorrhage is classified as either extraaxial or intraaxial. *Extraaxial hemorrhage* takes place outside the brain and includes epidural, subdural, and subarachnoid hematomas. *Intraaxial hemorrhage* occurs within the brain tissue itself and is called *intracerebral hemorrhage.* Intracerebral hemorrhage is further divided into intraparenchymal and intraventricular hemorrhages. Intracerebral hemorrhage is a serious medical emergency due to the increase in intracranial pressure. If left untreated, intracerebral hemorrhage leads to coma and death.

> **If left untreated, intracerebral hemorrhage leads to coma and death.**

Traumatic *intraparenchymal hemorrhage* is likely caused by penetrating trauma. However, this kind of hemorrhage can also be caused by depressed skull fractures and acceleration–deceleration trauma. The mortality rate for intraparenchymal hemorrhage is over 40 percent. The risk for death is especially high when the injury occurs within the brainstem. Bleeding in the medulla oblongata is even more lethal because breathing and circulatory mechanisms are controlled in this portion of the brain.

Intraventricular hemorrhage is characterized by bleeding into the brain's ventricular system, where cerebrospinal fluid is produced. This type of hemorrhage is found in 35 percent of adults with moderate to severe head injury. An extensive amount of force is necessary to create this injury; therefore, other associated injuries are common. The prognosis for intraventricular hemorrhage is fairly dismal because of increased intracranial pressure and the likelihood for the brain to herniate through the opening at the base of the skull.

Intracerebral hemorrhage is frequently associated with altered mentation. Altered levels of consciousness, as well as nausea and vomiting, are seen in nearly 50 percent of cases. Forty percent of patients also complain of a headache with intracerebral hemorrhage. Other signs and symptoms commonly seen in this injury include systolic hypertension, unequal pupils, neurologic deficits, and seizures.

Diffuse Axonal Injury

Diffuse axonal injury (DAI) is one of the most devastating types of TBI. The damage from this type of head injury occurs over a more widespread area of the brain rather than in a focal area.

DAI typically stems from traumatic acceleration–deceleration injuries. It is a pathologic process in which axons are stretched and twisted by rotational shearing forces that occur during rapidly changing movement. The damaged axons begin to swell and separate from each other, causing interference between the communication and transmission of nerve impulses throughout the brain. This injury is one of the major causes of unconsciousness and persistent vegetative state after head trauma.

DAI occurs in 50 percent of all cases of severe head trauma. It is commonly seen in victims of motor vehicle crashes, falls, and assault. Frequently, the outcome of this injury is coma. More than 90 percent of patients with diffuse axonal injury never regain consciousness. The few patients who do eventually wake up remain significantly impaired neurologically.

CONCUSSION *Concussion* is a milder form of diffuse axonal injury. It is a synonym for mild TBI, which is a head injury associated with a GCS score of 13 to 15. *Concussion* is defined as a trauma-induced alteration in mental status or other neurologic function that may or may not involve loss of consciousness. This injury is caused by an impulsive force transmitted to the head. The result is a rapid, short-lived impairment of neurologic function that resolves spontaneously. Concussive injuries produce structural injuries to the brain; however, they exhibit only temporary functional disturbances.

An average of 80 percent of the 1.5 million reported TBIs in the United States are mild. Mild head injury may result in cortical contusions from coup and contrecoup injuries. Milder degrees of axonal damage play a role in this TBI. It causes the hallmark signs and symptoms of confusion, retrograde and anterograde amnesia, and typically no preceding loss of consciousness. If loss of consciousness occurs, it is brief and does not recur.

Other signs and symptoms of concussion include headache, dizziness, lack of awareness, inability to concentrate, slurred speech, ataxia, nausea, and vomiting. Remember that these signs and symptoms are immediate after impact and subside gradually. Signs and symptoms that present several minutes after the original impact or worsen with time are indicative of a more serious head injury and not concussion.

Epidural Hematoma

Epidural hematoma is an accumulation of blood between the potential space of the dura and the bone of the skull (▶ Figure 43-1). This is considered to be the most serious complication of head injury and must be repaired quickly. Prognosis is excellent with aggressive treatment, including immediate surgical intervention. Therefore, the time required to diagnose this injury and transport the patient to an appropriate medical facility greatly affects the outcome.

Epidural hematoma complicates 2 percent of head injury cases, or approximately 40,000 cases per year. Alcohol and other intoxicating agents have been associated with increasing the incidence of these injuries. Morbidity and mortality are associated with level of mentation and location of the hematoma. The mortality rate for patients who are awake prior to surgery is nearly zero, for obtunded patients it is 9 percent, and for comatose patients it is 20 percent.

When looking at the location of the injury, patients with bilateral epidural hematomas have a 20 percent mortality rate. Those with epidural hematomas occurring in the posterior fossa of the

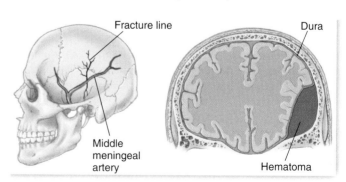

Figure 43-1 Epidural hematoma.

brain have an even higher mortality rate: 26 percent. Few epidural hematomas are located in the frontal or occipital portions of the brain. Men are more likely to incur this injury than women with a 4:1 ratio; however, there is no delineation between races.

Epidural hematoma originates from deceleration injuries or low-velocity impact to the head. Skull fractures are common with these injuries, occurring in 90 percent of adult patients. Epidural hematoma is frequently seen in the temporoparietal region, where the skull fracture crosses the path of the middle meningeal artery.

The bleeding takes place between the protective covering of the brain (dura) and the skull. The bleeding is profuse and rapidly expands within the space, causing a sudden increase in intracranial pressure (ICP). This rise in ICP causes the cascade of signs and symptoms, including decreased mental status, severe headache, fixed and dilated pupils, vomiting, altered or absent breathing, posturing, and systolic hypertension with associated bradycardia (Cushing reflex, which is a late finding). Among patients with an epidural hematoma, 20 percent have a lucid interval. The patient will suffer from a loss of consciousness and then a period of responsiveness. Shortly thereafter, his level of consciousness will deteriorate rapidly.

Subdural Hematoma

Subdural hematoma is a collection of blood over the surface of the brain, between the dura mater and arachnoid meninges (▶ Figure 43-2). Subdural bleeding is typically the result of deceleration injuries and low-pressure venous bleeding. The bleeding occurs as a result of shearing action along the subdural space and traumatic stretching of small bridging veins. This hematoma is frequently associated with trauma but can also occur spontaneously in patients who receive anticoagulant therapy such as warfarin (Coumadin) or have a coagulopathy condition (prolonged bleeding time).

Subdural hematoma is classified based on the time elapsed from the inciting event and diagnosis. The three phases are acute, subacute, and chronic. Signs and symptoms begin immediately in the acute phase. If left untreated, the subacute phase begins three to seven days after the injury, and the chronic phase begins two to three weeks later.

Subdural hematoma is the most common intracranial lesion, occurring in one-third of patients with severe head injury and a GCS of less than 9. Chronic subdural hematoma is reported in an average of 3 in 100,000 persons. It is more common among patients over 60 years of age due to the predisposition for cerebral atrophy and decreased resiliency of bridging veins.

The highest incidence, 7.35 in 100,000 patients, is among patients 70 to 79 years of age. These patients with chronic subdural hematoma often present with headache, personality changes, and ataxia, progressing over weeks. Subdural hematoma is also seen in child abuse cases and incidents involving shaken baby syndrome. The typical mortality rate for this type of hematoma is around 60 percent.

Manifestations of subdural hematoma can vary greatly, ranging from clinically silent to expansion large enough to cause brain herniation. Signs and symptoms of acute subdural hematoma include declining level of consciousness, abnormal or absent respirations, dilation of one pupil, weakness or paralysis to one side of the body, vomiting, seizures, increasing systolic blood pressure, and decreasing heart rate.

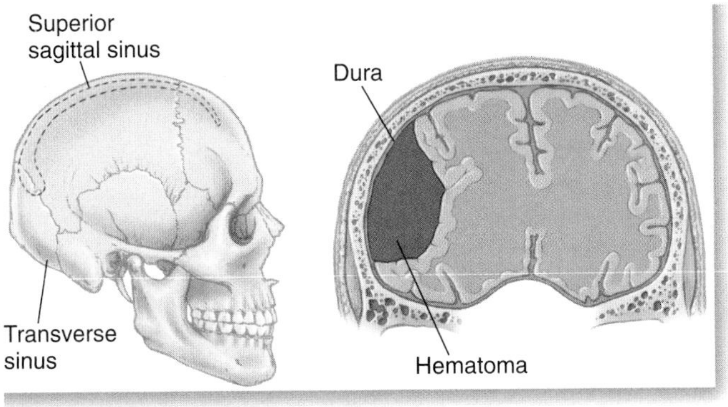

Subarachnoid Hemorrhage

Subarachnoid hemorrhage refers to an accumulation of blood in the subarachnoid space. Subarachnoid hemorrhage can be both traumatic and nontraumatic in nature. The most common cause is a spontaneous rupture of an aneurysm. (This nontraumatic form of subarachnoid hemorrhage is discussed further in Topic 18, "Neurology: Stroke.")

When looking at the traumatic causes of subarachnoid hemorrhage; it is seen that the elderly often incur this injury from a fall. Younger patients usually sustain this injury as a result of a motor vehicle crash. It is the most common intracranial hemorrhage as a result of blunt force trauma and is often associated with some other bleeding within the skull. Approximately 373,000 people are hospitalized with a subarachnoid hemorrhage each year. Of these patients, 56,000 succumb to their injuries, whereas 99,000 survive with permanent disabilities.

The immediate danger in subarachnoid hemorrhage is ischemia, in which portions of the brain that do not receive adequate blood and oxygen supply suffer irreparable injury. This can lead to permanent neurologic damage or death. The three most common complications that promote ischemia to the brain are vasospasm, hydrocephalus, and intracranial hypertension.

In vasospasm, blood vessels constrict in response to chemicals released when blood breaks down in the subarachnoid space. *Hydrocephalus* is an accumulation of fluid in the ventricles of the brain. This occurs in 15 percent of subarachnoid hemorrhage because cerebrospinal fluid cannot drain properly. Thus, pressure builds up on the brain, promoting further ischemic complications. Intracranial hypertension can lead to further bleeding and damage to the blood vessels. This complication is associated with a 70 percent mortality rate.

The classic symptom of nontraumatic subarachnoid hemorrhage is a thunderclap headache. It is described as the worst pain ever felt. The majority of studies have shown that patients progress from being pain free to experiencing severe excruciating pain in a matter of seconds. Loss of consciousness typically follows but can take several hours. Other signs and symptoms of subarachnoid hemorrhage include restlessness, confusion, motor and sensory dysfunction, vomiting, and

> **Epidural hematoma originates from deceleration injuries or low-velocity impact to the head.**

Figure 43-2 **Subdural hematoma.**

Superior sagittal sinus
Dura
Transverse sinus
Hematoma

seizures. Severe neurologic deficits develop and become irreversible within minutes.

ASSESSMENT FINDINGS

Assessment of head injury begins with your dispatch information and general impression. Information provided by the dispatcher can paint a picture of whether the patient is suffering from a traumatic incident or medical event. On arrival at the scene, evaluation of the mechanism of injury can help you ascertain whether a head injury is suspected. Obvious signs of a possible head injury include facial lacerations, scalp hematomas, a starred windshield, a cracked helmet, or evidence of a fall.

> **The classic symptom of subarachnoid hemorrhage is a thunderclap headache.**

Primary assessment of a patient suffering from a head injury begins with manual stabilization of the spine. The forces applied to the head that cause these head injuries have the potential of causing injury to the spine as well. Therefore, the airway should be opened using a jaw-thrust maneuver while maintaining manual stabilization of the spine. If necessary, clear the airway of any potential obstruction and keep suction available at all times.

Maintaining the airway and providing oxygenation to the brain are vital to preventing further neurologic demise. Provide oxygen via a nonrebreather mask with 15 lpm supplemental oxygen. Should the breathing be inadequate, administer positive pressure ventilation with supplemental oxygen via a bag-valve mask. Control any major bleeding as needed, as scalp lacerations have a tendency to bleed heavily.

> **A patient suffering from an injury to the head must have his mental status assessed and reassessed frequently.**

If the patient displays definite signs of brain herniation, where you suspect the brain is being pushed through the opening at the base of the skull, you should consider hyperventilating the patient with supplemental oxygen. (This remains somewhat controversial and may not be included in your specific protocol.) Signs of brain herniation include unequal pupils, fixed pupils, posturing, hemiplegia or hemiparesis, Cushing reflex, or a deteriorating GCS of two or more points. Begin positive pressure ventilation with a bag-valve mask and supplemental oxygen at a rate of 20 ventilations per minute. Do so with caution because ventilating at a rate greater than 20 can inversely cause a reduction of cerebral blood flow and worsen the head injury.

It is critical to maintain the systolic blood pressure above 90 mmHg in the TBI patient. A decrease in blood pressure will lead to a reduction in cerebral perfusion pressure and cerebral blood flow. Hypotension (systolic blood pressure < 90 mmHg) in the TBI patient is a devastating complication that leads to worsened outcomes. Therefore, you will initiate an intravenous line with a large-bore catheter and administer normal saline or lactated Ringer's to maintain a systolic blood pressure above 90 mmHg. Never use a fluid containing glucose, such as 5 percent dextrose in water (D_5W). A brain injury is a special situation in a trauma patient, when you must maintain the systolic blood pressure above 90 mmHg; avoid intentionally restricting fluid administration as in other trauma patients when you want to raise the systolic blood pressure no higher than 80 to 90 mmHg.

A patient suffering from an injury to the head must have his mental status assessed and reassessed frequently. The AVPU mnemonic (Alert, Voice, Pain, Unresponsive) is used to assess mentation. Keep in mind that the patient may be alert originally but then may decline according to the location and type of injury to the head.

During evaluation of the patient's response to pain, he may react in one of two ways: purposeful or nonpurposeful. The patient may attempt to remove the source of the pain or try to move away.

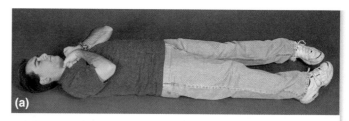
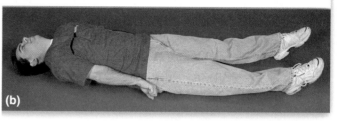

Figure 43-3 Nonpurposeful responses to painful stimuli include (a) flexion (decorticate) posturing and (b) extension (decerebrate) posturing.

These responses are considered purposeful and show a higher level of functioning in the brain. However, the patient may respond by inappropriately moving the extremities or parts of the body but with no effort to stop the pain. This is considered to be nonpurposeful movement and indicates a deeper level of unresponsiveness.

Nonpurposeful movement can be exhibited in one of two ways: decorticate or decerebrate posturing (▶ Figure 43-3). Decorticate posturing is evidenced by flexion of the arms across the chest and extension of the legs. Decorticate posturing is associated with an injury in the upper portion of the brainstem. On the other hand, decerebrate posturing is indicative of an injury in the lower portion of the brainstem. In decerebrate posturing, the patient extends both arms down at the side of the body with extension of the legs and arching of the back.

The patient is considered unresponsive when there is no response to verbal or painful stimuli. This is an ominous sign of head injury.

Be sure to document the patient's level of mentation accurately and often. A baseline level of mentation and continuous reassessment of mentation is crucial for determining if the patient is deteriorating. Further evaluation of mental status can be done by using the GCS. This assessment applies a numerical value to the patient's eye opening as well as best motor and verbal responses. To ensure accuracy, be certain that you are observing the patient's eye opening as you approach. Review the adult GCS as listed in Table 43-1 and the pediatric GCS found in Topic 45.

TABLE 43-1 — Glasgow Coma Scale

Eye Opening

Spontaneous	4
To verbal command	3
To pain	2
No response	1

Verbal Response

Oriented and converses	5
Disoriented and converses	4
Inappropriate words	3
Incomprehensible sounds	2
No response	1

Motor Response

Obeys verbal commands	6
Localizes pain	5
Withdraws from pain (flexion)	4
Abnormal flexion in response to pain (decorticate rigidity)	3
Extension in response to pain (decerebrate rigidity)	2
No response	1

During the secondary assessment, a physical exam paying particular attention to the brain and neurologic status is necessary. When evaluating the head, inspect thoroughly through the hair for abrasions, lacerations, and impaled objects (▶ Figure 43-4). Assess for deformities, depressions, and hematomas around the head and face. Use caution when palpating, though, as you do not want to cause further harm to any depressed areas of the skull.

Check the patient's pupils with a bright light for size, equality, and reactivity. If one or both pupils are fixed and dilated, increased intracranial pressure is likely. When you are evaluating the eyes, does the patient track and focus, as indicated by his looking at and following you with his eyes? Is there a purplish discoloration around the soft tissue of the eye? This "raccoon" sign may be indicative of an intracranial injury and is also a delayed sign of skull fracture. Finally, leakage of blood or CSF from the ears or nose can indicate a skull fracture or intracranial injury.

If the patient is awake and alert, you will want to assess his motor and sensory function. Begin by having the patient move his fingers and toes. Assess hand grasps for strength and equality. Have the patient push down on your hands with his feet and then pull up against your hands. When assessing dorsiflexion and plantar flexion, you are evaluating the strength and equality of this motor movement. You can assess sensory function by pinching the arm or touching a toe and having the patient identify which extremity is being touched.

Vital signs may be able to help you delineate between a head injury and some other disease process. Vital signs in head injury patients should be checked and recorded every 5 minutes. Variations in blood pressure, respiratory rate, and heart rate can also lead you to suspect impending deterioration of your patient (see Table 43-2).

History taking from bystanders at the scene can provide vital information about the mechanism of injury. As patients with head injury frequently have an altered mental status or loss of consciousness, bystanders can offer information that the patient is unable to provide.

The most crucial question is in regard to loss of consciousness. Determine how long the patient was unresponsive, when the loss of consciousness occurred in relation to the time of the injury, whether the loss of consciousness was sudden or gradual, and whether there was more than one episode of unconsciousness.

Ascertain where and how the incident took place and whether the patient was moved after the injury. Obtain complaints the patient may have had specifically relating to dizziness, numbness, weakness, tingling, and paralysis. Also, in addition to past medical history, ask whether the patient has a prior history of head injury and, if so, when it occurred.

EMERGENCY MEDICAL CARE

Unfortunately, head injuries can be severe and life threatening. Prompt recognition and treatment of these injuries is paramount for patient survival and limiting permanent disability. Head injuries require a standard systematic approach for treatment and include the following:

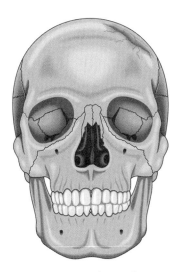

Soft area or depression.

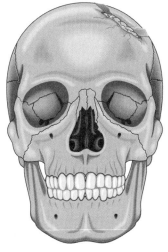

Open wound with bleeding and/or exposed brain tissue.

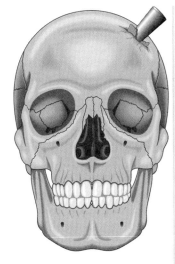

Impaled object in skull.

Figure 43-4 Examine the head for deformities, depressions, lacerations, or impaled objects.

TABLE 43-2　Implications of Changes in Vital Signs with Head Injuries

Vital Sign	Decreased	Increased
Blood pressure	Suspect hemorrhagic shock or head injury that has injured or compressed the brainstem	Suspect increased intracranial pressure
Respiratory rate	Respirations can be slow, shallow, or irregular with compression of the brainstem	Respirations can be fast, shallow, or irregular with compression of the brainstem
Heart rate	Suspect increased intracranial pressure or severe hypoxia	Suspect hemorrhage somewhere else in the body or early onset of hypoxia

- **Establish manual inline stabilization of the spine.**
  - Inline stabilization involves keeping the head, neck, and spinal column in alignment until the patient is fully immobilized to a backboard. This includes maintaining cervical stabilization even after a cervical collar is applied. Once immobilization including the head is complete, you may then release manual stabilization.
- **Maintain a patent airway.**
  - Use a manual jaw-thrust maneuver to open the airway.
  - Remove any foreign bodies in the mouth and suction any secretions that may compromise the airway.
  - The patient might vomit; therefore, protect him from aspiration. Keep suction available at all times,

and be prepared to log-roll the patient.
- **Assess the adequacy of respirations and provide oxygen therapy.**
  - If the respiratory status is adequate, administer oxygen at 15 lpm via a nonrebreather mask.
  - If the respiratory status is inadequate, provide positive pressure ventilation via a bag-valve mask with supplemental oxygen at a rate of 10 to 12 breaths per minute.
  - Maintain the SpO_2 reading at a level of 95 percent or greater.
  - Consider hyperventilation in patients with severe head injury and suspected brain herniation. (Note that the concept of hyperventilation in head injury is controversial. It may produce some short-term improvement but has no role in long-term

management of herniation or elevated ICP. Always follow your local protocol.)
- **Control bleeding, as head injuries are likely to bleed heavily.**
  - Dress and bandage open head wounds with sterile gauze.
  - Do not apply pressure to open or depressed areas of the skull.
  - Never remove a penetrating object from the head or face.
  - Do not stop the flow of any cerebrospinal fluid emitting from the ears or nose.
- **Transport the patient immediately to an appropriate medical facility.**
- **Initiate an intravenous line of normal saline or lactated Ringer's using a large-bore catheter.**
  - Infuse the fluid at a rate to maintain a systolic blood pressure above 90 mmHg.
  - Be careful not to be overly aggressive in fluid administration or make the patient hypertensive. Fluids can contribute to a worsened cerebral edema and increased intracranial pressure; however, maintaining an adequate mean arterial pressure is imperative in achieving adequate cerebral perfusion pressures and cerebral blood flow.
- **Be prepared for emergency care of seizures.**
- **Monitor the airway, breathing, circulation, and mental status continuously for any signs of deterioration, and treat appropriately.**

TRANSITIONING

REVIEW ITEMS

1. You believe your head injury patient is displaying the Cushing reflex. This is evidenced by _____.
   a. hypotension and bradycardia
   b. hypertension and bradycardia
   c. hypotension and tachycardia
   d. hypertension and tachycardia

2. Which head injury is commonly associated with a skull fracture in the temporal region of the skull near the meningeal arteries?
   a. intracerebral hemorrhage
   b. epidural hematoma

   c. subdural hematoma
   d. subarachnoid hematoma

3. What type of head injury interferes with the communication and transmission of nerve impulses throughout the brain?
   a. diffuse axonal injury
   b. epidural hematoma
   c. skull fracture
   d. intraventricular hemorrhage

4. A 15-year-old baseball player is hit in the head with a fly ball. He immediately drops to the ground and is unconscious. As

you approach his side, he immediately wakes up and is temporarily confused and amnestic to the event. As you continue to spend time with him, his mentation improves, and he begins to complain of a headache. Which type of head injury do you believe your patient has sustained?

   a. epidural hematoma

   b. subdural hematoma

   c. concussion

   d. intracerebral hemorrhage

5. Your 37-year-old male patient was sitting on the couch when he started complaining of a headache. He states that it is the worst headache he has ever felt in his life, and it is rapidly getting worse. This symptom is associated with which type of hemorrhage?

   a. epidural hematoma

   b. subdural hematoma

   c. subarachnoid hemorrhage

   d. intracerebral hematoma

6. A 42-year-old woman is on a skiing trip when she suddenly loses control and strikes a tree head-on. After a temporary loss of consciousness, the patient is awake and alert and complaining of a headache. She continues to act normally for a short time until suddenly she becomes lethargic and inappropriate. This lucid interval can be associated with which type of hematoma?

   a. epidural hematoma

   b. subdural hematoma

   c. subarachnoid hematoma

   d. intracerebral hematoma

APPLIED PATHOPHYSIOLOGY

1. Discuss fluid administration in the brain-injured patient and how it differs from fluid administration in other non-brain-injured trauma patients.

CLINICAL DECISION MAKING

You are dispatched for a 42-year-old lumberman who reportedly fell 30 feet from a tree. When you arrive on scene, you find the patient supine on the ground. He does not open his eyes, nor does he speak or groan. When you rub his sternum, he flexes his arms to his chest and extends his legs.

1. What is this patient's GCS score?

2. How would you open the patient's airway?

You open the patient's airway to find blood and vomitus in the mouth. The patient is breathing regularly at 6 times per minute. His SpO$_2$ reading is 74 percent.

3. How would you manage this patient's airway and breathing?

You observe a large pool of blood behind the head. On closer exam, you notice a depression in the occiput of the skull. His blood pressure is 76/40 mmHg, and his heart rate is 108 mmHg.

4. How would you control the bleeding from the head?

5. Does this patient require expeditious transport? Why or why not?

6. What treatment would you provide en route to the hospital?

7. Would you administer fluids? If so, what type and at what rate?

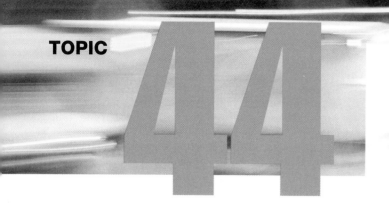

Standard Trauma

Competency Applies fundamental knowledge to provide basic and selected advanced emergency care and transportation based on assessment findings for an acutely injured patient.

COMPLETE AND INCOMPLETE SPINE AND SPINAL CORD INJURIES

TRANSITION *highlights*

- *Incidence with which spinal cord injury occurs, along with the predisposing factors of age, gender, and mechanism.*

- *Normal spinal cord anatomy, including important sensory and motor nerve tracts.*

- *Pathophysiology of spinal cord injury with basic mechanisms of injury, depending on amount of spinal cord involved:*
  - *– Complete spinal cord injury.*
  - *– Incomplete spinal cord injury.*
  - *– Spinal shock.*

- *Motor and sensory findings consistent with various types of incomplete spinal cord injuries:*
  - *– Central cord syndrome.*
  - *– Brown-Séquard syndrome.*
  - *– Anterior cord syndrome.*

- *Specific assessment tests that ascertain level of spinal cord involvement.*

- *General treatment strategies for the patient with a spinal cord injury.*

INTRODUCTION

Spinal cord injuries can be among the most traumatic injuries seen by the Advanced EMT. They may arise from a wide variety of causes—from motor vehicle crashes, diving accidents, falls, and sports injuries, to name just a few. The AEMT must be able to identify injuries that could damage the spinal cord or spinal column and to provide appropriate emergency care. Improper movement and handling of patients with spinal cord or spinal column injuries can lead to permanent disability or even death.

EPIDEMIOLOGY

An injury to the spinal cord could result in a catastrophic permanent disability to the patient. Approximately 11,000 new cases of spinal cord injury (SCI) occur each year in the United States. Most cases of SCI occur in men (80 percent), with an average age of 38 years. According to the National Spinal Cord Injury Database, the etiology of the majority of cases is associated with motor vehicle crashes, which account for close to half the cases, followed by falls, especially in the elderly; penetrating trauma; and sports and recreational activities.

Elderly patients are more prone to suffering from SCI from minor trauma due to degenerative vertebral disorders. In addition, elderly patients have become more active over the years; thus, the incidence of SCI in the elderly is on the rise.

SPINAL CORD ANATOMY

Understanding the basic anatomy of the spinal cord is important to adequately comprehend clinical assessment findings related to incomplete spinal cord injuries. The spinal cord is housed within the vertebral column and has 31 pairs of spinal nerves attached to it that exit at different levels. The spinal cord originates at the cervicomedullary junction inferior to the foramen magnum and terminates at the lower margin of the first lumbar vertebra (L1).

The most inferior portion of the spinal cord, known as the *conus medullaris*, narrows to a point and lies inferior to the lumbosacral enlargement. A series of nerve roots, referred to as the *cauda equina*, continues to extend inferiorly and exit through the lumbar and sacral vertebrae (▶ Figure 44-1). An injury below the level of the second lumbar vertebra (L2) is not necessarily considered a spinal cord injury because it involves segmental spinal nerves or the cauda equina. The dura mater, arachnoid, and pia mater meningeal layers extend from the brain to approximately the second sacral vertebra and provide protection to the spinal cord.

The spinal cord, like the brain, is composed of central nervous system tissue and requires a constant supply of oxygen and glucose. Blood supply to the spinal cord is provided by one anterior spinal artery and two paired posterior spinal

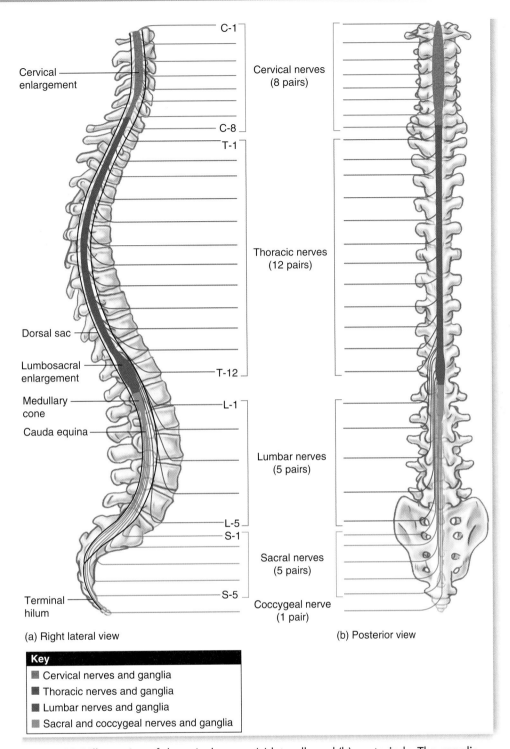

Cervical enlargement

Dorsal sac

Lumbosacral enlargement

Medullary cone

Cauda equina

Terminal hilum

C-1

Cervical nerves (8 pairs)

C-8

T-1

Thoracic nerves (12 pairs)

T-12

L-1

Lumbar nerves (5 pairs)

L-5

S-1

Sacral nerves (5 pairs)

S-5

Coccygeal nerve (1 pair)

(a) Right lateral view

(b) Posterior view

Key
- Cervical nerves and ganglia
- Thoracic nerves and ganglia
- Lumbar nerves and ganglia
- Sacral and coccygeal nerves and ganglia

Figure 44-1 Illustration of the spinal nerves (a) laterally and (b) posteriorly. The ganglia are detailed as well.

arteries. The anterior spinal artery supplies the anterior two-thirds of the spinal cord and extends the full length of the spinal cord. The posterior arteries supply the remaining posterior one-third of the spinal cord. An injury to the anterior spinal artery from laceration or compression by the vertebrae or a bony vertebral fragment may result in anterior spinal

cord damage and ischemia with neurologic dysfunction.

A cross section reveals that the cord is separated into a right and a left half by the anterior medial fissure and the posterior medial sulcus. The central portion of the cord contains gray matter that consists primarily of cell bodies of neurons and forms an "H" pattern. Surrounding the

gray matter is white matter that contains three major motor and sensory nerve tracts: (1) the dorsal or posterior column, which contains the gracile fasciculus and cuneate fasciculus; (2) the lateral pyramidal tract, which carries the corticospinal tracts; and (3) the anterior spinothalamic tract. Both the dorsal (posterior) column (gracile fasciculus and cuneate fasciculus)

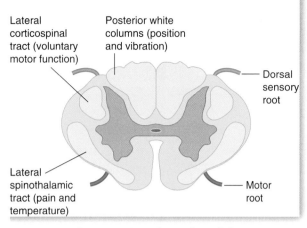

CROSS SECTION OF CERVICAL SPINAL CORD

Lateral corticospinal tract (voluntary motor function)

Posterior white columns (position and vibration)

Dorsal sensory root

Lateral spinothalamic tract (pain and temperature)

Motor root

Figure 44-2 Cross section of spinal cord showing corticospinal, spinothalamic, and posterior columns.

and anterior (spinothalamic) column contain sensory nerve tracts that carry information from sensory receptors up to the brain (▶ Figure 44-2).

The posterior (dorsal) column nerve tracts carry sensations of position (proprioception), vibration, and light touch from the skin, muscles, tendons, and joints to the brain. These posterior column nerve tracts cross over (decussate) at the cervicomedullary junction; therefore, the sensory impulse is carried by the ipsilateral (same side) portion of the spinal cord where the stimulus was received.

Thus, if light touch is applied to the right side of the body, the impulse is carried via the posterior column nerve tracts on the right side of the spinal cord. If an injury to the posterior column on the right side would occur, the patient would potentially lose the ability to feel light touch, vibration, and proprioception on the right side of the body below the site of the cord injury.

The spinothalamic nerve tracts carry pain, temperature, pressure, and crude touch sensations to the brain. Unlike the posterior column, these nerve fibers cross shortly after entering the cord and are carried on the contralateral (opposite side) of the spinal cord.

If an injury to the spinothalamic tract were to occur on the right side of the spinal cord, the patient would lose the ability to feel pain on the left side of the body; however, pain sensation would be preserved on the right. This may lead to some confusion in interpretation of the assessment findings for the emergency medical practitioner who is not familiar with the ascending nerve tracts and may be perceived as an indication that an injury to the spinal cord has not occurred, as the pain response is preserved even though light touch and motor findings may be absent on one side of the body and pain response absent on the opposite side.

The lateral pyramidal (corticospinal) tract is a motor nerve (descending) tract that carries impulses from the cortex of the brain down the spinal column to muscles that cause fine and voluntary muscle movement. Like the posterior column, these nerve tracts cross over in the medulla. Thus, an injury to the spinal cord on the right side would produce loss of motor function on the right or ipsilateral (same) side.

An easy mnemonic that one can use to remember the spinal tracts and the associated sensory and motor response is LMNOP. This refers to **L**ight touch, **M**otor, and **NO P**ain. This means that light touch sensation and motor impulses are carried by nerve tracts on the same side of the spinal cord, but the pain sensation is carried by pain tracts on the opposite side of the spinal cord.

PATHOPHYSIOLOGY

The spinal cord can be injured by a variety of mechanisms, including flexion, rotation, compression, hyperextension, lateral bending, distraction, and penetrating wounds. An actual complete anatomic transaction of the spinal cord is rare, whereas a physiologic or functional transaction is more common, leading to a loss of function below the level of injury. Primary injury is associated with direct injury of the cord as a result of compression, tearing, stretching, or laceration.

The primary injury to the spinal cord initiates a complex cascade of events that leads to secondary spinal cord injury that results from ischemic gray and white matter. Hypoxia, hypoglycemia, hypotension, hyperthermia, and improper immobilization can lead to more significant secondary injury to the patient. The complete or maximum neurologic deficit is most often not exhibited by the patient immediately following the injury. Typically, as the secondary injury progresses, the neurologic deficits continue to worsen.

Complete Spinal Cord Injury

Most EMS providers have been taught about complete spinal cord injury, which is defined as a total loss of motor or sensory function distal to the site of the cord injury. This condition is fairly easy to detect during the assessment, due to the complete bilateral loss of neurologic function. It is rare that neurologic function will be regained. However, a complete spinal cord injury could be mimicked by spinal shock, in which the patient presents with complete neurologic dysfunction following the injury but recovers motor and sensory function within 24 hours after the injury.

For the AEMT, management of the patient will be the same, regardless of whether spinal shock (discussed later in this topic) or complete spinal cord injury is suspected, and it will include complete spinal immobilization.

Incomplete Spinal Cord Injury

Incomplete spinal cord injury, which implies that only a portion of the spinal cord is injured, is more common than a complete spinal cord injury. Because of the undamaged spinal nerve tracts, the patient will not present with complete loss of motor or sensory function below the level of injury. Instead, the patient may present with partial neurologic function, which contributes to confusing assessment findings if incomplete spinal cord injuries are not well understood by the AEMT.

For example, if the anterior portion of the spinal cord is injured, where spinal tracts carry the sensation of pain, the patient will lose the ability to feel pain while maintaining the ability to move his extremities and feel the sensation of light touch. Likewise, if the lateral portions of the spinal cord are injured, where the motor tracts are located, the patient may retain the ability to feel pain and light touch; however, he would lose the ability to move his extremities below the level of injury.

> An injury to the spinal cord on the right side would produce loss of motor function on the right or ipsilateral (same) side.

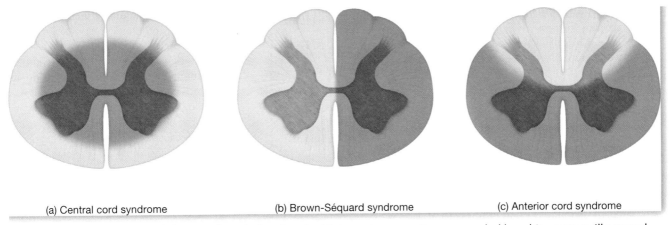

(a) Central cord syndrome   (b) Brown-Séquard syndrome   (c) Anterior cord syndrome

Figure 44-3 Cross sections of the spinal cord, showing the H-shaped gray matter surrounded by white matter. Illustrated here are the three most common types of incomplete spinal cord injury (the areas of the injury are highlighted in red): (a) Central cord syndrome results from injury to the central cord. (b) Brown-Séquard syndrome results from injury to the right or left half of the cord. (c) Anterior cord syndrome results from injury to the anterior cord.

These presentations conflict directly with the findings of complete spinal cord injury and may cause the AEMT to fail to provide complete spinal immobilization, especially if he was taught that all spinal injuries cause complete loss of motor and sensory function below the level of the spinal cord injury.

Specific presentations of incomplete spinal injury are central cord syndrome, Brown-Séquard syndrome, or an anterior cord syndrome in 90 percent of the incomplete injuries (▶ Figure 44-3). The most common is the central cord syndrome that is often associated with older patients with degenerative arthritis. Each syndrome results in different, distinct patient presentations (see Table 44-1).

CENTRAL CORD SYNDROME In central cord syndrome, the ligamentum flavum (▶ Figure 44-4) impinges on the central portion of the spinal cord, causing a concussion or contusion to the gray and inner portions of the spinal nerve tracts within the white matter. The sensory and motor tracts that innervate the lower extremities are located in the peripheral (outer) portions of the nerve tracts, whereas the upper extremities are controlled by the inner or central portions of the nerve tracts.

Thus, with central cord syndrome, the patient experiences weakness, paralysis, and sensory dysfunction in the upper extremities; however, the lower extremities have no or little neurologic dysfunction. This may appear confusing to many emergency care personnel because it is often thought that the sensory and motor dysfunction always occurs below the level of injury.

BROWN-SÉQUARD SYNDROME Brown-Séquard syndrome results from injury to only one side (hemisection) of the spinal cord, usually as a result of penetrating trauma. Because only one side of the cord is involved in the injury, the patient will exhibit loss of motor function and loss of light touch on the same side as the spinal cord injury; however, the pain response will be preserved to that side of the body. On the opposite side of the body, the patient will have motor function and light touch sensation but will have a loss of pain sensation.

ANTERIOR CORD SYNDROME Anterior cord syndrome results from injury to the anterior portion of the spinal cord from contusion of the cord, injury from bony fragments, and laceration or occlusion of the anterior spinal artery. Because the anterior portion of the cord is involved, the spinothalamic and corticospinal tract damage results in a loss of motor function and a loss of pain and temperature sensation below the level of injury. Because the posterior columns are not involved, the patient retains the ability to feel light touch.

Spinal Shock

Spinal shock is a temporary loss of neurologic function and autonomic tone distal to the injury to the spinal cord. The patient typically presents with the loss of motor and sensory function and urinary bladder incontinence. In addition, the patient may exhibit bradycardia, hypotension, and hypothermia.

Neurogenic hypotension may result from spinal shock. The loss of vasomotor

TABLE 44-1	Incomplete Spinal Cord Injury Syndrome Assessment Findings	
Incomplete Spinal Cord Injury Syndrome	Motor Findings	Sensory Findings
Central cord syndrome	Paralysis or severe weakness of the upper extremities, less severe or no motor dysfunction in the lower extremities	Loss of pain sensation in upper extremities, less pain dysfunction in the lower extremities
Brown-Séquard syndrome	Loss of motor function to one side of the body below the level of injury	Loss of light touch to the same side of the body as motor dysfunction, loss of pain sensation opposite the light touch, and motor dysfunction
Anterior cord syndrome	Loss of motor function to both sides of the body below the level of injury	Loss of pain sensation to both sides of the body below the level of injury; patient is able to continue to feel light touch

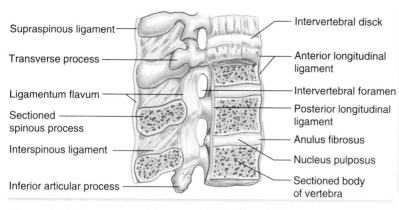

Figure 44-4 Ligaments and intervertebral disks of the spine. Lateral view of the spinal column (anterior to the right). The lower vertebrae have been cut sagitally to reveal the spinal canal and some of the ligaments.

TABLE 44-2		**Differential Assessment Findings: Hypovolemic Shock versus Neurogenic Shock**

Vital Sign Finding	Hypovolemic Shock	Neurogenic Shock
Blood pressure	Decreased	Decreased
Heart rate	Tachycardia	Bradycardia
Skin	Pale, cool, and clammy	Warm, dry, and flushed

control allows the vessels below the level of spinal cord injury to dilate, creating a distributive type of shock. Because the autonomic nervous system control to the body below the injury is blocked, loss of tone and vessel dilation remain unopposed. Blood begins to pool in the dilated vessels, causing a drop in the blood pressure. Administration of intravenous fluids may be the initial therapeutic measure to maintain adequate perfusion if the systolic blood pressure is below 90 mmHg. Vasoconstrictive agents may be added later in the patient's course by more advanced providers.

Typically, the heart rate would increase as a reflex response to the decrease in blood pressure, as seen in hypovolemic shock; however, interruption of the sympathetic trunk that fails to elicit an appropriate sympathetic response, including epinephrine release, does not allow an increase in the heart rate. Thus, the patient presents with hypotension and bradycardia. The hypotension tends to be mild, with systolic blood pressure maintained above 90 mmHg.

Because of the peripheral vasodilation and pooling of blood, the skin is initially flushed. The skin is also dry due to the lack of sympathetic stimulation of sweat glands. Most of these findings are totally opposite those associated with hypovolemic shock. If the patient presents with hypotension, tachycardia, and pale, cool, and clammy skin, always suspect blood loss and treat for hypovolemic shock (see Table 44-2).

ASSESSMENT FINDINGS

In assessment of the patient with a spinal cord injury, it is imperative to assess the various spinal tracts by testing for pain, light touch sensation, and motor function.

Testing for grip strength by having the patient squeeze one's fingers does not test the different nerve tracts and various levels of the spinal cord, and thus it is an incomplete and ineffective test.

A quick and effective method to test the corticospinal tract at various levels of the cord is to have the conscious patient perform the following motor function tests (see Table 44-3):

- Have the patient flex his elbows (tests C6).
- Have the patient extend his elbows (tests C7).
- Have the patient extend his arms with the hands out, palm down, fingers spread apart; have the patient resist as you squeeze the second and fourth fingers (tests T1).
- Support the patient's wrist and push on the extended hand while the patient resists (tests C7).
- Place your hands against the bottom of the feet and have the patient "push down" to test foot plantar flexion (tests S1 and S2).

TABLE 44-3		**Spinal Cord Motor Assessment and Level of Loss of Function**

Level of Spinal Cord	Motor Function	Assessment
C6	Flexion at elbow	Have the patient flex his arms at the elbows.
C7	Extension at elbow	Have the patient extend his arms at elbows.
C7	Resistance to downward motion with hand extension	Have patient hold his arms out with hand extended and palm down. Provide support under the wrist while you push downward on the hand.
T1	Flexion of fingers	Have the patient flex his fingers.
T1	Resistance to abducted fingers	With the arm and hand extended with the palm facing downward, have the patient abduct (spread apart) the fingers. Squeeze the second and fourth fingers, attempting to push them together.
T1–T12	Intercostal and abdominal muscles	Observe the patient for inadequate ventilation effort.
L5	Dorsiflexion of the foot	Place your hands on the top of the patient's feet; have the patient pull up against them.
S1–S2	Plantar flexion of the foot	Place your hands on the bottoms of the patient's feet; have the patient push down against them.

- Place your hands on top of the feet and have the patient pull up against your hands to test dorsiflexion (tests L5).

To test the posterior column (light touch), lightly touch each hand and foot while having the patient distinguish which hand or foot is being touched. To test the spinothalamic tracts (pain), pinch each hand and foot and have the patient distinguish which hand or foot is being pinched. One recommended method is to use a cotton swab with a wooden stick. Break the stick and use the cotton swab end to test for light touch and the broken wooden end of the stick to poke the patient to elicit a pain response.

Be sure the patient's eyes are closed during the light touch and pain testing. Redundancy is built into the assessment to identify any neurologic dysfunction that may indicate the potential for an incomplete spinal injury (see Table 44-4).

EMERGENCY MEDICAL CARE

Because spinal cord tissue is basically the same as brain tissue, it is essential to establish and maintain an adequate airway, ventilation, and oxygenation. If the SpO_2 reading is less than 95 percent,

administer supplemental oxygen. If the tidal volume or respiratory rate is inadequate, provide positive pressure ventilation.

In all the following instances, the patient must be immobilized regardless of the neurologic assessment findings:

1. A significant mechanism of injury is evident.
2. The patient has an altered mental status.
3. The patient complains of pain or tenderness to the vertebral column.
4. The patient is unreliable because of intoxication, head injury, stress reaction, or other distracting injury (fractures, abdominal injury).
5. Any sensory or motor dysfunction is found during the neurologic assessment.

En route to the medical facility, initiate an intravenous line of normal saline or lactated Ringer's. A large-bore catheter is recommended in case fluid must be administered

to maintain the blood pressure. Run the fluid at a rate to maintain the systolic blood pressure at 90 mmHg or above.

If there is any suspicion that the patient is hypoglycemic, check the blood glucose level using a glucose meter (glucometer). If the BGL is less than 60 mg/dL, administer 25 grams of 50 percent dextrose in water ($D_{50}W$).

TABLE 44-4 Level of Spinal Cord Injury Correlated to Loss of Sensory Function

Level of Spinal Cord	Level of Loss of Sensation
C4	Suprasternal notch
C5	Below the clavicle
C6	Thumb
C7	Index finger
T4	Nipple line
T10	Umbilicus
L1	Femoral pulse
L4	Knee
S1	Lateral aspect of foot
S2–S4	Perianal region

TRANSITIONING

REVIEW ITEMS

1. A patient presents with bilateral loss of motor and sensory function below the nipple line. You should suspect _____.
   a. central cord syndrome
   b. unresolved spinal shock
   c. anterior cord syndrome
   d. neurogenic spinal shock

2. A patient loses the ability to feel pain to the left side of his body. You should suspect an injury to the _____.
   a. right corticospinal tract
   b. left posterior column
   c. right spinothalamic tract
   d. left cauda equina

3. A patient who has an isolated spinal cord injury to the right posterior column would present with _____.
   a. an inability to move the right side of his body
   b. a loss of pain sensation to the left side of the body

   c. a loss of vibration sensation to the left side of the body
   d. an inability to feel light touch to the right side of the body

4. A suspected spinal cord injured patient exhibits sonorous sounds on inhalation and exhalation. This may result in _____.
   a. a worsened secondary spinal cord injury
   b. a decrease in circulating carbon dioxide
   c. the need for immediate advanced airway management
   d. application of continuous positive airway pressure (CPAP)

5. An elderly patient who was involved in a minor motor vehicle crash is walking around the scene when you arrive. Following your assessment, you note that the patient has noticeable weakness to both upper extremities; however, the lower extremities have normal motor function. The patient

is able to feel light touch and pain in all four extremities. You should _____.

    a. immobilize both upper extremities with splints to prevent further movement

    b. place the patient in a position of comfort, apply a non-rebreather mask, and transport

    c. place the patient in a lateral recumbent position to prevent aspiration of blood

    d. manually stabilize the spine until you can perform full spinal immobilization

APPLIED PATHOPHYSIOLOGY

1. List the major motor and sensory tracts in the spinal cord and the general location of each.

2. Describe how to assess each of the three major sets of tracts.

3. Explain why it would be necessary to test for pain in a patient who has the ability to feel light touch.

4. Why would the patient with spinal shock possibly develop hypotension?

5. Explain the difference in the pathophysiology between hypovolemic shock and spinal shock.

6. Describe fluid administration in the spinal cord-injured patient.

CLINICAL DECISION MAKING

You arrive on the scene at a construction accident and find a 43-year-old man who fell approximately 30 feet off scaffolding. The patient landed on his side and is still in that position as you approach him. The patient appears to be alert and talking.

1. What are your initial considerations when entering the scene and approaching the patient?

2. What injuries should you suspect based on the mechanism of injury?

Following the primary assessment, you determine that the patient is alert and oriented to person, place, and time. His airway is patent. His respiratory rate is 22/minute with adequate chest rise. His radial pulse is 92/minute. His skin is warm and dry. His SpO_2 reading is 98 percent on room air. His blood pressure is 84/56 mmHg.

3. Can you identify any life threats? If so, what are they?

4. What immediate emergency care should you provide based on the primary assessment?

5. What do the vital signs indicate?

During the secondary assessment, you note abrasions to the right temporal region and a contusion to the right lateral thorax. The pupils are equal and reactive, the nose and mouth are clear, and no evidence of trauma is noted to the neck. The trachea is midline, and the jugular veins are not distended or flat. The chest is rising and falling symmetrically, and no instability is noted on palpation. The breath sounds are equal and clear bilaterally. The abdomen is soft and nontender. The pelvis is stable. The right upper and lower extremities have abrasions and contusions. The peripheral pulses are present in all four extremities.

During the neurologic exam, you note that the patient is unable to move on the right side of the body below the nipple line; however, he is able to move his hands and feet on the left side of the body. He cannot feel light touch when applied to the right side of the body; however, he is able to feel the light touch to the entire left side of the body. The patient is able to feel a pinch to the right hand and foot. Although he is able to feel light touch to the left side of the body, he is unable to feel a pinch when applied to the left hand and foot. The patient has no pertinent past medical history, takes no medications, and has no known allergies. His last oral intake was approximately two hours earlier at lunch, when he ate a sandwich and drank a soda. He explains that his fall was a result of tripping and losing his balance.

6. What condition(s) have you ruled out in your differential field impression?

7. Do you suspect a spinal cord injury? If so, what specific type? Why?

8. Explain the reason for the conflicting neurologic findings.

9. Based on your differential field diagnosis, what emergency care should you provide?

10. Would you administer fluids in this patient? If so, what fluid, at what rate, and for what reason?

Standard Trauma

Competency Applies fundamental knowledge to provide basic and selected advanced emergency care and transportation based on assessment findings for an acutely injured patient.

TOPIC

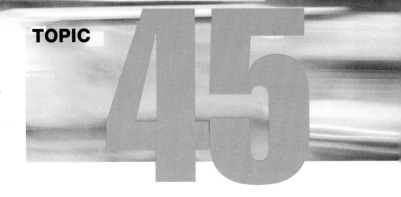

TRAUMA IN SPECIAL POPULATIONS: PEDIATRICS

INTRODUCTION

Trauma is the leading cause of death and disability in children. It is a difficult concept to grasp, but trauma is a *disease* with recognizable and predictable contributing factors, seasonality, high-risk populations and behaviors, and proven but not widely adopted prevention strategies. Injuries are responsible for more deaths of children than all other causes combined, but are only the tip of an iceberg that has huge financial and emotional effects on society from long-term disabilities. Most of the pediatric calls that EMS professionals get are because of trauma; thus it is critical to understand the anatomic and physiologic differences between children and adults.

Children have unique anatomic and physiologic characteristics that predispose them to an exaggerated and poorly adapted response to acute injuries. During the first hour following injury to a child—when poorer outcomes are significantly associated with the increasing time from injury to definitive therapy—the "golden hour" principle of adult trauma care is modified to the "platinum half-hour," which stresses the critical importance of (1) early recognition that children are less able than adults to cope with life-threatening stress and (2) the knowledge that the coping mechanisms children have are quickly exhausted.

Because of their smaller body mass and inability to withstand intense forces, children are more likely to suffer multiorgan system involvement and have multiple injuries, often including injuries to the central nervous system. In children, as in adults, the presence of shock and hypotension is the strongest predictor for increased mortality—the difference is that these two cardinal features have a quicker onset time in children and are more difficult to recognize than in adults, leading to costly treatment delays and worse outcomes.

Blunt abdominal or thoracic trauma, closed head injury, long bone fractures, or spinal cord injury can all result in severe hypotension and shock that, if unrecognized and inadequately treated, will lead to poorer outcomes, more quickly, and with higher morbidity (associated injuries and long-term disabilities) and mortality (death) compared with adults with similar injuries.

Establishing effective systems of triage, treatment protocols, and interfacility transfer policies to higher levels of care for injured children have all been shown to reduce the mortality

TRANSITION highlights

- Incidence of pediatric trauma and death.
- Normal physiologic differences between pediatric and adult patients that contribute to heightened morbidity and mortality in pediatric patients.
- Disease patterns and assessment findings common in pediatric patients.
- Maintaining the vital functions of airway, breathing, and circulation while managing pediatric trauma patients.
- Importance for the Advanced EMT to provide "organ-specific care" to the patient as well as care aimed at supporting lost function:
  - Cerebral blood flow.
  - Head, neck, and spine considerations.
  - Thoracic chest wall considerations.
  - Multiorgan system trauma.
  - Abdomen and pelvic considerations.
- General treatment strategies for the pediatric patient suffering from trauma.

and morbidity of pediatric trauma. Indeed, the outcome of a pediatric trauma victim is directly associated with the effectiveness of the trauma system he is in geographically, especially if that trauma system respects and has addressed the concept of the "platinum half-hour" with advanced prehospital pediatric emergency care, regional emergency departments equipped and trained in pediatric emergency care, and proximity to pediatric trauma centers, which may be children's hospitals with trauma care services and/or adult trauma centers with pediatric expertise.

In any event, it is essential that all EMS professionals understand and be able to identify the differences in pediatric expertise among the various hospitals in their service area.

EPIDEMIOLOGY

The burden of nonfatal injuries is enormous, with almost 10 million injuries in 2004 to the under-20-years-old population (www.cdc.gov/injury/wisqars/index.html). More than 300,000 children are hospitalized each year with trauma-related injuries. The cost of the associated morbidity on U.S. society is incalculable, as there are significant long-term rehabilitation issues, as well as neurologic impairments predisposing these children to increased risks of social and psychological sequelae. Ripple effects from acute and chronic conditions are significant and affect whole families, leading to higher divorce rates, financial burdens, and persistent behavioral concerns.

> **Because of their smaller body mass and inability to withstand intense forces, children are more likely to suffer multiorgan system involvement and have multiple injuries.**

Prevention is the most important strategy for controlling this epidemic of injury. Significant strides have been made with the adoption of mandatory seatbelt and helmet laws, increased fire safety, gun control, and education programs. Nonetheless, injury remains a significant killer and maimer of children.

Despite advances in prevention, detection, and resuscitation, the population of pediatric trauma patients continues to have the worst outcome. It is estimated that only 10 percent to 15 percent of traumatically injured children have life-threatening injuries. Despite that low figure, however, trauma is the leading cause of death for children, in no small part because medical care providers are not trained and equipped to provide a rapid and coordinated response focusing on the immediate threats to life and do not recognize the unique and sometimes subtle anatomic

> **Triage systems that pay attention to both physiologic criteria and mechanism of injury are important in the early management and referral of pediatric patients.**

and physiologic differences between children and adults.

The pattern of pediatric injuries varies with the mechanism. Because trauma encompasses everything from nonaccidental, inflicted injury to submersions and burns, the age-related differences in the incidence and outcomes vary considerably. Motor vehicle trauma accounts for the majority of injuries in the United States. Pediatrics is no exception, with more than 40 percent of injuries reported to the National Trauma Data Bank (www.facs.org/trauma/ntdb/index.html) stemming from motor vehicle crashes, 20 percent from falls, and another 10 percent from nonaccidental, inflicted injuries.

When considering motor vehicle-related trauma, pediatric patients can be either passengers or pedestrians. The term *restrained passenger* in reference to a pediatric patient is one that should be questioned closely, as it is estimated that only 15 percent of children in child safety seats are properly harnessed in correctly installed seats (www.cdc.gov/ncipc/factsheets/childpas.htm).

TRAUMA SCORING SYSTEMS AND OUTCOME

The introduction and spread of statewide trauma systems, the adoption of the American College of Surgeons' trauma center verification for hospitals, and the development of trauma registries and databases have allowed for categorization of trauma patients and increased attention to the necessary resources required for managing trauma, especially pediatric trauma.

Triage systems that pay attention to both physiologic criteria and mechanism of injury are important in the early management and referral of pediatric patients. Because trauma is a time-sensitive disease, early goal-directed therapy and prompt referral and transport of injured children to a higher level of care are critical to their survival and overall functional outcomes. In highly evolved trauma systems, triage and transport begin with prehospital EMS providers. Physicians and the public alike should insist on a high level of pediatric education and credentialing for EMS professionals, thereby creating an essential foundation that ensures optimal age-appropriate and competent resuscitation.

Trauma scoring systems are generally used for two purposes: as a tool for triage/treatment decision support or as a tool for predicting severity of illness or mortality. The triage tool should be simple and easy to calculate, but it must be accurate enough to include all patients who require a higher level of trauma services. The latter scoring system is usually more complex, using many variables, and is not considered relevant in the early resuscitation stages but is important for decision support later, for benchmarking, and for outcomes research. The most widely applied scoring system is the Glasgow Coma Scale (GCS). Modification of the GCS for pediatric patients has been an important advancement in the assessment of age-appropriate behavior in both verbal and preverbal children (see Table 45-1). As a gold standard in the rapid and early assessment of a trauma patient, it has outcome prediction value as well.

Reliability is experience dependent and can be difficult to obtain in an intubated patient; it is impossible to obtain in a sedated and/or paralyzed patient. Some studies have observed definite differences in outcome of patients with a low GCS (3–4) compared with higher (7–8) scores, whereas the middle–severe range (5–6) is less prognostic of outcome.

Multiple studies have shown that the admission GCS is more predictive of injury severity than field GCS, and the motor component has been found to be the best predictor of outcome. That said, one study observed a significant improvement in GCS in almost one-third of pediatric trauma patients who had initial GCSs between 6 and 8 following resuscitation, reminding us that (1) serial exams are more important than a single exam and (2) continual reassessment is important.

ASSESSMENT AND EMERGENCY CARE
Anatomic and Physiologic Differences in Children

"Airway, breathing, circulation" are the ABCs of resuscitation medicine and must be followed, in that order, every time. This is because children are more likely to have respiratory problems or airway complications from trauma that will respond to this approach. Failure to follow the ABCs, or "the basics," is a common error in medicine, especially in emergency and critical care, when a crisis situation may unexpectedly arise, and the untrained are

TABLE 45-1		Pediatric Glasgow Coma Scale		

		> 1 Year	< 1 Year	
Eye opening	4	Spontaneous	Spontaneous	
	3	To verbal command	To shout	
	2	To pain	To pain	
	1	No response	No response	

		> 1 Year	< 1 Year	
Best motor response	6	Obeys		
	5	Localizes pain	Localizes pain	
	4	Flexion—withdrawal	Flexion—withdrawal	
	3	Flexion—abnormal (decorticate rigidity)	Flexion—abnormal (decorticate rigidity)	
	2	Extension (decerebrate rigidity)	Extension (decerebrate rigidity)	
	1	No response	No response	

		> 5 Years	2–5 Years	0–23 Months
Best verbal response	5	Oriented and converses	Appropriate words and phrases	Smiles, coos, cries appropriately
	4	Disoriented and converses	Inappropriate words	Cries to pain
	3	Inappropriate words	Cries and/or screams	Inappropriate crying and/or screaming
	2	Incomprehensible sounds	Grunts	Grunts
	1	No response	No response	No response

caught unprepared. In the Pediatric Assessment Triangle, these ABCs have been modified to "appearance, [work of] breathing, and circulation" to incorporate the overall picture of the child as critical to one's early assessment and also to acknowledge the airway as a vital factor in the assessment of "breathing."

Understanding how blood loss can affect organ perfusion and cause shock, altered mental status, and cool and "clamped down" extremities in a pediatric patient is essential to providing responsive and lifesaving care to these patients, most of whom have injuries that are *not* life threatening initially but can rapidly become so if too much time is wasted between injury and presentation to health care providers.

Airway, Oxygenation, and Ventilation

Anatomic differences in the pediatric airway must be considered when assessing and controlling the oxygenation and ventilation of injured infants and children. The prominent forehead and occiput and relatively small midface (the area between the eyes and jaw) of the infant and child, the smaller jaw and relatively large tongue, narrow nares and lower airways that are prone to edema and secretions during injury, the high position of the vocal cords (glottis) at C2–C3 (as opposed to C5 in the adult) with anteroinferior slanting vocal cords, floppy epiglottis, and short neck all create a potentially very difficult airway to control, especially in the settings of gastric reflux, relative obesity, and aspiration.

Add to these anatomic concerns the high likelihood of traumatic brain injury, and one can easily envision how respiratory insufficiency can quickly progress to respiratory and then cardiorespiratory arrest. Thorough knowledge and appreciation of these anatomic differences in infants and children are essential for anyone managing a pediatric airway.

Breathing

Whether to control the pediatric airway with an endotracheal tube, a laryngeal mask airway, or another nonvisualized airway versus continuing with bag-mask ventilations is a hot topic in prehospital pediatric care. It cannot be overstressed that the AEMT has all the skills necessary to provide lifesaving care, and the data support the fact that good bag-mask skills are not just essential but possibly better than advanced airway skills.

As hypoxia and both hypo- and hypercarbia are major factors contributing to morbidity and mortality, patients with an altered GCS or rapidly deteriorating mental status should have their airway and

> In the Pediatric Assessment Triangle, the ABCs have been modified to "appearance, [work of] breathing, and circulation."

breathing continually assessed and their ventilation assisted. When in doubt that a pediatric patient is breathing adequately, understand that a GCS of less than 12 is not normal and that the patient may need assistance.

A GCS of 8 or 9 is an indication for endotracheal intubation by ALS providers (when allowed by protocol). Keeping your patient from deteriorating to that point will have more effect on the overall outcome than anything else you can do in the prehospital environment.

Recent literature on severely head-injured patients has shown a direct correlation between the adequacy of ventilation and survival with poorer outcomes seen on arrival to the emergency department in patients who were hyper- or hypoventilated to PETCO$_2$ < 30 or > 50 mmHg by EMS providers.

The dangers of hyperventilation are increasingly evident in the resuscitation literature; the only time it is recommended is in the setting of acute cerebral herniation. "Above all, do no harm" is our motto in medicine, and this is an important area in which to consider this. If you are assisting ventilations in your pediatric patient, be sure to keep an age-appropriate rate (infants, 0–1 year old: 30 breaths/minute; 1–6 years old: 25 breaths/minute; 6–12 years old: 20 breaths/minute; over 12 years old: 15 breaths/minute).

With assisted ventilation comes the transition from a spontaneously breathing patient to one who is now positive pressure (either mechanical or manual) ventilated. This commonly results in an alteration in the patient's cardiopulmonary status. In the hypovolemic condition commonly encountered in the traumatically injured patient, the application of positive pressure can result in a hemodynamic vise effect on the right atrium, leading to diminished atrial filling and decreased ventricular cardiac output. This vise effect, combined with overly aggressive airway pressures, can lead to pulseless electrical activity (PEA) or electromechanical dissociation (EMD), in which venous return, and thus cardiac output, is impeded from the tamponade effect of the high afterload on an underfilled right ventricle, due to high intrathoracic pressures.

The lack of pulmonary blood flow results in no left-sided filling or systemic cardiac output. The only treatment is to ensure that assisted breaths are giving just enough pressure to move the chest and to provide adequate oxygenation and ventilation while avoiding overdistention and the vise effect. In the hypotensive or potentially hemodynamically unstable trauma patient, this is essential to avoiding the "second hit" of hypotension and hypoxemia, which are major contributors to mortality and morbidity.

Circulation

The blood volume of children varies by age, with infants having up to 100 mL/kg; this figure decreases inversely with age until adolescence, when the adult 50 to 60 mL/kg blood volume is the rule. For a newborn, this volume is the equivalent of a 12-ounce can of soda; for a one-year-old child, a liter bottle of soda; for a six-year-old, a two-liter bottle.

It does not take much blood loss to put a young child in shock; early recognition of and response to shock saves more lives than anything else you can provide in the field. Once the pediatric patient is packaged safely, rapid transport to the hospital is the most important therapy we can offer in the prehospital setting.

Because the response to blood loss is to maintain cardiac output (Q) by increasing heart rate to compensate for the reduced preload, or stroke volume (the blood returning to the heart), the body must increase the vascular resistance to keep the pressure up. Putting it all together:

Blood Pressure (BP) = HR × Stroke Volume × Systemic Vascular Resistance (SVR)

To diagnose shock in the pediatric patient, one simply needs to record tachycardia above the age-related norms and recognize signs of poor perfusion (cool, pale extremities, weak pulses, altered mental status). Any child with an altered mental status—poor response to the environment, low tone, abnormal activity, weak or uncoordinated, unconscious—either has a closed head injury or, absent that possibility, is in shock.

Obtain IV access and administer up to three fluid boluses at 20 mL/kg or as directed in your protocols in response to the pediatric patient's presentation. Infants should receive boluses of 10 mL/kg. Use caution in fluid administration so the patient is not overloaded with fluid—something that is much easier done in pediatric patients than in adults. IV access should be obtained en route. Prompt transport to surgical intervention remains the definitive treatment in pediatric trauma for any level of EMS provider.

Organ-Specific Care: Cerebral Blood Flow

The acutely injured brain is highly susceptible to any second hit that disrupts perfusion and oxygenation. The same can be said for any organ; given the lack of regenerative properties of the central nervous system, however, this is the organ to target with our therapies.

Closed head injuries definitely disrupt regional (and potentially global) cerebral autoregulation, the unique ability of the cerebral vasculature to intrinsically constrict or dilate based on systemic arterial blood pressure to maintain a constant blood flow based on metabolic demands. In addition to this rheostatic autoregulation ability, cerebral vessels can constrict or dilate based on chemical influences, adjusting to carbon dioxide, oxygen, and pH levels.

The pressure-dependent autoregulation is usually the first to go in the setting of injury, and with that loss, the cerebral arterial vascular bed will either passively dilate as the blood pressure rises or constrict as the blood pressure falls. As the chemical regulatory properties usually remain intact except in areas of profound ischemia or necrosis, the need for maintenance of normoxia and normocarbia become even more important.

Head, Neck, and Spine

Pediatric pedestrians who are motor-vehicle trauma victims may suffer a pattern of injuries known as the Waddell triad, consisting of a femoral shaft fracture, intraabdominal and/or intrathoracic injuries, and a closed head injury that logically result from the three collisions that occur in succession: bumper versus leg, body versus hood, and head versus ground after being thrown. Although the incidence of all three injuries may be rare, a high index of suspicion should be maintained.

Given the disproportionately large head in children, the adage "Children lead with their heads" is an important one to remember when assessing the traumatically injured child. Head injuries are extremely common in children and may be difficult to assess. However, given that more than 80 percent of deaths from pediatric trauma are associated with severe traumatic brain injury, this needs to be at the top of any differential diagnosis of a child who is "not acting right."

An isolated closed head injury, combined with the limited developmental repertoire in children, makes these patients particularly difficult to assess. Therefore, thorough knowledge of age-appropriate developmental milestones coupled with a caretaker's report of the child's baseline functional status are the keys to accurate assessment. Use of the Pediatric Assessment Triangle, which focuses on appearance, breathing, and circulatory status, combined with the pediatric-modified GCS allows for an objective early and rapid assessment on which to base the need for intervention, consultation, and further testing.

Thermoregulation is an important factor in pediatric resuscitation; the head is a major source of this heat loss, contributing to stress and potentially affecting cardiovascular and coagulation properties. An increasing body of literature is now available regarding the use of controlled hypothermia in the setting of traumatic brain injury, but at this time no recommendations have been made for prehospital cooling in this population.

When the mechanism of injury is unknown or compatible with spinal cord injury, it is important to remember that the child's neck, being shorter and supporting a proportionately larger mass with less developed musculature, is particularly prone to spinal cord injury. For this reason, the AEMT should rapidly assess the child and the mechanism of injury, then proceed immediately with immobilization.

Spinal cord injury is more frequent in the upper cervical spine (C1–3) in children under eight years of age (as opposed to adults, in whom injury is more common in C5–7). Because of the relatively horizontal, nonstabilizing facet joints, active growth centers, and lax ligaments, lateral and rotational distraction injuries can occur without radiographic evidence (a condition called spinal cord injury without radiologic abnormality [SCIWORA]), making cervical and other spine injuries very difficult to diagnose.

Of the children presenting with spinal cord injury, half of them will have normal spine films. Thus, normal X-rays, though reassuring, cannot rule out spinal cord injury in the child. Complicating this is that when treating an unconscious or flaccid infant or child, the child must be assumed to have a high spinal cord injury until ruled out with physical exam and additional scans (MRI, helical CT). Because of the infant and young child's prominent occiput, every effort must be made to maintain neutral cervical alignment, avoiding hyperextension of the cervical spine during intubation or avoiding flexion when supine on a spine board.

Chest

An important characteristic of pediatric trauma is the fact that children can have significant solid and hollow organ damage with no external evidence or overlying fractures. The delayed ossification of the pediatric rib cage allows for blunt forces to be transmitted through the ribs onto the underlying organ, resulting in significant lung, cardiac, hepatic, splenic, or renal contusion with no radiographic findings of fractures and delayed plain radiographic findings of pulmonary contusion. For this reason, the mechanism of injury and a healthy amount of suspicion become important factors in the assessment, monitoring, and treatment of pediatric injuries.

It is well described that infants and children are 50 percent less likely to have rib fractures compared with adults, yet they are twice as likely to have intrathoracic (pulmonary or cardiac) injury with no bony abnormality, leading to twice the adult rate of lung contusion, pneumothorax, and hemothorax. This predisposes the pediatric patient to have early respiratory distress, hypoxia, and respiratory failure, given the child's anatomic differences, smaller lung volumes, and increased metabolic (energy) requirements. Early recognition and management with oxygen and rapid transfer are keys to survival and improved outcomes.

Multiorgan System Trauma

Injuries to the chest have been reported in 8 percent to 62 percent of children with multiorgan system injuries and usually result in immediate physiologic compromise, carrying a 25 percent mortality rate when associated with traumatic brain injury or abdominal trauma. Traumatic cardiac arrest holds the worst survival of all out-of-hospital arrests; there is no difference between adults and pediatric patients in this regard.

In a large sample of pediatric patients with traumatic arrests who received CPR, 24 percent survived and one-third of those survivors had a good neurologic outcome, as opposed to another study of out-of-hospital pediatric cardiac arrest in which only 8 percent survived, with only one-third of them having good neurologic outcomes. In the first study, pediatric patients who arrived with an undetectable pulse had poor outcome (4 surviving out of 269). Survival for patients with a detectable pulse and respirations on arrival to the emergency department (39 percent survival) was significantly better than survival of patients arriving apneic with a detectable pulse (19 percent).

In patients who survive long enough to arrive at the hospital alive, the injuries most highly associated with death are cardiac tamponade (70 percent), massive hemothorax (50 percent), direct cardiac injury (48 percent), injuries to the aorta and great vessels (42 percent), flail chest (40 percent), and tension pneumothorax (39 percent). Although these are often complicated by and confused with aspiration, the treatment is the same: supporting the ABCs with supplemental oxygen, assisting ventilation as needed, and close monitoring and observation.

Cardiac contusion and resulting myocardial irritability can give rise to EKG abnormalities and myocardial dysfunction that, if unrecognized, can progress rapidly to cardiovascular collapse. Hypotension that is unresponsive to fluid resuscitation may be the result of myocardial dysfunction or, due to the lax fixation of the mediastinum and propensity for more visceral shift, caused by compromise of preload or afterload. Commotio cordis is an entity that is increasingly reported as a cause of sudden traumatic cardiac

> **The AEMT should rapidly assess the child and the mechanism of injury, then proceed immediately with immobilization.**

arrest in children, caused by blunt sternal trauma and carrying a high mortality rate.

In the highly compliant chest wall of the child, the work of breathing can be amplified significantly, leading to subcostal, sternal, and supraclavicular retractions. The diaphragm is the major muscle of respiration in infants because of the lack of axillary and intercostal muscle development, but its muscle fibers are fatigue prone in the early stages of life, and its horizontal insertion is mechanically disadvantaged. Combine this with gastric distention, supine positioning, and narrow airways, and the infant is at significant risk for respiratory failure due to the increased work of breathing.

Because of the high chest wall compliance, infants and children are unable to maintain end-expiratory lung volumes, leading to lung collapse (atelectasis). Infants and children are much more prone to atelectasis than adults and, with the high potential for aspiration and/or lung contusion following trauma, their condition can change rapidly.

> **Internal abdominal injuries in the child can kill very quickly.**

It is well described that after these lung units have collapsed from underinflation (atelectasis), they require more pressure to open up once closed than they do to keep open once opened. An infant or child in distress, who is breathing rapidly and shallowly without any assisted positive pressure, is at high risk of atelectasis, especially when the condition is compounded by an altered mental status, lung contusion, and aspiration. The resulting atelectasis leads to worsening gas exchange with decreased oxygenation and ventilation (CO_2 removal).

The compensatory response to keep these lung units from collapsing is grunting, or laryngeal braking, and is an extremely costly sign of respiratory distress and an immediate precursor to respiratory failure. This anatomic mechanical disadvantage, coupled with the higher oxygen consumption per body mass, puts children under eight years of age at high risk for rapid progression to hypoxemia.

Abdomen and Pelvis

Internal abdominal injuries in the child can kill very quickly. Hepatic and splenic contusions from blunt trauma can be responsible for the child literally bleeding out into the peritoneum. Renal contusions involving the aorta and renal arteries can be quite severe as well, but most renal injuries are not as life threatening as intraperitoneal abdominal injuries.

In both peritoneal and retroperitoneal injuries, there may be no external sign of trauma (bruising, lacerations), but the patient's abdomen will be extremely tender, and there may be some abdominal distention. This can be a subtle sign, but it is a very important one that is not to be overlooked, as it means that a significant amount of fluid (blood, urine, intestinal contents) has collected already.

Abdominal distention is poorly tolerated by children because their diaphragms are so easily compromised, making the work of breathing even more difficult. Similarly, when assessing a child with suspected abdominal trauma, the child may be splinting and not taking adequate-size breaths, making it appear as if the child is in mild or moderate respiratory distress, which again is not a clue to be overlooked but instead is one to be

acted on: Transport the child as soon as it is safe to do so.

Eviscerating and penetrating trauma is fairly rare in pediatric patients but is treated as it would be in adults, with rapid assessment, stabilization, and transfer. Any vomiting of blood or bile should be a clue for significant abdominal trauma; the AEMT should suspect lower thoracic or lumbar spine injuries in children as well. Pelvic fractures can be quite severe and, because of the high risk for large vessel injuries (iliac and femoral arteries and veins), should be suspected in an immobile patient who has a high degree of pain with movement.

Because young children may be preverbal and unable to tell you where it hurts, it is critical that the AEMT be able to read their signs and interpret their actions and inactions, as those may be the only clues to what is bothering them. Diagnosing abdominal injury is one of the greatest challenges in pediatric medicine.

Skeletal Injuries

Skeletal injuries are the most common traumatic injuries to young and school-age children; they require medical attention even though they are rarely life threatening. The ability of a child to generate forces sufficient to cause a long-bone fracture is directly related to size and ability to get around. Toddlers are the youngest patients in whom accidental fractures are seen, as toddlers are ambulatory and can climb. Trauma in infants is very likely to be inflicted by others; therefore, the scene should be treated as a crime scene until proven otherwise. Keeping to fact-based, unbiased, and thorough documentation by the AEMT is of vital importance.

TRANSITIONING • • • • • • • •

REVIEW ITEMS

1. The leading cause of death of children is from trauma associated with _____.
   a. nonaccidental (inflicted) injuries
   b. falls
   c. motor vehicle crashes
   d. bicycle crashes

2. Factors associated with worse outcomes in pediatric trauma are _____.
   a. long-bone fractures (e.g., femur)
   b. abdominal injuries
   c. hypotension and hypoxia
   d. pelvic fractures

3. Children's lungs are more prone to collapse (atelectasis) because of children's _____.
   a. highly compliant chest wall
   b. retained secretions
   c. weak cough
   d. small airways

4. Abdominal trauma in children is poorly recognized primarily because _____.
   a. children cannot communicate their injuries to caretakers
   b. children can mask the signs and symptoms well
   c. children tolerate shock well
   d. medical providers are poorly trained to read the signs and symptoms

APPLIED PATHOPHYSIOLOGY

1. Explain the following equation:

$$BP = Cardiac\ Output \times SVR$$
$$where\ Cardiac\ Output = HR \times Stroke\ Volume$$

2. Describe the signs of shock in a child.

3. Describe the Pediatric Assessment Triangle.

4. Explain the signs of altered mental status.

CLINICAL DECISION MAKING

You are called for a 7-year-old male patient who is complaining of abdominal pain after hitting a tree while riding his bicycle. You suspect that his handlebars turned as he crashed. He has no head injury, no neck pain, and no loss of consciousness but is having trouble catching his breath, is tearful, and reports that his pain is the "worst ever felt." His heart rate is 170/minute, and his radial pulse feels thready. His respiratory rate is 35/minute. His arms are cool and skin looks mottled. He will not lie flat because of the pain in his "stomach."

1. Is this child in shock?

2. What do you suspect his injury is?

3. What is your priority in management of this condition?

The child's mother arrives on scene and offers more medical history: He had hernia surgery as an infant, has multiple environmental allergies, and recently has not been feeling well. During this time, your patient moves from a sitting position to lying down and seems to fall asleep. He becomes difficult to arouse, and you notice he is very clammy and pale. His abdomen is distended.

4. What is your priority now?

TOPIC

Standard Trauma

Competency Applies fundamental knowledge to provide basic and selected advanced emergency care and transportation based on assessment findings for an acutely injured patient.

TRAUMA IN SPECIAL POPULATIONS: GERIATRICS

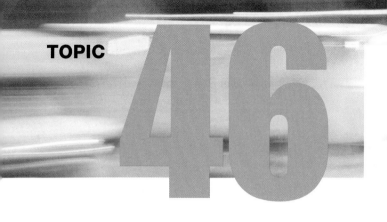

TRANSITION highlights

- Shifting population demographics of older Americans to an increasing size of the overall population.

- Incidence rates for geriatric trauma and death, as well as utilization of health care and EMS.

- Pathophysiologic changes that accompany injuries in the geriatric patient:
  - Brain trauma.
  - Neck trauma.
  - Spinal trauma.
  - Thoracic trauma.
  - Abdominal trauma.
  - Musculoskeletal trauma.
  - Burn trauma.

- Early and late assessment findings with various specific types of injury patterns in the geriatric population.

- Current treatment strategies for the geriatric patient suffering from trauma.

INTRODUCTION

Generally, when EMS providers receive a trauma call, almost automatically the first question in their mind is "What is the mechanism of injury?" as if the answer "penetrating trauma" or "blunt trauma" is the best descriptor of what to think or do. Although many times in EMS education we classify trauma this way, a more important criterion is, "How old is the patient?" If the answer is older than 65 years of age, then that becomes a much more important determinant of how and what is done for the patient than the type of trauma (or mechanism of injury) into which they best fit.

Age alone, however, may not be the best descriptor of a geriatric patient. Take, for example, a 60-year-old man with a history of chronic obstructive pulmonary disease (COPD). This patient will have a different response to thoracic trauma than a 60-year-old man without COPD. Therefore, beyond the patient's age, also consider the patient's ability to withstand trauma from a hemodynamic event and what ability the body has to repair itself.

Generally, if a patient has a chronic medical condition typically associated with the elderly (cardiovascular disease [CVD], hypertension, myocardial infarction [MI], COPD, congestive heart failure [CHF], osteoporosis, diabetes, and the like), or if a patient simply looks older than 65 because of difficult life experiences prior to this event, the AEMT may also want to treat that patient as a geriatric trauma patient. A single preexisting medical condition raises the mortality from any specific injury by 30 percent, and two or more preexisting conditions increase the expected mortality by 60 percent. Failure to make this distinction and failure to consider the special challenges of the geriatric population may lead EMS to cause more harm than good. Many times assessment and treatment steps are based on research done on younger adult patients, who anatomically and physiologically are not the same as geriatric patients.

Simply put, the Advanced EMT must reconsider the assessment approach and management techniques when faced with a geriatric trauma patient.

EPIDEMIOLOGY

Geriatric patients (those 65 years of age or older) numbered almost 40 million in 2008. This represented 12.8 percent of the U.S. population, or about one in every eight Americans. By 2030, this number will almost double, to more than 71 million elderly people. People over 65 years of age represented 12.4 percent of the population in 2000 and are expected to grow to 20 percent of the population by 2030.

Although the U.S. numbers are not universal, most other developed countries are seeing a similar trend. People over age 65 disproportionately use ambulance services and health care facilities. Even though the elderly are only roughly 12 percent of the population, they account for more than 36 percent of all

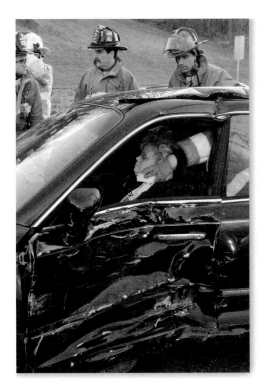

Figure 46-1 Motor vehicle collisions are the second-leading cause of accidental death, after falls, in the geriatric population. (© *Mark C. Ide*)

ambulance transports and 25 percent of hospitalizations.

Falls account for the majority of injuries in the geriatric population. The most common resulting injuries from falls are hip fractures, femur fractures, wrist fractures, and head injuries. Although falls do not produce serious injuries most of the time, geriatric falls account for 75 percent of all fall-related deaths.

Complicating the hospitalization, rehabilitation, and recovery from falls is *post-fall syndrome*. This is a sequence of events in which a geriatric patient falls and is admitted to the hospital for treatment and rehabilitation. On returning home, the patient loses confidence about moving around the home and assumes a more sedentary lifestyle. With this inactivity, muscles atrophy, bones weaken, joints become stiffer, and so on. This then leaves the patient at greater risk of a more serious fall in the future. In fact, the largest predictor of falls in the geriatric population is a history of a previous fall. The causes of falls are fairly evenly divided between intrinsic causes, such as dizziness or syncope, and extrinsic causes, such as tripping on a rug or slipping on ice.

Motor vehicle collisions (MVCs) are the second-leading cause of accidental death, after falls, in the geriatric population

(▶ Figure 46-1). Even though the elderly drive fewer miles than those in the younger age bracket and tend to drive closer to home, they have a death rate that is three times that of patients age 25 years per 100,000 population.

Following MVC deaths, the next most common cause of accidental death in the geriatric population is auto-versus-pedestrian accidents, which carry the highest fatality rate of any specific mechanism. Accidental burns (both contact and inhalation) account for about 8 percent of geriatric deaths, followed by penetration injuries (usually from attempted suicide).

PATHOPHYSIOLOGY

Topic 52, "Geriatrics," contains an important discussion of the changes in anatomy and physiology of the body due to aging. In tandem with this are the effects of pathologic conditions that further alter body physiology and the response of the body to trauma. All these variables must be taken into consideration when dealing with traumatized geriatric patients.

Head and Brain Trauma

Head trauma is of particular concern in the geriatric population. Beyond the briskness of hemorrhage from scalp lacerations that can bleed significantly because of poor vasoconstriction from vascular disease is the increased incidence of concurrent brain trauma. During the aging process the brain will atrophy, causing a void between the brain and skull within the cranium. This space will initially be filled with extra cerebrospinal fluid (CSF). Along with the shrinking brain tissue will be a stretching of the bridging vessels between the brain and skull.

When the geriatric patient sustains head trauma, the brain can actually shift within the cranial vault, which, in turn, tears blood vessels, resulting in epidural and, particularly, subdural hematomas. Unlike the younger patient with a cerebral bleed who will demonstrate symptoms more readily, in the geriatric patient the blood will continue to collect in the space left by the atrophied brain for a longer time before the patient becomes symptomatic for the head injury. In fact, enough time may pass between the initial injury and the symptoms of altered mental status or significant headache that the patient (and the family or care providers) may not recall the history of a fall or some other mechanism of injury.

In addition, assessment of the pupils may not yield reliable findings of brain herniation, as a large percentage of geriatric patients have a concurrent ophthalmic condition, such as cataracts, asymmetric pupils, or changes in light reflex from either ophthalmologic medications or other preexisting conditions. Complicating this in the geriatric patient as well may be organic brain syndromes, which will make gathering a reliable history of the patient's mental status more challenging.

> **Falls account for the majority of injuries in the geriatric population.**

> **Head trauma is of particular concern in the geriatric population.**

Neck Trauma

Neck injuries are also common in patients with a history of either head or chest wall trauma (▶ Figure 46-2). In geriatric patients sensory perception is diminished, and they may not complain of neck pain

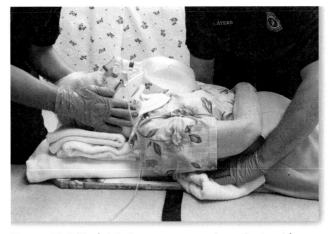

Figure 46-2 Neck injuries are common in patients with a history of either head or chest wall trauma.

> **The ribs become much more brittle and easier to break in the geriatric patient.**

despite the presence of an actual injury to the vertebrae. The absence of neck pain in a geriatric patient, with or without tenderness on palpation, is not a sufficient criterion for ruling out cervical trauma. It has been noted in the elderly population that high cervical fractures (i.e., C1 and C2) are possible, if not probable, with even a "minimal" mechanism of injury, such as a fall from a standing position. This fact should be recalled for any geriatric victim who is found in a lying position on the floor (or in a bed) when there is not a clear history of no traumatic incident.

Spinal Trauma

Degenerative changes in the spinal column from osteoporosis or spondylosis can alter the strength and structure of the vertebrae. Arthritic "spurs" can narrow the spinal canal and the exiting points for the spinal nerves, ultimately increasing the pressure on the nerves and the spinal cord itself. Further damage to the spinal column from trauma can easily shatter vertebrae, causing increased likelihood of cord trauma (compression or laceration) and spinal nerve root damage. The presence of kyphosis or scoliosis in the spine also increases the likelihood of spinal and cord trauma and poses an additional complication when trying to immobilize the patient properly. Anterior cord syndrome is seen almost exclusively in the elderly population.

As mentioned, because the geriatric patient commonly has diminished sensory capability, there may be either no complaint of pain despite an injury being present or a minimal amount of pain that is out of proportion with the significance of the injury.

> **Osteoporosis is the most common concurrent disease state contributing to bone weakness and fractures.**

Thoracic Trauma

The aging process is particularly hard on the thoracic cage and pulmonary system. The ribs become much brittler and easier to break in the geriatric patient

because of osteoporosis and the calcification of the costosternal and costovertebral joints. Furthermore, age-related changes to the underlying normal lung physiology result in diminished vital capacity, weaker respiratory musculature, and diminished efficiency at exchanging oxygen and carbon dioxide across the alveoli to the perialveolar capillary membranes. With what may seem to be a minimal mechanism of injury to the chest, the resultant rib fractures and pulmonary contusions can severely hamper the effectiveness of the respiratory system. The mortality for a geriatric patient with even a single rib injury can be as high as 12 percent.

Added to this are the detrimental effects of chronic lung conditions—emphysema, asthma, chronic bronchitis, cancer, and others—that are more common in the elderly. The resultant efficiency of the respiratory system may not have the compensatory mechanisms needed to overcome this pulmonary insult, and the patient's respiratory status can fail rapidly. The provision of positive pressure ventilation in the geriatric patient may also become problematic due to the lower airway pressures needed to cause barotrauma.

Abdominal Trauma

Because of the effects of aging and concurrent disease states, abdominal trauma is yet another condition that will likely present differently in the geriatric patient than it would in a younger patient. Because of the brittle nature of the ribs and the atrophy of abdominal musculature, the liver and spleen are more likely to be injured from blunt trauma because of a lack of protection. The resulting hemorrhage from these organs may go unnoticed because of the general lack of pain perceived by the geriatric patient and the inability of the cardiovascular system to mount a tachycardic response, which is common in younger patients suffering from internal bleeding.

Blood pressure, another measure that is used to gauge the efficiency of the cardiovascular system, may be misleading for internal bleeding because the systolic pressure may still be within a "normal" range, but in the geriatric patient this could actually represent hypotension because the patient's preinjury blood pressure may typically be higher because of a history of hypertension. Medications

(mainly beta blockers) may also diminish the heart rate response seen with blood loss. If the AEMT waits for either tachycardia or hypotension in the geriatric patient with abdominal trauma and internal bleeding, it could result in catastrophic consequences.

Musculoskeletal Trauma

In the geriatric patient, a drop in the amount of fat (adipose) tissue is relative to body weight, which leaves bones more susceptible to injury. Compounding this is the cartilaginous support of the skeletal system: With aging, it loses its adaptive capabilities and cannot flex as efficiently and, thus, is more likely to break when stressed. The presence of fat pads that are normally found around bony prominences diminishes and contributes not only to bedsores (pressure ulcers) in the bedridden patient but also to a higher likelihood of skeletal trauma with falls and other traumatic mechanisms.

As mentioned previously, falls account for a large percentage of the musculoskeletal trauma seen in the geriatric population. Osteoporosis, as a risk factor, is the most common concurrent disease state contributing to bone weakness and fractures. Hip fractures are the most common serious injury secondary to a fall, followed in significance and frequency by fractures of the femur, pelvis, tibia, and upper extremities. Even an isolated fracture can become life threatening to the geriatric patient, as the loss of tissue turgor and the negative effects of atherosclerotic changes to the vasculature can result in significant blood loss into the muscle compartment.

Burn Trauma

To provide a complete discussion of geriatric trauma, burn trauma must also be mentioned. As stated previously, burn trauma is the fourth-leading cause of death in the geriatric population. The effect of aging on the integumentary system plays a significant role in contributing to the seriousness of a burn. The geriatric patient has thinner epidermal and dermal layers of the skin, and with a diminution of the subcutaneous layer as well, with geriatric exposure to a heat load (be it thermal, chemical, electrical, or radiation), exponentially more damage occurs to the skin and underlying structures. There is a linear increase in mortality for burn injuries based on age only.

Burn shock, which results from the loss of intravascular proteins and fluid shifting, typically does not occur in the younger patient unless 20 percent to 25 percent of total body surface area is affected by either partial-thickness burns or full-thickness burns. In geriatric patients, however, the changes in physiology, compounded by the presence of underlying disease states, result in the development of burn shock with much lower body surface involvement.

The geriatric patient is also at greater risk of airway closure and respiratory failure from inhalation injuries. The elderly patient will develop significant edema around the glottic opening from inhalation of superheated air, causing airway closure, and will sustain tracheal, bronchial, and alveolar damage, which results in the inability to ventilate the alveoli and diminishes the exchange of gases at the alveolar level. The end result is early and rapid failure of the airway and pulmonary system. Naturally, the presence of chronic lung or cardiovascular disease states will only hasten and worsen the injury patterns seen.

ASSESSMENT FINDINGS

Assessment findings of trauma for geriatric patients exhibit some similarities, as well as some dissimilarities, with those for the younger adult. In remaining consistent with the aforementioned body location approach to geriatric trauma, Table 46-1 identifies common manifestations of trauma, with some delineation and differentiation on early versus late findings. In all the considerations listed in this table, the consistent feature assumed is that the AEMT has collected a detailed patient history and completed a thorough physical assessment to uncover these findings. Please remember that certain clinical conditions are very insidious in the geriatric patient, and the AEMT must remain vigilant during the assessment phase. Also remember that the older the patient and the more concurrent chronic conditions the patient has, the faster the progression from early clinical findings to late clinical findings and ultimate death.

Although Table 46-1 is not meant to be all-inclusive for all findings that may be present for each injury state, it is designed to provide a functional

TABLE 46-1	Common Manifestations of Trauma in Geriatric Patients	
Trauma Location	Earlier Clinical Findings	Later Clinical Findings
Head/brain trauma	• Scalp trauma • Facial contusions • Hematomas • Hemorrhage	• Headache • Altered mental status • Vital sign changes • Seizures
Neck trauma	• Limited motion • Discomfort • Vertebral deformity • Soft tissue trauma • Sensorimotor deficits • Hoarseness	• Vital sign changes • Expanding hematoma • Progressive paralysis • Dyspnea • Muscle spasms
Spinal trauma	• Vertebral deformity • Discomfort • Soft tissue trauma • Limited motion • Sensorimotor deficits	• Paralysis • Vital sign changes • Dyspnea • Altered mentation
Thoracic trauma	• Soft tissue trauma • Flailed segments • Tachypnea • Dyspnea • Unequal breath sounds • Decreased breath sounds	• Dyspnea/apnea • Decreased oximetry • Tachypnea/bradypnea • Unequal breath sounds • Absent breath sounds • Vital sign changes
Abdominal trauma	• Soft tissue trauma • Abdominal guarding • Expanding hematomas • Pain/discomfort • Dyspnea	• Abdominal rigidity • Abdominal guarding • Vital sign changes • Severe dyspnea • Distended abdomen
Musculoskeletal trauma	• Obvious deformity • Soft tissue trauma • Limited motion • Discomfort/pain	• Absent distal pulses • Absent sensory • Vital sign changes • Altered mental status
Burn trauma	• Superficial burns • Partial-thickness burns • Full-thickness burns • Discomfort/pain • Dyspnea (airway burn) • Dyspnea (chest burn)	• Loss of motion • Vital sign changes • Altered mental status • Stridor (airway burn) • Dyspnea or apnea • Vital sign changes • Pulmonary edema (ARDS)

knowledge base to enable the AEMT to ascertain the significance of the traumatic event. It is of utmost importance that the AEMT keep in mind that because of the effects of aging, pathologic findings, and concurrent medications, the presentation of trauma is different in the geriatric patient than in the younger adult. In addition, the relative absence of robust compensatory mechanisms in the elderly will allow the clinical progression from stable to unstable to occur extremely rapidly.

Although not an assessment step per se, part of recognizing and managing trauma in the geriatric population includes notification of the receiving facility as early as possible. Have a lower threshold for transporting a geriatric trauma patient to a trauma center. If transporting the patient to a facility with an in-house trauma team, consider activating the team. Aggressive management of the geriatric trauma patient is associated with minimized complications and overall improved outcomes. Consider the patient's mechanism of injury, the patient's age and concurrent medical conditions, the current clinical status of the patient, transport times, local protocols, and medical control when determining the receiving facility.

EMERGENCY CARE

The assessment and management of a geriatric trauma patient must be appropriate for the situation, specific for the injury, efficient in its rendering, and thorough in its completeness to realize the best possible scenario for the patient's survival. Geriatric trauma is often debilitating and too often fatal. The skills performed by the on-scene AEMT will have just as great an impact on survivability as any treatment that will be rendered in the hospital setting:

1. **Ensure inline immobilization.** Recall that kyphosis, scoliosis, and other skeletal anomalies may make the fitting of a cervical collar impossible. Be creative by using rolled towels and tape for a makeshift collar if necessary.

2. **Maintain patency of the airway.** Geriatric patients may have previous dental work that can complicate airway maintenance. Constantly assess and reassess the patency of the airway and provide suctioning as needed for secretions, vomitus, or hemorrhage. If sonorous airway sounds cannot be relieved by positioning or manual airway maneuvers, consider the insertion of an oropharyngeal airway or a nasopharyngeal airway to help keep the tongue off the posterior pharynx.

3. **Ensure adequacy of breathing.** Secondary to head, cervical, thoracic, or multisystem trauma, the breathing mechanics and strength of the respiratory muscles can easily fatigue and fail. Note the patient's speech patterns and quality of alveolar breath sounds if he is conscious to help guide the need for positive pressure ventilation (PPV). If the patient is unconscious, assess the chest wall excursion and quality of alveolar breath sounds to determine whether PPV is needed. Seal any open chest wounds with an occlusive dressing, and stabilize any flailed segment with a bulky dressing. If breathing is adequate, apply oxygen via a nonrebreather mask or nasal cannula, depending on the status of the patient. If breathing is inadequate, provide high-flow oxygen in conjunction with PPV (always ventilate gently to lower the chances for barotraumas). Provide supplemental oxygen to all geriatric trauma victims.

4. **Support cardiovascular function.** Any external hemorrhage should be treated immediately with direct pressure. Assess the quality of peripheral perfusion by the quality of the skin findings and peripheral pulses. The heart rate in a geriatric patient may not become tachycardic in response to hypoxia or hypovolemia because of cardiac disease and concurrent medications. Remember also that what may be a normal blood pressure in a younger adult may actually be hypotension in a geriatric patient with underlying hypertension. Management of hypoperfusion includes the administration of high-flow oxygen, proper patient positioning, and maintaining normothermia.

5. **Administer IV fluids according to protocol and patient presentation,** keeping in mind that geriatric patients may have preexisting conditions (e.g., congestive heart failure) that can be worsened by excess fluid administration. Administer fluids cautiously, and monitor lung sounds and respiratory status frequently during transport.

Management of other issues, such as soft tissue injuries, musculoskeletal trauma, and the like, should follow the same treatment principles as in other trauma victims. It is important to note again that full spinal immobilization of the patient may need to be modified because of the presence of skeletal deformity from kyphosis, scoliosis, osteoarthritis, and other skeletal diseases.

Constantly reassess the patient's airway, breathing, and circulatory components en route to the hospital, and ensure the quality of the ongoing interventions. Consider ALS backup with significant geriatric trauma patients, and notify the receiving facility as early as possible.

In conclusion, thousands of geriatric patients are victims of accidental trauma and traumatic injuries. The AEMT, always first on the scene, has the opportunity and responsibility to ensure that a rapid and thorough interview and assessment are performed so treatment decisions will have a positive impact on the patient and ensure an optimal patient outcome. To do this, the AEMT must remain abreast of changes in geriatric curricula, injury presentation, emergency management, and destination protocols to the appropriate facility.

TRANSITIONING

REVIEW ITEMS

1. Which of the following factors is most contributory to hip fractures in a geriatric fall victim?
   - a. osteoporosis
   - b. failing eyesight
   - c. joint stiffening
   - d. weight gain

2. A 78-year-old female patient has wrecked her car, has injured her sternum, and is complaining of respiratory distress. Of the following factors, which one would be most contributory should she go into respiratory failure?
   - a. weakening of the abdominal musculature
   - b. diminution of the number of functional alveoli
   - c. drop in carbon dioxide levels from hyperventilation
   - d. loss of strength and coordination of respiratory muscles

3. When providing mechanical ventilation to an elderly trauma victim in severe respiratory distress, why should the AEMT ventilate slowly with low airway pressures?
   - a. Failure to do so will result in inadequate oxygenation.
   - b. Geriatric patients are more susceptible to barotrauma.
   - c. It avoids the likelihood of wiping out the breathing reflex.
   - d. It prevents accidental overventilation.

4. An elderly female patient has been assaulted and beaten during a robbery. You find her unresponsive on the floor. Her vital signs are blood pressure 108/78, heart rate 94 beats per minute, and respiratory rate 26. She has two stab wounds to the abdomen, which is distended and rigid, and she has an open fracture of the radius and ulna, which is not actively bleeding. Pupils are unresponsive to light. The pulse oximeter reads 90 percent on room air. Of the following, which would be most contributory to acute deterioration?

    a. possible head injury

    b. the long bone fracture

    c. occult bleeding in the abdomen

    d. respiratory failure

5. Why would a geriatric patient be more likely than a younger adult to suffer a brain injury secondary to head trauma?

    a. because of atrophy of the brain and accumulation of blood in the subdural cavity

    b. because the geriatric patient is clumsier than the younger adult

    c. because medications that the geriatric patient is taking tend to make the brain bleed more easily

    d. because the geriatric patient is typically hypertensive, which makes the blood vessels rupture

6. A 78-year-old male patient has fallen in his bathroom while getting out of the shower, landing on his side on a tile floor.

Given this mechanism, what is the most likely significant injury he may sustain?

    a. fractured clavicle from falling on outstretched hand

    b. abdominal trauma with hidden internal bleeding

    c. pulmonary contusion with resultant dyspnea

    d. hip fracture or dislocation

7. Normal or expected early findings of hypoperfusion are typically absent in geriatric patients because _____.

    a. they typically cannot sustain tachycardia due to cardiac disease or medications

    b. owing to the effects of aging, geriatric patients are often hypotensive anyway

    c. it is too difficult to obtain accurate vital signs in the geriatric population

    d. the systolic pressure in geriatric patients tends not to decrease until significant blood loss has occurred

8. In a geriatric patient with a history of head trauma, the AEMT identifies unequal pupils. Why may this not be an accurate indication of a brain injury?

    a. because the geriatric pupil needs more intense light to respond

    b. because geriatric pupils normally do not constrict to light

    c. because of the possible presence of cataracts

    d. because of deterioration of the optic region of the brain

APPLIED PATHOPHYSIOLOGY

Family members have noticed that their elderly grandfather is not acting "normal." They summon EMS, and on your arrival you determine that the patient's mental status is diminished. Vital signs are normal, and the pulse oximeter is 97 percent on room air. The family stated that about a week ago they got home and found him lying on the floor, where he had fallen, in the kitchen. Because he was fine then, they didn't call for an ambulance.

1. What is the most likely cause for this patient's deterioration a week or so after the incident?

2. Discuss the problems with trying to obtain a good baseline mental status on geriatric patients.

3. Discuss why vital signs in a geriatric patient may not be truly representative of the underlying physiologic status.

4. For the following injuries, identify how the aging process changes the presentation of common injuries as seen in the geriatric patient.

    a. Head/brain trauma

    b. Thoracic trauma

    c. Neck and spinal trauma

    d. Musculoskeletal trauma

5. Why may pupil inequality found in a geriatric head trauma patient not be representative of the degree of actual brain injury present?

CLINICAL DECISION MAKING

You are called to an extended-care facility where a geriatric patient with Alzheimer disease was able to walk out an unlocked door and escape into the wooded area behind the facility. After about four hours, the patient was located by the local fire department at the foot of a ridge from which he apparently had fallen. The fire department personnel extricated the patient to your location using a Stokes basket. The patient is not currently immobilized, he appears unresponsive, his clothes look wet and cold, and dried blood is visible on the side of his head.

1. Based on this brief history, what would be at least three etiologies for this patient's unresponsiveness?

The primary assessment reveals the patient to be responsive to noxious stimuli with nonpurposeful motion. The airway is patent, but breathing is slow at 8 per minute, with minimal chest wall excursion and no alveolar breath sounds. The soft tissue trauma to the head is not actively bleeding anymore, and the pulse is found to be diminished peripherally with a rate of 89 beats per minute. The skin is cold to the touch, capillary refill is delayed, and you have noted that the patient's right leg is angulated awkwardly at the mid-femur location. The pulse oximeter reads 78 percent.

2. Would this patient be considered a high or low priority?

3. What action should the AEMT take to initially care for this patient?

After managing the situation described, you continue with your secondary assessment. You find the pupils to be unequal in size, but cataracts are present. A depressed right temporal skull fracture has an overlying laceration. The airway remains clear, breathing is now adequate, and peripheral perfusion has not changed. Your assessment of the injured leg reveals a suspected midshaft closed fracture of the femur.

4. How else could you confirm that the patient has a brain injury from the fall, as he also has cataracts?

5. Explain why the vital signs may be misleading regarding the degree of instability this patient may be experiencing.

6. Identify the appropriate treatment for this patient given his age, injuries, and present clinical status.

7. What would be key indicators of patient improvement with treatment?

8. What would be key indicators of deterioration with treatment?

Standard Trauma

Competency Applies fundamental knowledge to provide basic and selected advanced emergency care and transportation based on assessment findings for an acutely injured patient.

TOPIC

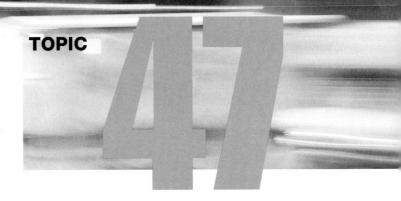

47

TRAUMA IN SPECIAL POPULATIONS: PREGNANCY

INTRODUCTION

Pregnant patients who are involved in trauma pose a special challenge in that Advanced EMTs must care for two patients at one time. Trauma to a pregnant woman, whether severe or minor, can have significant effects on both maternal and fetal health.

EPIDEMIOLOGY

Trauma occurs in approximately 6 percent to 7 percent of all pregnancies and is the leading cause of death for pregnant women. The morbidity and mortality of the patient depend in part on the mechanism of injury, gestational age of the fetus, and severity of the trauma. It is estimated that 1 percent to 3 percent of minor traumas involving pregnant women result in fetal loss and that 41 percent of fetuses die when the mother suffers a life-threatening injury. Approximately 8 percent of pregnant female trauma patients do not know they are pregnant.

Motor vehicle collisions account for more than 50 percent of all the injuries sustained by pregnant trauma patients. Maternal death is the primary cause of fetal death following a motor

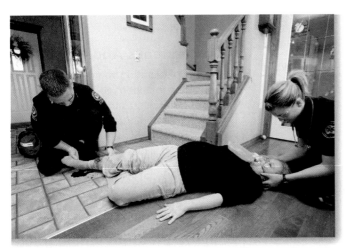

Figure 47-1 Pregnant women may sustain all types of trauma and are especially susceptible to falls and physical abuse.

TRANSITION highlights

- Incident rates at which pregnant females are traumatized, and the most common mechanisms of injury causing the trauma.

- Normal anatomic and physiologic variations in the pregnant woman.

- Complications that can occur from trauma in the pregnant woman:
  - Uterine contractions.
  - Preterm labor.
  - Spontaneous abortion.
  - Abruptio placentae.
  - Uterine rupture.
  - Penetrating trauma.
  - Pelvic fractures.
  - Hemorrhage and shock.
  - Cardiopulmonary arrest.

- Assessment findings with various specific types of injury patterns in the traumatized pregnant patient.

- Current treatment strategies for the pregnant patient.

vehicle collision. Pregnant women, especially those after their 20th week, are prone to falling because of physiologic changes they experience (▶ Figure 47-1). About 2 percent of pregnant women sustain repeated blows to the abdomen because they have fallen more than once. Approximately 4 percent to 17 percent of pregnant women will experience physical abuse, which is most often initiated by their husbands or boyfriends.

Gunshot wounds and stab wounds are the most frequent causes of penetrating trauma to this population. Penetrating trauma to the abdomen alone accounts for approximately 36 percent of overall maternal mortality. Penetrating trauma directly to the uterus has a 67 percent fetal death rate.

ANATOMY AND PHYSIOLOGY

Various anatomic and physiologic changes occur during pregnancy (▶ Figure 47-2). These changes can influence how the patient presents in the prehospital environment.

> **The most common complication resulting from traumatic injury in the pregnant patient is uterine contractions.**

Several cardiovascular changes occur in the pregnant woman. The total blood volume is increased by about 25 percent. There is a decrease in the patient's total peripheral resistance during the first two months of pregnancy. This change precipitates a gradual decline of about 2 to 4 mmHg in the systolic pressure and a decline of 5 to 15 mmHg in the patient's diastolic pressure. The woman's blood pressure will return to almost a normal prepregnancy level by the third trimester.

An increase in estrogen levels results in a 10- to 15-beat-per-minute increase in the patient's heart rate, as well as a 30 percent to 50 percent increase in cardiac output. Blood flow to the pregnant patient's uterus increases from 60 mL/min prepregnancy to 600 mL/min by the third trimester. These cardiovascular changes can mask the signs of shock in the trauma patient.

Other anatomic and physiologic changes occur in the pregnant woman's other body systems. The diaphragm gradually elevates 4 cm upward into the thoracic cavity, which contributes to an increase in oxygen consumption and may result in hyperventilation. The abdominal viscera are pushed upward and stretched, making injury to the bowel more likely. This change may also desensitize the patient's perception of pain, despite the severity of an abdominal injury. A decrease in gastrointestinal motility and an increase in acid production make the patient prone to aspirating and vomiting.

The uterus grows throughout the pregnancy and rises out of the pelvis into the abdominal area. The woman's bladder is also displaced into the abdominal cavity. The renal blood flow is also increased. The pelvic joints are loosened, and the woman's center of gravity changes, which can make her prone to accidents and falls.

The patient's presentation may be influenced by the gestational age and size of the fetus. The growing uterus and fetus can compress the patient's vena cava, which may result in supine hypotensive syndrome. When the compression of the vena cava occurs, the patient's cardiac output can be decreased by 28 percent, which causes a reduction in the patient's systolic blood pressure of about 30 mmHg. This reduction in venous blood flow can lead to signs and symptoms of shock if left untreated.

COMPLICATIONS OF TRAUMA

Some of the most frequent complications resulting from traumatic injury to the pregnant patient are described here.

Uterine Contractions

The most common complication resulting from traumatic injury in the pregnant patient is uterine contractions. These contractions may progress into preterm labor. The frequency, strength, and duration of these contractions should be assessed, monitored, and documented.

Preterm Labor

Preterm labor is defined as labor occurring before the 37th week of gestation. For a fetus to be viable, it must be at least at 24 weeks of gestation. The longer the fetus remains in the mother, the better are its chances of survival.

Spontaneous Abortion

Blunt or penetrating traumatic injuries can result in spontaneous abortion if the injury occurs before the 20th week of gestation. The most common signs and symptoms include abdominal pain or cramping as well as vaginal bleeding.

Abruptio Placentae

Abruptio placentae, resulting mostly from blunt trauma experienced during pregnancy, accounts for 50 percent to 70 percent of fetal losses. Abruptio placentae is the

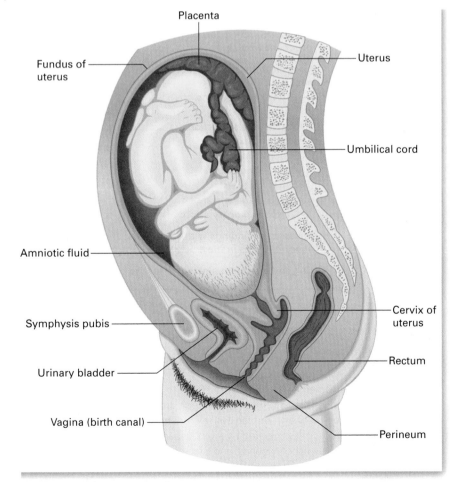

Placenta
Fundus of uterus
Uterus
Umbilical cord
Amniotic fluid
Cervix of uterus
Symphysis pubis
Rectum
Urinary bladder
Vagina (birth canal)
Perineum

Figure 47-2 The anatomy of pregnancy.

separation of the placenta from the uterine wall and can be either partial or complete in nature. The gas exchange between the mother and fetus is inhibited, and intrauterine hemorrhaging can occur with—or, more commonly, without—external hemorrhaging. Signs and symptoms associated with this condition are maternal abdominal pain, uterine tenderness, vaginal bleeding, and hypovolemia.

Uterine Rupture

Uterine rupture occurs in less than 1 percent of pregnant trauma victims. The most common cause is severe blunt force trauma to the abdomen. Uterine rupture often presents with maternal shock and palpable fetal parts inside the abdomen. It is one of the most fatal complications for the mother and fetus.

Penetrating Trauma

Penetrating trauma also can result in fetal injury or death. The size of the uterus may help shield the mother against some abdominal injuries, but it puts the fetus at greater risk for injury. The location of the penetrating trauma has a direct impact on the patient's outcome. Bowel and abdominal injuries occur more frequently in the upper abdomen and can cause injury to the mother, whereas direct trauma to the lower abdomen can result in more injuries or death to the fetus.

Pelvic Fractures

Pelvic fractures in pregnant patients result most frequently from blunt trauma to the abdomen. The patient may experience significant hemorrhaging and may sustain bladder, urethral, or intestinal injuries. Pelvic fractures are associated with a 25 percent fetal mortality rate.

Hemorrhage and Shock

Hemorrhage is a common finding associated with trauma during pregnancy and can result in shock. It can result from any of the conditions previously described in this section or as a result of another injury. Hemorrhaging, both internal and external, should be suspected after trauma. Shock is a frequent cause of death to both the fetus and the mother. It should be anticipated and managed aggressively. It is possible for a pregnant patient to lose 30 percent of her blood volume before normal signs and symp-toms of shock begin to appear. If the traditional signs of hypovolemic shock appear, the fetal mortality can be as high as 85 percent.

Cardiopulmonary Arrest

Cardiopulmonary arrest in the pregnant trauma patient poses a significant threat to the viability of the fetus. Although the chance of the fetus surviving maternal cardiopulmonary arrest because of trauma is poor, resuscitative attempts should be provided for pregnant patients in their third trimester, unless instructed otherwise. Rapid transport to a medical facility is imperative.

ASSESSMENT FINDINGS

The prehospital assessment and management of the pregnant trauma patient are focused on identifying, ensuring, maintaining, and supporting the vital functions of the patient's airway, breathing, and circulation. Unlike other traumatic emergencies, two patients must be considered by the AEMT. The best way to help both the mother and fetus involved in trauma is to take a proactive approach and to treat the mother aggressively. All pregnant women who have suffered an injury, regardless of the severity of the injury, should be evaluated by a physician in the emergency room.

The assessment of the pregnant trauma patient should be conducted in basically the same fashion as other trauma assessments. However, you should pay particular attention to the abdomen and uterus. The uterus will be palpable above the iliac crest after the 12th week of pregnancy. It will continue to grow and progress upward throughout the pregnancy. The normal uterus will be firm and round. When contractions occur, the uterus will usually harden. If the uterus is asymmetrical or irregular in shape, it may suggest a uterine rupture.

In addition to the usual trauma assessment, it is important to obtain information related directly to the pregnancy, if possible. Questions may include asking about the pregnancy, due date, gestational age, fetal movement, contractions, and previous obstetric history.

EMERGENCY MEDICAL CARE

The management of a pregnant trauma patient includes the following:

- **Spinal immobilization** is required for pregnant patients suspected of having spinal injury. Once the pregnant patient who is more than 20 weeks pregnant is secured appropriately, the backboard must be tilted to the left side, and this position must be maintained throughout the duration of your care. This will help prevent supine hypotensive syndrome.
- **Establish and maintain an open airway.** Use mechanical devices as appropriate. Anticipate vomiting with pregnant patients and have suction readily available. Airway compromise is more likely when the patient is pregnant.
- **Determine whether the patient is breathing adequately** and whether bilateral breath sounds are present. If the patient's breathing is inadequate, provide positive pressure ventilation with supplemental high-flow oxygen. If breathing is adequate, provide oxygen via nonrebreather or nasal cannula so you maintain the patient's oxygen saturation at 100 percent. Remember that the fetus is very vulnerable to any reduction in oxygen and will require as much oxygen as possible to prevent hypoxia, even if signs of maternal hypoxia are not present.
- **Assess the patient's circulation and check for major bleeding.** If vaginal bleeding is present, absorb the blood flow with a pad but do not pack the vagina. Anticipate, prevent, and treat shock.
- **Start at least one large-bore IV en route to the hospital** and run fluids according to patient presentation and local protocols.
- **Perform a visual exam at the vaginal opening** to assess for crowning or bleeding. If labor occurs as a result of the trauma, additional resources will be needed to help care for both patients.
- **Treat and manage any other injuries.**
- **Transport the patient to a medical facility that preferably has obstetric capabilities.** Consider air medical transport for major traumas. Inform the trauma center as soon as possible that the patient is pregnant.

The best method of caring for the fetus is by anticipating injuries and shock and aggressively managing the mother.

REVIEW ITEMS

1. A pregnant trauma patient who is in her third trimester presents with a palpable fetus in her upper abdomen. Based on that finding, you should suspect _____.
   - a. eclampsia
   - b. uterine rupture
   - c. abruptio placentae
   - d. pelvic fracture

2. A 26-weeks-pregnant trauma patient is suffering from supine hypotensive syndrome. After properly securing the patient to a backboard, the board must be _____.
   - a. tilted downward
   - b. tilted upward
   - c. tilted to the right
   - d. tilted to the left

3. What is the most common complication resulting from traumatic injury in the pregnant patient?
   - a. uterine rupture
   - b. uterine contractions
   - c. pelvic fractures
   - d. abruptio placentae

4. Which of the following mechanisms of injury account for more than half of all injuries sustained by pregnant patients?
   - a. falls
   - b. gunshot wounds
   - c. stab wounds
   - d. motor vehicle collisions

5. What percentage of fetal loss is accounted for by abruptio placentae due to mostly blunt trauma?
   - a. 10–25 percent
   - b. 25–45 percent
   - c. 50–70 percent
   - d. 1–10 percent

APPLIED PATHOPHYSIOLOGY

1. Explain how the physiologic changes experienced during pregnancy may mask the signs and symptoms of shock resulting from trauma.

2. Why is maximum oxygenation important in the management of a pregnant trauma patient?

3. Why can fetal growth influence the patient's perception of abdominal pain?

4. Explain how gas exchange between the mother and fetus is inhibited if the patient has abruptio placentae.

CLINICAL DECISION MAKING

You are dispatched to a residence for a patient who fell. When you arrive, a teenager emerges from the residence and states that his aunt has fallen while in the shower. You determine the scene is safe, and you approach the 26-year-old female patient, who is lying in the bathtub.

1. Based on the scene size-up characteristics, list the possible conditions you suspect the patient may be experiencing.

The primary assessment reveals that the patient is anxious, alert, and oriented. She states she slipped on some shampoo left inside the tub. She is complaining of severe abdominal pain. Her respiratory rate is 22/minute with adequate chest rise and fall. Her radial pulse is strong and regular at a rate of 112 beats per minute. You note no external bleeding. Her skin is warm and still very wet from the shower. The SpO$_2$ reading is 97 percent.

2. What are the life threats to this patient?

3. What immediate emergency care should you provide based on the initial assessment?

4. What conditions have you ruled out from your initial considerations in the scene size-up?

5. What conditions are you still considering as the possible cause? Would you add any conditions as a possible cause?

During the secondary assessment, the patient continues to complain of severe abdominal pain and cramping. She states that she is 24 weeks pregnant. In addition, she has a headache and her lower back hurts. Her abdomen is tender, her pelvis is stable, and no deformities or trauma to the extremities are evident. You note no crowning or external bleeding. The peripheral pulses are all present. The patient is allergic to aspirin, has a history of depression, and takes no prescription medication aside from her prenatal vitamins. She had lemonade and a turkey sandwich about 30 minutes prior to your arrival. Her blood pressure is 112/66 mmHg, her heart rate is now 112 beats per minute, and her respirations are 18 per minute.

6. What conditions have you ruled out in your differential field diagnosis? Why?

7. What should your emergency care include?

8. Why is it important to anticipate shock in this patient?

Standard Trauma

Competency Applies fundamental knowledge to provide basic and selected advanced emergency care and transportation based on assessment findings for an acutely injured patient.

TOPIC

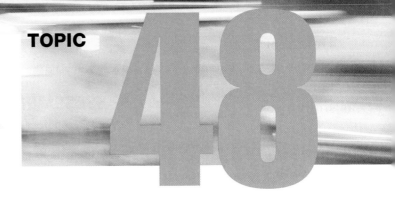

DIVING EMERGENCIES: DECOMPRESSION SICKNESS AND ARTERIAL EMBOLISM

INTRODUCTION

According to the Divers Alert Network (DAN), between 1.5 and 3 million people scuba dive commercially or recreationally each year. The popularity of this sport means that many of our friends, neighbors, colleagues, and, potentially, patients will have participated in compressed air diving. Many of these people will dive in deep water. Although the vast majority of these participants will dive safely, a small portion of diving excursions will result in decompression-related injuries and air emboli. As an Advanced EMT, you must be prepared to recognize and treat these injuries properly.

EPIDEMIOLOGY

Until recently, the incidence of diving-related injuries has been difficult to track. Between 1998 and 2002, DAN reviewed more than 50,000 dives and found that recompression treatment was required 28 times. Although these are perhaps the best data we have, there may be many more unreported incidents. Again, according to DAN, as many as 500,000 divers will take their first dive each year. That means that at any moment, up to nearly a quarter of the scuba diving population is relatively novice.

Given that most decompression-related injuries occur because of incorrect diving procedures or mistakes, it is reasonable to expect a potentially higher rate of injuries. On the other hand, we do know that severe injuries and death resulting from decompression injury and air emboli are rare. A U.S. military study estimated death rates among compressed air dives to be quite rare, with a ratio of roughly 1.3 deaths per 100,000 dives.

PATHOPHYSIOLOGY

Dysbarism

Dysbarism, or decompression sickness, results from expanding pressures between diving depths and the surface. Divers who fail to employ safe ascending techniques expose themselves to the risks of nitrogen bubbles and rapid gas expansion. Dysbarism is best described by relating it to the physics of diving.

DIVING AND PHYSICS   Four laws of physics play an important role in decompression-related injuries:

TRANSITION *highlights*

- Overview of the popularity of diving (including recreational), and documented occurrence of dive-related emergencies.
- Causes of dysbarism, and the laws of physics that contribute to it:
  – Boyle law.
  – Dalton law.
  – Henry law.
  – Charles law.
- Common assessment findings when caring for a patient with a dive-related emergency.
- Types of decompression sickness (type I and type II).
- Current treatment strategies for diving emergencies.

Boyle law. *At a constant temperature, the volume of a gas varies inversely with the pressure.* For example, at the pressures of 50 feet of depth, the volume of air in the lungs is roughly half of what it would be on the surface. If a diver were to ascend rapidly without the necessary safety precautions, gases in gas-filled organs such as the lungs would quickly expand and potentially rupture. Pressure changes can also damage air-filled structures, such as the eardrum and sinus cavities.

Dalton law. *The total pressure of a mixture of gases equals the sum of the partial pressures of the individual gases that make up the mixture.* Simply put, the total pressure of the air we breathe is made up of a series of individual pressures of gases. These individual pressures change as the external pressure changes. For example, nitrogen comprises about 78 percent of total pressure of the air we breathe. If you were to descend to a depth of 50 feet, the ambient pressure

> **The effect of every 50 feet of depth is similar to the intoxicating effects of one alcoholic beverage.**

would significantly increase and therefore increase the pressure of nitrogen.

At high pressures (greater depths) the increased pressure of nitrogen can cause higher levels of nitrogen to dissolve into the bloodstream. This can cause a central nervous system disturbance called *nitrogen narcosis*. It has been said that the effect of every 50 feet of depth is similar to the intoxicating effects of one alcoholic beverage.

Henry law. *At a constant temperature, the amount of gas dissolved in a liquid is proportional to the surrounding pressure.* For example, at high pressures (great depth), gases, especially nitrogen, dissolve into the blood and tissues of the body. If a diver were to ascend too rapidly, pressure would quickly increase, and nitrogen would be returned to a gaseous state while still in the blood and tissues.

This gaseous nitrogen forms bubbles in fats and other body tissues and can cause tissue damage and severe pain. Compression from these bubbles harms tissue and can cause nerve and blood vessel disruption. The immune system often responds to the presence of nitrogen bubbles and can cause allergy-related symptoms. In addition, nitrogen bubbles can cause clotting-related problems in the form of obstructions called *emboli*.

Charles law. *The volume of a gas is proportional to the temperature.* Cold temperatures cause the volumes of gases to decrease. As temperatures increase rapidly, as in a rapid ascent from the cold depths, the volume of gas will increase rapidly. This increased volume can cause trauma to gas-filled organs.

Arterial Emboli

In severe cases of decompression sickness, barotrauma in the lungs can lead to air entering the pulmonary vein. Air bubbles, also called air emboli, are then returned to the left side of the heart and are potentially distributed to the arterial side of the cardiovascular system. When the bubbles reach small arterioles, they can result in an obstruction to flow and impair perfusion to tissues beyond the obstruction.

ASSESSMENT FINDINGS

Mechanism of injury will be the most important finding when assessing a diving injury. Although many of these injuries will be acute onset and therefore obviously diving injuries, some will not. If your patient is wearing a wetsuit, you would suspect a diving injury, but remember that symptoms of diving injuries can be delayed.

Also remember that decompression injuries are exacerbated by air travel. Even though your current location might not include diving venues, be sure to investigate recent history when symptoms point you in the direction of decompression sickness. Remember also that dysbarism occurs in divers of all skill levels, not just in first-time novices.

Important considerations with decompression sickness include the following:

- History of diving
- Use of compressed air (scuba)
- What types of compressed air mixtures were used
- Depth of diving
- Recent air travel after diving
- Any complications during the dive (entrapment, injuries, etc.)

Complicated Diving Injuries

When assessing a diving injury, remember that these injuries often involve more than one significant problem. Although we have been discussing dysbarism exclusively, the overwhelming number of fatalities associated with diving result from drowning. Keep in mind that decompression sickness often results from the rapid ascent used to escape another injury or problem. For example, the diver might have had to ascend rapidly because of an injury, entanglement, or equipment failure.

Always be sure to consider the entire picture and not just the decompression sickness. Complete a thorough primary assessment, consider spinal immobilization (when indicated), and look for other associated injuries.

Assessing Decompression Sickness

The signs and symptoms of dysbarism/decompression sickness are typically divided into two categories.

Type I decompression sickness is most commonly typified by pain. Often referred to as *the bends*, this pain is typically dull, achy, and worst in major joints, such as the shoulder. This pain is most commonly caused by nitrogen bubbles in the blood and tissues and can come on rapidly or more chronically. Occasionally pain will worsen with time (especially if the diver flies too soon after deep-water diving). Skin rash and irritation are also common complaints.

Type II decompression sickness is the more severe variant and can affect a number of body systems:

- **Respiratory system.** Pulmonary air emboli are rare but potentially life threatening. Symptoms include respiratory distress, bloody sputum, and acute-onset chest pain. Decompression sickness in the lungs, also called *the chokes*, can also be life threatening. These symptoms can be immediate or delayed 12 to 48 hours and include burning sensation on inhalation and a nonproductive cough. Nonspecific symptoms also include pallor, cyanosis, low oxygen saturations, and accessory muscle use.
- **Circulatory system.** Decompression sickness can cause fluid to shift out of the blood vessels and can, thereby, cause hypovolemia. This disorder is characterized by the signs and symptoms of shock, including tachycardia and low blood pressure. Coagulation disorders can also lead to clot formation and perfusion-related problems.
- **Nervous system.** The brain and spinal cord can be affected by nitrogen bubbles and small emboli. Nitrogen narcosis, compression damage, and perfusion problems can cause neurologic symptoms such as altered mental status, vision disturbance, weakness, numbness and tingling, and even loss of bowel and bladder control. Air emboli can cause strokelike problems and include similar symptoms, including seizures, motor and sensory deficits, and pupil changes.

Arterial emboli are related to decompression sickness but may exist independently. Recall that barotrauma in the lungs can cause air to enter the arterial bloodstream. Emboli then obstruct the flow of blood and cause perfusion deficits to tissue. In the extreme, this can cause a pulmonary embolism, but it can also cause more local signs and symptoms. Always assess for signs of barotrauma, including the following:

- Shortness of breath
- Use of respiratory accessory muscles
- Pallor, cyanosis, and low oxygen saturation
- Subcutaneous emphysema (air trapped beneath the skin, especially in the neck area)
- Bleeding from the ears
- Vertigo

Signs of pulmonary air embolism include the preceding signs and symptoms plus chest pain, blood-tinged sputum, and cardiac arrest. Signs of localized emboli include increasing pain, especially in the joints.

While assessing a person with a potential dive injury, also consider that certain conditions make decompression sickness more likely. Predisposing risk factors include the following:

- Flying too soon after diving (typically sooner than 12 to 24 hours)
- Not following standard safety procedures while diving

- Diving at extreme depths (or prolonged exposure to extreme depths)
- Manual exertion (work) while diving
- Cold water
- Obesity
- Age
- Dehydration
- Prior heart/cardiovascular conditions

EMERGENCY MEDICAL CARE

As stated, decompression sickness may be only one of a variety of concerns when responding to a diving accident. Consider spinal precautions where indicated, and treat life threats based on the findings of your primary assessment.

When treating decompression sickness, consider the position of the patient. When spinal injury is not a consideration, place the patient in a lateral recumbent position. Do not place the patient in a Trendelenburg or head-down position.

As always, treat airway and breathing problems aggressively. High-flow oxygen is exceptionally important because it diminishes the effects of nitrogen.

Obtain venous access as a precautionary measure en route to the hospital. Administer fluids per protocol.

Appropriate Transport

Aside from oxygen, few prehospital treatments are therapeutic in decompression sickness. As a result, rapid transport may be the most important therapy. When you identify a patient with type II decompression sickness and/or signs of arterial embolism, rapid transport to an appropriate facility is the highest priority.

When making a transport decision, consider that the treatment of severe decompression sickness often requires the use of a decompression chamber. It may be advisable to facilitate transport to a facility with this type of capability. That may mean alternative transport methods, such as air medical transport. You should advise the crew that diving-related accidents are being considered so that the crew will fly at the lowest possible altitude (and/or the cabin will be appropriately pressurized). Always follow local protocol.

TRANSITIONING • • • • • •

REVIEW ITEMS

1. Which of the following would be a diving injury associated with the Boyle law?
    a. ruptured alveoli from increased air volumes
    b. nitrogen bubbles in the fatty tissue
    c. nitrogen narcosis
    d. nitrogen emboli

2. Which of the following would be a diving injury associated with the Dalton law?
    a. nitrogen bubbles in the fatty tissue
    b. ruptured alveoli from increased air volumes
    c. air emboli in arteries
    d. ruptured eardrum

3. A diver working in cold water ascends quickly and now complains of ear pain and bleeding from his ears. This would best be an example of a problem associated with the _____.
    a. Charles law   b. Henry law
    c. Dalton law   d. Boyle law

4. A deep-water diver ascends but is now acting confused and has difficulty answering questions. He has no other complaints. Which of the following conditions might best explain his altered mental status?
    a. nitrogen narcosis
    b. barotrauma
    c. pulmonary emboli
    d. the chokes

5. A deep-water diver had an equipment failure and had to ascend at an unsafe rate. He now complains of shortness of breath, coughing up blood, and chest pain. The most likely cause would be _____.
    a. pulmonary embolism
    b. nitrogen narcosis
    c. hyperventilation
    d. pneumonia

APPLIED PATHOPHYSIOLOGY

1. Describe the effects of type II decompression sickness on the following systems:

   a. Respiratory system

   b. Circulatory system

   c. Nervous system

2. Describe how barotrauma might result in an arterial gas embolism.

3. Describe why high-flow oxygen is important in treating type II decompression sickness.

CLINICAL DECISION MAKING

You are called to the local airport. Dispatch tells you that a man has just been taken off an arriving plane. Prearrival questioning indicates that the patient is complaining of severe pain in his back, arms, and knees. He also is complaining of shortness of breath. No other passengers have had similar complaints. Dispatch notes that airline staff will meet you in the terminal.

On arrival you find a 35-year-old man seated in a wheelchair. He is restless and in obvious distress from pain. You notice that he is also tachypneic and has a cough. Airport staff tell you he was fine when he got on the plane but now is "very sick."

1. As you begin to consider a differential diagnosis, what are some potential causes for this patient's pain and shortness of breath?

2. What immediate assessment steps should you take?

Your primary assessment notes a patent airway and somewhat labored breathing. His respiratory rate is 36/minute, and he has crackles in the bases of his lungs. His pulse is also fast at 128. His skin is slightly pale and moist. He is alert but agitated. He tells you he is in severe pain. His knees, shoulders, and back "are killing him."

3. What other questions might you ask to better make a differential diagnosis?

The patient tells you he was just returning from a scuba weekend. He has been diving all weekend but now needs to get home for work on Monday. He tells you it was a great "party weekend," but he "may have overdone it."

4. What elements of the history of the present illness might indicate decompression sickness?

5. Does this patient have predisposing factors that might make decompression sickness likely?

6. What are the most important elements of treatment for this patient?

Standard Special Patient Populations

Competency Applies a fundamental knowledge of growth, development, aging, and assessment findings to provide basic and selected advanced emergency care and transportation for a patient with special needs.

TOPIC

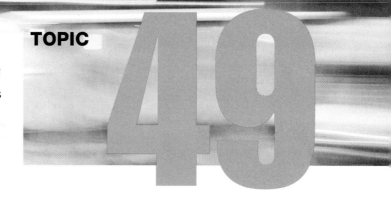

OBSTETRICS (ANTEPARTUM COMPLICATIONS)

INTRODUCTION

Antepartum refers to the period of pregnancy before the onset of labor. Therefore, antepartum emergencies entail obstetric complications that can occur any time between conception and delivery of the fetus. These emergencies carry a variety of clinical manifestations that can be as subtle as abdominal cramping and as life threatening as massive hemorrhage. Antepartum emergencies can pose a significant risk not only to the pregnant patient, but also to the fetus. These complications require the Advanced EMT to maintain a keen level of awareness to protect the lives of the mother and her unborn child.

EPIDEMIOLOGY

Pregnancy is a natural process that can result in complications over the course of nine months. Four percent of pregnancies develop complications during the third trimester alone. Of that 4 percent, placenta previa occurs 22 percent of the time and abruptio placentae 31 percent of the time. In other cases, a cause for these complications cannot be identified. Further epidemiology of placenta previa, abruptio placentae, ectopic pregnancy, preeclampsia, ecclampsia, and abortion is discussed in the next section.

PATHOPHYSIOLOGY

Placenta Previa

Normal implantation of the placenta should occur in the posterior portion of the fundus, or top portion of the uterus. In *placenta previa*, the placenta implants over the internal cervical os (or opening; ▶ Figure 49-1). The three variants of this condition are complete, partial, and marginal. *Complete* placenta previa covers the entire cervical os, *partial* covers the os to some extent, and *marginal* approaches the border of the os.

In placenta previa, placental implantation is initiated by the embryo adhering to the lower end of the uterus. As the placenta grows, it may cover a portion of the cervix. Then when the cervix thins for impending labor, the placental attachment is disrupted, which leads to bleeding at the implantation site.

The uterus is unable to contract properly to stop the flow of blood from the open blood vessels. Thrombin releases from the bleeding sites, causing further uterine contractions and thus a vicious cycle of bleeding, contractions, and worsening separation of the placenta. Generally, the abdomen is not tender between contractions. Placenta previa can occur in the first trimester of pregnancy; however, it is more typical to present in the second and third trimesters.

Placenta previa complicates 5 out of every 1,000 pregnancies and is responsible for 0.03 percent of maternal deaths. The incidence for placenta previa increases by 10 percent after a woman has had four or more Caesarean births. The risk of neonatal mortality is higher for placenta previa babies than for those not exposed. A great majority of maternal deaths are related to uterine bleeding and complications from disseminated intravascular coagulopathy.

Several risk factors are associated with placenta previa. Women younger than 20 years of age and those over 35 years of

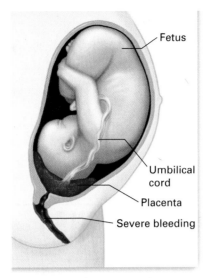

Figure 49-1 Placenta previa.

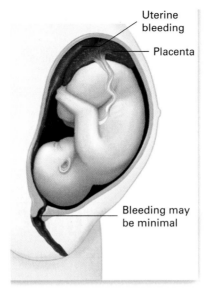

Figure 49-2 Abruptio placentae.

age are at the greatest risk. Other factors include multiparity (more than two deliveries), multiple gestation (more than one fetus), rapid succession of pregnancies, recurrent abortions, infertility treatments, residence at a higher altitude, and cocaine and cigarette use.

Vaginal bleeding occurs 80 percent of the time in placenta previa. The classic presentation of placenta previa is painless, bright red vaginal bleeding; however, the color of the blood should not preclude the consideration of placenta previa. Bleeding starts slowly and may increase in flow as the separation continues. On abdominal examination, the uterus will appear soft, nontender, and relaxed. The absence of abdominal pain and uterine contractions is used primarily to distinguish between placenta previa and abruptio placentae.

However, up to 10 percent of women may experience painful uterine contractions. In addition, bright red blood is not always present, and the blood may be dark or an intermediate color. Any vaginal bleeding occurring after 24 weeks gestation should be a consideration for placenta previa, as it is a major cause of third trimester hemorrhage.

Abruptio Placentae

Abruptio placentae, or placental abruption, is an obstetric catastrophe in which the placental lining separates from the uterus prematurely. It is referred to as a separation that occurs after 20 weeks gestation and before birth. Incidence of abruptio placentae peaks at 24 to 26 weeks gestation. It is a common cause of late-term pregnancy bleeding in women, occurring in 1 percent of pregnancies worldwide. In the United States, placental abruption complicates 1 in 100 births and results in stillbirth in 1.2 of every 1,000 deliveries. Abruptio placentae carries a fetal fatality rate of 20 percent to 40 percent and is also a significant contributor to maternal mortality.

Abruptio placentae begins with avulsion of the anchoring placental villi from the expanding lower uterine segment (▶ Figure 49-2). This leads to bleeding into the tissue between the uterine wall and the placenta, which in turn pushes the placenta away from the uterus, causing further bleeding. In addition to severe maternal blood loss, abruptio placentae initiates a cascade of events that results in reduced maternal–fetal oxygen and nutrient exchange, membrane rupture, uterine contractility, and clotting abnormalities. Clinical manifestations include abdominal pain, vaginal bleeding (80 percent), premature contractions, and fetal distress or death.

Abruptio placentae can present in one of two types: complete or partial. In *complete* abruption, the placenta separates completely from the uterine wall. This type carries a 100 percent fetal mortality rate. *Partial* placental abruption is an incomplete or partial separation from the uterine wall. Because the placenta is partially attached and functioning, it is associated with a lower fetal mortality rate, rather than 100 percent.

There are several risk factors for placental abruption. Maternal hypertension is responsible for 44 percent of all abruptions. Other risk factors include maternal trauma, short umbilical cord, prolonged or premature rupture of membranes, previous abruption, infection, and toxins such as cocaine intoxication and cigarette smoking. Another major risk factor for placental abruption is maternal age. Pregnant women younger than 20 years of age and older than 35 are at an even greater risk.

Patients with placental abruption display specific signs and symptoms. Painful, dark vaginal bleeding is ominous in abruptio placentae. However, vaginal bleeding does not always take place, nor is the blood always dark in color. Bleeding can transpire internally, causing the uterus to appear disproportionately enlarged. Be watchful for hypovolemic shock, as evidenced by tachycardia, hypotension, and signs of poor perfusion. Contractions are commonly painful and palpable on exam. They may be so frequent as to seem continuous. Tenderness in the abdomen, as well as pain in the uterus, are also frequent findings in abruptio placentae.

Abruptio placentae with greater than 50 percent separation is considered to be severe. The presence of severe abruption causes both maternal and fetal compromise. Unfortunately, the amount of vaginal bleeding does not correlate with the degree of placental separation and is a poor indicator to the extent of impending compromise.

In summary, there are no clinical findings that definitively suggest placenta previa or placental abruption; however, bleeding in the second or third trimester requires expert evaluation.

Ectopic Pregnancy

Ectopic pregnancy is a complication of pregnancy in which the ovum implants outside the uterine cavity (▶ Figure 49-3). Ninety-eight percent of ectopic pregnancies occur in the fallopian tube; therefore, they are called *tubal pregnancies*. Implantation, although unlikely, can occur in other places, such as the cervix, ovaries, or abdomen. Almost 100 percent of ectopic pregnancies end in fetal death. Furthermore, ectopic pregnancy can be very dangerous for the mother because of the risk of internal bleeding. Hemorrhage from ectopic pregnancy is still a leading cause of pregnancy-related maternal death in the first trimester.

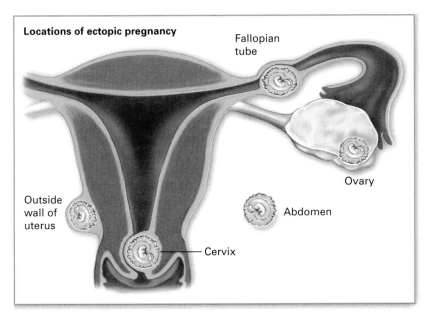

Locations of ectopic pregnancy

Fallopian tube

Ovary

Abdomen

Outside wall of uterus

Cervix

Figure 49-3 Ectopic pregnancy.

In a typical ectopic pregnancy, the embryo does not reach the uterus and instead adheres to the lining of the fallopian tube. The implanted embryo burrows into the tubal lining and invades the blood vessels of the tube, which causes bleeding. The pain from an ectopic pregnancy is caused by the release of prostaglandins at the implantation site and free blood in the peritoneal cavity. Fifty percent of ectopic pregnancies that are left untreated will resolve without treatment.

Overall, the incidence of ectopic pregnancy increased during the mid-20th century. It plateaued at 20 per 1,000 pregnancies and an average of 7 percent of all pregnancy-related deaths. At present, ectopic pregnancy occurs in 1 out of every 44 pregnancies in the United States. For unclear reasons, there is a seasonal incidence for ectopic pregnancy, with increasing frequency between June and December.

There are many risk factors for ectopic pregnancy, including pelvic inflammatory disease, infertility, the use of an intrauterine device, previous ectopic pregnancy or tubal ligation, adhesions from surgery, and smoking. However, nearly half of all ectopic pregnancies are found to have no risk factor identified.

Early signs and symptoms of ectopic pregnancy are extremely subtle, or even absent. Early findings include pain in the lower abdomen, pain while urinating or during a bowel movement, and mild vaginal bleeding. Patients with a late ectopic

pregnancy or rupture of the fallopian tube typically experience pain and hemorrhage. Hemorrhage will be both vaginal (external) and internal. The vaginal bleeding is cause by the falling progesterone levels, and the internal bleeding comes directly from the affected fallopian tube. Severe internal bleeding may be evidenced by low back pain, abdominal pain, and referred shoulder pain from free blood irritating the diaphragm.

Preeclampsia and Eclampsia

Preeclampsia is a medical condition that may develop after 20 weeks gestation, in which hypertension, edema, and protein in the urine develop during the pregnancy. Diagnostic criteria for hypertension include blood pressure greater than 140/90 mmHg in two consecutive measurements four hours apart. If the patient has preexisting hypertension, then a systolic pressure more than 30 mmHg over the patient's baseline and diastolic pressure more than 15 mmHg over the baseline are considered diagnostic.

In addition to hypertension and proteinuria, other diagnostic clinical manifestations include visual disturbances, headaches, edema, and scant urine output. Patients having hypertension as described with no other associated signs and symptoms are diagnosed with pregnancy-induced hypertension. Once the patient develops these signs and symptoms, preeclampsia is diagnosed. *Eclampsia*

refers to the development of generalized tonic–clonic seizures in women with pregnancy-induced hypertension or preeclampsia, when the seizures cannot be attributed to another cause.

In preeclampsia, abnormal formation of placental arteries causes susceptibility to vasoconstriction. The vasoconstriction causes hypoperfusion to the placenta. This, in turn, promotes ischemia and even infarction of the placenta. Once this occurs, a release of vasoactive substances causes a cascade of events, including inflammatory response, vasoconstriction, clotting disorders, and increased capillary permeability. All these responses present the clinical manifestations of preeclampsia and eclampsia.

Preeclampsia occurs in approximately 5 percent to 8 percent of all pregnancies in the United States. Ten percent of preeclampsia cases occur at less than 34 weeks gestation. It is the third-leading cause of pregnancy-related death, with hemorrhage being the first cause and embolism the second. Preeclampsia is estimated to cause 790 maternal deaths out of 100,000 live births.

Preeclampsia is more common among women under 20 years of age and over 35 years of age. The frequency varies across race and ethnicity; however; African-American women have a higher mortality rate than other groups. A history of preeclampsia is also a strong risk factor for recurrence. Other risk factors include a history of diabetes, heart disease, kidney problems, preexisting hypertension, first pregnancy, or multiple gestations.

Several signs and symptoms are specific to preeclampsia. Mild cases can present very subtly and sometimes even go unnoticed. Common signs and symptoms of preeclampsia include hypertension, sudden increase in edema, angioedema (facial swelling), proteinuria, complaint of sudden weight gain, headache, nausea and vomiting, and visual disturbances. In severe cases and development of eclampsia, the patient will present with generalized tonic–clonic seizures.

> **Preeclampsia is the third leading cause of pregnancy-related death, with hemorrhage being the first cause and embolism the second.**

TABLE 49-1 Types of Abortion

Type	Description
Spontaneous (unintentional)	Involuntary termination of the pregnancy before viability, 20 weeks gestation
Threatened	Abdominal cramping and lower back pain with light spotting; cervix remains closed with no products of conception passed
Inevitable	Increased vaginal bleeding and abdominal cramping; cervix dilates
Incomplete	Vaginal bleeding, abdominal cramping; dilation of the cervix with partial passage of products of conception
Complete	Passage of all the products of conception; cervix closes, vaginal bleeding stops
Missed	Fetus dies in utero but is not expelled; uterine growth stops
Recurrent	Two or more consecutive spontaneous abortions
Induced (intentional)	Voluntary termination of the pregnancy before viability, 20 weeks gestation
Therapeutic	Intentional termination of the pregnancy to preserve the health of the mother
Elective	Intentional termination of the pregnancy for reasons other than preserving the health of the mother (e.g., fetal anomaly)

Hypertension, as described, should be greater than 140/90 mmHg or, with pre-existing hypertension, more than 30/15 mmHg over the patient's typical blood pressure. Edema in pregnancy is not uncommon. However, a sudden increase in edema or angioedema is consistent with preeclampsia and should not be considered normal.

Proteinuria is a very specific sign of preeclampsia; however, at present there is no means of testing for it in the prehospital environment. Weight gain is also expected in pregnancy. If a pregnant patient expresses a gain of more than 2 pounds in a week or 6 pounds in a month, you should suspect preeclampsia. In the first trimester of pregnancy, nausea and vomiting are extremely common; however, a sudden onset of nausea and vomiting in the second or third trimester is another indicator of preeclampsia when accompanied with other associated signs and symptoms.

Spontaneous Abortion

Also known as miscarriage, *spontaneous abortion* is a loss of pregnancy before the age of viability. A pregnancy is considered viable at 20 weeks gestation. Abortions can be spontaneous or induced. Spontaneous abortions are unintentional, are involuntary, and occur because of a wide variety of natural causes. Induced abortions are intentionally performed for medical reasons (therapeutic) or personal reasons (elective).

Spontaneous abortion is extremely common in early pregnancy. Fortunately, the frequency for miscarriage decreases with increasing gestational age. As many as 20 percent of clinically recognized pregnancies under 20 weeks gestation will have vaginal bleeding, and 10 percent will have a spontaneous abortion. Abdominal cramping or pain and vaginal bleeding are common in miscarriage. The further along the gestation, the heavier the bleeding. Refer to Table 49-1 for the various types of abortion and patient presentation.

Maternal causes for spontaneous abortion include structural problems, incompetent cervix, infection, poor nutrition, substance abuse, smoking, and trauma. Maternal age is also a significant maternal risk factor. Women over 40 years of age have a 40 percent risk of miscarriage, and women over 50 years of age have an 80 percent risk of miscarriage. Abnormal placental implantation and placental separation are abnormalities involving the placenta that are capable of inducing abortion. Also, abnormal genetics and fetal implantation complications can both result in spontaneous abortion.

ASSESSMENT

Antepartum emergencies can be extremely stressful not only for the patient, but also for the AEMT. Anxiety and stress can inhibit the accuracy of information communicated among everyone involved. Use your dispatch information as well as scene size-up to help you determine the extent of the emergency at hand.

Once you ensure proper Standard Precautions and scene safety, perform a primary assessment. Your primary assessment should thoroughly evaluate the patient's airway, breathing, and circulation, as well as mental status. Use the same assessment and treatment techniques for a pregnant patient as you would for a patient who is not pregnant.

Use the history and secondary assessment to determine specific information about the patient and her pregnancy. Keep in mind that not all patients are aware that they are pregnant at the time of your interview and that those who are may not be accurate in the gestational age. In some cases, the patient's current emergency may be her first sign of pregnancy. Include the following questions as appropriate:

- When was your last menstrual period?
  - Was your last period normal for you (color and amount)?
  - Have your periods been regular?
  - Have you missed a period?
  - Have you experienced breast tenderness, nausea, vomiting, or fatigue?
- Have you been pregnant before?
  - How many times have you been pregnant (gravida)?
  - How many live children did you deliver (para)?
  - How many births were vaginal? Caesarean?
  - What complications did you have with your pregnancy?
  - Have you had a spontaneous or therapeutic abortion?
- Are you experiencing any pain or discomfort?
  - What is the quality of your pain (sharp, dull, achy, or crampy)?
  - Is the pain constant or intermittent?
  - Did the pain come on suddenly or gradually?

TABLE 49-2 Antepartum Complications and Associated Signs and Symptoms

Complication	Signs and Symptoms
Placenta previa	Painless, bright red vaginal bleeding; soft, relaxed uterus with minimal uterine contractions
Abruptio placentae	Painful, dark vaginal bleeding; firm, tense uterus with frequent uterine contractions
Ectopic pregnancy	Abdominal cramping or pain that can be associated with voiding; vaginal bleeding, usually early in the pregnancy
Preeclampsia	Hypertension and proteinuria; edema, weight gain, headaches, nausea and vomiting, usually later in pregnancy
Eclampsia	Hypertension and proteinuria with the onset of generalized tonic–clonic seizures not associated with another cause
Abortion	Abdominal cramping and vaginal bleeding; possible passage of tissue or blood clots

– Does anything make the pain better or worse?
– Does the pain radiate anywhere?
– Can you point to the pain with one finger?
– Do have any other associated symptoms, such as nausea or vomiting?
• Are you experiencing any vaginal discharge?
– What color is it?
– How much was discharged (pad count)?
– Does it have an abnormal or foul odor?
• If the patient knows she is pregnant, ask the following:
– Have you had any prenatal care?
– When is your due date?
– How many babies are you expecting?
– Are you having a high-risk pregnancy?

Assessment of the abdomen during the secondary assessment may reveal very valuable findings related to an antepartum condition. Inspect for abnormal distention or signs of injury. Palpate the abdomen to determine where the patient's pain is located. Assess for guarding, tenderness, and abnormal masses. Obtain a baseline set of vital signs and reassess frequently looking for a trend, especially one pointing to hemorrhage and shock.

Pregnancy is a natural process. Should the patient experience complications, however, she will typically present with one or more of the following signs and symptoms: abdominal pain, vaginal bleeding, passage of tissue or clots, weakness or dizziness, nausea and vomiting, edema, hypertension, and even seizures. Table 49-2 summarizes the signs and symptoms you may see on assessment of a patient with an antepartum emergency.

Remember, these are considered classic or hallmark signs and symptoms that are typically seen in these emergencies. They are not absolutes, and patients do not present in this manner 100 percent of the time. Use these hallmark signs and symptoms to accurately diagnose your patient and treat her according to her presentation.

EMERGENCY CARE

Prehospital emergency care for antepartum complications is primarily supportive. When providing emergency care to the pregnant patient you must always consider the status of the fetus. Although the pregnant patient may appear to be relatively well, especially in the early stages of shock and hemorrhage, the fetus may be severely compromised.

Emergency care of antepartum emergencies should include the following:

• **Establish and maintain a patent airway.**
– Altered mental status, seizures, and coma are possible findings in these

emergencies. It may be necessary to manually maintain the airway or use an airway adjunct, such as an oropharyngeal or nasopharyngeal airway, to maintain a patent airway.

• **Establish and maintain adequate oxygenation and ventilation.**
– Determine the patient's SpO_2 reading and assess for evidence of hypoxia. The pregnant patient is one situation in which, regardless of the SpO_2 reading, a high concentration of oxygen should be administered via a nonrebreather mask at 15 lpm. Application of high-concentration oxygen maximizes oxygenation to the fetus, as hypoxia due to vasoconstriction is possible. If the patient's respiratory rate and tidal volume are inadequate, provide positive pressure ventilation with high concentrations of oxygen delivered via the ventilation device.

• **Place the patient in a left lateral recumbent position.**
– Left lateral recumbent positioning prevents supine hypotensive syndrome during the later phases of pregnancy by displacing the gravid uterus off the maternal aorta. This will prevent any further reduction of placental perfusion and help increase fetal oxygenation.

• **Provide supportive care for seizures.**
– Maintain airway management, adequate oxygenation and ventilation, and circulation in a patient having seizures. Maternal seizures cause hypoxia to the fetus. Ensure adequate oxygenation and ventilation to prevent the increasing hypoxic state of the fetus.

• **Initiate expeditious transport.**
– Antepartum complications can pose a serious risk to the mother. In some circumstances, definitive treatment is delivery of the fetus and placenta. Choose a medical facility that is capable of managing acute obstetric compromise.

• **En route, establish an intravenous line of normal saline.**
– If the patient is exhibiting signs and symptoms of shock, run the fluid at a rate to maintain perfusion. If no signs of hemorrhage or shock are present, run the fluid at a to-keep-open rate.

REVIEW ITEMS

1. During your secondary assessment of a 32-year-old woman with abdominal pain, the patient explains that her physician terminated her pregnancy because the fetus had a genetic anomaly. What kind of abortion is this?

   a. spontaneous abortion

   b. inevitable abortion

   c. therapeutic abortion

   d. elective abortion

2. Who has the higher mortality rate in ectopic pregnancy?

   a. mother

   b. fetus

3. A blood pressure of 140/70 mmHg with associated signs and symptoms is indicative of preeclampsia.

   a. true

   b. false

4. Implantation of the placenta near the edge of the cervical os is what kind of placenta previa?

   a. complete   b. partial

   c. marginal   d. minimal

5. External vaginal bleeding is always present in abruptio placentae.

   a. true

   b. false

CRITICAL DECISION MAKING

You and your partner are dispatched for a 42-year-old pregnant patient with abdominal pain. She is 32 weeks pregnant with a history of seven pregnancies, two miscarriages, and one stillbirth.

1. What are the patient's gravida and para?

On exam, you observe a round, distended abdomen. The patient states that her abdomen appears larger than usual. There is no vaginal bleeding, but she is having contractions.

2. What is your diagnosis?

3. Why is the patient's abdomen expanding?

The patient's vital signs include blood pressure 90/50 mmHg, heart rate 124 beats/minute, respiratory rate 20/minute, and SpO$_2$ 94 percent.

4. Would you administer oxygen to this patient? If so, how much and why?

5. Why is the patient hypotensive and tachycardic?

6. What emergency care would you provide to this patient?

Standard Special Patient Populations

Competency Applies a fundamental knowledge
of growth, development, and aging and assessment
findings to provide basic and selected advanced
emergency care and transportation for a patient with
special needs.

TOPIC

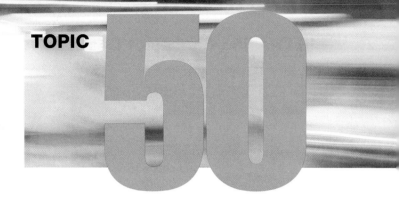

NEONATOLOGY

INTRODUCTION

From the time we are born, our lives are guided by the
need to cope with the stressors nature throws at us. To
be unable to cope with these stresses is to not survive—
and life is survival.

In utero, the fetus can see, feel, hear, and breathe, although
he is totally dependent on the mother for protection, warmth,
oxygen, nutrition, waste removal, and immune function. After
birth, the infant must begin to fend for himself by breathing air,
must depend on his own circulatory and respiratory systems for
an adequate cardiac output and oxygen delivery, must be capable of feeding effectively to allow for rapid growth, and must
develop an immune system that can protect him from the many
bacterial, viral, and fungal pathogens that he will encounter from
the moment of birth.

When one considers how complex our development is, from
embryo to neonate, the true miracle in life is that anyone comes
out able to survive at all. The spectrum of birth defects, either
passed on through the genes or acquired from insults during
pregnancy, fills textbooks and is growing every day as new ones
are discovered from unlocking the human genetic code. Most
women carrying fetuses with congenital anomalies spontaneously abort or miscarry in the first trimester (3 months) of pregnancy. Many, however, go on to be born prematurely or even at
full term; it must be the assumption of every medical professional who approaches a neonate that the baby *may* have a
congenital anomaly.

The most important advice to the EMS professional is that
(1) you can never trust or assume that an ill infant does *not* have
an anomaly and (2) the diagnosis, management, and ultimate
treatment of that anomaly will require specialized practitioners
found at children's hospitals.

EPIDEMIOLOGY

Not all infants are born equipped to cope with the stresses
and huge changes, both anatomic and physiologic, that occur
with the transition from an intrauterine to an extrauterine environment. Congenital anomalies—birth defects or anatomic
maldevelopments affecting one or more organ systems—are

TRANSITION *highlights*

- *Incidence and morbidity/mortality of neonatal complications as well as rates that illustrate the commonality
with which the neonate will need additional resuscitation following birth.*

- *Leading causes of death according to age brackets
from < 1 year of age to > 65 years.*

- *Assessment format for a newborn child, including critical care interventions at each step.*

- *Mnemonic to assist the Advanced EMT in remembering
the steps and interventions when caring for a neonate.*

the leading cause of death in the pre- and postnatal periods
(▶ Figure 50-1).

It is estimated that about 20 percent to 30 percent of perinatal deaths are the result of congenital anomalies and that they
are present in 2 percent to 5 percent of all live births. About half
are due to genetic or inheritance causes, and the other half are
either unknown or caused by teratogenic or uterine factors—
injuries that occurred during the pregnancy itself from exposure
to toxins (alcohol, drugs, and the like) or maldevelopment of
the placenta.

About 10 percent of all newborns will require some medical
interventions at birth, mostly to help them
begin to breathe effectively. Of those, about
10 percent (or 1 percent of all newly born
infants) will require resuscitation to survive
the immediate neonatal period. Resuscitative measures include, but are not limited to,
assisted bag-mask ventilations with oxygen,
chest compressions, and even administration of medications.

Having the appropriate equipment and
skill set to provide temperature control,

**About 10 per-
cent of all
newborns
will require
some medical
interventions
at birth.**

10 Leading Causes of Death by Age Group-2001

Rank	<1	1–4	5–9	10–14	15–24	25–34	35–44	45–54	55–64	65+	Total
1	Congenital Anomalies 5,513	Unintentional Injury 1,714	Unintentional Injury 1,283	Unintentional Injury 1,553	Unintentional Injury 14,411	Unintentional Injury 11,839	Malignant Neoplasms 16,559	Malignant Neoplasms 49,562	Malignant Neoplasms 90,223	Heart Disease 582,730	Heart Disease 700,142
2	Short Gestation 4,410	Congenital Anomalies 557	Malignant Neoplasms 493	Malignant Neoplasms 515	Homicide 5,237	Homicide 5,204	Unintentional Injury 15,945	Heart Disease 38,399	Heart Disease 62,486	Malignant Neoplasms 390,214	Malignant Neoplasms 553,768
3	S1DS 2,234	Malignant Neoplasms 420	Congenital Anomalies 182	Suicide 272	Suicide 3,971	Suicide 5,070	Heart Disease 13,326	Unintentional Injury 13,344	Chronic Low Respiratory Disease 11,166	Cerebro-vascular 144,466	Cerebro-vascular 163,536
4	Maternal Pregnancy Comp. 1,499	Homicide 415	Homicide 137	Congenital Anomalies 194	Malignant Neoplasms 1,704	Malignant Neoplasms 3,394	Suicide 6,635	Liver Disease 7,259	Cerebro-vascular 9,608	Chronic Low Respiratory Disease 106,904	Chronic Low Respiratory Disease 123,013
5	Placenta Cord Membranes 1,018	Heart Disease 225	Heart Disease 98	Homicide 189	Heart Disease 999	Heart Disease 3,100	HIV 5,867	Suicide 5,942	Diabetes Mellitus 9,570	Influenza & Pneumonia 55,518	Unintentional Injury 101,537
6	Respiratory Distress 1,011	Influenza & Pneumonia 112	Benign Neoplasms 52	Heart Disease 174	Congenital Anomalies 505	HIV 2,101	Homicide 4,268	Cerebro-vascular 5,910	Unintentional Injury 7,658	Diabetes Mellitus 53,707	Diabetes Mellitus 71,372
7	Unintentional Injury 976	Septicemia 108	Influenza & Pneumonia 46	Chronic Low Respiratory Disease 62	HIV 225	Cerebro-vascular 601	Liver Disease 3,336	Diabetes Mellitus 5,343	Liver Disease 5,750	Alzheimer's Disease 53,246	Influenza & Pneumonia 62,034
8	Baderial Sepsis 698	Perinatal Period 72	Chronic Low Respiratory Disease 42	Benign Neoplasms 53	Cerebro-vascular 196	Diabetes Mellitus 595	Cerebro-vascular 2,491	HIV 4,120	Suicide 3,317	Nephritis 33,121	Alzheimer's Disease 53,852
9	Circulatory System Disease 622	Benign Neoplasms 58	Cerebro-vascular 38	Influenza & Pneumonia 48	Influenza & Pneumonia 181	Congenital Anomalies 458	Diabetes Mellitus 1,958	Chronic Low Respiratory Disease 3,324	Nephritis 3,284	Unintentional Injury 32,694	Nephritis 39,480
10	Intrautenine Hypoxia 534	Cerebro-vascular 54	Septicemia 29	Cerebro-vasoular 42	Chronic Low Respiratory Disease 171	Liver Disease 387	Homicide 2,467	Septicemia 3,111	Septicemia 25,418	Septicemia 32,236	Septicemia 32,236

Note: Homicide and suicide counts include terrorism deaths associated with the events of September 11, 2001, that occurred in New York City, Pennsylvania, and Virginia, A total of 2,926 U.S. residents lost their lives in these acts of terrorism in 2001, of which 2,922 were classified as (transportaion-related) homicides and 4 were classified as suicides.
Source: National Center for Health Statistics, (NCHS) Vital Statistics Systems.
Produced by : Office of Statistics and Programming, National Center for Injury Prevention and Control, CDC.

Figure 50-1 Ten leading causes of death by age group. Courtesy of the Centers for Disease Control and Prevention.
Source: Morbidity and Mortality Weekly Report, Vol. 58, No RR-1 (2009)

airway suctioning, assisted ventilations, chest compressions, and glucose monitoring are among the most important aspects of neonatal resuscitation. This topic will focus on those lifesaving skills.

TERMINOLOGY RELATED TO NEWBORNS

Before discussing how to assess and treat a newborn, one must start with the terminology used by health care professionals to describe the stages of development.

The fetal or *in utero* period is the prenatal (literally, before birth) development of the human. The average duration of fetal development—called the *gestational period*, which begins with conception—is 9 months, or around 40 weeks; this is referred to as the baby's *gestational age*, measured in weeks.

Babies born before 37 weeks gestational age are considered *premature*, those born within the 37-to-40-week period are called *term* infants, and those born after 40 weeks are considered *late term* gestations. For many reasons, premature infants are at especially high risk for complications; any EMS call to one should be considered a true emergency.

The term *perinatal* is used to define the immediate period around labor and delivery, which includes the late *prenatal* into the immediate *postnatal* times. The *neonatal period* refers to the first 30 days of life.

Infancy refers to the first year of life following the neonatal period (ages 1–12 months).

Having an understanding of this sometimes confusing terminology can help one both communicate with other health care professionals and understand why issues in one period of time can affect the infant in others.

Understanding the anatomic and physiologic transition from in utero to the extrauterine environment is crucial to appropriate assessment and management of the neonate or infant requiring medical attention. Those changes are the subject of introductory textbooks and will not be discussed in depth here, the assumption being that the AEMT should already have a working understanding of these changes.

Because the infant is so fragile and dependent on his environment for survival, seemingly little things, such as ambient or room temperature, can make the difference between successful and failed resuscitation efforts. Because our assessment and interventions require physical examination of a naked infant and because infants are at such high risk for hypothermia, we must ensure normal body temperature when infants are well, but even more so when they are ill.

This is important to mention at the outset, as it is something the AEMT needs to think about and be prepared for ahead of time (e.g., while en route to the call, warm up the back of the ambulance). For this reason, forethought and preparation are keys to good treatment. In no other population is attention to detail more important than in the care of the neonate.

ASSESSMENT AND EMERGENCY CARE

The most obvious and dramatic transition for neonates is going from an amniotic fluid-filled, "underwater" environment to an oxygen-rich, aerated (and colder) environment in which they are no longer able to receive oxygenated blood from their mothers via the placenta but are totally dependent on their lungs opening up to (1) the air they now need to breathe and (2) the pulmonary blood flow from the heart. The lungs need to literally open with air and redistribute the watery amniotic fluid, drying out in a way, and allowing the alveoli to begin gas exchange (CO_2 for O_2) for the first time.

If this amniotic fluid that was filling their lungs contained any of the meconium (or stool) that they have been producing in utero, their lungs may not function properly; they will quickly develop respiratory distress and then respiratory failure, characterized by cyanosis (blueing of the skin from deoxygenated blood), tachypnea, grunting, retractions, and even apnea. Cardiorespiratory failure and arrest are soon to follow if appropriate interventions are not taken.

If the newborn infant has a structural defect in the heart that does not permit adequate blood flow to the lungs or to the body, he will develop similar signs and symptoms. If the newborn develops an infection from delivery because his immune system is inadequately developed, he will present with the same signs and symptoms of respiratory distress, impending respiratory failure, and ultimately cardiorespiratory arrest. Respiratory failure can occur quickly—within minutes to hours—and requires immediate attention. Any deterioration must be acted on without delay.

Having the right equipment is the first rule of rescue for the neonatal and pediatric populations. There is no excuse for not having appropriately sized resuscitation equipment, from oral and nasal airways, to bag-valve masks, to suctioning equipment.

One of the most important pieces of airway equipment (and the one most often overlooked) is something that gives you the ability to suction the airway. For the neonate and infant, a bulb suction may be all that is necessary to clear the airway and allow the infant to breathe.

Because infants are obligate nose breathers (meaning they are literally hard-wired by their nervous systems to breathe through their noses and do not yet know how to breathe through their mouths), infants with upper respiratory infections that cause swelling and mucus production of the already narrow nasal passages can present in respiratory distress. Simple suctioning with saline drops can open an airway very effectively.

possible craniofacial abnormalities (e.g., Pierre-Robin sequence), placing them prone may open their airways and allow for better air movement if they are breathing spontaneously.

Use of soft, red rubber nasopharyngeal airways may be necessary to help keep the airway open if these infants are not breathing spontaneously. Use of an appropriately sized oral airway in the apneic infant can be very important in keeping the tongue forward enough to allow for adequate ventilation.

Remember that the infant's head, neck, and airway anatomy is significantly different from that of the older child: The head is proportionately much larger and heavier, with a prominent occiput and small midface (the part between the eyebrows and the chin) and a large tongue with limited mobility; the neck cannot support the head unassisted in the neonatal age range and must be supported by the caretaker; the airway structures of the neck—being collapsible, tracheal rings—are incompletely formed and flexible; and the entire airway, from nostrils to alveoli, is much smaller, easily blocked by secretions and highly resistant to airflow when edematous.

The soft tissue and joint laxity of the neonate and infant allow for easy manipulation, and it should be obvious that overly vigorous resuscitative efforts (such as jaw lift or neck extension) could cause harm. Because of the large occiput of the infant, it is important to be familiar with

how to position the infant supine and to use warm, dry towels to aid in positioning for the neck/shoulder roll.

Just as flexing the head (chin to chest) or even inadequate head extension (chin away from chest but not far enough) can close the airway because the tongue can cause occlusion, overextension of the head and jaw can actually compress the upper trachea and lead to more airway resistance, making ventilation more difficult. Find the middle ground between not enough extension and too much by listening with your stethoscope to the inspired (or delivered) breaths along the infant's neck.

BREATHING   When the airway patency has been established, assisted ventilation should be performed in any neonate with respiratory distress, apnea, or significant hypotonia (i.e., a floppy baby) and at a rate of 40 to 60 breaths per minute for a newborn or 30 to 40 per minute for an older neonate. High airway pressures during bag-valve-mask (BVM) ventilation can lead to trauma in the lungs and should be avoided.

Having the appropriately sized manual resuscitator bag is also important. The AEMT should seek to use only

> **Having the right equipment is the first rule of rescue for the neonatal and pediatric populations.**

ABCs: "In That Order, Every Time"

AIRWAY   The use of bag-mask ventilation in a neonate should never require force or much strength. Keeping a good facial-mask seal and avoiding pressure on the infant's eyes is easy if the appropriate mask size is available (▶ Figure 50-2). Use of an adult mask covering the infant's entire face may be required if an appropriately sized mask is not available—but this may require two rescuers for an adequate seal and to provide breaths.

Avoid pressure on the trachea, as it is not rigid and can easily collapse. Light downward pressure on the face with the mask, together with a corresponding light upward pressure from a one-fingered chin lift, is usually all that is required to maintain a good seal and open the airway. For infants with small jaws and

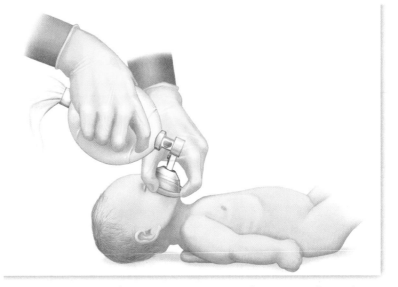

Figure 50-2 To provide positive pressure ventilation, use a bag-valve mask. Maintain a good mask seal. Ventilate with just enough force to raise the infant's chest. Ventilate at a rate of 40–60 per minute for 30 seconds, then reassess.

size-appropriate tidal volumes (15–25 mL for a newborn, 25–50 mL for neonates up to 1 month of age) during assisted ventilation. The best rule is "just enough to move the chest" but no more than that because of the risk for causing a pneumothorax.

In the heat of the resuscitation, it is easy to forget these little things—once again reinforcing the need for attention to details as the key to successful resuscitation. Whenever possible, a manometer on the BVM apparatus should be used, and peak inspiratory pressures kept below 30 cm H_2O. Aggressive use of positive end-expiratory pressure (PEEP) is usually not necessary because of the very compliant lungs and chest walls of the infant.

The efficacy of assisted ventilation will be obvious during a physical exam of the newborn or infant. One should see a rapid improvement in color and perfusion. If the infant was bradycardic when manual ventilations began, you should see an increase to normal or elevated heart rates if your ventilations are successful. An apneic infant will usually begin spontaneous respirations once adequately oxygenated and not overventilated.

Allowing the infant to continue breathing on his own is advised, but do not trust him to not become apneic again and require more assistance. According to the 2010 American Heart Association Guidelines for Cardiopulmonary Resuscitation and Emergency Cardiovascular Care, a blended mix of oxygen and air should be titrated to achieve a targeted preductal SpO_2 after birth at 60 to 65 percent after 1 minute, 65 to 70 percent after 2 minutes, 70 to 75 percent after 3 minutes, 75 to 80 percent after 4 minutes, 80 to 85 percent after 5 minutes, and 85 to 95 percent after 10 minutes. If the heart rate is less than 60 bpm after 90 seconds of resuscitation, the oxygen concentration should be increased to 100 percent until the heart rate increases to more than 100 bpm.

Although the AEMT is an advanced provider with some advanced airway skills and modalities available, in the absence of extenuating circumstances (e.g., significant meconium staining or inability to ventilate with a BVM), careful and efficient basic airway management is preferred over advanced techniques.

CIRCULATION   In the infant with persistent bradycardia (heart rate less than 60 bpm and not increasing) and signs of poor perfusion (cool extremities, mottling, capillary refill time more than 3 seconds, cyanosis) after 1 minute of adequate assisted bag-mask ventilation, chest compressions should be delivered. Review of the technique is important to prevent injury.

With two hands encircling the chest, and using the thumbs to depress the inferior half of the sternum, this so-called thumb technique is very effective if the rescuer's hands are large enough, and it is not as fatiguing as the two-finger technique (▶ Figure 50-3). If the rescuer is unable to encircle the chest with his hands, the "two-finger" technique is recommended. Two fingers of one hand compress the chest while the other hand is used to support the infant's back. In both techniques, the depth of compression should be one-third of the anterior-to-posterior diameter of the infant's chest, the thumbs or fingers should not be lifted off the chest but full recoil allowed, and chest expansion should be allowed.

The compression:breath ratio is 3:1 with a total 2-second cycle time such that the rescuer providing compressions counts "one-and-two-and-three-and-BREATHE." In one minute, there should be 90 compressions and 30 breaths delivered. Practicing this is important to ensure good timing when and if the real need arises.

For the infant who has a perfusing rhythm, circulation is a critical part of the exam, as shock in infants is so poorly tolerated and blood pressure can either be difficult to obtain or normal in the setting of shock. Accounting for the environmental temperature, capillary refill time in the newborn or infant should always be brisk. In the setting of an adequate cardiac output, the extremities will be warm to at least the wrists and ankles, and the capillary refill time immediate. The presence of cool extremities and/or mottling of the skin with any delay of the capillary refill over two seconds is cause for concern and is a true emergency.

Because the infant's heart is relatively immature and stiff, any drop in cardiac output is compensated for by an increase in heart rate. Having a thorough knowledge

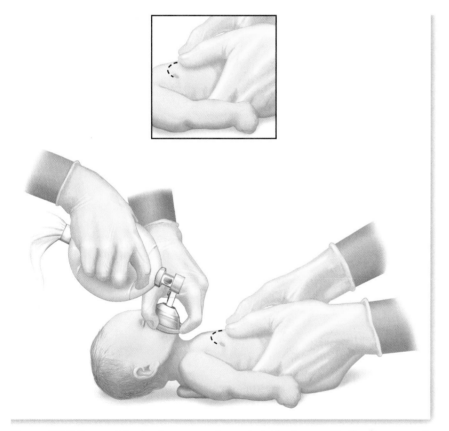

Figure 50-3 To provide chest compressions, circle the torso with the fingers and place both thumbs on the lower third of the infant's sternum. If the infant is very small, you may need to overlap the thumbs. If the infant is very large, compress the sternum with the ring and middle fingers placed one finger's depth below the nipple line. In the newborn, compress the chest one-third the depth of the chest at the rate of 120 per minute and a ratio of 3:1 compressions to ventilations.

of age-related normal (and abnormal) vital signs is crucial to appropriate triage and management of this population. In any suspected ill or injured infant, tachycardia (HR > 180 bpm) is never good until proven otherwise. Heart rates over 220 bpm usually signify a problem with the heart's conduction system and represent a true emergency requiring ALS intervention.

Blood pressure is probably the trickiest vital sign to obtain on an infant. Often the monitors are not sensitive enough because the infant is moving (or the ambulance is) or rescuers do not have the appropriate-sized cuffs. Because studies show that blood pressure is "the last to go" (unlike in adults, in whom shock is present when the systolic BP is less than 90 mmHg), a low-for-age BP is not necessary for the diagnosis of shock in infants and children. The presence of tachycardia and poor perfusion are all that is necessary. For this reason, it is crucial that the AEMT perform a thorough physical exam and pay attention to the other vital signs (heart rate, respiratory rate, capillary refill time, mental status/activity level, and muscle tone).

For newborns, a mean systolic blood pressure equal to or greater than the gestational age in weeks is considered acceptable, but again, this is in an otherwise healthy-looking infant. In the first month of life, a systolic BP less than 60 mmHg is considered hypotensive, in the infant (1 month–1 year) it is 70 mmHg, and up to 10 years of age the lower acceptable systolic limit is 70 + (2 × age in years).

Assessing the blood volume (i.e., hydration status) of a newborn or infant is probably one of the most challenging skills in all of medicine. Because the infant cannot communicate thirst or discomfort other than by crying, we must (again) rely on the details of the history, physical exam, and impressions of caretakers and rescuers together. A history of poor feeding, vomiting, copious diarrhea, decreased number of wet diapers that day, any fever, sweating, or respiratory difficulties during feeding should all clue you in to the fact that the infant may be dry.

On exam, as mentioned, look for resting tachycardia, tenting of the skin, absence of tears, and most important but latest to show, a lethargic infant with mottling and cool extremities, reflecting the increased systemic vascular resistance (SVR) required to maintain blood pressure in the setting of a decreased cardiac output from a low stroke volume due to dehydration. Remember that:

$$BP = SVR \times Cardiac\ Output,\ and$$
$$Cardiac\ Output = Heart\ Rate \times Stroke\ Volume$$

Thus, the increase in heart rate is the first and most subtle sign of a diminished cardiac output and will precede frank shock by hours in many cases.

IV access in the neonate is challenging. If fluid or medications (e.g., $D_{10}W$) must be administered, attempt peripheral vascular access. Intraosseous access may be considered based on protocol if peripheral IVs are unsuccessful. Use a buretrol whenever fluids are to be administered to a neonate to prevent overhydration, which occurs rapidly in this population.

What Comes after ABC? DEFG—"Don't Ever Forget Glucose!"

Because the fuel stores of glycogen in infants are so quickly exhausted by their rapid metabolic rates, hypoglycemia is a very frequent finding in the ill or injured infant. Just as it is impossible to resuscitate a cold infant, so is it impossible to resuscitate a hypoglycemic one. All key metabolic pathways rely on rapid uptake and utilization of glucose, especially the brain, and it is crucial to remember that infants are at higher risk for this than any other age group. If the AEMT does not consider hypoglycemia in the differential diagnosis, he will never think to check it. Because oral glucose can be rapidly absorbed, failure to check and treat for hypoglycemia is an unfortunately common mistake.

Feeding for newborns and infants is their exercise. It can be exhausting for a sick infant to feed, to coordinate the muscles of respiration and those of swallowing. This is especially true for premature or fragile infants with medical conditions. For this reason, questions about the infant's feeding (amount, duration, frequency, and whether there was any emesis, sweating, or frequent coughing) can be very important clues to the underlying problem. In a sense, the newborn infant's "day" can be reduced to four-hour cycles of sleeping, crying to communicate discomfort, feeding, and some period of alertness before sleeping again.

Understanding this routine, asking the caretaker about it, and paying particular attention to any deviations from it are crucial tips to getting a good history. Any lethargic infant with a history of poor feeding should be assumed to be hypoglycemic, and his blood sugar should be checked as soon as possible.

If glucose is to be administered to a neonate, $D_{10}W$ should be used at a dose of 5 to 10 mL/kg IV over 20 minutes. Follow local protocols.

> Heart rates over 220 beats per minute usually signify a problem with the heart's conduction system and represent a true emergency requiring ALS intervention.

H Is for Hypothermia

Once again, it cannot be overemphasized how important attention to the environmental temperature is to the care of an infant. Even the best resuscitation skills and efforts will fail if the infant is cold. A corollary to the old EMS adage, "They're not dead until they're warm and dead," is that the infant will not survive until he is warm.

The inability of the neonate to generate enough heat is directly related to heat loss from the head's large surface area, the lack of insulating fat, and the high proportion of metabolically active brown fat—called "brown" because of the high density of energy-producing mitochondria that, when in a condition of inadequate fuel (oxygen and/or glucose) are unable to produce heat to keep the infant warm.

I Is for Infection

Infection is a major killer of neonates and can have a very rapid presentation. Sometimes the history is only of a fussy baby who was not feeding very well, whose breathing became more labored and then would stop occasionally (apnea) and have episodes of turning blue (cyanosis). This is the common introduction to the story of a potentially very sick and dying neonate and cannot be overlooked or discounted by health care professionals.

Any history of fever in an infant, any cyanosis, any apnea, and any history of rapid or shallow breathing requires immediate transport for evaluation. *Any* history of poor feeding, decreased urine output from the usual number of wet diapers per day, vomiting, or sweating, which all can lead to dehydration, requires that the infant be seen by a pediatric professional. *Any* history of blood in the stool, urine, or emesis and *any* rash beyond "baby acne"—especially a petechial rash, which is not raised and is nonblanching because it is, in fact, ruptured capillaries just under the skin and associated with severe infections (i.e., meningitis)—requires evaluation by a pediatric professional.

> **Any infant who is "not acting right" requires examination and is assumed to be ill until proven otherwise.**

In short, any infant who is "not acting right" requires examination and is assumed to be ill until proven otherwise. Because the ways infants have to tell us that something is wrong are so few, we must be looking for the clues and pay attention to the little details—this can literally mean the difference between life and death.

No other patient age group encountered by EMS professionals will require such basic resuscitative care and yet have such a high potential for recovery and good outcome. That said, these calls are rare and highly stressful. Seeking out and receiving additional training such as that offered through the American Academy of Pediatrics' Neonatal Resuscitation Program is a good way to develop the confidence and skill set necessary to care for this most fragile population.

Safe Transport of the Infant

Every EMS provider should be familiar with how to safely transport a patient of any size and age. Entire chapters in EMS textbooks are devoted to lifting, packaging, and moving adult patients, but only a paragraph or two are given to safely packaging and transporting the most tenuous and fragile pediatric patient. Transporting an infant or child in the arms of a properly restrained caretaker is absolutely unacceptable. The force generated by a 10-pound patient on the arms of the parent involved in a 30-miles-per-hour crash is beyond anyone's ability to achieve.

Having a convertible child passenger restraint system (car seat) with two belt paths and a five-point harness system that can be adjusted to the size of the child is standard of care. Transporting the neonate in an isolette is ideal, as the chamber can be heated. In the absence of that, a car bed that lies across the stretcher and is strapped down using the stretcher's harnessing is next best. Few EMS systems have these, however, and most may not even have car seats (although that should change).

Unfortunately, most neonates (< 5 kg) may not fit properly in these car seats. The restraining straps may not fit their shoulders and/or the seat may cause their heads to fall forward and obstruct their airways. For this reason, having a tested system that can be readily available for use during a neonatal emergency is crucial to our ultimate goal: safely transporting that patient to the hospital. Resources exist to help train EMS services in proper restraint of neonatal and pediatric patients, and they should afford themselves those opportunities.

TRANSITIONING

REVIEW ITEMS

1. What percentage of newborns will require resuscitation with delivery?
   - a. 1 percent
   - b. 3 percent
   - c. 5 percent
   - d. 10 percent

2. You are transporting an infant who is having periods of apnea, but you don't have the appropriate-size mask to provide assisted ventilations. Before starting mouth-to-mouth/nose-assisted ventilations, what else could you try?
   - a. a nonrebreather mask on high-flow oxygen, using the reservoir bag to assist ventilations
   - b. an oral airway, blowing through it instead of using mouth-to-mouth/nose
   - c. an adult-size mask, creating a seal over the infant's entire face
   - d. nothing, just stimulating the baby to breathe

3. What is the normal range of heart rates for an awake newborn infant?
   - a. 60–80/minute
   - b. 80–100/minute
   - c. 100–120/minute
   - d. 120–140/minute

4. The recommended breath-to-compression ratio for infant CPR is _____.
   - a. 3:1
   - b. 2:1
   - c. 1:2
   - d. 1:3

5. For the past two days, according to the mother's report, a three-week-old infant is sleepier than usual, has been fussing continually when awake, cries when picked up but then falls quickly to sleep, has had some fever, and has not had the normal number of wet diapers per day. What is your assessment?
   - a. This is normal for three-week-old infants—because of their rapid growth, they frequently need more fluid and are more tired.
   - b. This is not normal but happens frequently, and the infant should be evaluated in the next couple of days.
   - c. This is not normal, and the infant should be transported immediately to a facility capable of managing the infant.

APPLIED PATHOPHYSIOLOGY

1. Describe the proper positioning for performing chest compressions on a newborn.

2. Explain how to assess for an altered mental status in a neonate.

3. Describe the signs of respiratory distress in a newborn.

4. Explain transitional circulation in the newborn.

CLINICAL DECISION MAKING

You are called to the home of a two-week-old infant who turned blue for 20 seconds. according to her 16-year-old mother. She has been feeding poorly for the past few days but has had no fever. You notice that the infant looks tired, has low muscle tone but is working to breathe, and is showing signs of respiratory distress (tachypnea, grunting, nasal flaring, subcostal and sternal retractions) with a respiratory rate of 80–90, heart rate 220 beats/minute, and unpalpable distal pulses.

1. What is your major concern about this patient?

2. Could this represent congenital heart disease? Infection? Dehydration?

3. What are normal vital signs (heart rate and respiratory rate) for a two-week-old?

The mother reports that the baby is looking better and that she does not want to go to the hospital, stating that she will call her baby's doctor or take her into the clinic.

4. Is this acceptable for her to do?

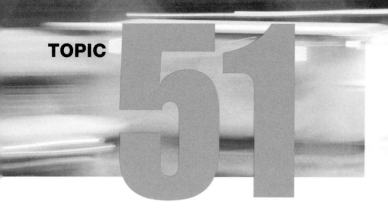
Standard Special Patient Populations

Competency Applies a fundamental knowledge of growth, development, and aging and assessment findings to provide basic and selected advanced emergency care and transportation for a patient with special needs.

PEDIATRICS

TRANSITION highlights

- Personal, EMS system, and health care system resources necessary to manage pediatric patients.

- How to approach the pediatric patient, and how to incorporate the primary caregiver's needs/wants/fears into the Advanced EMT's assessment and treatment plans.

- The Pediatric Assessment Triangle (PAT) and its ability to help guide the Advanced EMT into a thorough assessment.

- Common underlying pathology for disturbances in the pediatric airway, breathing, and circulatory functions.

- Current treatment standards when caring for a patient with a pediatric emergency.

INTRODUCTION

Before responding to any pediatric calls, one needs to look into three mirrors: one reflects yourself, your attitudes and beliefs; the second reflects your EMS service's unique abilities and weaknesses (whether from an educational, resource, or equipment standpoint) for handling pediatric patients during an emergency; and the third requires looking at your capabilities from a regional prehospital and hospital-based *systems* perspective: Does your region have the needed elements in place to fully care for critically ill and injured children? This topic will discuss these three views that need to be examined to best care for our most precious resource—our children.

Ask yourself, "What would I want if it were my child?"

INTO THE LOOKING GLASS: PERSONAL PERSPECTIVE

Few EMS calls provoke more anxiety than the pediatric cases. Most AEMTs would prefer *any* sick adult to a screaming, ill, or injured child. The reasons cited for this are many ("I can't talk to them," "I'm afraid of hurting them," "They always fight me when I'm trying to help," "I can never remember what are normal vital signs," "The parents always try to tell us what to do," "We don't carry the right-size equipment"), and if you fall into this majority of EMS professionals, doing some self-analysis to discover your reasons is very important—ideally before that call comes in.

If we do not examine and address those reasons, we will seek to avoid these calls, discount them when they do not go as well as they should, and blame others, and—fundamentally—we will not perform as well as we could for our patients, for our professional colleagues, and for ourselves.

When you can understand the reasons why caring for children provokes anxiety in you, you can begin to work with them to better suit the environment and the patient. Asking yourself, "What would I want if it were my child?" will help guide you to become the best pediatric EMS professional you can be.

Pediatric calls present unique challenges, for a wide variety of reasons, and most EMS educational curricula do not adequately address our fears about caring in these situations for the most dependent and fragile members of our society.

APPROACHING THE CHILD: FIRST IMPRESSION

The first step in caring for children is to be able to get down to their level, both figuratively and quite literally. Standing above a child, as an adult stranger in a uniform with equipment and a squawking radio, is terrifying to any child. First impressions matter more to children because they cannot make the assumptions about you, based on your appearance, that adults can—from your gender, hairstyle, uniform, type of footwear, height, tone of voice, and demeanor—because children do not yet have the experience to make such judgments.

The way you approach the child initially will determine how the next few minutes will go. Getting down to the child's eye level,

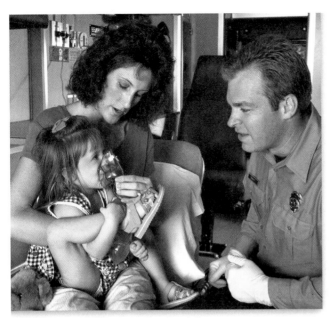
Figure 51-1 Approach a young child on the child's level, with the caregiver present.

which may mean crouching or sitting on the ground near him, while keeping your distance initially until the child "lets you in," is crucial to engaging that child and making a good first impression (▶ Figure 51-1).

Ideally, the initial assessment of a child is done as you approach him. Any child with "attitude" is one you need to take some time getting to know. The critically ill or injured child, for whom you need to intervene right away, will not care about your approach and interventions or will have little energy to spare to fight or disagree with you. For other children who are not so time-critical, a slow and respectful initial approach is critical to establishing that relationship.

For any conscious, alert child over six months of age, you are a potential threat until you prove that you aren't. Even though you may not be able to adequately treat his pain from an injury or relieve his respiratory distress right away, you can provide reassurance by reading his signs and respecting them.

Even an infant has signs or cues that, if you are looking for them, will alert you to when you are being too imposing, aggressive, or frightening; when it is okay to approach him; and when it is okay to touch him. This becomes even more important as the child grows and develops the autonomy to self-determine and control his environment. Illness and injury threaten that autonomy by stressing the child and his environment, including his parents or caretakers, and this puts an added dimension of stress back on the child.

Although you know you are there to help, the child does not and may need some convincing. Putting aside some of your need to hurry (i.e., your desire to minimize on-scene time) to spend an extra minute or two engaging the child is time well spent and may afford you an opportunity to learn something that could affect the course of that child's treatment.

Many children perceive looking them in the eyes, talking to them loudly, and reaching out to touch them all at once as threats. This approach can quickly overwhelm the scared child and cause him to retreat, to cry inconsolably, and to fight any further advances. Limiting your approach to just talking to him but not looking at him, or talking to the parent while visually assessing the child from a distance, can help the child adjust to your presence and give him time to assess you. The child will take many cues from the parent's response to the EMT.

Working with the child by respecting his space, addressing him by name, and asking permission to examine him cannot be underestimated or overemphasized. Using toys or stuffed animals to approach the child is a good tactic, and they can also be used to help quiet and distract a crying child, allowing you to auscultate breath sounds or heart tones.

Be careful not to try to trick the child or lie to him—if you are caught, you will lose his trust. For example, do not tell the child that something will not hurt when it will, do not tell him medicine tastes good when it will not, and do not distract him with a toy and check a finger stick glucose without offering a warning.

PARENTS AND CARETAKERS

Certainly caretakers understand that you are there to help, but they will place their trust in you even more quickly if they see that you respect their child and value the child's cues. Respecting the child is respecting the parent and has an added benefit for working with the child: When the child sees that his caretaker trusts you, he will look at you differently, less as a stranger, and will be more likely to open up to you.

To further help this process, understanding the stress the caretakers are under will allow you to help them cope with what is likely one of the biggest crises in their life: having to call for emergency help because of a sick or injured child. "Value passion wherever you find it" is a phrase that EMS personnel should always remember when dealing with parents and caretakers of sick and injured children. Valuing passion refers to the fact that they care most about their child, and during the stress from an illness or injury, nothing else matters as much to them—not you, not the doctors or nurses, not the police.

Furthermore, if you betray the caretakers' trust or do not align yourself with them in caring for and respecting their child, you have in essence betrayed them. When seen in this light, it becomes clear that allying yourself with parents or caretakers is much easier than not doing so and having them turn against you. Sometimes we must swallow our pride and be humble with stressed parents, but this is a sign not of weakness but of compassion.

Medical professionals have coined the term *difficult parents* to refer to parents who are stressed by a having a sick or injured child, who are having trouble coping, and who feel that the environment that is supposed to be caring for their child is instead uncaring, hostile, and unsafe. These parents can be bossy, very directive, and rigid and will sometimes order health care professionals around or be oppositional.

As professionals, it is our first responsibility to the patient and family members to make them feel safe and cared for, to always communicate with respect. Taking the time to listen to them and to address their fears and concerns honestly (saying "I don't know" when you do not is acceptable and preferable to making something up) is as important as

> **Work with the child by respecting his space, addressing him by name, and asking permission to examine him.**

performing a good history and physical exam.

ASSESSMENT OF THE PEDIATRIC PATIENT

For the reasons discussed in the preceding section, the physical assessment of a child is more art than science and requires a high degree of personal investment, professionalism, and expert communication skills. The knowledge base required is an understanding of the developmental and physical differences among infants and children of different ages.

Even within the first year of life (infancy), significant changes occur physically, neurologically, emotionally, and cognitively. Parents are well aware of these changes in their own children and are also aware of unique or subtle differences if their child has a chronic medical condition.

It is crucial to your assessment to use the parents' knowledge of these differences and, in so doing, build that bond of trust with the parent. Once you have an understanding of the growth and development of children through the first 12 to 15 years, age-related differences in vital signs and equipment become second nature, instinctual, and easy to remember.

Adult-oriented physical exam skills have limited applicability in assessing the ill or injured child. In terms of appearance, when one understands what should be the child's baseline normal activity, attitude, and appearance, one can quickly assess an altered mental status, a depressed level of functioning, or abnormalities in gait, posture, or coordination that make the difference in diagnosis and management.

> **Adult-oriented physical exam skills have limited applicability in assessing the ill or injured child.**

Vital sign differences are sometimes misinterpreted and can lead to delays in management and outcome. Knowing, for example, that the response of an infant or child to shock is to increase cardiac output through a dramatic increase in heart rate and systemic vascular resistance allows one to know to look for tachycardia and delayed capillary refill time, mottling, and low urine output (a decrease in the number of wet diapers when asked of the parent on history taking), which will prompt you to intervene quickly, without waiting for the low blood pressure of decompensated shock.

As delays in resuscitation of the child in shock are an independent variable increasing mortality rates by more than 20 percent, early intervention in pediatric shock has a proven benefit to the child's ultimate outcome.

Pediatric Assessment Triangle

No contribution to our assessment armamentarium is more important than the Pediatric Assessment Triangle (PAT; ▸ Figure 51-2), which modifies the traditional ABCs of airway–breathing–circulation to appearance–breathing–circulation, incorporating the adult-focused *airway* into pediatric *breathing* and elevating the importance of *disability*, which is sometimes forgotten, into *appearance*.

Outside the Apgar scoring system for neonates, the PAT has allowed for a more objective and reproducible set of criteria for assessing the ill or injured child than any other system to date. It also follows the logical progression of the AEMT as he or she enters the scene: Looking at the child's appearance, level of activity, and "attitude" can be done from across the room; assessing breathing requires one to be a bit closer to the child to look and listen for signs of increased work of breathing (grunting, stridor, nasal flaring, retractions, and an increased respiratory rate); and the assessment of circulation requires a hand on the child's extremity to assess warmth and capillary refill time and to check the heart rate either by pulse or monitor.

Thinking of your assessment and triage as starting from the moment you enter the room or arrive on scene allows you to quickly determine the life support decisions you need to make:

Do you have time to further assess the awake and screaming infant, or do you need to call for ALS intercept or medical control for interventions for the unresponsive toddler lying in front of you? The paradigm is intuitive to those experienced in pediatric assessment and should be the cornerstone of your assessment, triage, intervention, and reassessment strategy for pediatric care.

APPEARANCE Because of the high metabolic requirements of the infant and child (think in terms of the body's energy production and utilization, oxygen delivery and consumption, and carbon dioxide production), significant disturbances in the child's health from illness or injury will manifest themselves early and profoundly in the child's appearance. For this reason, appearance is the most important and first of the ABCs in pediatric assessment.

Recognizing an abnormal appearance in a child requires a more detailed system than the traditional AVPU used in adult-oriented care. The TICLS mnemonic has proven itself over time and can help detect subtle but crucial deficits in the child's appearance and behavior:

- Tone
- Interactiveness
- Consolability
- Look/gaze
- Speech/cry

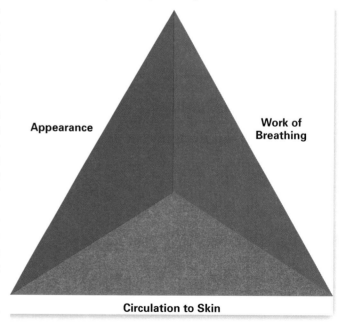

Figure 51-2 The Pediatric Assessment Triangle (PAT). (Used with permission of the American Academy of Pediatrics.) *Source:* General Approach to Pediatric Assessment

It is important to evaluate one's own contribution to the child's appearance, as a rapid and loud entry of the EMS team can, as previously mentioned, lead to an agitated and difficult-to-console child. Even though it should be somewhat reassuring that the child has this much attitude and is not likely to be critically ill, bear in mind that children do have effective, though somewhat limited, compensatory mechanisms.

A good rule of thumb is to not trust the child: His clinical condition can change very quickly as his limited ability to compensate is overwhelmed by the underlying illness or injury. This requires continued observation and reassessment, especially if transport times are long. On the other hand, a lethargic child who cannot muster the energy to cry is one to be very worried about: He needs immediate evaluation in a hospital equipped to resuscitate children and thus triggers a true "load and go" response.

Abnormal appearance is never good and can be caused by shock from inadequate perfusion, hypoglycemia, respiratory distress leading to respiratory failure and hypoxemia, hypercarbia and acidosis, neurologic compromise from a closed head injury, or poisoning.

BREATHING The process of *respiration* actually refers to our cellular engines (*mitochondria*) in which the consumption of oxygen and fuels (carbohydrates, fat) and production of energy and carbon dioxide (exhaust) allow us to cope with our environment and to grow and thrive. Cellular respiration requires homeostasis (balance and health), sufficient fuel intake, delivery (cardiac output and hemoglobin), and adequate mechanisms for getting oxygen in (oxygenation) and carbon dioxide out (ventilation) through the lungs (breathing).

The respiratory systems of the infant and child are poorly designed to handle an increased workload and thus are at a unique disadvantage when it comes to the mechanics of breathing when the lungs are sick. The AEMT should have a thorough knowledge and understanding of why that is, as this will allow for early recognition and management of pediatric respiratory distress and failure, which are the leading cause of hospitalization and the second-leading cause of death and disability in children. The significantly higher metabolic requirements of the infant and child make them unique from adults and more prone to fatigue and failure, with less ability to communicate their needs.

To elucidate the issues, consider the following case:

> **Respiratory distress and failure are the leading cause of hospitalization and second-leading cause of death and disability in children.**

CASE STUDY

A three-month-old boy develops viral bronchiolitis during the winter, acquired from his two-year-old sister, who attends day care; it starts with nasal congestion. With small nares with swollen mucosal lining and secretions, the increased resistance of breathing through his smaller nasal passages takes more energy. Because he is an obligatory nose breather and is literally not "wired" neurologically to be able to breathe through his mouth, this nasal congestion keeps him from being able to bottle-feed or breast-feed well. He becomes more tired as his energy stores are depleted and begins to get mildly dehydrated, which is made worse by his low-grade fever.

Both his heart and respiratory rates increase, requiring more energy from him. This leads to a vicious cycle, as his metabolic requirements for fuel, oxygen, water, and carbon dioxide removal all increase, placing larger and larger requirements on his already stressed cardiorespiratory system. He becomes more tired and begins to look lethargic, unable to cry or interact for very long. His wet diapers are much fewer in number, and he doesn't seem as interested in feeding.

As the viral infection moves down his respiratory tract, he begins to have trouble breathing because of the secretions and inflammation that are now affecting his bronchiolar tree. His coughing spells lead to more exhaustion, and his work of breathing increases even more to compensate. As his respiratory rate increases, so does his effort to inhale, as his lungs become heavier with mucus and fluid, and his compliant chest wall does not give him any mechanical advantage the way a rigid, adultlike rib cage would.

His diaphragm-dependent breathing causes his sternum to retract because his ribs and sternum are mostly cartilaginous and are unable to expand in diameter with each inspiratory effort in the way adult rib cages do. In addition to the softer rib cage, infants' chests lack the normal bucket-handle movement of the adult rib cage, which also translates into an increase in thoracic and lung volumes in the adult.

His diaphragm has fatigue-prone muscles, as he will not develop a majority of type II, fatigue-resistant diaphragmatic muscles until he is as old as his sister. His accessory muscles (intercostals, shoulder girdle, and neck strap muscles) are also poorly developed, as he is not yet sitting up unassisted and only uses his shoulder and neck muscles with gravity from a supine position, not being old enough to roll over yet. His lung congestion worsens from the airway inflammation and mucus production, making him have to pull harder to get an adequate tidal volume.

His chest wall retracts with each breath, and he begins to laryngeal brake or "grunt" (it is impossible to do this quietly), closing off his glottis or vocal cords at the end of inhalation, bearing down with a Valsalva maneuver briefly before quickly exhaling and breathing in again. It is an extremely inefficient and only temporarily effective way of keeping his lung units from collapsing at the end of every breath.

This method of breathing—faster than normal, using what accessory muscles he has (mostly nasal flaring), sternally retracting and grunting—causes his normal oxygen requirements for breathing to go up by a factor of 5 to 10, leaving little oxygen reserve for anything else, such as attitude, interaction, crying, or physical activity.

The end result is an infant in severe respiratory distress and impending respiratory failure, with hypoxemia, hypercarbia, tachycardia, and tachypnea, resulting in respiratory and metabolic acidosis from dehydration. The infant will, from across the room, appear lethargic with decreased activity and tone, and without any attitude, and on exam will have all the preceding signs of increased work of breathing—until he cannot hold on anymore.

CIRCULATION Assessment of a child's circulatory system involves consideration of three essential elements that are in constant communication with each other: the pump (heart), the pipes (vasculature), and the fluid filling them (the blood volume). Dysfunction in any one of these will lead to the other two needing to compensate for it. The principles of circulation follow strict laws of nature. Most important is the Ohm law, in which Pressure = Flow × Resistance, which is the equation for blood pressure (BP = Cardiac Output × Systemic Vascular Resistance [SVR]), incorporating the three components (Cardiac Output = Heart Rate [HR] × Stroke Volume).

Volume Loss Take the most common form of shock, hypovolemic shock from bleeding or dehydration, as an example: Because the blood volume is low, the vasculature will clamp down to increase SVR, which will temporarily increase BP and the venous return to the heart (preload), which increases stroke volume and cardiac output. At the same time, the heart will pump faster to further increase cardiac output and maintain delivery of oxygen and life-sustaining nutrients to the tissues.

If these mechanisms are inadequate to compensate for the primary problem, the body will begin to shut down blood flow to nonvital organs, starting with the peripheral muscle beds of the arms and legs, by further increasing SVR until these extremities are cool to the touch, mottled in appearance, and pale. End-organ perfusion is affected with the findings of dry mucous membranes and low or no urine output. Because BP might be preserved, the rapid assessment of shock in a child involves tachycardia and these signs of compensatory increases in SVR.

A normal BP in a child with these findings is called *compensated shock*; this child requires emergent transport and advanced life support interventions. *Decompensated shock* refers to the late and preterminal phase when the BP starts to drop. Never wait for hypotension to begin rapid transport and intervention.

Pump Failure Primary pump dysfunction from a cardiomyopathy will lead to findings of increased heart rate and SVR, along with poor end-organ perfusion. When the cardiac output is inadequate to keep up with the demands, these compensatory mechanisms ironically make matters worse. Increasing the metabolic needs of an already sick heart by increasing the rate and force with which it pumps while also increasing the load against which it has to pump (afterload) is a vicious cycle.

Cardiomyopathy can result from prolonged tachydysrhythmias such as supraventricular tachycardia (SVT), from viral infections of the myocardium, or from congenital heart disease. Because the myocardium is stiff and poorly contractile, increasing preload gently is important, but aggressive fluid management is dangerous; decreasing heart rate and SVR is critical, but requires specially trained pediatric practitioners.

Children with this form of shock require immediate care available in a children's hospital. As our ability to surgically treat congenital heart disease improves, more and more of these children are living to older ages and will be patients you will see.

Low Vascular Tone In this last example—distributive shock from sepsis, anaphylaxis, or a neurogenic etiology associated with a spinal cord injury—the problem is one of low vascular tone in which the body's catecholamines are unable to increase the SVR so vital to maintaining BP, perfusion, and preload to the heart. The heart rate will increase immediately (except in cases of spinal trauma), which is always the first sign and is never good, but the blood volume cannot increase by itself and will be distributed in a larger vascular bed, resulting in hypotension, a widened pulse pressure, and, paradoxically, skin that appears warm and well perfused.

In this situation, the child's appearance will be consistent with shock in that he will be lethargic, tachycardic, and tachypneic but not in respiratory distress, which is the child's attempt to remove carbon dioxide and compensate for the acid production from inadequate perfusion.

Rapid assessment of a child's circulation requires consideration of the three components of the circulatory system: the pump, the pipes, and the fluid in them. In all these categories, rapid transport and resuscitation are critical to outcome.

TREATMENT GUIDELINES AND PROTOCOLS

Thorough knowledge and understanding of pediatric emergency care will be reflected in an EMS service's patient care protocols. Although many protocols and guidelines are available on the Internet, going through the process of developing one's own set of protocols can be highly educational and empowering. Color-coded, length-based resuscitation tapes can form the foundation of color-coded guidelines for patients of different sizes and ages.

For advanced EMS providers, vascular access may be required on the pediatric patient. Access may be obtained through IV catheters or intraosseous (IO) insertion. Although IO is now widely used in the adult population, not long ago it was limited to the pediatric patient. The IO route is used in the critical patient when IV access cannot be obtained or would cause delay in care in the critically ill or injured pediatric patient. Fluid challenges are used in shock and are recommended at 20 mL/kg (10 mL/kg in infants). Follow local protocols for vascular access and fluid challenges.

Although ideally the EMS medical director should take the lead in the development and implementation of these guidelines, frequently this is not the case. EMTs and advanced providers should insist on some minimum treatment guidelines to handle the majority of pediatric calls: trauma (accidental and non-accidental), respiratory distress, asthma, seizures, hypoglycemia, poisonings, cardiopulmonary arrest, environmental emergencies, and shock.

An essential component of any high-quality service is the use of quality improvement and case review strategies to analyze areas of weakness in education, equipment, systems of care, and other resources. It is important to ensure that the pediatric communities of interest, from the families to the hospital-based providers, are involved in the review process.

Pediatric Champion

It is recommended that an EMS service designate a "pediatric champion" who can serve as a resource for others in the department, keep an eye on the latest developments in prehospital pediatric management, serve as a liaison with the state Emergency Medical Services for Children (EMSC) program and the local community, develop and maintain treatment guidelines, and help facilitate continuing pediatric education.

TRANSITIONING

REVIEW ITEMS

1. The Pediatric Assessment Triangle refers to what ABCs?
   a. attitude, behavior, consolability
   b. activity, breathing, cardiovascular
   c. appearance, breathing, circulation
   d. appearance, behavior, cuddliness

2. The equation for blood pressure is _____.
   a. BP = Stroke Volume × Heart Rate
   b. BP = Systemic Vascular Resistance × Heart Rate
   c. BP = Systemic Vascular Resistance × Stroke Volume
   d. BP = Systemic Vascular Resistance × Cardiac Output

3. The main reason that infants and children are poorly equipped to handle respiratory distress is because _____.
   a. their lungs are immature and airways are small
   b. after infancy, their immune systems are poorly developed
   c. their chest walls are so compliant that they cave in with the increased work of breathing
   d. they do not know how to cough effectively

4. Signs of respiratory distress in a child include _____.
   a. tachypnea   b. retractions
   c. nasal flaring   d. grunting (laryngeal braking)
   e. all of the above

5. Children with special health care needs are especially challenging primarily because _____.
   a. they frequently have conditions that require ALS to manage
   b. their parents are often difficult to work with
   c. they are medically complex and frequently have baseline conditions that are very abnormal
   d. they cannot tell the AEMT what is wrong with them

6. The pediatric airway is different from the adult airway because _____.
   a. the child's tongue is proportionately smaller than the adult's
   b. the adult's head is bigger and neck is longer than the child's
   c. the child's airway structures are proportionately smaller
   d. the child produces more secretions

APPLIED PATHOPHYSIOLOGY

1. Differentiate between the Pediatric Assessment Triangle (PAT) and the adult primary assessment.

2. Explain why blood pressure is not the most critical finding in determining a shock state. Explain what vital signs are more important to assess in determining shock.

3. Explain the vicious cycle associated with respiratory distress that leads to failure in the pediatric patient.

4. Describe the signs and symptoms of respiratory distress.

5. Explain the difference between the presentations of respiratory distress and respiratory failure. What is the difference in emergency care?

6. Explain why children with special health care needs are most challenging to manage.

7. Explain the difference between the pediatric airway and the adult airway.

CLINICAL DECISION MAKING

You are called to the home of a three-year-old child with croup. She is sitting in her mother's lap and breathing quickly, with a respiratory rate of 50/minute, with audible inspiratory stridor. She is calm until you approach her, but when you get to within six feet of her, she begins to cry, and her breathing becomes more audible and labored. She appears warm and well perfused, and her mother says she has had good liquid intake today but is not interested in solid foods. She has had some upper airway congestion but no fever. Her past medical history is unremarkable.

1. How would you describe her clinical condition? Stable? Urgent? Emergent?

2. Is her behavior normal for her age?

3. Is she in respiratory distress? Respiratory failure?

4. What are your treatment priorities?

Because her agitation makes her respiratory condition worse and her mother can calm her, you decide to let her mother hold her in her lap en route to the hospital. You secure her mother to your stretcher and have her hold her daughter in her arms.

5. Is this an appropriate arrangement in which to transport the child and mother?

TOPIC

Standard Special Patient Populations

Competency Applies a fundamental knowledge of growth, development, and aging and assessment findings to provide basic and selected advanced emergency care and transportation for a patient with special needs.

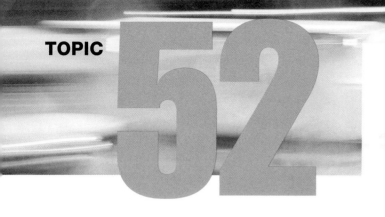

GERIATRICS

TRANSITION *highlights*

- How the U.S. population is aging, and what percentage of the geriatric population uses health care services; incident rates for common chronic conditions as it pertains to the geriatric population.

- Pathophysiologic body changes that occur to geriatric patients:
  - Cardiovascular.
  - Respiratory.
  - Nervous.
  - Gastrointestinal.
  - Endocrine.
  - Musculoskeletal.
  - Renal.
  - Integumentary.

- Common assessment findings in geriatric patients and how to use a differential diagnosis process to determine the most likely field impression of the patient's emergency.

- Current treatment strategies for the geriatric patient with emphasis on supporting lost function.

INTRODUCTION

As you know, a significant number of EMS calls you receive as an AEMT involve geriatric patients—understandably so, given that people over the age of 65 constitute the fastest-growing segment of population, and the largest group of users of health care, in the United States today. Therefore, it is important that you understand the characteristics of geriatric patients and how to tailor your assessment and treatment to their special needs.

Geriatric patients differ from their younger counterparts in many ways, largely due to changes in physiology from lifestyle and aging. The geriatric patient often has very different signs and symptoms of an acute illness or traumatic injury as compared with younger patients. Compounding this is the fact that geriatric patients often have one or more coexisting long-term condition(s) that require multiple medications, which also affects how problems present.

The key to remember is that geriatric patients may not display common presentation patterns for emergency conditions that AEMTs are called on to treat; as such, always maintain a high index of suspicion.

EPIDEMIOLOGY

Although it is not news that we are constantly aging, it is interesting to see *how* the population of the United States is aging. The elderly (those 65 years or older) numbered almost 40 million in 2008. This represented 12.8 percent of the U.S. population, or about one in every eight Americans. By 2030, this number will almost double, to more than 71 million elderly people. People over age 65 represented 12.4 percent of the population in 2000 but are expected to grow to 20 percent of the population by 2030.

Cardiovascular diseases, primarily heart attacks, are the leading cause of death in the elderly. Cancer is a close second, and strokes and COPD disorders comprise cause numbers three and four, respectively. The fifth-leading cause of death in the elderly is accidental injuries. The death rate per 100,000 population is three times higher for elderly victims of trauma than that for young adults, despite the fact that trauma is thought of as a "young person's disease." Other chronic conditions present as well, but collectively they account for a minority of geriatric mortality. In addition, the elderly commonly have more than one chronic condition, and they use one-third of all prescription medications—an elderly patient takes, on average, 4.5 medications per day (▶ Figure 52-1).

The lesson to be learned is that elderly patients comprise a very significant percentage of calls seen by EMS providers. It behooves the AEMT to be familiar with the effects of aging on the body and how these effects manifest themselves during instances of injury or illness.

PATHOPHYSIOLOGY

The human body changes with age. As a person ages, cellular, organ, and system functioning changes. This change in physiology—which typically starts around age 30—is a normal

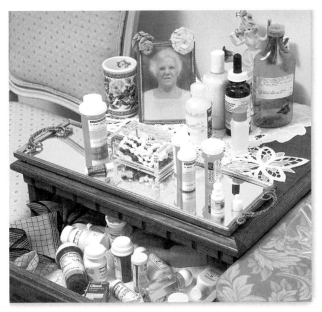

Figure 52-1 Elderly patients often take multiple medications.

part of aging. Although people may try to slow the aging process by diet, exercise, health care, and so on, it cannot be stopped entirely. To further compound the picture, most elderly patients will have not one but a combination of different disease processes in varying stages of development. Unfortunately, the aging body has fewer reserves with which to combat disease, and this ultimately contributes to the incidence of acute medical and traumatic emergencies.

It is important for the AEMT to understand and recognize changes in geriatric body systems so that appropriate care for elderly patients can be provided. Remember that the physiologic effects (summarized in Table 52-1 and ▶ Figure 52-2) result from the normal aging process, not from disease progression per se. However, any disease or injury the patient experiences will only worsen—or be made worse by—these changes.

Cardiovascular System

With age, degenerative processes affect the ability of the heart to pump blood. Calcium is progressively deposited in areas of deterioration, especially around the valves of the heart. Damage to the valves of the heart caused by this degeneration can result in different problems.

TABLE 52-1	Effects of Aging on Body Systems
Cardiovascular	The heart grows weaker even though it must pump against a higher resistance in the arteries, there may be abnormal heart rates or rhythms, the systolic blood pressure may start to rise because of increased arterial resistance to blood flow, and the blood vessels will not react as efficiently in response to brainstem stimulation that complicates blood pressure regulation during times of stress or emergency. Maximum cardiac output drops by 1 percent every year after age 35.
Pulmonary	The net effect of pulmonary changes in an elderly patient is that the body is less able to detect hypoxia or hypercapnia, less air enters and exits the lungs, less gas exchange occurs, the lung tissue loses its elasticity, and many of the muscles used in breathing lose their strength and coordination.
Nervous	As the nervous system fails, sensory functions diminish, reflexes become slower, proprioception diminishes, autoregulation of vegetative functions begins to fail, eyesight begins to fail, and pain perception diminishes, which can contribute to unrecognized injury or illness (such as heart attacks).
Gastrointestinal	Degeneration of the intestinal lining causes nutrients to be not as readily absorbed, which contributes to malnutrition. Fecal impaction and constipation are common because smooth muscle contractions of the large intestine diminish. Degeneration of the rectal sphincter muscle can also cause loss of bowel control. The liver does not function as effectively in metabolizing medications.
Endocrine	Changes to the endocrine system may cause fluid imbalance (resulting in either fluid retention or dehydration) and can alter the blood pressure (resulting in high or low blood pressure); changes in insulin secretion and effects may cause the blood sugar level to be elevated higher after a large meal and take longer to return to normal.
Musculoskeletal	The elderly are more prone to falls because of general weakness, worsening balance, and a loss in joint mobility; unfortunately, because of the changes in bone structure, these falls commonly result in skeletal fractures that take longer to heal than in younger people and may also contribute to medical emergencies.
Renal	Declining kidney function typically leads to a secondary disturbance in fluid balance and electrolyte distribution; because many drugs are filtered out by the kidneys, it is common for the elderly to suffer from drug toxicity if they take too much medication or take it too frequently. The geriatric renal system may be functional enough to meet the demands of the body on a day-to-day basis, but as a result of acute illness or injury the elderly patient's renal system may fail.
Integumentary	With injury, generation of new skin cells occurs less rapidly, so wounds heal slowly. Less perspiration is produced, and the sense of touch is dulled. As the skin ages, sores and tearing injuries tend to occur. This diminishes the effectiveness of the skin as a protective barrier in keeping microorganisms out of the body. Less subcutaneous fat leads to less protection against hypothermia.

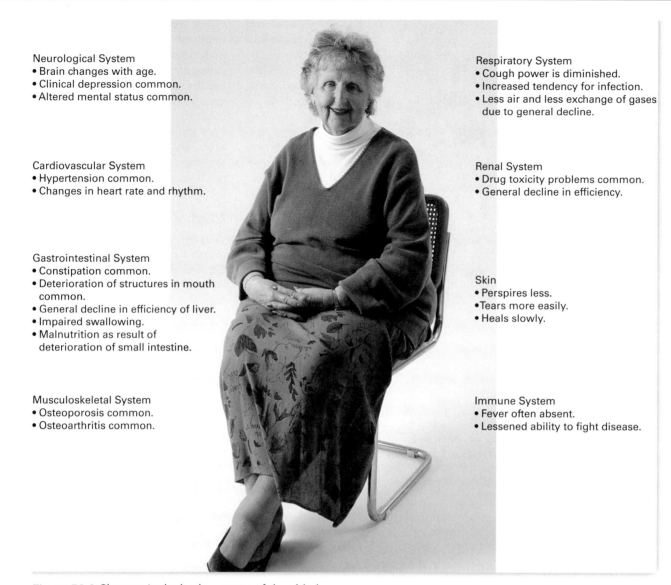

Neurological System
• Brain changes with age.
• Clinical depression common.
• Altered mental status common.

Cardiovascular System
• Hypertension common.
• Changes in heart rate and rhythm.

Gastrointestinal System
• Constipation common.
• Deterioration of structures in mouth common.
• General decline in efficiency of liver.
• Impaired swallowing.
• Malnutrition as result of deterioration of small intestine.

Musculoskeletal System
• Osteoporosis common.
• Osteoarthritis common.

Respiratory System
• Cough power is diminished.
• Increased tendency for infection.
• Less air and less exchange of gases due to general decline.

Renal System
• Drug toxicity problems common.
• General decline in efficiency.

Skin
• Perspires less.
• Tears more easily.
• Heals slowly.

Immune System
• Fever often absent.
• Lessened ability to fight disease.

Figure 52-2 Changes in the body systems of the elderly.

One problem is *stenosis* (narrowing of the valve opening); another problem occurs when the valve fails to seal correctly, causing regurgitation (backward flow of blood).

> **As the body ages the arteries lose their elasticity, which creates greater resistance against which the heart must pump.**

With aging, fibrous tissue also begins to replace muscle tissue throughout the cardiovascular system. The walls of the heart generally become thickened without any increase in the size of the atrial or ventricular chambers. This thickening of the heart walls is known as *cardiac hypertrophy*. It causes a decrease in the stroke volume of the heart (because the heart is unable to hold as much blood), resulting in less blood being ejected from the heart with each contraction and a consequent decrease in cardiac output.

Another cardiovascular change that occurs as the body ages is that the arteries lose their elasticity (their ability to constrict and dilate easily), which creates greater resistance against which the heart must pump. Widespread hardening of the arteries, or *arteriosclerosis*, tends to occur with age, which causes the arteries to become stiff and leads to further increases in the pressure the heart must pump against—and reducing cardiac output.

This also leads to an increase in the systolic blood pressure with increasing age.

Compounding the stiffness of the arteries is a drop in baroreceptor sensitivity, which monitors the body's blood pressure. With a drop in baroreceptor sensitivity, it becomes harder for the geriatric patient to regulate blood pressure under normal circumstances as well as during emergencies.

Respiratory System

Changes in the aging respiratory system occur mainly as a result of alterations in the respiratory muscles and in the elasticity and recoil of the thorax. Specifically, the size and strength of the muscles used for respiration decrease, and calcium deposits begin to form where the ribs join the sternum, causing the rib cage to become less pliable and increasing lung compliance. Diffusion of oxygen and carbon dioxide across the alveolar membrane decrease progressively as more and more alveolar surfaces degenerate.

Chemoreceptors located in the aortic arch, in the carotid bodies, and on the surface of the brainstem that monitor the levels of carbon dioxide and oxygen in the blood become less sensitive over time. This results in a relative inability to detect oxygen depletion (hypoxia) or increased carbon dioxide levels (hypercapnia) in the blood and tissues.

Airflow into and out of the lungs changes as well. In a younger person, the smaller airways (bronchioles) are supported by smooth muscle, which allows the bronchioles to keep their open shape so oxygen is easily inhaled with each incoming breath and carbon dioxide is easily exhaled with each exiting breath. With aging, both the number and size of these smooth muscle fibers that support the smaller airways decrease. The result is turbulent airflow, which diminishes air delivery to the terminal alveoli during inspiration and can result in air trapping during exhalation.

A number of pathologic diseases (such as COPD) aggravate this pulmonary decline. These factors become further exaggerated with the heightened respiratory activity needed during episodes of stress, shock, or pulmonary dysfunction from acute illness or injury (▶ Figure 52-3).

The ability of the lungs to inhibit or resist disease and infection is also diminished with age. The cough reflex, which helps eliminate inhaled particles from the airway, may not trigger as readily, and the resulting cough may be less forceful because of the weakening muscles. The hairlike projections (cilia) that line the airway and help remove foreign particles trapped in the mucous lining are less able to move the material up and out of the airway. In addition, the nose and breathing passages secrete less of an antibody substance, which protects the body from viruses, into the mucus. Dehydration, common in the elderly, increases the tendency for respiratory infection as well.

Nervous System

The neurologic (nervous) system also becomes impaired by the normal effects of aging. Nerve cells (neurons) begin to degenerate and die as early as the mid-20s, and this ultimately impedes the ability of the body to adapt rapidly to changes within and outside the body. Reflexes slow, proprioception (sensing of one's body position) falters, sight diminishes (especially at night), and although hearing loss is not inevitable, the ability to discern higher-frequency sounds may slowly be lost.

The mass and weight of the brain actually decrease (atrophy), resulting in an increase in the amount of cerebrospinal fluid (CSF) to occupy the extra space in the skull. As brain neurons degenerate, waste products can collect in tissues, causing abnormal structures called plaques and tangles to form. As these changes from atrophy, plaques, and tangles take place, the overall ability of the brain to operate as it did when the person was younger becomes increasingly impossible (e.g., the ability of the elderly brain to control many of the body's processes becomes less efficient).

Because of changes that occur in the brainstem and other neurologic regulatory centers, the ability to perceive hunger and thirst are altered. The ability of the brain to monitor and regulate vital functions such as the rate and depth of breathing, heart rate, blood pressure, and core body temperature can become impaired and not operate with the same efficiency during stressful times as in the younger patient.

Sensory perception, as mentioned, tends to diminish as well over time; this includes everyday senses such as auditory, visual, olfactory, touch, pain, hot and cold sensations, and body position. Changes in both vision and balance lead to an increased incidence of falls in the elderly. Diminished tear production leads to eye irritation from inadequate moisture.

Another neurologic disorder is peripheral neuropathy (which is sometimes just called neuropathy); this is a generic term for any type of deranged or abnormal function of the peripheral motor, sensory, and autonomic nerve tracts. It could be diffuse, involving multiple neurons and nerve tracts that affect many parts of the body, or focal, involving neurons that affect a single, specific nerve and part of the body.

Gastrointestinal System

The sense of taste and smell is reduced in elderly patients, resulting in decreased food enjoyment (and possibly causing the person to stop eating regularly). Structures in the mouth deteriorate; periodontal

> **Sensory perception tends to diminish over time.**

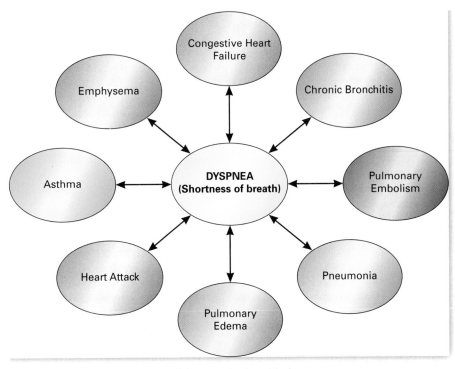

Figure 52-3 Common causes of dyspnea in the elderly.

disease can cause a loss of gum tissue and consequent tooth loss. Salivary flow lessens from degeneration of the salivary glands.

The smooth muscle contractions of the esophagus decrease, and the opening between the esophagus and the stomach loses tone, which can result in chronic heartburn as gastric acid enters the esophagus from the stomach.

The amount of hydrochloric acid secreted into the stomach also drops. This contributes to less efficient breaking down of ingested food before it enters the small intestine.

The liver decreases in size, weight, and function; this in turn decreases hepatic enzymes, causing a loss in the liver's ability to aid in digestion and metabolize certain drugs. This is further hampered by the drop in blood flow that occurs over time to the liver. Smooth muscle contractions (peristalsis) throughout the rest of the gastrointestinal tract slow; therefore, it takes much longer for food to move through the system.

Because the lining of the small intestine degenerates, nutrients are not as readily absorbed, further contributing to malnutrition. Fecal impaction and constipation are common because smooth muscle contractions of the large intestine diminish. In some patients, degeneration of the rectal sphincter muscle can cause loss of bowel control.

Endocrine System

The progression of age-related changes of the endocrine system is unique. For most people, the changes in the endocrine system have no noticeable effect on overall health, but in some the changes may increase the risk of health problems (e.g., the changes in insulin effectiveness increase the risk of type 2 diabetes). Both hormone levels and target organ response are altered in the aging endocrine system.

Levels of certain hormones that elevate blood pressure (e.g., norepinephrine and vasopressin) can increase and contribute to hypertension, whereas other hormones that help regulate the body's fluid balance (such as renin and aldosterone) become deranged and contribute to fluid imbalance.

Furthermore, target organ response to beta adrenergic (sympathetic) stimulation in the heart and vascular smooth muscle decreases because of a loss of sensitivity of receptor cells. Aging produces mild carbohydrate intolerance and a minimal increase in fasting blood glucose levels from a drop in receptor cell responsiveness to insulin. Atrial natriuretic hormone (ANH) from atrial muscle tissue acts to help regulate water, sodium, potassium, and fat. The serum level of this hormone is also typically increased in the elderly and contributes to fluid imbalance. Aging also decreases the metabolism of thyroxine, a hormone that influences overall metabolic activity of the body.

Musculoskeletal System

The most significant musculoskeletal change resulting from aging is a loss of minerals in the bones, which is known as osteoporosis. This makes the bones more brittle and susceptible to fractures and slows the healing process. The disks located between the vertebrae of the spine start to narrow, which causes the characteristic curvature of the spine, seen in two out of every three elderly patients, known as kyphosis.

Joints begin to lose their flexibility with aging. The cartilage that covers the articular surfaces where joints meet begins to thin. The synovial fluid that surrounds these joints starts to thicken, causing joint stiffness. The ligaments that provide joints with stability start to weaken as well.

Renal System

The normal aging process also affects the renal system. The kidneys become smaller in size and weight because of a loss of the functional parts of the kidney, the nephrons. The effect is a decrease in the surface area of the kidney available to filter blood. The arterial system supplying the kidneys is also subject to the changes in the cardiovascular system, which results in a drop in renal blood flow. In combination, these changes result in a lesser amount of blood per minute passing through the kidneys for filtration, in addition to the decrease in available filtration surface area.

Because the kidneys play a vital role in fluid and electrolyte balance, kidney malfunction or injury typically leads to a secondary disturbance in fluid balance and electrolyte distribution. Because many drugs (including antibiotics) are filtered out by the kidneys, it is common for elderly patients to suffer from drug toxicity if they take too much medication or take it too frequently.

Integumentary System

Aging results in tremendous changes in the integumentary system (the skin). The skin becomes thinner from a deterioration of the subcutaneous layer, and less attachment tissue separates the dermis (inner layer) and epidermis (outer layer). An elderly person's skin is much more prone to injury than is the younger person's skin. Replacement cells are produced less rapidly, so wounds heal more slowly, and skin is slow to replace itself. Less perspiration is produced, and the sense of touch is dulled. In addition, the loss of subcutaneous fat results in less insulation against the cold and a higher incidence of hypothermia in the elderly. As the skin breaks down, sores and tearing injuries tend to occur. This diminishes the effectiveness of the skin as a protective barrier in keeping microorganisms out of the body.

ASSESSMENT FINDINGS AND DIFFERENTIAL CONSIDERATIONS

Because of the general decline in body systems, the elderly are prone to certain traumatic and medical emergencies that can cause rapid deterioration. As stated, aging may change the individual's response to illness and injury. For example, pain may be diminished or absent, and consequently the patient or AEMT may underestimate the severity of the patient's condition.

It is important that the AEMT be able to recognize these emergencies and provide appropriate emergency care. Having an understanding of what is occurring physiologically in these emergencies will help in recognizing and providing prompt, appropriate care. Table 52-2 is designed to assist you in interpreting several common complaints of the geriatric patient and differential field impressions that are consistent with them as you are completing your assessment. In addition, refer to the special considerations for scene size-up (Table 52-3) and for primary assessment (Table 52-4).

EMERGENCY MEDICAL CARE

Remember, a geriatric patient's condition can deteriorate rapidly. Therefore, it is critically important to anticipate problems

TABLE 52-2	Potential Differential Diagnoses Based on Clinical Findings in Geriatric Patients		
Clinical Finding	**Changes Due to Altered Physiology**	**Common Assessment Findings**	**Potential Differential Diagnosis**
Chest pain	• Altered pain perception, from neuropathies • Difficulty maintaining heart rate and regularity, from heart disease • Cardiac output lowered, from hypertrophy • Inability to maintain blood pressure regulation, from cardiovascular disease • Concurrent finding of dyspnea, from rapid onset of pulmonary edema • Acute decompensation, from failing body systems	• Severe, mild, or no chest pain • Respiratory distress • Weakness • Fatigue • Confusion • Dizziness • Nausea/vomiting • Aching shoulders • Abdominal pain	• Myocardial infarction (MI) vs. angina • Pleuritis • Pneumonia • Congestive heart failure (CHF) • Hypertensive disorder • Chronic obstructive pulmonary disease (COPD) • Pulmonary embolism • Gastrointestinal dysfunction • Possible recent thoracic injury or trauma
Dyspnea	• Failure to detect hypoxia or hypercapnia as readily because of failing chemoreceptors • Diminution in alveolar exchange cause by lowered tidal volume • Loss of alveoli decreases actual gas exchange • Weakening respiratory muscles contribute to rapid development of inadequate breathing	• Inability to speak in full sentences • Loss of alveolar breath sounds • Decreasing pulse oximetry • Vital sign changes • Crackles or wheezing • Possible fever • Altered mental status • Tachypnea, orthopnea • Tripod positioning • Sharp chest pain • Prolonged bed rest • Recent trauma • Gradual or rapid onset	• Asthma • Emphysema • Pneumonia • Pleurisy • Pulmonary emboli • Pulmonary edema • Chronic bronchitis • Spontaneous pneumothorax • Acute MI
Altered mental status	• Altered memory recall • Slowing of the reflexes • Global diminishing of the senses • Development of neurologic plaques and tangles that slow mental processing • Poor proprioception • Altered nutrition and thirst perception	• Mild to significant changes in mental status • Unresponsiveness • Headache • Changes in muscle coordination • Inequality of pupils • Changes in vital signs • Altered speech patterns • Seizures • Sensory loss • Changes in blood glucose level	• Cerebrovascular accident (CVA, or stroke) or transient ischemic attack (TIA) • Syncope • Alzheimer disease • Drug overdose • Brain tumor • Hypertensive crisis • Seizure disorder • New/old brain injury • Electrolyte imbalance • Diabetic emergency • Dementia versus delirium • Thyroid disorder
Seizure	• Lowered seizure threshold with certain concurrent medical conditions • Increased risk of stroke or TIA • Changes in renal function cause electrolyte disturbance	• Tonic–clonic muscular activity • Tongue biting • Incontinence • Unresponsiveness • Changes in blood glucose level • Focal muscle spasms or hypertonicity	• Seizure disorder • CVA/TIA • Renal failure • Traumatic brain injury • Drug overdose • Infections • Electrolyte imbalance
Syncope	• Loss of normal autoregulation possibly leading to poor cerebral perfusion with sudden standing • Drop in cerebral perfusion caused by effects of drugs/meds	• Passing out after standing suddenly • History of strong emotional event • Possible loss of bowel/bladder control	• Seizure disorder • CVA/TIA • Drug overdose • Massive MI • Diabetic emergency • Cardiac arrhythmia

TABLE 52-2 (Continued)

Clinical Finding	Changes Due to Altered Physiology	Common Assessment Findings	Potential Differential Diagnosis
Drug toxicity (or) overdose	• Delayed gastric emptying • Forgetfulness regarding medication compliance • Renal and hepatic dysfunction lead to elevated blood levels	• Altered mental status • Seizures • Nausea • Vomiting • Vital sign changes • Diarrhea • Abdominal pain	• Diabetic emergency • CVA/TIA • Gastrointestinal emergency • Liver or kidney failure
Hypoperfusion	• Diminished cardiovascular performance • Failing pulmonary system • Hydration status usually diminished • Minor trauma can afflict multiple body systems negatively • Inability to aggressively counter acute illnesses or injuries from weak compensatory mechanisms • Side effects of medications	• Diminished orientation • Tachycardia • Normal to low blood pressure • Dyspnea • Poor peripheral perfusion • Diminished muscle tone • Tachypnea • Capillary refill > 4 seconds • Skin cool and diaphoretic • Possible increased temperature (septic shock)	• Cardiogenic shock • Hypovolemic shock • Distributive shock

and to continually reassess the patient. In the geriatric patient, the injury or failure of one body system can rapidly cause the failure of others. The following are key considerations and emergency care steps for the geriatric patient:

1. **Maintain a patent airway.** Geriatric patients often wear dentures; if these dentures become dislodged, they can create an airway obstruction.

If necessary, suction and clear the airway immediately before assessing the breathing status. If the neck is stiff and not flexible enough to perform a head-tilt, chin-lift maneuver, perform a jaw thrust to establish a patent airway.

2. **Insert an airway.** If the patient is unable to maintain his own airway because of injury or altered mental status, insert an oropharyngeal

airway. If the patient cannot tolerate an oropharyngeal airway, insert a nasopharyngeal airway. Use advanced airways as indicated and allowed by protocol.

3. **Assess and be prepared to assist ventilations.** If the rate or depth is inadequate, initiate positive pressure ventilation immediately. Be careful not to ventilate the patient with

TABLE 52-3 Clues to Illness Found in the Scene Size-Up

Clues	May Indicate
Bucket next to bed	The patient suffers from nausea and vomiting.
Hospital bed	The patient has no or limited mobility and a preexisting chronic illness.
Nebulizer setup	The patient has a chronic respiratory disease process.
Oxygen tank setup or oxygen concentrator	The patient has a chronic respiratory or cardiac disease.
Medications found at the scene	These may provide a clue as to the patient's preexisting condition(s).
Washcloth on the patient's forehead or near the patient	The patient has a severe headache or fever.
Patient in nightclothes in the middle of the afternoon	The patient has been sick all day.
Tripod position	The patient has significant respiratory distress.
Patient propped up on pillows	The patient has difficulty breathing when lying flat, commonly because of congestive heart failure.
A hot room temperature in the summer months	The patient has a possible heat emergency caused by dehydration or hyperthermia (elevated core body temperature).
A cold room temperature in the winter months	The patient has a possible cold emergency, hypothermia (decreased core body temperature).

TABLE 52-4	Special Considerations in the Primary Assessment of the Geriatric Patient
Chief complaint	The elderly patient may not complain of pain because of a preexisting central nervous system condition, such as stroke. However, any complaint of pain in the elderly must be taken seriously.
	Some elderly patients will not experience pain when suffering a serious condition, such as a heart attack, because of a disease process that affects the nerve endings. This is common in diabetic patients.
	Prickling and burning-type pain is usually caused by a condition affecting the superficial structures of the body, whereas an aching-type pain usually indicates that an organ is involved in the condition.
	Changes in the peripheral nerves in the skin can affect the elderly patient's ability to distinguish between hot and cold.
	A sudden loss of vision in one eye is not normal in the elderly and generally indicates a retinal artery occlusion or retinal detachment.
	Depression in the elderly is a serious complaint and must be managed properly. A depression state may cause the patient to not report or to minimize significant symptoms. The rate of suicide is high among the elderly.
	Alcohol abuse is more common in the elderly. Keep a higher index of suspicion and look for evidence of alcohol abuse in the scene size-up.
	Side effects of medications or interactions with other medications may cause the presenting signs and symptoms.
	Fainting may be a serious complaint associated with conditions affecting the brain, lungs, heart, or circulatory system, such as heart attack, pneumonia, blocked pulmonary artery (pulmonary embolism), shock, head injury or stroke, or congestive heart failure.
Mental status	Hypoxia causes agitation and aggression. High levels of carbon dioxide cause confusion and disorientation.
	A sudden onset of an altered mental status is not a normal part of aging and is not considered to be dementia. It is usually an indication of a serious illness or injury.
	Altered mental status may be caused by inadequate perfusion to the brain, hypoxia in the brain, dehydration, electrolyte disturbances, change in the blood glucose level, infection, cold emergency (hypothermia), stroke, head injury, tumors, drugs, or alcohol intoxication.
Airway	A reduction in the patient's reflexes may cause a high incidence of choking and aspiration of food or other substances.
	Cervical arthritis may make performing an effective head-tilt, chin-lift maneuver difficult because of the stiffness of the neck structures. A jaw-thrust maneuver may provide a better manual airway.
	Loose dentures may cause an airway obstruction. If the dentures are loose or poorly fitted, remove them. If the dentures are well fitted and snug in place, do not remove them. In a patient without dentures or teeth, it is much more difficult to get an effective mask seal if ventilation needs to be performed.
Breathing	Elderly patients have higher resting respiratory rates. A resting respiratory rate greater than 20 per minute may be completely normal.
	Elderly patients have lower tidal volumes. This can lead to early onset of hypoxia.
	Retractions are less likely to occur in the elderly because of the less elastic and compliant chest wall muscles.
Circulation	Elderly patients have higher resting heart rates, typically greater than 90 beats per minute, unless they are taking beta blockers.
	An irregularly irregular pulse (no regular rhythm or pattern) may be normal in an elderly patient.
Skin	The skin will normally appear to be dry and less elastic. Assessment of skin turgor in the elderly is not a reliable test of skin hydration. Inspect the inside of the mouth or under the lower eyelid to check for hydration status.
	Cold skin may indicate hypothermia, even when the elderly patient is found in the home. This is referred to as "urban hypothermia." A reduction in subcutaneous fat and skin vessel response may cause the body core temperature to decrease faster.
	Hot skin may indicate a heat emergency, such as heat stroke. Elderly patients are more prone to heat emergencies because of their inability to dilate the vessels to assist in cooling the body.
	Fever is less common in the elderly patient, even with serious infections.

excessive pressure or volumes, which could cause lung injury. Although loose dentures could cause an airway obstruction, if they are still firmly seated in the elderly patient in need of positive pressure ventilation, it may be advisable to leave them in place. The dentures will help support the soft tissues around the mouth on which the mask of the ventilation device will be seated.

4. **Establish and maintain oxygen therapy.** Be sure to provide supplemental oxygen with positive pressure ventilation if the patient's breathing is inadequate. If the patient has adequate respirations, administer oxygen if the SpO_2 is less than 95 percent or signs of hypoxia are present.

5. **Position the patient.** Exercise extreme caution when preparing the patient for transport, based on the type of emergency as outlined in the following guidelines:

   • If the emergency is medical in nature and the patient is alert and able to protect his own airway,

place the patient in a position that is comfortable for him. This is typically a Fowler (sitting up) position.

   • If the patient has an altered mental status and is unable to protect his own airway, he should be placed in a left lateral recumbent position (recovery position) to prevent aspiration.

   • If spinal injury is suspected, the patient needs immediate stabilization of the spine during primary assessment, followed by immobilization to a long backboard. One limitation, however, is the geriatric patient with severe curvature of the spine caused by kyphosis. You may need to be creative and construct the cervical immobilization devices out of blankets to accommodate the curvature of the spine.

   • If the patient is unresponsive, assume a possible cervical spine injury and immobilize the patient fully as a precautionary measure.

6. **Obtain intravenous access if the patient has any signs of instability or potential instability.** Obtaining access may be more challenging in the geriatric patient because of smaller, more fragile veins. Patients on warfarin may develop bleeding and hematomas at the IV start site. Finally, use caution when administering fluid boluses to patients with existing cardiac conditions, especially heart failure. IV access should be obtained en route in many cases.

7. **Transport.** Reassess the patient en route to the hospital, remembering that the geriatric patient's condition can rapidly deteriorate without warning.

To ensure appropriate care, reevaluate the geriatric patient frequently. The length of time spent with the patient or the condition of the patient will assist in establishing how to and how often to repeat the reassessment phase. Repeat and record the assessment at least every 15 minutes for a stable patient. If the patient is unstable, repeat and record at a minimum of every 5 minutes.

TRANSITIONING

REVIEW ITEMS

1. An elderly patient presents with a sudden onset of weakness, nausea and vomiting, dyspnea with inspiratory crackles, and an irregular heartbeat. This collection of findings may be representative of _____.

   a. a heart attack
   b. hypoglycemia
   c. seizures
   d. stroke

2. An elderly patient has fallen down three steps, which has resulted in a compound fracture of his left femur with heavy bleeding. On assessing the patient you find a blood pressure of 96/70, a heart rate of 88 beats per minute, respirations 22 per minute, and a pulse oximetry reading of 94 percent. Which of these described assessment findings *is not* consistent with hypovolemic shock but *is* consistent with geriatric trauma?

   a. blood pressure
   b. heart rate
   c. respiratory rate
   d. pulse oximetry reading

3. Failure of the chemoreceptors would lead to what disturbance in the geriatric patient?

   a. diminished perception of hypercapnia
   b. overproduction of insulin by the pancreas
   c. poor autoregulation of the systolic blood pressure
   d. increased intracranial pressure and diastolic hypertension

4. Which of the following is *not* an effect of aging that would contribute to the increased incident of falls in the elderly population?

   a. loss of proprioception
   b. kyphosis of the spine
   c. limited night vision
   d. atrophy of the brain

5. What medical emergency may present atypically in the elderly patient as a result of being diabetic with peripheral neuropathy?

   a. seizures
   b. syncope
   c. vertigo
   d. myocardial infarction

APPLIED PATHOPHYSIOLOGY

An elderly male patient was attempting to cross the street when he was stuck by a car traveling at a low rate of speed. The patient was thrown back about 4 feet and landed on his side. Given the changes in the cardiovascular, pulmonary, nervous, and musculoskeletal systems, discuss how the patient may be at risk for significant trauma.

1. Discuss the differences in presentation that may occur in an 87-year-old patient suffering a heart attack compared with a 45-year-old suffering a heart attack.

2. Identify how the failure or dysfunction of the following bodily systems may cause an altered mental status in a geriatric patient:

   a. Cardiovascular system

   b. Pulmonary system

   c. Nervous system

CLINICAL DECISION MAKING

You are called for an "unknown unresponsive" elderly woman found by the driver for the meal-delivery service for the elderly. On your arrival, the police escort you into the house, where you find the patient lying unresponsive on the couch. It is midday, the ambient temperature is warm, and no sign of struggle is evident. The patient is alone, and no family members or friends from whom to gather information are present.

1. Based on the scene size-up characteristics, describe possible ways to learn about the patient's medical history.

2. For each body system (nervous, respiratory, cardiac, vascular, endocrine, etc.) list at least one differential diagnosis that could cause this unresponsiveness.

The primary assessment reveals the patient to be unresponsive to external stimuli. There is vomitus in the airway, breathing is slow and shallow, the heart rate is about 44 beats per minute and peripherally absent, and the skin is cool to the touch. The SpO_2 reading is 74 percent.

3. Of what life threats to the patient are you currently aware?

After managing and supporting the patient's lost function, further assessment reveals the pupils to be pinpoint, blood glucose level of 111 mg/dL, and the pulse oximeter increased to 94 percent with treatment. Breath sounds are bilaterally equal. No clinical findings of trauma are anywhere on the body. Your partner returns from the kitchen with a prescription bottle of Percocet (a narcotic pain medication) and a bottle of metoprolol (beta blocker), which was filled two days earlier. Both bottles are empty.

4. What conditions have you ruled out from your initial consideration in the scene size-up?

5. What conditions are you still considering as the possible cause? Would you add any conditions as a possible cause?

6. Explain the pathophysiologic cause for the following:

   a. Unresponsiveness

   b. Vomitus in the airway

   c. Poor peripheral perfusion but slow heart rate

During the secondary assessment, you learn from a family member who just arrived on scene that this patient had been upset the past week because of the recent death of her spouse. The pain pills, the person explains, were for a hip injury the patient suffered a few days earlier.

7. What conditions have you ruled out in your differential field diagnosis? Why?

8. What conditions are you considering as a probable cause? Why?

9. Based on your differential diagnosis, what are the next steps in emergency care? Why?

10. Explain how you came to a differential field diagnosis based on specific history and physical assessment findings.

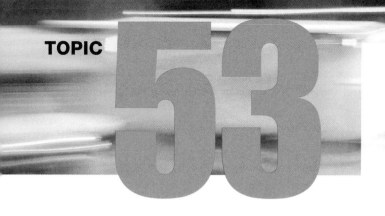

Standard Special Patient Populations

Competency Applies a fundamental knowledge of growth, development, and aging and assessment findings to provide basic and selected advanced emergency care and transportation for a patient with special needs.

SPECIAL CHALLENGES

TRANSITION *highlights*

- Complexity of problems when people are living at home with medical technology or are victims of abuse.
- Pathophysiology of certain special challenges the patient may have, which necessitated the call to EMS:
  - Abuse (children and the elderly).
  - Mental illnesses.
  - Disabilities:
    - Paralysis.
    - Obesity.
    - Traumatized patients.
  - Technology assistance/dependency:
    - Apnea monitors.
    - Tracheostomy tubes.
    - CPAP and BiPAP.
    - Home mechanical ventilators.
    - Vascular access devices.
    - Dialysis.
    - Feeding tubes.
    - Intraventricular shunts.
- Current treatment strategies for the specially challenged or technology-assisted patient.

INTRODUCTION

Because of changes in medicine and lifestyle, the life span of Americans is increasing. Despite this, however, some people are still born with congenital defects, and some suffer significant trauma or endure critical illnesses that leave residual deficits.

In today's world, though, advances in medical care and medical technology allow people with certain deficits, who previously could only have been properly cared for within an extended care facility, to live at home (either independently or with family). Deficits that are compensated by medicine and technology could be as minimal as hearing impairment, or as advanced as mechanical ventilators for people who have lost the ability to breathe spontaneously.

There may be a mixing of lost function as well. For example, a patient who experienced severe brain trauma may be paralyzed on one side of the body and also may be unable to feed himself normally, so a feeding tube may be inserted into the abdominal wall.

Common causes of impairments include, for example, aging, birth defects, chronic illnesses, traumatic accidents, abuse, and/or neglect.

In your EMS career thus far, you have almost certainly encountered patients who have special medical challenges or whose lives are dependent on medical technologies. When their preexisting special challenges worsen, their medical devices fail, or they experience some other emergency independent of the chronic condition, EMS is the first one called to intervene.

The challenge to the Advanced EMT is determining how to properly assess, intervene, and transport a patient with special challenges—especially in light of medical equipment or conditions that further complicate the situation—while still focusing on and treating the initial call for help.

EPIDEMIOLOGY

Trying to determine the number of people living in the United States with some type of special challenge is next to impossible because there is neither a common registry for these individuals nor a unified definition of what a "specially challenged" patient is. The number is large, however, as evidenced by the more than 74 million "hits" received in response to a recent Internet search for the term *specially challenged patient*.

Underreporting of abuse is also widespread. Many times, especially when the abused person lives at home with others, the victim is unable to report abuse to the authorities because the person's physical or mental conditions prohibit a call for help. Although this is not a total picture, it is known that more than 3 million children are victims of abuse annually, more than 560,000 cases of elder abuse are reported in the United States every year, and 3 to 4 million people are victims of spousal or partner abuse annually.

Underreporting of abuse is widespread.

Finally, more than 8 million disabled patients are receiving health care from professional providers, and it is estimated that millions of others receive care from family members or volunteers. In sum, given these numbers, this is not a statement of "*if* you will have a specially challenged patient" but rather "*when* you will."

PATHOPHYSIOLOGY

A person may be receiving care at home for any of multiple reasons. Perhaps the patient's condition is not severe enough to warrant admission into a hospital or rehabilitation center. Perhaps the patient's status or condition is expected to improve over time, and he wants to be with his family. Some patients, however, have conditions that will not improve, but they want to live at home, and with the help of medical technology, they can do so with the greatest degree of normalcy possible.

Although the patient's primary care providers are usually knowledgeable about the equipment or technology being used, they may not be as well versed in what to do if that equipment fails or the patient's status begins to deteriorate.

Although it is impossible to discuss everything that you may encounter regarding special needs patients, this topic is intended to provide you with the knowledge and the mental processing required to meet the needs of abused patients, mentally retarded patients, and patients with disabilities. Tertiary care hospitals that care for such patients often maintain an on-call person for specialized conditions and/or equipment.

Abuse

Child abuse occurs when a child falls victim to abuse or neglect. In fact, child abuse has been the only major cause of infant and child death to increase in the past 30 years. It ranges from actual physical and emotional harm to neglect of the body's basic needs. The abuser is not necessarily the parent and can be a babysitter, foster parent, sibling, stepsibling, stepparent, or anyone else responsible for the child's care.

Generally, child abuse falls into one of three categories: physical abuse (which can include neglect), emotional abuse, and sexual abuse. *Physical abuse* occurs when improper or excessive action is

taken that injures or causes harm. *Neglect* is the provision of inadequate attention or respect to someone who has a claim to that attention. *Emotional abuse* occurs when a child is regularly threatened, yelled at, humiliated, ignored, blamed, or otherwise emotionally mistreated. *Sexual abuse* occurs when a child is subject to an older child or adult's advances of a sexual nature and can include both contact and noncontact events.

Elder abuse may occur in care centers and other medical institutions, but it can also occur at home. Any elderly person is especially at risk if he is cared for by someone who is under stress from other sources. Abuse of the elderly can occur in many forms and can include neglect, physical abuse, sexual abuse, financial abuse, and/or emotional and mental abuse. At highest risk are elderly patients who are bedridden, demented, incontinent, frail, or experiencing disturbed sleep patterns (▶ Figure 53-1).

Elder abuse in the form of neglect is similar to pediatric neglect: It is the care provider's withholding of attention or medical care to which the victim is entitled. This type of neglect could occur passively or actively, the difference being the intent of the care provider. In situations of *active neglect*, the care provider intentionally fails to meet the obligations to the elderly victim.

In *passive neglect*, the failure is said to occur unintentionally and is often the result of the care provider feeling overwhelmed by the needed tasks. Regardless of the reason, this type of neglect could be manifested as failure to provide adequate nutrition or hydration, to provide medications or access to medical services when warranted, or to care for personal hygiene. The development of bedsores because the care provider is not turning the patient as needed to prevent the breakdown of the skin is also a form of passive neglect.

Physical abuse can involve the hitting, restraining, shaking, or shoving of an elderly patient. Because of elderly patients' frail status, the injuries sustained from these attacks can be significant.

Sexual abuse is said to occur when unwanted or unwarranted advances of a

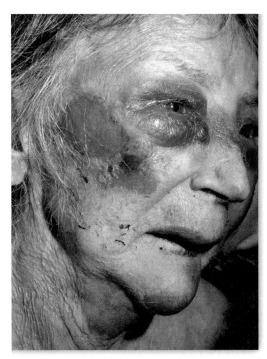

Figure 53-1 Physical abuse of an elderly person can have dire consequences because of the patient's frailty.

sexual nature (either through body contact or exposure) are made to which the older person does not or cannot consent.

Financial abuse consists of the care provider exploiting the material possessions, property, credit, or monetary assets of the elderly patient for his own personal gain.

With *emotional/mental abuse*, psychological distress or mental harm is inflicted on the elderly patient through verbal assaults, verbal insults, threats of physical harm, or simply ignoring the patient.

Mental Illnesses

Mental (or emotional) illnesses can present as unique challenges to the AEMT. The impairment that the patient demonstrates may range from being so mild that it is almost imperceptible to being significant enough that communicating with the patient is almost impossible. Generally, though, the term *mental retardation* encompasses disabilities that affect the nervous system and typically have a negative impact on intelligence level and how the person learns. These disabilities may also cause problems such as speech impediments, behavioral disorders, language difficulties, and some movement disorders. Table 53-1 describes some of the more common causes of mental retardation.

TABLE 53-1   Causes of Mental Retardation

Down syndrome	This is a disorder in which the patient is born with an extra 21st chromosome. The disability usually results in characteristic facial features well as learning disabilities and multiple physical problems (heart, vision, intestinal, lung).
Fragile X syndrome	This disorder is the second-most-common inherited form of mental retardation. The result is the body's inability to produce a certain protein needed for normal brain growth and development. Patients with fragile X syndrome also have characteristic facial features and severe mental retardation. Over time, the person may also present with cardiac, behavioral, speech, and motor abnormalities.
Autism	Autism is a genetic-based developmental disorder of the brain, which results in mild to significant impairment of social interaction and communication skills. Although the cause is still being debated, it is usually suspected by the parents when the child fails to reach developmental milestones.
Fetal alcohol syndrome	This is caused by excessive alcohol consumption by the mother during pregnancy. It is occasionally confused with Down syndrome, as patients with both syndromes have similar facial features. A patient with this disorder often displays mental disabilities, hyperactivity, and delayed physical growth.
Phenylketonuria (PKU), hypothyroidism	These are both metabolic disorders that can affect how the body processes materials needed for functioning. In both these conditions, the abnormal metabolic activity of the body results in mental retardation and other cognitive and behavioral deficits.
Rett syndrome	This syndrome, which afflicts females almost exclusively, is characterized by a genetic mutation of the X chromosome. The child usually displays normal early development, but this is followed by progressive loss of purposeful motion, inability to speak, behavioral disorders, abnormal skeletal growth, and loss of motor skills previously acquired.

Disabilities

The term *disabilities* is often used as an encompassing label that includes impairments, activity limitations, and participation restrictions. The medical model for "disabilities" views it as a problem of the patient that was caused by disease, trauma, inheritance, or other factors that necessitate sustained medical care for the individual. As such, trying to discuss all the disabilities known to medicine far exceeds the intent of this topic.

As an alternative, what will be discussed are the more common disabilities that can or may result in acute deterioration of the patient or leave him dependent on medical technology—either way, the patient's deterioration or equipment malfunction necessitates the summoning of EMS to treat the patient. In these situations, the intent is not to diagnose the disability and provide curative care but rather to recognize the dysfunction caused by

the disability and provide supportive care to the body system that is failing.

Paralysis refers to the complete loss of function in one or more groups of muscles. Paralysis is caused by damage or dysfunction of the nervous system (especially the spinal cord) or the brain. Common causes for paralysis include trauma to the head, spinal cord, or vertebral column. Strokes can also cause residual paralysis when the area of the brain that controls certain muscle groups is damaged.

Neuromuscular diseases can also result in paralysis that typically originates in the extremities and progressively causes weakness and paralysis to the muscles of the trunk and respiratory system. Common diagnoses include amyotrophic lateral sclerosis, Guillain-Barré syndrome, muscular dystrophy, poliomyelitis, myasthenia gravis, and multiple sclerosis.

Patients who are paralyzed are susceptible to multiple other problems as well.

For example, if the paralysis involves the respiratory muscles, the patient may be ventilator dependent. Patients with paralysis also have frequent respiratory infections resulting from the inability to cough and clear out inhaled debris from the airway. They also are susceptible to urinary tract infections (totally paralyzed patients are routinely catheterized).

In addition, because they are wheelchair confined or bedridden, paralyzed patients may develop pressure necrosis (bedsores) over the bony areas of the body. If a feeding tube is inserted, the insertion site may become infected or the tube may become occluded. Secondary emergencies from this can include sepsis, dyspnea, chest pain, open soft tissue deterioration, unrecognized injury, and many other problems.

Obesity is a definite concern in the United States today. It is estimated that more than 40 percent of people in the United States are obese. In addition, obesity is the second-leading cause of preventable death today, after smoking. Long-term body deterioration from obesity can result in coronary heart disease, type 2 diabetes, immobility, sleep apnea, and hypertension, to name a few problems—all of which can reduce the life span of the patient should no corrective measures be taken (see Table 53-2).

Obesity can occur for a number of reasons. Whereas the short explanation is that the patient is consuming more calories than he is burning (i.e., overeating with a sedentary lifestyle), obesity can be caused by physiologic problems as well. For example, a patient with hypothyroidism may have a lowered metabolic rate, which means he burns calories more slowly.

Some medications, such as CNS depressants and anticonvulsant medications, can lower the metabolic rate and contribute to weight gain. Genetic factors have been cited as contributing to obesity in some people as well. It has also been noted that obese people tend to form relationships with each other, and their children are often obese as well (be it from genetics, predisposition, or lifestyle).

Traumatized patients are another type of specially challenged patient that the AEMT may be called on to care. Head trauma (or more specifically, brain trauma) in patients can easily result in a multitude of residual disabilities. The disability may be mild, such as changes in speech pattern or mild cognitive changes, or can be

TABLE 53-2	Effects of Excess Weight on Organ Systems
Organ System	**Disease State**
Cardiovascular	Hypertension, coronary artery disease, congestive heart failure, cerebrovascular accident
Respiratory	Obstructive sleep apnea, asthma, chronic obstructive pulmonary disease
Endocrine and reproductive	Diabetes mellitus, infertility, birth defects, menstrual disorders
Gastrointestinal	Esophageal reflux, liver disease
Musculoskeletal	Osteoarthritis, gout, back injuries, immobility
Psychological	Depression, suicide

so severe as to leave the patient unresponsive to external stimuli and dependent on ventilators for breathing; feeding tubes for nutrition; and care providers for day-to-day washing, turning, and bedding changes. Most previous head injury patients, though, fall somewhere between those two extremes.

Trauma to the brain can occur at any age and may result in permanent damage, as evidenced by changes in cognition, learning abilities, emotional abilities, and/or muscle weakness or paralysis.

Technology Assistance/ Dependency

Whereas some medical equipment is designed to enhance the quality of life and allow patient independence (e.g., feeding tubes or urinary catheters), other medical equipment found in the home setting actually sustains life (e.g., mechanical ventilators). As an AEMT, you must remain abreast of current home medical care and equipment, as it is common for the AEMT to be summoned to a patient whose home medical equipment has failed or is no longer able to support the patient's vital functions.

Apnea monitors are designed to constantly monitor the patient's breathing status and then emit a warning signal should breathing cease. Some are also designed to monitor the heart rate, as changes in the heart rate may signal failure of the respiratory system. This type of equipment is commonly found in a home with an infant, especially a newborn who was born prematurely. These devices will emit a loud piercing sound to signal a problem and often will emit a series of

beeps indicating how long the machine has been alerting.

Tracheostomy tubes (▶ Figure 53-2) are used when it becomes necessary to provide a new surgical opening for the airway in patients with certain medical and/or traumatic conditions. More specifically, a tracheostomy is a surgical opening through the anterior neck and into the trachea that serves as an alternative site for air entry and exit from the body (bypassing the mouth and nose). The site for this surgical opening is usually the inferior trachea, somewhere near the second through fourth tracheal rings anteriorly.

A tracheostomy may be used as a permanent opening and is then referred to as a *stoma*. This technique is commonly performed for patients who have either long-

term upper airway problems or medical conditions that result in long-term dependence on mechanical ventilation.

Continuous positive airway pressure (CPAP) and *bi-level positive airway pressure (BiPAP)* machines are both designed to provide a therapeutic back-pressure during exhalation via an airway circuit attached to a mask that covers the mouth and/or nose. Whereas the CPAP device provides a constant positive pressure during the entire ventilatory cycle, the BiPAP machine provides a higher pressure during inhalation and a lower pressure during exhalation.

The primary therapeutic goal of both devices is to keep the small bronchiole airways open during exhalation, which in turn improves both oxygenation and ventilation; it also lowers the work of breathing. These devices are commonly used on patients with sleep apnea or certain chronic lung diseases. Some CPAP and BiPAP machines also allow the administration of oxygen during use.

> **Head trauma can easily result in a multitude of residual disabilities.**

Home mechanical ventilators are designed to assist a patient who cannot breathe adequately on his own. The patient may have any one of several reasons to be dependent on a ventilator, but these causes typically center around either the brain's inability to initiate a

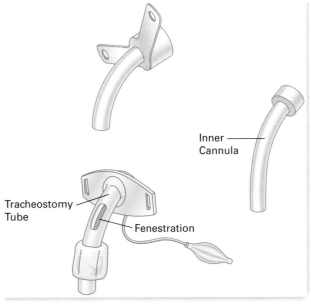

Figure 53-2 A tracheostomy tube for older children and adults has an outer cannula and an inner cannula.

Tracheostomy Tube

Inner Cannula

Fenestration

spontaneous breath, a structural defect of the thorax or lungs that prohibits or greatly diminishes normal gas exchange, or a disease process that renders the respiratory muscles of the body useless, most commonly spinal cord injury.

Commonly, the AEMT will learn the exact reason for the ventilator dependency while ascertaining the patient's medical history. Causes include (but are not limited to) a history of a debilitating stroke, brain damage following head trauma, long-term pulmonary problems (e.g., COPD or lung cancer), and neuromuscular diseases.

The two types of ventilators are negative pressure ventilators and positive pressure ventilators. *Negative pressure ventilators*, such as the "iron lung," encircle the patient's chest and generate a negative pressure around the thoracic cage. The negative pressure created by the devices draws out the rib cage, which, in turn, creates a negative intrathoracic pressure, thereby causing air to be drawn into the lungs.

The most commonly encountered mechanical ventilators, though, are *positive pressure ventilators*, which push air into the airway (i.e., positive pressure), much like the EMS provider who squeezes a bag-valve mask. Exhalation then ensues when the positive pressure stops, and the chest wall and lungs recoil.

Home ventilation units typically have two or three controls: one is for the ventilatory rate, one is for adjusting the size of each breath (i.e., tidal volume), and some units may have one control that adjusts the amount of oxygen that is provided during ventilation if so required by the patient. Tidal volume in most ventilators is adjustable, whereas the ventilatory rate and oxygen supply (if so equipped) may be either fixed or adjustable. The ventilator is attached to the patient by large-diameter tubing, referred to as the ventilator circuit.

Ventilators may also have several alarms that help the primary care provider identify whether the ventilator is functioning properly. In fact, the AEMT may be summoned to care for a patient when one of these alarms alerts a warning. Because of

> **Ventilators may have alarms to help the primary care provider identify whether the ventilator is functioning properly.**

variances in the device, the particular ventilator your patient uses may or may not have the following alarms:

- **High-pressure alarm.** A high-pressure alarm is activated when the pressure needed to cause lung inflation exceeds the present value. This can be from increased airway resistance caused by increased secretions (mucus plugs) occluding the tracheostomy tube, kinking of the ventilator circuit, movement of the tracheostomy tube, bronchospasms, or the patient coughing during inspiration. The alarm can also be triggered by decreased lung compliance. Causes of decreased lung compliance include the development of a pneumothorax, progressive pneumonia, acute pulmonary edema, or alveolar collapse (atelectasis).

- **Low-pressure alarm.** The low-pressure alarm is usually set to activate when the tidal volume falls 50 to 100 mL below the set tidal volume. This usually indicates a problem in the breathing circuit, such as a disconnected segment or a leak in the cuff of the tracheostomy tube.

- **Apnea alarm.** A patient on a ventilator may still have some respiratory effort, but it is inadequate to sustain life. As such, the home ventilator may not trigger a breath until the patient starts to breathe in. In these models, the apnea alarm sounds when the patient stops breathing. Causes are usually physiologic and include decreased mental status, overmedication, and respiratory muscle fatigue.

- **Low FiO₂.** A low FiO_2 alarm will occur when the oxygen source is disconnected or depleted.

Vascular access devices (VADs) are devices that are used when a patient is in need of ongoing intravenous medications. Usually VADs are placed in a surgically created pocket under the surface of the skin in patients who are in need of medication for longer than seven to ten days, but they may also be needed on a long-term basis as well (▶ **Figure 53-3**). The type and duration of use of the device is largely dependent on the medical needs and disease process for which the patient is being treated.

Annually, more than 500,000 devices of this nature are in use. They are typically placed in patients who have ongoing chemotherapy, peritoneal dialysis, hemodialysis, total parenteral nutrition (TPN), and antibiotic therapy needs.

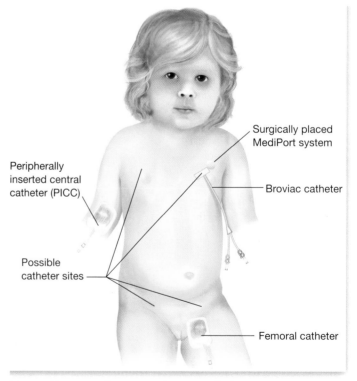

Peripherally inserted central catheter (PICC)

Surgically placed MediPort system

Broviac catheter

Possible catheter sites

Femoral catheter

Figure 53-3 Vascular access devices include central IV catheters such as a PICC line, central venous lines such as the Broviac catheter, and implants ports such as the MediPort system.

Although the AEMT is able to administer some medications by IV, vascular access devices require specific devices and needles for access and training in their use. Do not use one of these devices for vascular access unless you have been specifically trained and this is allowed by protocol. Do not initiate an IV in an arm that contains a vascular device (shunt).

Dialysis is a medical procedure designed to support the lost function of the kidneys, although total replacement of all renal functions is not possible. Dialysis removes the buildup of toxins that occurs when the kidneys can no longer filter out these toxins. *Hemodialysis* is the type of dialysis in which blood is extracted from the body and sent through a dialyzer. The *dialyzer* filters the blood from the body via a membrane that also uses a dialysate fluid to help cleanse the blood. Following the cleansing process, the blood is returned to the body.

The process takes anywhere from 2 to 5 hours for ongoing removal of blood for filtration, followed by the filtered blood being returned to the body. Dialysis typically occurs in a dialysis center and must be repeated two or three times per week.

Peritoneal dialysis is another type of dialysis that is done in the home or the extended care facility. With this type of dialysis (which the AEMT is more likely to encounter), dialysate fluid that contains glucose and minerals is instilled via gravity into a port that leads into the peritoneal cavity. The fluid then surrounds the intestines, where it interacts with the body to remove waste products. After a specific amount of time, the fluid is removed from the abdominal cavity and replaced with fresh fluid.

Because this form of dialysis is not as effective as hemodialysis, it must be repeated several times a day. However, due to current technology, the procedure is relatively easy for the patient to perform and, thus, allows the patient greater freedom in daily activities because he is not bound to several long appointments a week at the dialysis center.

Feeding tubes are medical devices that provide nutrition to patients who cannot chew and/or swallow because of medical conditions or trauma resulting in paralysis or unconsciousness. Patients receiving their nourishment this way are said to be receiving *enteral feeding* or *tube feeding*. The device is typically a flexible tube that is long and small in diameter. It is named according to the site of insertion. If it is inserted through the nose and ends in the stomach, it is a *nasogastric tube*, or *NG-tube*. If the tube is inserted through the mouth and to the stomach, it is an *orogastric tube*, or *OG-tube*. Some feeding tubes are inserted through the skin into the stomach (G-tubes) or jejunum (J-tubes).

Intraventricular shunts are used mainly in pediatric patients who have medical illnesses or anatomical defects that result in either the overproduction of cerebrospinal fluid (CSF) in the brain, inadequate reabsorption of CSF, or irregular flow of CSF through the ventricles and/or meningeal layers. When excess CSF accumulates, the patient is said to have *hydrocephalus*.

Regardless of the reason for the hydrocephalus, because the skull is a fixed size and cannot expand to accommodate the extra fluid, the pressure within the skull (intracranial pressure [ICP]) builds, which can then result in compression of brain tissue. To alleviate the rising ICP, a *shunt* (a long, hollow, tubelike device) is surgically placed. It originates within a ventricle of the brain and extends to a blood vessel in the neck, heart, or abdomen to drain extra CSF and keep the ICP within an acceptable level. In some patients, the AEMT may also find a reservoir on the side of the skull, placed beneath the scalp, which collects the excess CSF for laboratory testing purposes.

ASSESSMENT AND MANAGEMENT

Unless you are caring for the patient in some type of medical facility, specialized residential facility, or group home, if the patient is unresponsive it may be difficult to recognize or get information regarding many of the aforementioned conditions or types of medical equipment. If the patient's clinical status is mild, however, then you can usually obtain a history and complete your physical exam because the patient can still communicate with you.

If, however, during your assessment of the patient, you start to identify some of the developmental or cognitive problems discussed previously, or if the patient is relying on medical equipment and is noncommunicative, you will need to rely on the patient's primary care provider (be it family or professional heath care) for your information.

It is important for the AEMT to remember that it is impossible to cover all types and makes of medical technology used in the home; therefore, the AEMT should always approach the patient or caregiver and ask the following questions to help determine the best course of action for ongoing assessment and care:

- Where would I get the best information regarding this piece of equipment?
- What does this device do for the patient?
- Can I replicate its function should the device fail? Remember that the most important support is to the airway or ventilation.
- Will this equipment have an effect on how I assess the patient or on the findings I may discover?
- Has this problem ever occurred previously, and if so, what fixed it?
- Has anyone attempted already to remediate the problem?
- Are there specific considerations I need to make when deciding how to best prepare the patient for movement and transport him?

You may also need to rely on the care provider to obtain the patient's medical history and information about any care that has been provided thus far relative to the current emergency. During your assessment of the patient with special challenges, incorporate the following treatment interventions as appropriate:

1. **Ensure scene safety.** Although not a patient care step per se, the AEMT must always ensure the safety of himself and his crew when responding to any call.

2. **Consider spinal immobilization.** The patient with special challenges may have fallen; therefore, immobilization may be warranted. Because the patient may have other skeletal abnormalities (e.g., kyphosis) that preclude normal immobilization techniques, be sure to use padding to align and secure the patient to the best of your ability.

3. **Assess the airway.** Carefully assess the airway to ensure that it is clear of any blood, vomitus, heavy secretions, or other fluids. Sometimes people with special challenges cannot chew food or swallow well, and

the AEMT may find partially chewed food occluding the airway. If this is the case, progressively treat the airway occlusion until it is removed (suctioning, manual techniques, simple mechanical techniques, advanced mechanical techniques). In obese patients, extra adipose tissue in the cheeks, lower jaw, and anterior neck places pressure on the tongue and airway structures, causing closure. Position these patients with a towel behind the shoulder blades to facilitate an open airway (if no cervical problems are suspected). If the patient has a stoma, use a French catheter to suction it out should it be occluded with mucus or secretions.

4. **Assess the breathing.** The critical question here is to ascertain whether the patient is breathing adequately. Assess for chest rise and fall, listen to alveolar breath sounds, and note the patient's speech patterns (if the patient is able to talk). A patient who has good alveolar breath sounds, has normal chest excursion, and is speaking in full sentences is still breathing adequately. If the patient is on a mechanical ventilator, use the same parameters (chest excursion and breath sounds) to ascertain whether it is still ventilating properly. If it is not, consider using your own mechanical ventilator if you are equipped with one, or use a bag-valve-mask (BVM) device to replace the ventilator. Exercise extreme caution to ensure that you are ventilating at an appropriate rate and depth. If the patient has a stoma, use a pediatric mask attached to the BVM and ventilate over the stoma. If a tracheostomy tube is placed in the stoma hole, attach the BVM directly to this (▶ **Figure 53-4**). You may need to seal the mouth and nose should the glottic opening still be patent.

5. **Assess central and peripheral circulation.** Assess the patient for adequate or inadequate peripheral perfusion following normal assessment techniques. Also assess for indications of hemorrhage if the patient is a victim of trauma or is relying on some medical equipment (e.g., urinary catheters or VAD devices) that has somehow dislodged, causing local trauma or bleeding. Treat the patient with a hemorrhage as you normally would, consider any patient with indications of poor peripheral perfusion to be unstable, position him appropriately, and keep him warm. Consider the patient with hypoperfusion to be in need of ALS backup. In the meantime, support any lost function.

6. **Complete the secondary assessment.** After managing any lost function to the airway, breathing, and circulation in the specially challenged patient, complete a secondary assessment to note whether any other minor conditions are present (treating them appropriately as well). During the secondary assessment, note any signs of abuse and learn as much as you can about any medical technology on which the patient is reliant. Be careful when preparing the patient

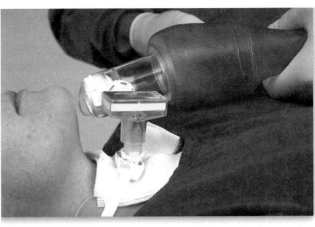

Figure 53-4 The AEMT can ventilate a patient with a tracheostomy by attaching the bag-valve device to the tracheostomy tube's 15/22 mm adapter.

for movement to the ambulance, and make allowances for proper handling of the patient's medical equipment. Typically, your on-scene time with specially challenged patients is longer than for nonchallenged patients because of the additional time needed for assessment and proper packaging for transport.

Overall, the care you render for specially challenged patients will depend on the condition(s) for which you were summoned. Most tertiary centers have a program to educate local EMS on special needs patients who are released to the community (e.g., VAD patients) and have consultative services for these patients. Always remember, though, to maintain an open and patent airway, ensure that breathing remains adequate, and make sure peripheral perfusion is intact. Consider summoning ALS for a patient who is critically unstable or deteriorating. Become familiar with the medical technology on which the patient may be relying, and provide careful and expedient transport to the hospital.

TRANSITIONING • • • • • • • •

REVIEW ITEMS

1. You arrive on scene for a patient with an altered mental status. You note during your physical exam that the patient has a VAD placed beneath the skin in the upper left thoracic region. Knowing this, what can you conclude about the patient's medical history?

   a. The patient has a pulmonary dysfunction.
   b. The patient is suffering from cancer.
   c. The patient is likely terminal and probably has a DNR order.
   d. The patient's medical condition warrants ongoing medication injections.

2. A two-year-old male patient has a history of hydrocephalus, and the parents state that the boy's mental status has been continually deteriorating over the past 8 hours. What might be a cause for this?

    a. There is likely bleeding into the brain tissue.

    b. The shunt is probably blocked and the ICP is increasing.

    c. Because of the medical history, the child's electrolytes are deranged.

    d. The child may be suffering from ongoing child abuse.

3. A morbidly obese patient is found supine and unresponsive in his home. You hear loud sonorous airway sounds with each breath. What action should you take next?

    a. Position some folded towels between the shoulder blades.

    b. Provide endotracheal intubation with an appropriate-size ET tube.

    c. Initiate positive pressure ventilation at 12/minute with 100 percent oxygen.

    d. Suction out the airway with a rigid-tip catheter, then provide positive pressure ventilation.

4. Your patient has a history of a traumatic injury that has left him completely paralyzed. What type of medical equipment will he most likely be dependent on for survival?

    a. VAD   b. apnea monitor

    c. peritoneal dialysis   d. mechanical ventilator

5. A patient who uses a CPAP or BiPAP machine will likely have what type of medical history?

    a. sleep apnea

    b. renal failure

    c. traumatic brain injury

    d. neuromuscular disease

APPLIED PATHOPHYSIOLOGY

A patient has been diagnosed with a neuromuscular disease that has left him dependent on care providers for ongoing care. The patient is ventilator dependent, has a feeding tube inserted and has a urinary catheter placed.

1. Given this history, what other clinical conditions is he at risk for developing that may result in the summoning of EMS?

2. Discuss the problems with airway and ventilation maintenance in a patient with morbid obesity who is found unresponsive and apneic.

3. Discuss how morbid obesity can also have a detrimental effect on the following body systems:

    a. Cardiovascular

    b. Pulmonary

    c. Musculoskeletal

    d. Psychological

CLINICAL DECISION MAKING

You are called for a "medical equipment alarm" at a residential address. On arrival you are met by an elderly female who seems very distressed. She explains that her husband came home from the hospital the previous day, after suffering a major stroke a month ago. He is now reliant on a mechanical ventilator for breathing through a tube placed in his neck. She tells you that the ventilator's alarm keeps sounding.

1. Based on this brief history, what would be at least two etiologies for the ventilator alarm to be sounding?

The primary assessment reveals the patient to be responsive to noxious stimuli with nonpurposeful motion. You note that the ventilator alarm is indicating "high airway pressure," and you note heavy secretions to the stoma placed in the anterior neck. The pulse oximeter reading is 93 percent, and the heart rate is 110 beats per minute.

2. Is this patient suffering from an airway disturbance or a ventilatory disturbance?

3. What action should you take to initially care for this patient?

After managing the situation described, you continue your assessment. You find that the pupils are midsize and responsive, the airway remains patent, peripheral pulses are present, capillary refill is <2 seconds, the skin is warm and slightly diaphoretic, the blood pressure is 138/86, the heart rate is now 88 beats per minute, and the pulse oximeter reads 96 percent. After placing the patient back on the ventilator, the ventilator resumes functioning without any alarms sounding.

4. How could you confirm clinically that the ventilator's operation is actually resulting in adequate ventilations for the patient?

5. What conditions are you still considering as the possible cause? Would you consider any other conditions as a possible cause?

6. Explain why this patient is at a greater risk for:

    a. Respiratory infections

    b. Sepsis

    c. Pressure ulcers

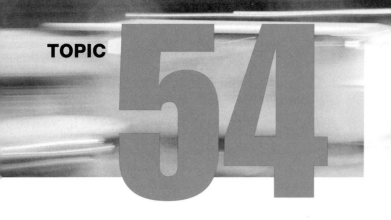

TOPIC

54

Standard Special Patient Populations

Competency Applies a fundamental knowledge of growth, development, aging and assessment findings to provide basic and selected advanced emergency care and transportation for a patient with special needs.

BARIATRIC EMERGENCIES

TRANSITION *highlights*

- Incidence of obesity in the general population.
- Effect of obesity on organ systems.
- Types of bariatric surgeries.
- Complications associated with postoperative bariatric surgical patients.
- Assessment issues specific to the bariatric patient.
- Issues with emergency care of the bariatric patient.

TABLE 54-1	Examples of BMI for a Person 5 Feet 9 Inches Tall	
Weight	**BMI Value**	**Interpretation**
≤ 124 pounds	Below 18.5	Underweight
125–168 pounds	18.5–24.9	Normal weight
169–202 pounds	25.0–29.9	Overweight
≥ 203 pounds	30.0 or higher	Obese

person's BMI is greater than 30 kg/m^2, the term "obese" is used. As an example, Table 54-1 shows various body mass index values for a person 5 foot 9 inches tall.

Ours is a nation that has become obsessed with weight—not only for its unhealthy effects on the body, but also for its detrimental effects on how a person (and society) views what is attractive or unattractive. To this end, there have been significant increases in various weight loss programs, including dieting, the use of herbal supplements or medications claiming to reduce one's weight, and the most recent development, the use of surgery as a corrective remedy.

Bariatrics, as this branch of medicine is known, is the focus for this chapter, as the patient who has undergone bariatric surgery not only may suffer complications from his excessive weight prior to surgery, but also may have postsurgical complications that may result in the summoning of EMS. Obesity and bariatric surgery are on the rise in the United States with no real end in sight; it is just a matter of time until you encounter one of these patients in your practice of prehospital medicine.

INTRODUCTION

To understand what bariatric medicine is about, one first must understand obesity. Beyond the common layperson's interpretation of what "obese" or "overweight" means, there is actually a medical interpretation of this condition and its effects on the body. More so, obesity has become a national health care concern, as it is ranked as one of the top reasons of preventable death in the United States today.

Obesity, as described by the Centers for Disease Control and Prevention and by the U.S. Department of Health and Human Services, is a condition in which the individual is of a weight that is considered "unhealthy" for that person. Simply put, the effect of extra weight on the body is detrimental to the body systems, often leading to disease, disability, and, ultimately, death.

Obesity can be defined by a body mass index (BMI) of 30 kg/m^2. This BMI calculation considers both the height and weight of the person and allows for fluctuations due to the patient's body size rather than being a standard size/weight formula designed to fit all. According to this formula, a person is overweight if his BMI is between 25 and 29.9 kg/m^2; if the

Obesity can be defined by a BMI of 30 kg/m^2.

EPIDEMIOLOGY

Obesity is a national epidemic that is becoming pandemic across all modern industrialized countries. In fact, one of the only areas on earth that is *not* seeing increased obesity levels is some sub-Saharan regions in Africa. The United States currently ranks number one for the highest level of obesity of all developed

TABLE 54-2 — Effects of Excess Weight on Organ Systems

Organ System	Disease States
Cardiovascular	Hypertension, coronary artery disease, congestive heart failure, stroke
Respiratory	Obstructive sleep apnea, intrinsic asthma, COPD
Endocrine	Diabetes mellitus, dyslipidemia, cancer
Gastrointestinal	GERD, cholelithasis, nonalcoholic fatty liver disease
Musculoskeletal	Osteoarthritis, gout, back injuries
Psychological	Depression

nations—a trend that is likely not going to change soon. From a monetary perspective, more than 80 billion dollars in public and private health care money is spent each year on combating obesity and its associated disease states.

Data from 2007 indicate that 33 percent of males and 35 percent of females are obese, with an ethnicity disproportion of up to 50 percent in African-American women. In addition, obesity levels in children are still climbing and present a cause for alarm. Further research reported in the *Journal of the American Medical Association* in 2010 has found that obesity levels have started to plateau for American women over the past decade, with minor increases in men and children. Although it is pleasing to see the increasing trend slow, the fact still remains that from a "bird's-eye view" (or a prevalence rate), 65 percent of the U.S. population is overweight or obese, and obesity still contributes to more than 300,000 deaths per year.

As mentioned, one remedy for obesity that has been on the rise is bariatric surgery. Surgical techniques have improved, it is more publicly accepted, and some insurance companies even will pay for the surgery if it will improve the health of the patient. One current estimate from 2008 indicated that more than 220,000 bariatric surgeries were being performed yearly, of which about 10 percent resulted in postsurgical complications, with nearly 5 percent having serious or life-threatening complications.

PATHOPHYSIOLOGY

The problem of weight control has been well published for many years. Whereas the physical and emotional problems associated with obesity are important concerns, the morbidity and mortality associated with this disease are readily recognized by health care practitioners. The major disease states that are often caused by weight gain are diabetes mellitus, hypertension, coronary heart disease, obstructive sleep apnea, dyslipidemia, nonalcoholic fatty liver disease, and depression. Table 54-2 details the effects of excess weight on the major body organ systems.

Bariatric surgery is a prevalent and popular treatment for patients who are classified as morbidly obese (BMI between 40 and 49.9 kg/m^2). In these patients, often their size and/or their comorbidites inhibit effective weight loss through diet and exercise; thus, a surgical procedure may be performed. To be considered for a surgical procedure, the patient must be classified as morbidly obese *and* have one or more of the previously discussed comorbidites.

Prior to surgery, the patient will also be subjected to a battery of psychological and physiologic testing to be cleared for surgery. Psychological counseling is focused on lifestyle modifications that need to be made both before and after the surgery. To ensure that the patient is physiologically stable enough to endure the surgery, physiologic testing is done and may include a cardiac stress test, diagnostic heart catheterization, pulmonary function test, diabetes testing, endocrine testing, and others.

After the patient has completed these first steps, the surgeon decides what type of surgical procedure to perform. There are basically two types of surgical procedures, those that confine the size of the stomach so the patient does not eat as much (restrictive procedures), and those designed to lessen the length of the GI system, which in turn reduces its ability to absorb nutrients (malabsorption procedures).

Restrictive surgical procedures restrict the size of the stomach, thereby not allowing the person to eat as much food (hence lower caloric intake). This type of surgery has two common variations. The first and most common is the *adjustable-banded gastroplasty* (ABG). It can be performed laparoscopically, which decreases the potential complications often associated with the opening of the abdominal cavity. The surgery involves placing an inflatable cuff around the upper portion or cardiac region of the stomach. The cuff is supplied with an inflation line that is connected to a reservoir embedded subcutaneously in the abdominal wall. The reservoir can be injected with saline, which would fill the cuff and increase the pressure exerted by the band. Pressure exerted by the band causes a feeling of "fullness" by the patient and lessens the stomach size, which, combined with smaller portions, should result in a decreased caloric intake.

A subtype of this procedure is a *vertical-banded gastroplasty*, which can also be performed laparoscopically. This procedure involves stapling a portion of the stomach closed and banding the remaining portion, resulting in the same feeling of fullness by the patient after only a few bites of food.

Malabsorption surgical procedures are more complicated, as they require the surgical opening of the abdominal cavity. Opening of the abdomen is required because the procedures involve dissection of the normal GI tract and rerouting of the stomach and portion of the small intestines. The common feature of these remedies is they decrease the length and absorption capabilities of the GI tract, resulting in fewer calories. The most common procedure is the *Roux-en-Y* bypass, which involves partitioning off a small portion of the upper stomach by stapling, and then connecting (anastomosing) it to the distal jejunum. By rerouting the lower GI tract to the stomach and avoiding the pyloric sphincter, oral intake will pass into the lower small intestine and large intestine more rapidly, without much chance for the body to absorb nutrients.

Variations of this procedure involve different sites of anastomosing to the jejunum, various lengths of jejunum used, and pouch size created by the stapling of the stomach. Other types of malabsorptive

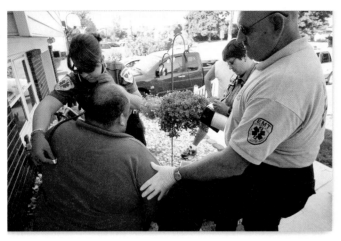

Figure 54-1 Assessment and care of the obese patient follows a normal format, but modifications may be required because of the patient's size. (© *Mark C. Ide*)

surgical procedures include the biliopancreatic diversion and the biliopancreatic diversion with a duodenal switch. Both these surgeries require a section of stomach to be removed (making it smaller) and the lower small intestine reattached to the stomach (the former surgery bypasses the pyloric sphincter, whereas the latter surgery does not bypass the pyloric sphincter, as the duodenum is connected to the lower part of the small intestine).

Although numerous types of surgical and nonsurgical procedures have been used (with various degrees of success) in the management of obese patients, the common theme with these procedures is the minimizing of the nutritional intake by the patient. It is done either by minimizing the food intake or minimizing the absorption through the gastrointestinal tract.

> **Bariatric patients often need special wheeled stretchers capable of holding their weight.**

Despite the goal being restriction of caloric intake, another issue occurs as a result of these procedures: the minimization of absorbing other necessary nutrients and vitamins that the body needs. To counter this, the patient who has bariatric surgery will remain on various dietary supplements for the rest of his life.

Complications Associated with Bariatric Surgery

Bariatric surgery is considered major surgery; therefore, it is associated with a number of postoperative complications that you might see in the prehospital setting. Emergencies may include the following:

- Patients may develop a pulmonary embolism associated with a deep vein thrombosis (DVT). Patients are often put on heparin to prevent DVT occurrence or may receive daily heparin injections for three to four weeks following surgery if they are at high risk. Look for a sudden onset of shortness of breath, chest pain, and syncope.

- Gastrointestinal tract leak may occur where the bowel and stomach are stapled, causing the contents of the bowel to leak in the abdominal cavity. This may lead to a serious abdominal infection. This complication usually occurs within two weeks following the surgery. The patient will likely complain of abdominal pain associated with fever, tachycardia, dyspnea, and malaise.

- Bowel obstruction may occur from scar tissue or kinking of the bowel early after surgery—or months to years following the procedure. The patient would likely complain of abdominal pain, nausea, and vomiting.

- Stricture often occurs as a result of an excessive formation of scar tissue where the stomach is connected surgically to the bowel. This complication usually occurs within two months after surgery. The patient often complains of a decreased tolerance of food, including liquids, and vomiting.

- Bleeding can occur wherever stapling was done or tissue removed. The blood loss may be within the gastrointestinal tract or in the abdominal cavity. The patient may present with abdominal pain, hematemesis, or blood clots in the stool. Severe bleeding may lead to hypovolemia. Patients on heparin to prevent DVT are at a greater risk of bleeding complications.

ASSESSMENT FINDINGS

Assessment findings for a bariatric patient share some similarities with other adults, as well as having some dissimilarities (▶Figure 54-1). First, during the scene size-up, the AEMT should always use Standard Precautions. Another consideration that the AEMT needs to rapidly assess and develop a course of action for is how to move the patient safely. It is better to call for additional help early for lifting and moving, and it is best to get more backup than you would likely need (having too many people and not needing them is always better than finding out you need more people than you have).

Bariatric patients often need special wheeled stretchers capable of holding their weight. In addition, many EMS systems have a specially designed bariatric ambulance equipped with a winch system that will pull the patient into the ambulance via ramps, rather than having EMS providers attempt to lift them (▶ Figure 54-2). Again, the goal is to call for these services

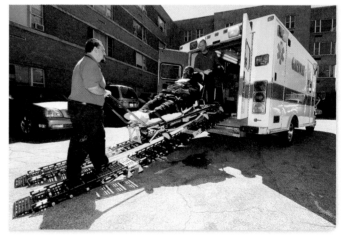

Figure 54-2 Bariatric devices include special cots designed to support the greater weight of an obese patient and loading devices such as ramps and winches that interface with specially designed ambulance cot-locking systems. (© *Ray Kemp/911 Imaging*)

as soon as possible and to not put yourself or your crews at risk of injury.

During the primary assessment, assess the patient's chief complaint while noting the patient's mental status, airway patency, breathing mechanics, and circulation adequacy. Although bariatric surgery does not involve manipulation or surgical removal of airway/breathing/circulatory components, the patient's body habitus can present a challenging situation for EMS providers.

Obese patients commonly have "extra" skin and adipose tissue around the face, chin, neck, and on the posterior surface of the upper thorax. When the patient is standing or sitting forward, the extra tissue does not usually interfere with normal breathing; however, when the patient is placed in or assumes a supine position, problems can develop. The extra adipose tissue places pressure on the tongue and on vital airway structures, including the glottic opening and trachea. Additional airway closure can result from the fat pad or "buffalo hump" sometimes seen between a patient's shoulder blades.

The obese patient may also use a noninvasive continuous positive airway pressure (CPAP) or a bilevel continuous airway pressure (BiPAP) device when he sleeps, thus underscoring the patient's inability to maintain his own airway while supine.

Airway occlusion can be prevented by proper positioning of the patient, a simple maneuver that is often overlooked. If the patient is conscious, allow the patient to assume a position of comfort, usually sitting upright or in a slightly reclined position. If the patient is obtunded or unable to protect his airway, the providers must ensure that the airway is maintained in a neutral position and remains patent. Multiple towels or blankets can be placed under the shoulder blades and behind the neck (if no cervical injury is suspected), providing atlanto-occipital extension. This will align the laryngeal and pharyngeal axes to improve the airway patency.

To anteriorly displace the tongue mechanically, an oropharyngeal or nasopharyngeal airway can be used. Remember that the oral airway can stimulate vomiting if placed in a patient with an intact gag reflex. If that is the case, a nasopharyngeal airway should be used. Along with an artificial adjunct airway, the AEMT may need to provide a modified jaw thrust to move the jaw and tongue and prevent a partial airway obstruction.

If the patient requires endotracheal intubation, thorough preparation is necessary, as well as a plan on what to do if the intubation is unsuccessful (a failed airway plan). If the patient's condition allows, evaluate the potential intubation difficulty by using the Mallampati classification or the "3-3-2" assessment. If, on assessment, the patient is either a Grade I or Grade II Mallampati, the intubation should not be that difficult. However, with a Grade III or Grade IV Mallampati, the AEMT may wish to consider an alternative airway maneuver, device, or technique.

With the 3-3-2 assessment—which is a better technique at predicting airway difficulty—the assessment should yield (hopefully) at least three fingerbreadths between the central incisors, three fingerbreadths between the thyroid cartilage (Adam's apple) and the anterior apex of the mandible, and two fingerbreadths between the top of the larynx and the floor of the chin. Distances less than those stated have been associated with poor laryngoscopic view.

When considering endotracheal intubation, a number of precautions/options should be considered. Do you have enough providers to assist with a two-person bag-valve mask (BVM) if needed, provide the backward upward rightward pressure (BURP) maneuver, and perform intubation? If the patient is still conscious, the prudent technique would be to allow the patient to breathe on his own and assist the ventilations with a BVM.

A caution to any EMS system in which the AEMT is working with a paramedic and the decision is made to use sedative or paralytic agents with obese patients: Loss of muscle tone could completely occlude the patient's airway and make it improbable or impossible to intubate or ventilate the patient.

Most important, have rescue airway devices set out and ready to use. Obese patients tend to desaturate rapidly because they have a decreased functional reserve capacity. If the patient desaturates during the intubation procedure, pull out and immediately ventilate the patient with a BVM. Failure to ventilate the patient adequately manually should prompt the provider to insert a rescue airway (be it a single- or double-lumen airway device) and resume ventilations.

Once the airway is secure, the provider should turn his attention to the oxygenation and ventilation of the patient. If the

patient presents postoperatively (less than 6–8 weeks postsurgery), he may have still have a large bulky dressing extending from the abdomen to the lower chest and/or may still have drains in place. Ventilation in these patients may be impaired by the patient's body habitus itself or from splinting due to surgical site pain or wound dehiscence (opening of the surgical site).

Remember also that it is anatomically difficult for the patient (and the provider) to ventilate the obese patient while he lies supine. In the supine position, the posterior thoracic wall has limited mobility, and the anterior thoracic wall is now under direct pressure from the patient's own adipose tissue. Rapid fatigue of the intercostal muscles and sternocleidomastoid muscle may leave the diaphragm as the final muscle preventing respiratory failure.

In an attempt to compensate for decreased respiratory effort, the patient's respiratory rate may be tachypneic. But with tachypnea comes hypopnea (shallow breathing), so the provider must always remember that a breathing patient does not equal an *adequately* breathing patient.

If the patient needs ventilatory assistance or requires mechanical ventilation, the patient's size must be taken into account. It is significantly more difficult to ventilate a patient weighing 185 kg than a patient weighing 85 kg. Common causes of ventilation/perfusion deficits that may result in respiratory distress include abdominal splinting because of pain, pneumonia related to decreased ventilatory effort, decreased ventilatory rate as a result of the use of prescribed narcotic pain medications, decreased thoracic cavity expansion because of increased intraabdominal pressure, increased capillary permeability caused by any underlying hypertension, and decreased pulmonary perfusion resulting from a pulmonary embolism.

After the airway is secured and oxygenation and ventilation have been established, a rapid circulatory assessment can be performed. An early sign of inadequate circulation and perfusion or hypercapnia is a change in mentation. Alterations in heart rate and blood pressure can cause cerebral hypoxia. Another dysfunction that can affect the circulatory status is an infection leading to sepsis. In fact, the most common cause of mortality within the first 12 weeks postsurgery is an intraabdominal infection from a leaking anastamosis.

Even before the body responds by resetting the hypothalamus temperature switch and raising the core temperature, pain and anxiety will cause an increase in heart rate. Thus, any patient presenting with an elevated heart rate should be evaluated thoroughly, treated appropriately, and transported to the hospital. Other circulatory signs of infection include an increase in temperature and redness at the wound site.

Another common postoperative problem associated with bariatric surgery is nausea and vomiting. As stated previously, the goal of the surgery is to decrease the patient's absorption of food and/or fluid that is placed in the body. As such, the patient's ability to absorb fluid will be greatly decreased as a result of the surgery. As the GI tract adapts to the new "arrangement" of organs and physiology, an expected response is nausea and vomiting. Intense nausea and vomiting, accompanied by "dumping syndrome" (caused by an inability to absorb fluid as it rapidly passes through the GI tract, resulting in watery diarrhea/bowel movements), can lead to profound dehydration. This dehydration can present with tachycardia, warm dry skin and pallor to the mucosal membranes, and decreased urinary output.

Fluctuations in blood pressure can also be expected in the first few months postsurgery. Most morbidly obese patients have a preoperative diagnosis of hypertension and are usually treated with a number of medications. Immediate postoperative pain and anxiety can cause sharp increases in the patient's blood pressure. In addition, the patient's blood pressure may fluctuate because of the patient not being able to digest the medication as a result of postoperative nausea and vomiting.

Another cause of cardiovascular dysfunction seen postoperatively is an infective process. Infections of the abdominal cavity are often associated with the release of bacterial endotoxins, resulting in peritonitis and encompassing the entire body in a septic presentation. This infection usually is borne from a leaking anastamosis. Signs of localized infection include erythema at the surgical site and an increase in the patient's temperature.

EMERGENCY CARE

The assessment and management of a bariatric patient must be appropriate for the situation, specific for the emergency, efficient in its rendering, and thorough in its completeness to realize the best possible scenario for survivability of the patient. The following are some important considerations whenever the AEMT is caring for a bariatric patient.

1. **Ensure inline immobilization.**
   Because of the patient's size, immobilization can become a challenge if the bariatric patient is injured. Be creative by using pillows or blankets for posterior support. You may also need rolled towels and tape for a makeshift collar if necessary.

2. **Maintain patency of the airway.**
   This is perhaps the most difficult part of the management. Remember to use body positioning and padding to your advantage. Use of a two-handed jaw thrust with an OPA or NPA may be necessary to keep the airway open. If intubation is warranted, consider the use of a straight blade for better visualization, and constantly monitor the patient during the intubation procedure to prevent hypoxia. If the patient is not easy to intubate, consider using a rescue device rather than multiple attempts at intubation (ventilating the patient is always more important than intubating the patient).

3. **Ensure adequacy of breathing.** If the patient is conscious, note the patient's speech patterns and quality of alveolar breath sounds to help guide the need for positive pressure ventilation (PPV). If the patient is unconscious, assess the chest wall excursion and quality of alveolar breath sounds to determine whether PPV is needed. If breathing is adequate, apply oxygen via nonrebreather mask or nasal cannula, depending on the status of the patient. If possible and protocol allows, the use of CPAP may be beneficial for the bariatric patient.
   If the patient's breathing is inadequate, provide high-flow oxygen in conjunction with PPV (always ventilate gently to lower the chances for barotraumas). Use a two-handed, two-person technique. Finally, never insert an orogastric or nasogastric tube for gastric decompression, as the change to the stomach size and bowel can easily cause perforation if a tube is inserted blindly.

4. **Support cardiovascular function.**
   Treat any external hemorrhage immediately with direct pressure, and assess any present drains for hemorrhage. Dumping syndrome can easily lead to dehydration, and the propensity for infection can cause overwhelming peripheral vasodilation and hypoperfusion. Determine the quality of peripheral perfusion by the quality of the skin findings and peripheral pulses. Intravenous access should be obtained using a large-bore, short-length IV catheter and administering a crystalloid solution. Lactated Ringer's or 0.9 percent normal saline can be used, administered with controlled boluses of 250 to 500 mL each time. After each bolus the patient's pulse, blood pressure, respirations, mentation, and lung sounds should be assessed to guide further fluid therapy.
   Current literature and research recommend not increasing the systolic blood pressure too rapidly in an attempt to correct and obtain the patient's "normal" pressure. Systolic blood pressures of 80 to 90 mmHg correlate to adequate perfusion of the body's vital organs (heart, brain, lung, kidneys). Finally, maintain normothermia.

Other management, such as soft tissue injuries, musculoskeletal trauma, and the like, should follow the same treatment principles as for other trauma victims. Likewise, the treatment of medical conditions such as hypoglycemia, myocardial infarctions, or respiratory distress generally follows normal treatment parameters.

In conclusion, the likelihood of the AEMT having to care for obese and bariatric patients is only going to rise in the foreseeable future. The challenge the AEMT will have with each bariatric patient, regardless of why the patient called EMS, is how to best move the patient safely, maintain the airway, support inadequate breathing, and preserve peripheral perfusion. It is only after tackling these parameters that the AEMT will be able to turn his attention to the rest of the problems the patient may be experiencing.

REVIEW ITEMS

1. Which of the following medical conditions will help identify the bariatric patient who may deteriorate with supine positioning?

   a. sleep apnea
   b. hypertension
   c. hypoglycemia
   d. congestive heart failure

2. You are caring for a bariatric patient with respiratory distress. Of the following findings, which one best identifies that the patient is not breathing adequately?

   a. pulse oximetry of 95 percent
   b. anxiousness and irritability
   c. use of accessory muscles to breathe
   d. absence of vesicular (alveolar) breath sounds with auscultation

3. When providing mechanical ventilation to a bariatric patient in severe respiratory distress, why should the AEMT ventilate slowly with low airway pressures?

   a. It prevents causing accidental overventilation.
   b. Failure to do so will result in inadequate oxygenation.
   c. Higher airway pressures may cause gastric insufflation.
   d. It avoids the likelihood of wiping out the patient's breathing reflex.

4. An obese patient recently had bariatric surgery and has now summoned EMS for severe nausea. During the assessment of the patient, you note that one of the insertion points for a drain is reddened. The patient is noted to have a fever and is mildly dehydrated. This presentation is most suggestive of what problem?

   a. low blood sugar
   b. respiratory failure
   c. dumping syndrome
   d. probable abdominal infection

5. Which of the following bariatric patients would likely be the most difficult to intubate?

   a. patient with a Mallampati Grade II
   b. patient with a Mallampati Grade IV
   c. patient who weighs more than 600 pounds
   d. patient who has a normal 3-3-2 assessment

APPLIED PATHOPHYSIOLOGY

You are called by the family for an obese patient who underwent adjustable-banded gastroplasty surgery two weeks earlier. On your arrival, you estimate the patient's weight to be about 210 kg. The patient is complaining of severe nausea with vomiting for the past few days. On closer assessment, the patient presents with a fever, is tachycardic, and says he is very "uncomfortable." You call for backup to help move the patient, but they are still 20 minutes away from your location.

1. Discuss what types of problems you may encounter in moving the patient.

2. What type of preparation, considering both equipment to use and skills to employ, should the AEMT incorporate into the assessment, management, and movement of the patient?

3. For the circumstances listed below, discuss how the assessment and management of bariatric patient would be dissimilar from those for the nonobese patient.

   a. Airway management
   b. Provision of PPV
   c. Treatment of dyspnea
   d. Patient positioning

CLINICAL DECISION MAKING

You are called to the home of a 30-year-old male patient who is complaining of respiratory distress. On arrival to the home, you are escorted into the living room, where you see an obese patient lying on a hospital bed. Your primary survey reveals that the patient is in acute respiratory distress, with shallow breathing. The patient has an altered mental status, the pulse is tachycardic, peripheral perfusion is poor, and your partner reports no alveolar breath sounds on auscultation. The pulse oximeter displays a reading of 82 percent on room air.

1. Based on this brief history and presentation, would this patient be classified as a high or low priority? Support your answer with facts taken from the scenario.

2. What would be at least two critical interventions the AEMT should take now, before continuing on with the assessment of the patient?

After initiating care, you gather the SAMPLE history from the family and learn that the patient was released from the hospital five days earlier after bariatric surgery. The patient is also an insulin-dependent diabetic with a history of hypertension. He has been taking his insulin, but because of a recent history of nausea with vomiting, he has been unable to keep his oral antihypertensive or any food down. Ongoing ventilatory assistance only produces breath sounds in the upper and middle lobes with minimal sounds to the lower lobes. Your partner reports that it is hard to keep a good seal with the BVM during ventilations.

3. What could be done to help your partner better ventilate the patient?

4. Is this patient a candidate for CPAP therapy by EMS? Why or why not?

5. What other bedside diagnostic should be obtained, given this patient's medical history and recent medical problems?

The secondary assessment reveals that one of the patient's drain appears infected. In addition, the pulse oximetry has only improved slightly with PPV and oxygen. The vitals are currently blood pressure 102/80, pulse rate 110, and pulse oximetry is 92 percent with oxygen and PPV. Blood sugar is 42 mg/dL. The patient's temperature is 101.7°F. The patient is morbidly obese, weighing 180 kg. The findings during the balance of the secondary exam were benign and noncontributory.

6. What intravenous solution should be initiated?

7. Should this patient receive D_{50} or oral glucose? Why or why not?

8. What additional techniques could be employed to make the PPV more effective?

9. What would be key indicators of patient improvement with treatment?

10. What would be key indicators of deterioration with treatment?

Standard EMS Operations

Competency Knowledge of operational roles and responsibilities to ensure patient, public, and personnel safety.

TOPIC

55

MULTIPLE-CASUALTY INCIDENTS AND INCIDENT MANAGEMENT

INTRODUCTION

A multiple-casualty incident (MCI) is any event that places a great demand on personnel or equipment. MCIs range from vehicle collisions with a few injured passengers to major disasters. Although most large-scale incidents require more time, resources, and support from other agencies, the principles for managing any MCI are fundamentally the same, regardless of the size of the emergency.

To manage any MCI effectively, the following must be accomplished:

- Enough help and resources, both personnel and equipment, must be obtained.
- Emergency vehicles must respond to and have access to the emergency scene.
- The appropriate emergency medical care must be provided to every patient.
- Patients requiring care must be transported to hospitals for treatment.
- Effective communication must be ensured.
- Follow-up care for both the patients and rescue personnel must be received.

The Department of Homeland Security developed and administers the National Incident Management System (NIMS). NIMS provides a framework to guide all levels of governmental, nongovernmental, and private agencies to work together to prevent, protect against, respond to, recover from, and mitigate the effects of incidents, regardless of cause, size, location, or complexity, in order to reduce the loss of life and property and harm to the environment.

NIMS is composed of five major components that are designed to work together:

- **Preparedness** involves a combination of assessment; planning; procedures and protocols; training and exercises; personnel qualifications, licensure, and certification; equipment certification; and evaluation and revision.
- **Communications and Information Management** utilizes the concepts of interoperability, reliability, scalability, and

TRANSITION highlights

- *Review of what a multiple-casualty incident is.*
- *The NIMS framework.*
- *How the Incident Command System within NIMS is to be deployed during an MCI.*
- *The START triage format.*
- *The psychological stress that may arise in EMS secondary to an MCI.*

portability, as well as the resiliency and redundancy of communications and information systems.

- **Resource Management** defines mechanisms and establishes the process to identify requirements, order and acquire, mobilize, track and report, recover and demobilize, reimburse, and inventory resources.
- **Command and Management** is designed to provide a flexible structure based on three key organizational constructs: the Incident Command System, Multiagency Coordination Systems, and Public Information.
- **Ongoing Management and Maintenance** is facilitated through two components: the National Integration Center (NIC) and Supporting Technologies.

The Incident Command System (ICS) is a subset of the NIMS. It is based on successful business practices and decades of lessons learned in the organization and management of emergency incidents. The ICS is a flexible, cost-effective system that can be used to match the complexities and demands of a single or multiple incidents. It is applicable across all disciplines and is legally required to be used during some incidents, such as those involving hazardous materials. The ICS is structured to facilitate activities in five major functional areas:

- **Command:** Establishes and prioritizes objectives and has overall responsibility at the incident.

- **Operations:** Develops the tactical objectives and directs the use of tactical resources to carry out the plan.
- **Planning:** Prepares and documents the plan, collects and evaluates information, and maintains resource status and documentation for incident records.
- **Logistics:** Provides support, resources, and other services needed to meet the incident needs.
- **Finance/Administration:** Monitors costs related to the incident. Provides accounting, procurement, time recording, and cost analyses.
- **Intelligence and Investigation:** Sometimes added as a sixth area.

> **Every agency that responds to a disaster is required to be NIMS compliant.**

Every agency that responds to a disaster is required to be NIMS compliant. Various levels of incident management training are available to emergency personnel. The courses "FEMA IS-700: NIMS, An Introduction" and "ICS-100: Introduction to ICS," or their equivalents, are required for Advanced EMTs; however, particular organizations and positions might require additional training.

The initial training helps emergency responders understand the systems, use common terminology, communicate effectively with other agencies, identify the objectives to be accomplished during the incident, designate organizational resources, and manage the various spans of control and accountability throughout an incident.

AEMTs can better prepare themselves to respond to large-scale incidents by receiving additional training, participating in training activities, and using the principles of these systems in smaller-scaled incidents based on their protocols.

BRANCH UNITS

The incident commander (▶ **Figure 55-1**) may establish a number of branches to implement the plan effectively. The commander may assign a unit leader who will supervise the activities within the unit. Common units used for EMS personnel include triage, treatment, staging, transport, and communications. Many EMTs also participate in the care provided following the incident.

Triage

The triage unit sorts patients by criticality and assigns priorities for emergency care and transport. As an AEMT, you may be directed to assist in or may be completely responsible for accurately and efficiently triaging the patients at a multiple-casualty incident. Triage is one of the first functions performed at the scene, and it directly affects all the other aspects of the operation.

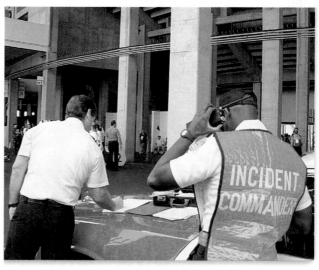

Figure 55-1 The incident commander directs the response and coordinates resources. Wearing reflective vests makes it easier to identify personnel.

There are typically two types of triage: primary and secondary. *Primary triage* occurs immediately on arrival of the first EMS crew. It is usually performed by the most knowledgeable and experienced EMS personnel first on the scene. Primary triage is used on the scene to rapidly categorize a patient's condition as one of the following:

- **Red/Highest Priority/Immediate/ Priority 1: Treatable Life-Threatening Illness or Injuries.** This category is assigned to patients with the most critical injuries who may be able to survive the incident with quick treatment and transport. Most of the treatable problems in this category correlate with the primary assessment. Patients in this category may have airway and breathing difficulties, uncontrolled or severe bleeding, decreased mental status, severe medical problems, shock, and/ or severe burns.

- **Yellow/Second Priority/Delayed/ Priority 2: Serious But Not Life-Threatening Illness or Injuries.** This category is assigned to patients who are suffering severe injuries but still have a good chance of survival. The treatable problems in this category usually correlate with the findings identified during a rapid trauma assessment, such as burns without airway problems, major or multiple bone or joint injuries, and back injuries.

- **Green/Lowest Priority/Minor/ Priority 3: "Walking Wounded."** This category is assigned to patients who are capable of walking. Patients in

this category have injuries that will not reduce their chance of survival, such as fractures and soft tissue injuries without life-threatening bleeding.

- **Black/Deceased/Priority 4 (sometimes called Priority 0): Dead or Fatally Injured.** This category is assigned to patients who, despite the provision of emergency care, will not survive or who are already dead. Examples include patients with exposed brain matter, in cardiac arrest, or decapitated, and those who are incinerated.

Secondary triage is used for patient reevaluation after the patient is moved to the treatment area. Depending on the size of the incident, it may be necessary to retriage and reassign a patient to a different group based on the patient's presentation. Various techniques and systems are used to triage a patient, so it is necessary to be familiar with your local procedures and protocols. The Centers for Disease Control and Prevention (CDC) guidelines and START (Simple Triage and Rapid Transport) systems are two of the most commonly used.

START TRIAGE The START triage is performed primarily to initially categorize older children and adult patients for priority movement to the triage unit. It should not take more than 30 seconds per patient to complete. The assessment in START includes the following:

- **Respiratory status.** Any patient who is able to walk is considered low priority and is tagged "green." The AEMT should assess the respiratory status of

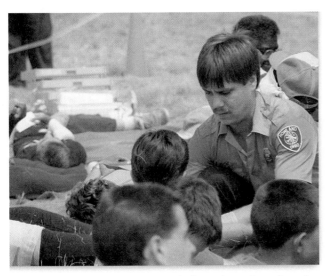

Figure 55-2 Patients are treated after triage, in order of priority.

those who cannot walk. If the patient is not breathing, the AEMT should open the patient's airway. If the patient remains apneic, tag him "black." If the patient's respiratory rate is greater than 30 per minute or inadequate, tag him "red." If it is less than 30 per minute, assess his perfusion status.

- **Perfusion status.** The AEMT should then assess the patient's radial pulse and capillary refill. If the patient has a radial pulse and his capillary refill is less than 2 seconds, the EMT should then proceed to the mental status examination. If the patient's capillary refill is greater than 2 seconds or the radial pulse is absent, tag the patient "red."
- **Mental status.** The AEMT should ask the patient to squeeze his fingers. If the patient follows the command, tag him "yellow." If the patient is not alert, does not obey the commands, or is unresponsive, tag him "red."

After the patients are tagged appropriately, they can be identified, sorted, treated, and transported according to their criticality by rescue personnel at the incident.

Treatment

The treatment unit provides emergency care based on the priority assigned to the patient. Patients should be fully immobilized, if needed, and moved from the triage unit to the treatment unit in order of their priority (▶ Figure 55-2). The treatment area should be a safe distance from the incident and close to the area where the ambulances arrive. Larger-scaled incidents may require use of more than one treatment unit. A morgue should be established and used appropriately. Follow local protocol.

Staging

The staging unit holds ambulances, helicopters, and additional equipment until they are assigned to a particular task. The staging unit leader monitors, inventories, and directs the available ambulances to and from the treatment area. The staging unit leader should also provide the responding EMS personnel with maps to the appropriate receiving facilities.

Transport

The transport unit leader ensures that ambulances are accessible and that transportation does not occur without the direction of the incident commander. Patients should be transported based on their priority. The transport unit leader must consider the following when making decisions on where to transport each patient:

- Distribution of patients to each medical facility
- Surge capacity of each hospital or medical facility
- Need for transport to a specialty medical facility, such as a burn unit or pediatric emergency department
- The need for constant coordination and communication

The transport unit leader should radio the hospital and provide a brief patient report and estimated time of arrival. Ambulatory patients may be transported via bus with adequate personnel and supplies once the more critical patients have been transported. Deceased casualties should be transported to the morgue.

Communications

Emergency management is dependent on effective communication among all those involved. Without efficient communication, an AEMT should anticipate problems throughout the incident. Many communication problems, such as dead spots, frequency unavailability, and channel gridlock, are usually identified early but may still be encountered during an MCI. To reduce communication problems during an MCI, the details of a communication system should be established prior to an incident and should be incorporated into disaster drills. A communication plan should include the following:

- Incident-related policies and standards
- Systems and equipment to be used
- Training necessary to achieve integrated communications
- Responsibility assigned to those operating the system and equipment
- A reliable backup system

Follow-Through

After all the patients have been transported from an incident scene, the emergency personnel assist hospital personnel in follow-through care if necessary. If an AEMT's assistance is needed, the facility's incident manager will provide instructions to the EMT. If the AEMT's assistance is not needed at the hospital, the AEMT should prepare to respond to other emergency calls.

PSYCHOLOGICAL STRESS

Psychological stress often affects the rescuers, as well as the patients, at the scene of a multiple-casualty incident. Personal safety, crying, anger, guilt, numbness, preoccupation with death, frustration, fatigue, and burnout are common concerns encountered by EMS personnel. Effective stress management should be considered prior to and incorporated into the relief efforts of any MCI. Stress management plans and activities should emphasize the following actions:

- Ensure that personnel are appropriately trained and aware of their specific tasks.
- Provide nourishing food and water.
- Ensure rest at regular intervals, maybe as often as once every 1 to 2 hours.
- Monitor personnel for signs of physical exhaustion, stress, or breakdown.
- Encourage rescue workers to talk to their colleagues about their experiences.
- Provide trained counselors to talk with personnel throughout and after the incident.
- Treat and transport immediately any rescuer who is injured or becomes ill during rescue operations.

REVIEW ITEMS

1. Which of the following is *not* used when making decisions on where to take each patient involved in a MCI?
   a. the need for transport to a specialized facility
   b. the ability of each patient to pay for services from the receiving medical facility
   c. the distribution of patients to each medical facility
   d. the surge capacity of each hospital or medical facility

2. Which of the following activities is performed first at an MCI?
   a. triaging patients based on their presentations
   b. treating a patient's minor secondary injuries
   c. transporting all deceased patients to the morgue
   d. transporting all patients to a hospital as soon as you reach them regardless of the severity of their conditions

3. When using the START system, which of the following should be assessed first?
   a. mental status
   b. perfusion status
   c. respirations
   d. Glasgow Coma Scale

4. Which branch unit is responsible for holding the ambulances, helicopters, and additional equipment until they are assigned to a particular task?
   a. triage unit
   b. transport unit
   c. staging unit
   d. treatment unit

5. Which of the following NIMS component responsibilities includes ensuring that rescue personnel meet specific qualifications?
   a. Command and Management
   b. Preparedness
   c. Communications and Information Management
   d. Ongoing Management and Maintenance

APPLIED KNOWLEDGE

1. List and describe the branch units frequently used during an MCI.

2. Explain the process of triage.

3. What is the purpose of the incident management system?

4. How should START triage be used to assign priority to and properly tag a patient?

5. Discuss the importance of effective communications during an incident.

6. Discuss ways to help reduce responder stress throughout an incident.

7. Differentiate between primary and secondary triage.

CLINICAL DECISION MAKING

You and your partner are the first on the scene of a motor vehicle collision. Dispatch has advised you that, because of another major incident, you are the only unit available. Dispatch advises that backup will not be able to arrive on the scene for approximately 10 minutes. As you approach the scene, you note that three vehicles are involved, one of which is a motorcycle that appears to be missing a driver.

1. What concerns do you have as you approach the scene?

2. What information do you need to obtain?

After you determine that the scene is safe, you approach the vehicles. You are met by a patient who approaches you and states that he and his wife were inside vehicle 1. Their vehicle is an SUV with minor front-end damage. The driver, a 25-year-old man, states that they were on their way to the hospital because his wife is in labor when a man on a motorcycle passed them and hit the car ahead of them. The woman, who is 27 years old and obviously pregnant, states she is having contractions that are 10 minutes apart. She states says her abdomen is hurting, but she has never been in labor before. Her husband denies any pain or complaints. Both patients are alert and oriented, deny any loss of consciousness, and state they were restrained.

3. As the most experienced AEMT on scene, what should you do now?

4. What should you instruct your partner to do?

After reassuring the patients in vehicle 1, you proceed to vehicle 2, as your partner begins to look in the nearby ditch for the driver of the motorcycle. Vehicle 2 is a minivan with extensive damage to the front passenger side. The driver of the vehicle is a 60-year-old woman who is alert and oriented. She is complaining of neck pain. She denies any loss of consciousness and says she was the only passenger in her vehicle.

Your partner states that he found the motorcycle driver, who was ejected into the ditch. The patient appears to be a teenage boy who is currently unresponsive, has a weak radial pulse, and has multiple abrasions and deformities to his upper and lower extremities.

5. Based on the scene size-up characteristics, what resources do you need?

6. What priority status would be assigned to each patient? Why?

7. What would your plan be for this incident?

8. Once additional units arrive, in what order would you have the patients transported? Why?

9. Despite your arrival first on the scene, explain why you and your partner will be the last to leave.

56

ADVANCED SKILLS FOR THE AEMT

TRANSITION *highlights*

- Application of partial end-tidal CO_2 monitoring and capnometry.

- Clinical applications of capnometry in the prehospital setting.

- Interpretation of capnometry tracings and LED readings.

- Indications for initiation of an intraosseous cannulation with an EZ-IO in the adult patient.

- Appropriate sites for intraosseous cannulation in the adult patient.

- General procedure for intraosseous cannulation.

- Procedure for establishing a saline or heparin lock.

- Preparation of medications for administration.

- Six rights of medication administration.

- Administration methods by container type:
  - Glass ampule.
  - Single and multidose vials.
  - Nonconstituted drug vial.
  - Prefilled syringe.
  - Intravenous infusion (IV piggyback).

INTRODUCTION

One consistent facet of EMS is that it evolves constantly. Many skills once thought unimaginable in the prehospital arena have been adopted as common practice for current emergency care providers across the United States. The information contained within this topic is no different. Given the climate of EMS provision in many states, it is now being recognized that Advanced EMTs can be used to assist their ALS partners (paramedics) with many advanced life support skills that are employed during patient management. Although this topic will provide the AEMT with the necessary knowledge for performing these important interventions, actually performing them should occur only after there has been a structured educational component to include knowledge testing, skill practice, and technique mastery.

Because no EMS provider can function without appropriate medical direction, the AEMT who reads this topic must also remember that the EMS system of which he is a part must possess appropriate medical control and treatment protocols permitting these techniques. Furthermore, the EMS system should have an established quality assurance program to ensure that the skills performed by the AEMT are meeting both internal EMS standards and patient expectations.

Finally, all EMS providers, regardless of certification or licensure level, are encouraged to constantly strive for bettering both their skills as providers and the delivery of emergency services as a whole. The weight of any emergency medical service system rests squarely on the shoulders of those who perform these skills on a daily basis. The authors hope that this topic will help emergency care providers continue to achieve this purity of purpose.

This topic is one that is based in patient care skills, not on a specific clinical entity. Although training curricula and scope of practice documents have been developed at the national level, EMS practice is determined at the state level. Thus, the use of individual skills is determined by state authority. Each AEMT is responsible for knowing which of these skills are permitted within his state.

As an example, IV therapy has always been an exclusive skill for the AEMT or paramedic according to the educational standards. However, in some states the EMT-Basic is allowed to start an IV after proper training and appropriate medical oversight. The lesson is that the patient care skills permitted for the AEMT will always be dynamic and ever-changing. It would be best for the AEMT to stay abreast of this by constantly reviewing and improving his own skill sets.

The skills discussed in this topic for the AEMT will include capnometry and waveform capnography, saline/heparin locks, setting up IV medications (IVP and infusions), basic 3-lead ECG recognition, and how to acquire a 12-lead ECG.

CAPNOMETRY

End-tidal carbon dioxide ($ETCO_2$) monitoring is a noninvasive method of measuring the levels of carbon dioxide (CO_2) in the exhaled breath. Recordings or displays of exhaled CO_2 measurements are called *capnography*. Various terms have been applied to capnography; a review of them may help you to understand the material in this section. These terms include:

- **Capnometry.** Capnometry is the measurement of expired CO_2. It typically provides a numeric display of the partial pressure of CO_2 (in torr or mmHg).
- **Capnography.** Capnography is a graphic recording or display of the capnometry reading over time.
- **Capnograph.** A capnograph is a device that measures expired CO_2 levels.
- **Capnogram.** A capnogram is the visual representation of the expired CO_2 waveform.
- **End-tidal CO_2 ($ETCO_2$).** End-tidal CO_2 is the measurement of the CO_2 concentration at the end of expiration (maximum CO_2).
- **$PaCO_2$.** The $PaCO_2$ represents the partial pressure of CO_2 in the arterial blood.

Capnometry provides a noninvasive measure of $ETCO_2$ levels, thus providing medical personnel with information about the status of systemic metabolism, circulation, and ventilation. The use of capnography has become a standard in the operating room, in the emergency department, and in the prehospital setting.

The body is continuously producing waste products as a result of ongoing metabolism. The waste byproducts of aerobic metabolism are hydrogen ions (strong acid) and carbon dioxide (weak acid). In fact, if the concentration of hydrogen ions rises, the body will convert this excess hydrogen into more carbon dioxide via the blood buffering system (see Topic 5, "Anatomy and Physiology: Cellular Metabolism") so it can be eliminated via the lungs during normal ventilation. This constant elimination of carbon dioxide through the lungs is the basis for noninvasive carbon dioxide monitoring. Understanding CO_2 production and elimination in the body is integral to understanding the carbon dioxide level reading.

As mentioned, CO_2 is a normal end-product of metabolism and is transported by the venous system to the right side of the heart. It is then pumped by the right ventricle into the pulmonary artery for delivery to perialveolar capillaries. There, according to its partial pressure gradient, it diffuses into the alveoli and is removed from the body throughout the exhalatory phase of ventilation, where it can then be sampled by the monitoring device. If there is a change in the $ETCO_2$ waveform (capnogram) or the numeric level (capnometry), the change must be interpreted in light of the factors that can influence carbon dioxide levels. These factors are:

- **Changes in ventilation:**
  a. If the patient's minute ventilation increases and the alveoli are better ventilated, more carbon dioxide will be eliminated, and the $ETCO_2$ level will drop.
  b. If the patient's minute ventilation decreases and the alveoli are poorly ventilated, then less carbon dioxide will be eliminated and the $ETCO_2$ level will rise.
- **Changes in perfusion:**
  a. Because the heart delivers blood to the lungs via the pulmonary circulation, changes in blood volume or changes in blood flow from a failing right ventricle will lower $ETCO_2$ levels.
  b. If there is an increase in perfusion to the lungs because of an increase in right-sided cardiac output (i.e., the patient has had return of spontaneous circulation [ROSC] from arrest, volume deficits are corrected), more carbon dioxide will be delivered to the lungs by the right side of the heart, and $ETCO_2$ levels will rise back to normal.
- **Changes in metabolic activity:**
  a. If there is a drop in metabolic activity (e.g., hypothermia), there is less overall carbon dioxide in the bloodstream, and the $ETCO_2$ levels tend to drop.
  b. If there is an increase in metabolic activity (think about hyperthermia, seizures, stimulatory drugs), more carbon dioxide will be produced by the cells and delivered to the lungs via the heart. As such, the $ETCO_2$ level will increase.

When metabolic production and circulation are normal, $ETCO_2$ levels change with ventilation and are a reliable estimate of the partial pressure of carbon dioxide in the arterial system ($PaCO_2$). As a general rule, the $ETCO_2$ is 3 to 4 mmHg less than the $PaCO_2$.

When first introduced into prehospital care, $ETCO_2$ monitoring was used exclusively to verify proper endotracheal tube placement in the trachea with a colorimetric device (▶ Figure 56-1). The presence of adequate CO_2 levels following intubation confirms that the tube is in the trachea through the presence of exhaled CO_2.

> **Capnometry is the measurement of expired CO_2.**

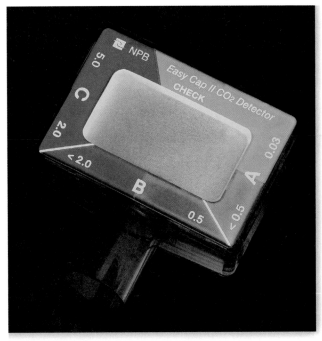

Figure 56-1 Colorimetric end-tidal CO_2 detector. (*Reprinted by permission of Nellcor Puritan Bennett LLC, Pleasanton, CA*)

Colorimetric devices are not designed to detect hypercarbia and have limited usefulness in detecting hypocarbia. If gastric contents or acidic drugs (e.g., endotracheal epinephrine) contact the paper in the device, subsequent readings may be unreliable. Although this type of $ETCO_2$ monitoring is appropriate for BLS providers, ALS providers should be using waveform capnography whenever possible.

The use of waveform capnography is rapidly becoming the standard for ALS providers. Along with breath-to-breath waveform monitoring, the provider can also track CO_2 concentrations over time with the waveform capnography device. With these devices, the waveform of the breath reflects the exhalatory phase characteristics, and the numeric value of the $ETCO_2$ represents the carbon dioxide level present in the exhaled gas. Both are necessary for full interpretation.

Although interpreting the $ETCO_2$ number is straightforward, interpreting capnography requires understanding the $ETCO_2$ waveform itself. The following is an explanation of a normal waveform as it is typically divided into four phases (▶ Figure 56-2).

- **Phase I.** Phase I (AB in Figure 56-2) is the respiratory baseline. It is flat when no CO_2 is present and corresponds to the late phase of inspiration and the early part of expiration (in which dead-space gases without CO_2 are released).
- **Phase II.** Phase II (BC in Figure 56-2) is the respiratory upstroke. This represents exhalation of a mixture of dead space

gases and alveolar gases from alveoli with the shortest transport time.

- **Phase III.** Phase III (CD in Figure 56-2) is the respiratory plateau. It reflects the airflow through uniformly ventilated alveoli with a nearly constant CO_2 level. The highest level of the plateau (point D in Figure 56-2) is called the $ETCO_2$ and is recorded as such by the capnometer.
- **Phase IV.** Phase IV (DE in Figure 56-2) is the inspiratory phase. It is a sudden downstroke and ultimately returns to the baseline during inspiration. The respiratory pause restarts the cycle (EA in Figure 56-2).

Clinical Applications

In a very simple sense, the use of capnography can be indicated for each and every patient you encounter. Two types of sampling lines that provide the exhaled gases to the monitor for interpretation: those used on the mechanically ventilated patient and are placed between the bag-valve mask (BVM) and the airway adjunct (▶ Figure 56-3), and those used for the spontaneously breathing patient, in which a sampling line is applied like a nasal cannula (▶ Figure 56-4). It will sample the exhaled gas while the patient is breath-

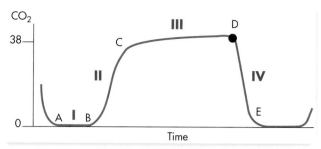

Figure 56-2 Normal capnogram. AB = *Phase I:* late inspiration, early expiration (no CO_2). BC = *Phase II:* appearance of CO_2 in exhaled gas. CD = *Phase III:* plateau (constant CO_2). D = highest point ($ETCO_2$). DE = *Phase IV:* rapid descent during inspiration. EA = respiratory pause.

ing (this type of adapter for the breathing patient will also typically allow for the administration of low-flow oxygen simultaneously).

Before we discuss the steps of setting up the $ETCO_2$ monitoring device, we will first discuss changes to the waveform. Whenever the AEMT identifies a change to either the $ETCO_2$ value or the waveform, he should recall the three influences that can change the $ETCO_2$:

1. Is the change due to the lungs?
2. Is the change due to perfusion to the lungs?
3. Is the change due to some metabolic derangement?

It is important to understand the cause of the change, as your treatment to correct the underlying problem will be based on the underlying derangement. To determine this, the AEMT must know how to assess each of the components that can

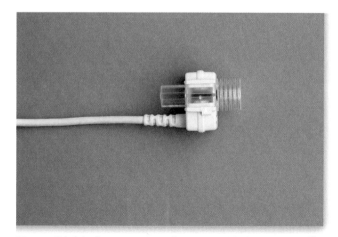

Figure 56-3 In-line capnography sensor. (© *Scott Metcalfe*)

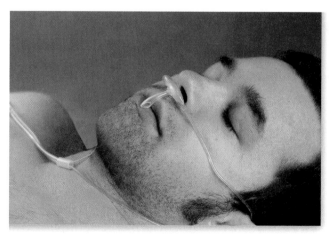

Figure 56-4 Spontaneously breathing patient with a sampling line for CO_2 measurement.

TABLE 56-1   Changes to the CO_2 Waveform

CO_2 Waveform Etiology of Change	How to Assess	How to Correct
Respiratory change	Alveolar breath sounds and speech patterns if patient is conscious. Alveolar breath sounds and chest excursion if patient is unconscious. *If the patient has good alveolar ventilation, at an appropriate rate and depth, then the cause of disturbance is likely not ventilation.*	If the patient has a low $ETCO_2$ and increased alveolar ventilation, assess for hypoxia and provide oxygen. Consider coaching the patient to slow his breathing. If the patient has a high $ETCO_2$ level with diminished alveolar ventilation, consider initiating PPV to increase alveolar ventilation. Continue to administer oxygen. If the patient has either a high or low $ETCO_2$ level, and alveolar ventilation is normal (i.e., normal rate and depth), the lungs are not at fault. Continue your assessment to determine whether the perfusion is at fault.
Perfusion change	Determine the quality of the cardiac activity. Assess the heart rate, ECG, central perfusion, and peripheral perfusion. *If the patient has appropriate perfusion findings, is neither extremely tachycardic nor bradycardic, and has no findings consistent with hypovolemia, the cause of disturbance is not likely perfusion.*	If the patient has a low $ETCO_2$ value and has finding consistent with poor perfusion, employ corrective measures to improve cardiac output (fluid therapy, heart rate control, MI management). If the patient has a rising $ETCO_2$ level, and you note that the perfusion status is improving from your initial assessment, this is actually a good finding, indicating that the patient's overall status is improving. Continue care. If the patient has either a high or low $ETCO_2$ level and the lungs and perfusion findings are within normal limits, continue your assessment for metabolic activity findings.
Metabolic change	Assessing metabolic activity is the most challenging to do in the prehospital environment because there is no test or evaluation finding that directly represents it. Consider the patient's history and associated findings when considering a metabolic cause. *If a patient has a metabolic derangement, consider factors such as hypothermia, hyperthermia, stimulant or depressant drug overdose, seizure activity, or toxicology. In any instance, the determination of these conditions is part history findings and part assessment findings.*	If the patient has a high $ETCO_2$ level and neither the lungs nor the heart is at fault, consider metabolic causes like temperature (high), toxicology (stimulants), or seizure activity. Provide corrective treatment per protocol for etiology. If the patient has a low $ETCO_2$ level and neither the lungs nor the heart is at fault, again consider metabolic causes such as temperature (low) or toxicology (depressants). Provide corrective treatment per protocol for etiology. If the patient has either a high or low $ETCO_2$ level and the lungs, heart, and metabolic causes are ruled out, consider equipment malfunction or misinterpretation of the $ETCO_2$ findings by the AEMT. Correct as appropriate.

influence the waveform (discussed in Table 56-1).

As you assess for the reason the waveform changed, always remember that the lungs are the *most common* cause for change seen in the prehospital environment. If the lungs are not at fault, the next most common reason for waveform change is perfusion to the lungs. If the AEMT determines that neither the lungs nor the heart is at fault, the next thing to consider as the cause is metabolic activity (which is rarely the cause in acute situations). Last, if it is not the lungs, heart, or metabolic activity,

consider that there may be an equipment failure. To simplify things, use the following "blame formula" for determining the cause:

1. *Blame the patient:*
   a. Blame the lungs first
   b. Blame the perfusion second
   c. Blame the metabolic activity third

2. *Blame the equipment:*
   a. Are all fittings tight?
   b. Is sampling line plugged with mucus or fluid?
   c. Are all lines properly attached to the equipment?

3. *Blame yourself:*
   a. Do you know what a normal waveform looks like?
   b. Do you recall what the normal carbon dioxide level is?
   c. Are you properly evaluating the waveform and the patient's condition?

Although these findings, assessments, and treatments of $ETCO_2$ can largely be made based on the numeric representation of the $ETCO_2$ level, the AEMT's interpretation of the waveform is also part of the picture. This is best

TABLE 56-2   **Waveform Changes**

Waveform Capnography	Explanation of Findings
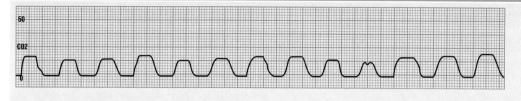	If the patient has increased alveolar ventilation and a lowering numeric level of ETCO$_2$, consider that the patient is hyperventilating (this happens only for a reason). Find the reason and treat it.
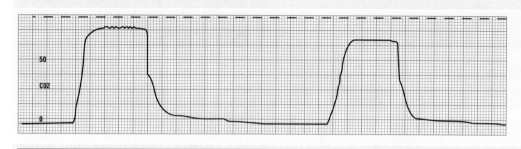	If the patient has decreased alveolar ventilation due to a slow respiratory rate, ETCO$_2$ will rise. Treat by improving alveolar ventilation (i.e., mechanical ventilation).
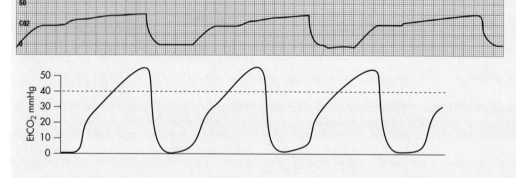	The important thing to note with this waveform is the depressed upward slope and the sharper increase in the alveolar plateau. This is consistent with bronchoconstriction, and is often called a "shark fin" capnogram. The actual ETCO$_2$ reading will be a function of how well the patient is diffusing and ventilating. Treatment will include bronchodilators, oxygen, and PPV if the carbon dioxide levels remain high.
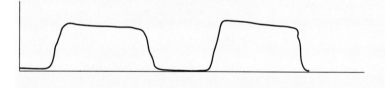	The AEMT will notice in this capnogram that the alveolar plateau is reversed. This is common to disease processes that result in alveolar destruction, such as emphysema. The waveform may be taller or shorter based on CO$_2$ levels, but the basic shape will not change with treatment, only the CO$_2$ level will.
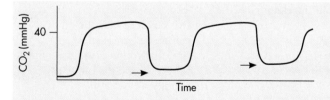	With this waveform, the AEMT should note that the baseline is increasing (it should always be at zero). This could be seen in a patient with no ventilatory, circulatory, or metabolic reasons for the change; rather, it could be from rebreathing of carbon dioxide due to equipment malfunction or high levels of PEEP or CPAP.

TABLE 56-2   Waveform Changes (*Continued*)

Waveform Capnography	Explanation of Findings
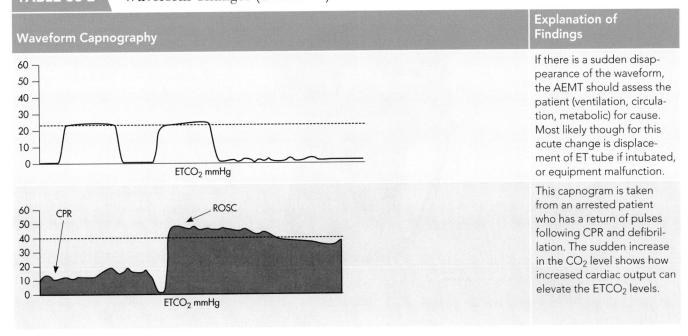	If there is a sudden disappearance of the waveform, the AEMT should assess the patient (ventilation, circulation, metabolic) for cause. Most likely though for this acute change is displacement of ET tube if intubated, or equipment malfunction.
	This capnogram is taken from an arrested patient who has a return of pulses following CPR and defibrillation. The sudden increase in the CO_2 level shows how increased cardiac output can elevate the $ETCO_2$ levels.

discussed by showing various waveforms and offering explanations for the change (Table 56-2).

INTRAOSSEOUS ACCESS INITIATION WITH AN EZ-IO IN THE ADULT

One skill with which the AEMT is already familiar is the establishing intravenous (IV) access or cannulation. Because it is known that the vascular system transports many chemicals, proteins, and fluids throughout the body, gaining access to the vascular system can allow the AEMT to deliver medications and fluids into the body in times of physiologic instability. Some of the common reasons for gaining intravenous access are:

- Need for fluid replacement (hypovolemia)
- Obtaining venous blood samples
- Administration of medications
- As a precaution for a stable patient who may deteriorate

IV access, like endotracheal intubation, can be established by multiple techniques. As discussed earlier in this topic, the most common way to access venous circulation is by peripheral vein cannulation. However, also as noted earlier, many patient complications may make peripheral IV access difficult, if not impossible, in the prehospital

environment. To that end, medical research and technology have produced another way to gain access to venous circulation—intraosseous (IO) cannulation. Used often in the prehospital environment for intravenous access in infant and pediatric patients, IO access is gaining popularity for use in adult patients as well.

IO involves the insertion of a rigid needle into the medullary cavity of a bone (usually long bones or the sternum). These bones have a richly vascular medullary cavity that is capable of accepting large volumes of fluid or drugs and rapidly transporting them to the venous system and central circulation. Comparisons of IO and IV infusion and distribution rates have shown that medications and fluids given by either route reach central circulation in a similar concentration in the same amount of time.

Any solution or drug that can be administered intravenously, by either bolus or infusion, can also be administered by the IO route. Use of IO access is indicated in emergency situations in which intravenous access is required but unobtainable or presumed difficult, such as in cardiac arrest, severe trauma patients, or even significant medical emergencies. Remember, though, the decision to use the IO route should be based on the patient's clinical condition, not on whether he has a specific diagnosis. Generally speaking, IO cannulation should be considered in any unstable

patient in whom peripheral access is essential and IV access cannot be established in two tries or 90 seconds.

The difficult part of IO access is getting the needle through the hard outer cortex of the bone. Although a manually inserted IO needle is sufficient to use in infants and pediatric patients because of their thinner cortex, the thicker bone of the adult usually bends the needle. To overcome this, the EZ-IO® device is a small battery-operated drill that places the needle into the bone (▶ Figure 56-5). The driver is reusable, and the needle length is selected based on the characteristics of the patient. Studies have shown that vascular access can be established with this device in as little as 10 seconds.

Three needle sizes accommodate intraosseous access in patients larger than 3 kilograms:

- 15-mm Needle Set (pink hub) Designed for use in patients weighing 3 to 39 kilograms, and for patients with minimal tissue over insertion sites.
- 25-mm Needle Set (blue hub) Designed for any patient weighing more than 39 kilograms, or for patients who

Any solution or drug that can be administered intravenously can also be administered by the IO route.

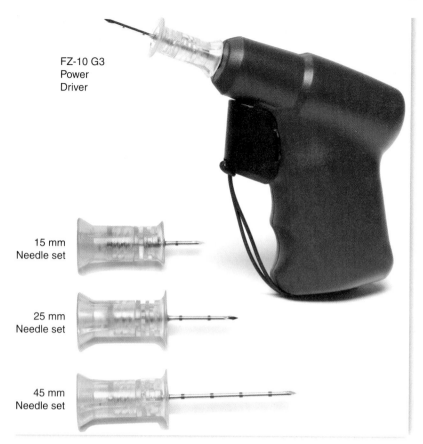

FZ-10 G3
Power
Driver

15 mm
Needle set

25 mm
Needle set

45 mm
Needle set

Figure 56-5 EZ-IO device with needles.

have too much tissue over the insertion site for the 15-mm needle to be used.

- 45-mm Needle Set (yellow hub) Designed for patients weighing more than 39 kilograms who have excessive tissue over the targeted insertion site (e.g., edema, large musculature, obesity). The 45-mm needle is ideal for the humerus site in patients weighing more than 39 kilograms.

▶ Figure 56-6 further demonstrates how to properly select the appropriate needle. The AEMT should ensure that the 5-mm mark should be visible above the skin. If it is, this provides the assurance that after insertion, the tip will make it through the bony cortex and into the medullary cavity.

Common sites for IO insertion in adults include long bones, such as the proximal and distal tibia and proximal humerus (▶ Figure 56-7). The proper landmarks are found as follows:

1. **Proximal tibia:** In adults, palpate the tibial tuberosity and move two fingerbreadths below this point. Rotate the leg slightly externally and insert the

needle on the broad flat surface of the tibia.

2. **Distal tibia:** For adults, measure two fingerbreadths' width proximal to the tip of the medial malleolus—this is your insertion site.

3. **Proximal humerus:** With the arm positioned on the cot or ground, palpate the anterior midshaft humerus and continue palpating proximally up the anterior surface of the humerus until the greater tuberosity is met. Palpate the coracoid and acromion, then imagine a line between them. The insertion point is about 2 cm down from its midpoint.

As with any other intravenous skill, the AEMT must use Standard Precautions at all times while performing intraosseous cannulation. All blood and body fluids should be considered potentially infected with HIV or HBV. Wash your hands before and after working with IO equipment and immediately after coming into contact with blood or body fluids during the procedure. At a bare minimum, wear gloves while establishing IO access and dispose of them in an appropriate waste receptacle after use. Use eye protection, mask, and a gown if there is a risk of splashing or spraying of blood or other body fluids. Place used IO needles into an approved sharps container immediately after use.

The insertion procedure is straightforward and should be followed with each attempt at IO access. Failure to do so will likely increase the possibility that the needle will be placed improperly in the medullary cavity, and the access site will fail to flush or flow fluids. Whereas the specific procedure depends on the device and

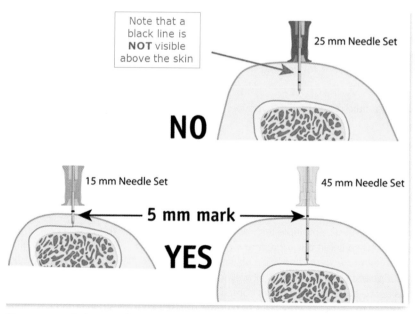

Note that a black line is **NOT** visible above the skin

25 mm Needle Set

NO

15 mm Needle Set

45 mm Needle Set

← 5 mm mark →

YES

Figure 56-6 Selecting the appropriately sized EZ-IO needle.

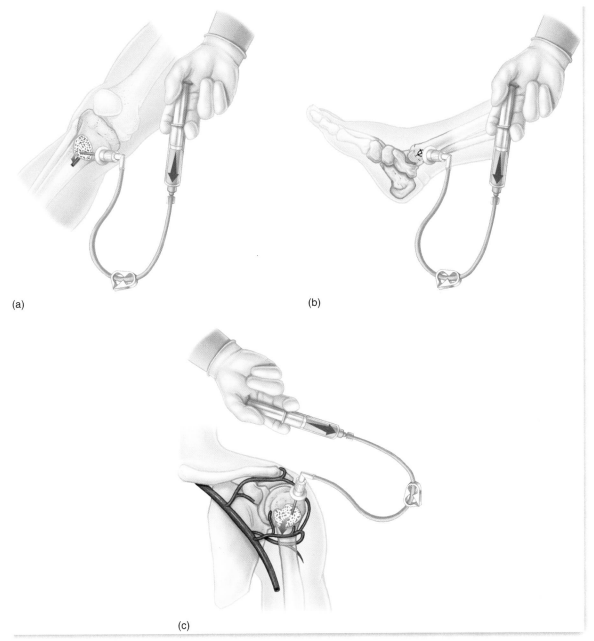

(a)

(b)

(c)

Figure 56-7 IO needle insertion sites depend on the device being used and include (a) the proximal tibia, (b) the medial malleolus of the distal tibia, and (c) the humeral head.

location used, the general procedure is as follows:

1. Determine the need for IO access and employ appropriate Standard Precautions.
2. Assemble and check all equipment.
3. Position the patient as appropriate for the intended insertion site.
4. Locate the access site and identify all landmarks.
5. Cleanse site with alcohol or Betadine. Start at the intended puncture site and work outward in an expanded circular motion.

6. Perform the puncture using the device manufacturer's instructions.
7. Remove the trocar, attach the syringe, and attempt to aspirate bone marrow. Easy aspiration of bone marrow and/ or blood indicates correct placement in the medullary cavity.
8. Attach IV administration and/or extension set if required. Then set and confirm fluid flow.
9. Secure the needle at the insertion site with bulky dressings or a commercially available device that accompanies the IO needle.

Even though this technique is simple and fast to perform, this does not suggest that it comes without limitations, precautions, or contraindications. If a patient has a recent fracture of the insertion site bone, or a proximal bone in that extremity, the AEMT should select another site. In addition, if there is a known history of osteoporosis or osteogenesis imperfecta, the procedure should not be attempted. Furthermore, insertion should be avoided through areas of cellulitis, infections, burns, or other skin disorders.

Caution should also be taken to avoid more common complications: if too large a needle is used or if it is inserted forcefully, the bone may fracture (more common in the very young and very old). If the hole created by the gun is too large as a result of movement of the AEMT during insertion, fluid may infiltrate into the surrounding tissues. When the incorrect needle is used, it may not penetrate the medullary cavity (too short), or go all the way through the bone (too long).

Finally, there is a slim chance that a fat, bone, or bone marrow embolus may enter the vascular system and travel to the heart and lungs. Even though this is rare, the AEMT should always be alert for signs and symptoms of pulmonary embolism after IO insertion. Whenever the IO line fails to flow (either during insertion or after placement), attempt to flush the needle with a few milliliters of intravenous solution. If the flush fails to restore flow, discontinue use of that IO site.

ESTABLISHMENT OF A HEPARIN LOCK OR SALINE LOCK

There will be times when the AEMT wishes to obtain vascular access, but may not necessarily want to administer fluids. For these situations, a heparin lock or saline lock may be used. A heparin lock is a peripheral IV port that does not use a bag of fluid attached to the cannula. Like a typical IV start, placement of a heparin lock requires an IV cannula to be placed into a peripheral vein; however, instead of

IV administration tubing with a bag of fluid attached to it, it has an attached short tubing with a clamp and a distal medication port (▶ Figure 56-8).

For shorter-term use, a saline lock may be used. Whereas the aforementioned cannula is still placed for either, instead of a lock containing heparin being attached to the cannula, the lock has sterile saline injected into it to help keep the intravenous cannula patent. Initiating a heparin or saline lock requires the following equipment:

- IV cannula
- Heparin lock or saline lock
- Syringe with 3- to 5-mL sterile saline or commercial saline injection device
- Tape or commercial securing device
- Venous blood drawing equipment
- Venous constricting band
- Antiseptic swab (Betadine, alcohol, or other cleansing agent)

To place a heparin or saline lock, follow these steps:

1. Use Standard Precautions.
2. Prepare the saline lock by attaching it to a syringe containing 4 to 5 mL of saline, and flushing out the air. Leave at least 2 mL in the syringe for use later.
3. Select the venipuncture site.
4. Place the constricting band proximal to the puncture site.
5. Cleanse the venipuncture site with antiseptics.

6. Insert the IV cannula into the vein as described for a traditional IV.
7. Slide the catheter into the vein.
8. Carefully remove the metal stylet and promptly dispose of it into the sharps container. Remove the venous constricting band.
9. Attach the lock tubing to the angiocatheter hub.
10. Cleanse the medication port and inject 2 to 3 mL of sterile saline into the lock. Easy flow of the saline without edema at the puncture site indicates patency. If you encounter resistance or if edema forms, restart the procedure with new equipment.
11. Apply antibiotic ointment to the site and cover with an adhesive bandage or other commercial device. Secure the tubing to the patient.

If fluid administration becomes necessary, you can either remove the lock and place the intravenous administration set directly to the intravenous catheter, or you can attach the administration set to the lock itself (be sure to use the appropriate equipment for a needle versus needleless system). Periodically flush the lock with sterile saline or heparin to prevent clot formation and occlusion at the intravenous catheter's distal end.

PREPARATION OF MEDICATIONS FOR ADMINISTRATION

As an AEMT, your EMS system may allow you to help prepare medications that your paramedic partner needs to administer. Examples include patients in cardiac arrest, those undergoing a rapid sequence induction (RSI) procedure, or even patients with complicated MIs who require multiple medication administrations by the paramedic. In these situations, it would be a benefit to your partner if these medications could be prepared and readied to be administered when the time comes. This would save time during patient care management and allow both EMS providers to focus on specific lifesaving skills.

If you become responsible for this, you must always be certain that you correctly prepare all medications as intended. Failure to do so may result in a medication overdosage or underdosage, with possibly disastrous outcomes. You and your partner

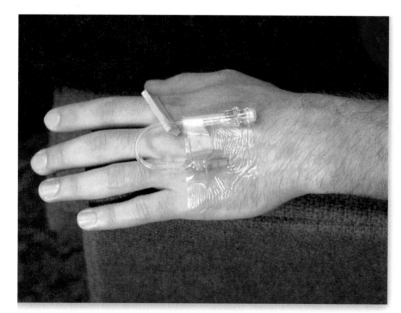

Figure 56-8 A heparin or saline lock regulates IV flow and decreases the risk of accidental fluid overload or electrolyte derangement.

can attain effective drug therapy and eliminate medication errors by following the "six rights" of drug administration:

- Right person
- Right drug
- Right dose
- Right time
- Right route
- Right documentation

If you ever doubt the type or dosage of a medication requested by your paramedic partner for you to assemble, clarify that with your partner immediately. You must repeat back, or echo, all drug preparation requests issued made by your paramedic partner. For example, if your partner asks you to assessable and prepare 100 mg of lidocaine for intravenous push, you would echo back, "OK, I am going to prepare 100 milligrams of lidocaine for intravenous push." By echoing, you confirm your reception and understanding of the order. Another benefit of this is if your paramedic partner has requested an inappropriate medication or dosage, this echoing of the order back to him may bring it to light and elicit an immediate correction:

Medications come packaged in a variety of containers with which you must be familiar because obtaining medication from each type requires a different procedure. Common types of medication containers include

- Glass ampules
- Prefilled syringes
- Nonconstituted drug vials
- Single and multidose vials
- Intravenous medication fluids

Before opening a drug package and assembling the medication for patient administration, the AEMT must first select the correct drug and know how to read the packaging label. Here is an overview of the traditional information found on a medication label:

- **Name of medication:** The label lists both the generic and trade names of the medication. Always ensure that you have selected the right medication.
- **Expiration date:** All medications have an expiration date after which they cannot be used. Never use an expired medication.
- **Total dose and concentration:** The total dose of drug is the total weight

(g/mg/mcg) of medication in the container. The concentration represents the weight of the drug per volume of fluid. For example, if 10 mg of a drug were packaged in 5 mL of fluid, the total dose would be 10 mg, and the concentration would be 10 mg/5 mL or 2 mg/mL. Use caution, though, as identical drugs can be packaged in different dosages and concentrations. For example, you may recall that 1 mg of epinephrine can be packaged in 1 mL (1:1,000 epinephrine), or 1 mg in 10 mL (1:10,000 epinephrine).

These labels are printed directly on the vial, ampule, prefilled syringe, or IV medication bag. Always use them to confirm the correct medication.

An *ampule*, or amp, is a breakable glass container that contains liquid medication (▶ Figure 56-9). It has a cone-shaped top with a thinner neck, and circular tubular base that houses the medication. The thin neck is scored to make it a weaker spot so the EMS provider can intentionally break off the cone-shaped top and retrieve its contents with a syringe. Amps usually range in volume from 1 to 5 mL of solution. Commonly, each ampule contains only single doses of medication.

To obtain medication from a glass ampule, you will need a syringe and needle, and follow this technique:

1. Confirm the medication order from your partner.
2. Confirm the ampule label (medication name, dose, and expiration).
3. Hold the ampule upright and tap its top to dislodge any trapped solution.
4. Place gauze around the thin neck and snap it off with your thumb.
5. Place the tip of the hypodermic needle inside the ampule and withdraw the medication into the syringe. Take care not to injure yourself against the broken edge of glass.

6. Provide your paramedic partner with the medication when asked for it, verbally confirming with him the drug name and concentration found in the syringe.
7. Dispose of the needle, syringe, and broken glass ampule properly after use.

Single and *multidose vials* can be plastic or glass containers with self-sealing hubs at the top (▶ Figure 56-10). Obviously, from their name, vials can contain either single doses or multiple doses of a medication. The self-sealing rubber top prevents leakage from needle punctures and permits multiple accesses with a needle and syringe. The medication inside the vial is packaged in a vacuum. To obtain medication from a vial, you will need a syringe and needle, and then follow these steps:

1. Confirm the medication order from your partner.
2. Confirm the vial label (name, dose, and expiration).
3. Determine the volume of medication to be administered (see Topic 12, "EMS Pharmacology").
4. Prepare the syringe and hypodermic needle (try to use a syringe one size larger in milliliters than the contents of the vial).
5. Because the vial is vacuum packed, you will have to replace the volume of medication removed with air to maintain equilibrium in the vial. Withdraw the plunger to draw a volume of air into the syringe equal to the volume of medication to be administered.
6. Cleanse the vial's rubber top with an antiseptic alcohol preparation.
7. Insert the hypodermic needle into the rubber top and inject the air from the syringe into the vial. Then withdraw the appropriate volume of medication.

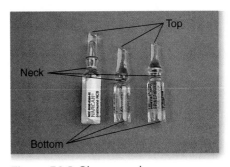

Figure 56-9 **Glass ampules.**

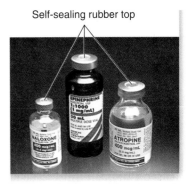

Figure 56-10 **Glass medication vials.**

8. Provide your paramedic partner with the medication when asked for it, verbally confirming with him the drug name and concentration found in the syringe.

9. Dispose of the needle, syringe, and vial properly.

The *nonconstituted drug vial* is a packaging system used when the medication has a short shelf life or is unstable in liquid form (▶ Figure 56-11). The nonconstituted drug packaging system consists of two vials, one containing the powdered medication and one containing a liquid mixing solution (or dilution solution). To administer the drug, you must first mix it (or reconstitute it) by withdrawing the dilution solution from its vial and placing it in the powdered medication's vial. To prepare a medication from a nonconstituted drug vial, you will need a needle and syringe, then use the following technique:

1. Confirm the medication order from your partner.

2. Confirm the vial's label (name, dose, expiration date).

3. Remove all solution from the vial containing the dilution solution, using the same procedure as you would to withdraw medication from a single or multidose vial.

4. With an alcohol prep, cleanse the top of the vial containing the powdered drug and inject the mixing solution.

5. Gently agitate or shake the vial to ensure complete mixture.

6. Determine the volume of newly constituted medication to be administered.

7. Cleanse the medication vial's rubber top with an antiseptic alcohol preparation, and withdraw the appropriate amount of fluid to provide the needed dose of medication.

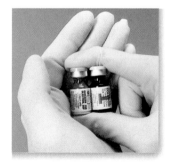

Figure 56-11 The nonconstituted drug vial actually consists of two vials, one containing a powdered medication and one containing a liquid mixing solution.

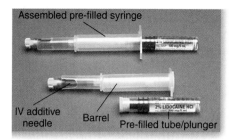

Figure 56-12 Prefilled syringes.

Assembled pre-filled syringe
IV additive needle   Barrel   Pre-filled tube/plunger

8. Provide your paramedic partner with the medication when asked for it, verbally confirming with them the drug name and concentration found in the syringe.

9. Dispose of the needle, syringe, and vials properly.

A *prefilled syringe* (or *preloaded syringe*) has two components, a drug cartridge (glass or plastic) and a plunger (▶ Figure 56-12). Because the syringe is prefilled, you do not need to draw the medication from another source. Generally, prefilled syringes contain standard dosages, thus decreasing the chance of dosage error.

To use this packaging system, the AEMT need only to remove the protective cap(s) and then screw the plunger into the prefilled drug cartridge securely (finger tight). While holding the needle end of the prefilled syringe upright, push on the plunger to engage the two together and expel any air that is in the drug cartridge before leveling the plunger at the beginning of the graduations (normally labeled

as zero). Follow these steps to administer a medication from a prefilled syringe:

1. Confirm the medication order from your partner.

2. Confirm the prefilled syringe label (name, dose, and expiration date).

3. Assemble the prefilled syringe by removing the pop-off caps and screwing the two together.

4. Expel any air in the drug cartridge and level the plunger to "zero" or the beginning of the mL graduations.

5. Provide your paramedic partner with the medication when asked for it, verbally confirming with him the drug name and concentration found in the syringe.

6. Dispose of the prefilled syringe properly after use.

Some drugs are administered as an *IV infusion* (or *IV piggyback*). IV infusions deliver a steady, continual dose of medication through an existing IV line (▶ Figure 56-13). Paramedics may use IV infusions for either loading doses of drugs (e.g., dopamine) or for maintenance doses after the loading dose has been given by IV bolus (e.g., lidocaine).

Piggybacking IV infusions through an existing IV line gives the EMS provider more specific control of medication dosing, as many medications delivered this way affect the autonomic nervous system and require a high degree of precise regulation. When used, IV infusions are always given as a "piggyback" into a primary

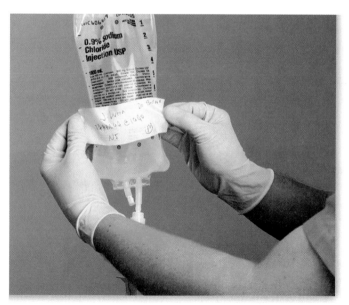

Figure 56-13 IV piggyback medication. (© *Scott Metcalfe*)

IV line. IV infusions should never be established as the primary line. If the IV infusion is premixed, then the AEMT will only have to attach a microdrip administration set to the medication bag, flush the line, and attach it to the primary line through the medication port (the AEMT should *never* actually establish the IV medication drip rate; this can be done only by your paramedic partner). The AEMT can ensure, however, that the following information appears on the label of the medication bag:

- Name of medication (generic and trade name)
- Total amount of drug premixed in bag
- Concentration (amount of drug per single mL)
- Expiration date

If the medication desired is given via IV infusion, but the infusion is not premixed, the AEMT may be required to prepare the medication and set it up for administration. To do so, the AEMT will have to use multiple skills already discussed, such as drug math calculation; using a vial, ampule, or prefilled syringe; flushing of intravenous lines; and documentation. Although none of these skills is especially hard, they all must be done correctly to administer the appropriate amount of drug. Use the following technique to set up an IV infusion when you need to premix the bag yourself:

1. Establish a normal primary IV line and assure patency.
2. Confirm the medication order from your partner.

3. Prepare the medication infusion bag:
   a. Ask your paramedic partner how much to draw up and place into the IV infusion bag. Then draw up the appropriate quantity of medication from its source with a syringe.
   b. Cleanse the IV bag's or bottle's medication port with an alcohol antiseptic wipe.
   c. Insert the hypodermic needle into the medication port and inject the medication.
   d. Gently agitate the bag or bottle to mix its contents thoroughly.
   e. Label the bag or bottle with the added drug's name, amount, new concentration, date and time added, and your initials.

4. Connect the administration tubing to the medication bag or bottle and fill the drip chamber to the fluid line (most infusions require microdrip tubing).

5. Place a hypodermic needle (usually a 20-gauge needle) on the end of the administration set if using a needle system; do not do this if using a needleless administration set.

6. Flush the administration set of all air by opening the flow control and allowing the premixed medication to flow through the tubing.

7. Cleanse the medication administration port on the primary line with alcohol and attach the secondary line from the medication bag.

8. Secure the secondary administration line with tape or another securing device to the primary line. Do *not*

establish a flow rate; this is the responsibility of the paramedic.

9. Dispose of any used sharps equipment properly.

When the infusion is complete, shut down the secondary line with the flow regulator or a clamp. Open the primary line and adjust it to the appropriate drip rate. Remove the IV piggyback administration set from the primary line and dispose of all contents properly.

Remember that assisting with medication administration is a fundamental skill used in the treatment of the sick and injured. Assisting your paramedic partner with this procedure can save precious time. For medications to be effective, however, they must be safely delivered into the body by the appropriate route. If you are allowed to perform these skills in your EMS system, it is solely your responsibility to be familiar with all equipment and techniques needed for safely employing them. You will use some medication assist skills often (prefilled syringes), and some types of administration very infrequently (IV drug infusions)—and these will quickly fade from memory. Nonetheless, someone's well-being may depend on your ability to properly use these techniques in an emergency. Therefore, periodic review of these skills is highly recommended.

> **Piggybacking IV infusions through an existing IV line gives the EMS provider more specific control of medication dosing.**

TRANSITIONING

REVIEW ITEMS

1. You have attached end-tidal CO_2 monitoring to your patient. In interpreting the findings, you recall that the normal $ETCO_2$ value should be _____.
   a. 25–35 mmHg
   b. 35–45 mmHg
   c. 45–55 mmHg
   d. 55–65 mmHg

2. When establishing a saline lock on a patient, when should the extension set be primed with fluid?
   a. after the IV cannula is placed
   b. after the saline lock has been attached to the cannula

   c. prior to the attachment of the saline lock to the cannula
   d. it can be flushed at any time prior to or after attachment to the cannula

3. What information should be placed on the label that is going to be affixed to the medication bag while setting up an intravenous medication infusion?
   a. the AEMT's name and the date it was prepared
   b. the amount of medication added to the intravenous bag
   c. the medication added, the date added, and your initials
   d. the medication added, the date, your initials, and the new concentration

4. While monitoring the ETCO$_2$ level in an intubated patient receiving mechanical ventilation, you observe a reading of 24 mmHg. What does this mean?
   a. This is a normal value of ETCO$_2$.
   b. The patient is probably being overventilated.
   c. The patient is probably being underventilated.
   d. The patient needs IV fluids to restore blood volume.

5. What should the AEMT do prior to withdrawing medication from a multidose vial?
   a. Use an alcohol prep to clean the tip of the needle first.
   b. Tap the top of the vial to displace trapped solution.
   c. Shake the vial to ensure the medication is evenly mixed.
   d. Inject the same volume of air into the vial as the volume of solution being withdrawn.

APPLIED PATHOPHYSIOLOGY

You are called to back up another ALS unit for a patient who is unresponsive from a narcotic drug overdose. The patient is currently receiving PPV with an oropharyngeal airway placed, and the paramedic on scene is initiating an IV line of normal saline. While he is doing so, he asks you to prepare a 2-mg dose of naloxone (Narcan). The medication is packaged in a vial.

1. List the equipment needed to perform this medication setup.

2. What are the six "patient rights" that should be applied to this episode of drug administration?

3. If the vial of naloxone contains 2 mg of drug in 5 mL of solution, what is the exact concentration of medication, and how many milliliters will you withdraw to achieve the ordered dose of 0.8 mg?

CLINICAL DECISION MAKING

You are called to the scene of an elderly patient in cardiac arrest. The patient was found in bed by family members after he didn't wake up for breakfast. On your arrival, the family had already taken the patient from the bed and started compressions for CPR on the floor, according to EMD directions given to them from the EMS dispatcher. While you move to the patient's head to start ventilations with a BVM, your partner attaches the monitor to see the presenting rhythm, which is ventricular fibrillation.

1. Based on this brief history and presentation, would this patient be classified as a high or low priority? Support your answer with facts taken from the scenario.

2. What would be at least two critical interventions the AEMT should take now, before continuing on with the assessment of the patient?

Following a successful defibrillation at 200 joules, the patient is now in a bradycardic rate at 42 beats per minute, with a blood pressure of 70/palpation. The patient is now intubated, and the ETCO$_2$ adapter is placed and attached to the monitor. You are ventilating the patient at 8 times a minute and getting a good rise with each ventilation.

3. Given the ETCO$_2$ reading, what should the AEMT do, if anything, about how the patient is being ventilated?

4. The paramedic on scene has attempted intravenous access twice without success. Is this patient a candidate for intraosseous cannulation with the EZ-IO gun?

After several minutes, the patient has been secured to a backboard for movement. Intravenous cannulation has been completed, and the first round of drugs has been administered to the patient. After loading the patient into the ambulance, your paramedic partner asks you to ride with him in the back to continue patient care while an on-scene firefighter drives you to the hospital.

5. Your paramedic partner states he needs another milligram of atropine. He asks you to get this ready. If atropine comes packaged in a 1-mg prefilled syringe, briefly describe how you would prepare the medication.

6. The paramedic attempts to administer the atropine IV push through the IO site; however, it fails to push properly. Identify how the AEMT should try to reestablish flow. When should the IO line be abandoned and another initiated?

7. If the waveform on the capnography suddenly went almost flat and the numeric display started reading a value of 12 mmHg, what should the AEMT do to confirm that the readings are accurate (or discover why they may be inaccurate)?

After the ETCO$_2$ reading issue is corrected, the NIBP is found to still be 70 mmHg systolic with a heart rate of 82/min. The patient is being ventilated at 10/minute, and the ETCO$_2$ reading is 39 mmHg. The patient's skin is still cool peripherally with no palpable radial pulse. Per protocol, the paramedic is to initiate a dopamine infusion by placing 400 mg of drug into a 500-mL bag of D$_5$W. Dopamine comes in large glass ampules of 200 mg each.

8. Briefly describe how you will withdraw the medication from the ampules and place it in the D$_5$W, and then discuss how to finish preparing the IV piggyback for administration.

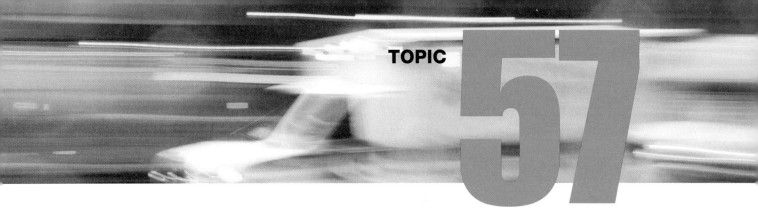

ADDITIONAL PHARMACOLOGY FOR THE AEMT

INTRODUCTION

As prehospital care advances in the 21st century, so has the use of pharmacology in the prehospital environment. Historically, Advanced EMTs have had a somewhat limited scope of practice regarding the pharmacologic agents that they could administer. With the evolution of the AEMT's scope of practice, however, medical directives for the AEMT have been expanded to drugs beyond the traditional use of oxygen, intravenous fluids, and epinephrine for allergies. As a result, the AEMT now has a tremendous task in staying current with new pharmacologic treatments in the care of the critically ill or injured patient.

In Topic 12, "EMS Pharmacology," the AEMT will find specific information about common drugs given according to the AEMT Educational Standards. The intent of this topic, however, is to discuss additional medications that go beyond the Educational Standards that the AEMT may administer according to specific medical direction authorization. In any situation the AEMT faces when drug therapy is warranted, one must remember that understanding a drug's indications, dose, and route are all important—but the understanding of how a drug works in the body (on a cellular level) is absolute essential knowledge the AEMT must have.

AEMTs should not (and cannot) become complacent and rely exclusively on charts or pocket references to guide drug therapy during patient management. Books and charts cannot interpret special circumstances that exist in every patient encounter, nor can they offer all the differential approaches to drug therapy that may be required. That is not to say that having reference material immediately available is inappropriate, just that relying on a reference chart to make your drug therapy decisions is not the intended purpose of these guides.

Proper patient management will occur only when the AEMT understands the pathophysiology behind the patient's condition, understands the physiologic actions of the drugs, and then integrates this information together to provide the appropriate drug therapy for the patient. Reference charts or books should be used only to augment this decision-making process.

To aid in the learning process, the information contained within this topic is presented in a logical, concise, and easy-to-read

TRANSITION highlights

- **Generic name, trade name, mechanism of action, indications, and administration of additional medications by the AEMT:**
  - Activated charcoal.
  - Atropine sulfate.
  - Benzodiazepines:
    - Diazepam.
    - Lorazepam.
    - Midazolam.
  - Diphenhydramine.
  - Ipatropium bromide.
  - Thiamine hydrochloride.
  - Ondansetron.

- **Recommended medication use:**
  - Ingested poisoning.
  - Organophosphate poisoning.
  - Seizure activity.
  - Mild allergic reaction.
  - Respiratory distress (COPD).
  - Malnutrition/thiamine deficiency.
  - Nausea and vomiting.

format. It will take an investment of time on the part of the reader, however, to comprehend and apply the information.

One word of caution is essential. Do not simply try to "memorize" drug indications, side effects, contraindications, and so forth. Information learned by rote memory is often lost because of a lack of use and context, or during the stress of an emergency—it cannot be recalled. Instead, take the time to thoroughly understand how a drug works. If you are familiar with how a drug works in the body, the indications, contraindications, and side effects become obvious. Thus the

Take the time to thoroughly understand how a drug works.

only thing left to memorize is the specific drug dose—and there is no shortcut to memorizing drug doses.

The drugs presented in this chapter include activated charcoal, atropine, diazepam, diphenhydramine, ipratropium, lorazepam, midazolam, thiamine, and zofran.

EPIDEMIOLOGY

Appreciating the commonality of drug administration in the prehospital setting would certainly help the AEMT understand how often it really occurs. But perhaps what is more important than how often you give a drug (because this is a skill) is how often the situation presents in which the drug may be necessary. The best way to describe that is to assess the frequency in which these disease processes and emergencies occur. Remember too, though, that the decision to administer a drug is only half the picture—the other half is the decision of when *not* to use a drug.

A poison is anything that can kill or injure the tissues of the body through its chemical actions. The AEMT will encounter many situations in which the patient has been purposely or accidently poisoned. The word *poison* comes from the Latin word *potare*, which means "to drink," but poisons can also enter the body in other ways, such as injection, inhalation, and absorption. The most common mechanism for poisoning, however, is the ingestion, or swallowing, route. This route accounts for about 80 percent of all poisoning episodes seen in the emergency department. Activated charcoal is a common medication that is used under appropriate circumstances for ingested poisons.

In keeping with poisonings, greater emphasis has been placed on the use of atropine for organophosphate overdoses in agricultural settings, or as a nerve agent antidote for certain weapons of mass destruction (WMD)-type exposures. Atropine counters the ill effects of excessive cholinergic stimulation caused from organophosphate poisoning. Even though it is fortunate that the incidence of organophosphate poisoning has been decreasing since 1995 due to the EPA phasing this agent out of household and agricultural applications, there were still more than 96,000 calls to poison control centers relating to pesticide exposures, many of which included organophosphate agents and 2-PAM.

Benzodiazepines (BZDs) are a drug class of medications with a common chemical structure and wide applications to EMS care. Benzodiazepines are often used for their CNS calming effects and the ability to control seizure activity. Seizures often arise from epilepsy, which afflicts some 4 million people in the United States, and BZD drugs are a common first- or second-line agent to treat or prevent these seizures. As an anxiolytic (reduce anxiety), BZD drugs are almost exclusively the first-line agent.

In Topic 21, "Immunology: Anaphylactic and Anaphylactoid Reactions," the AEMT learned more about the incidence, assessment, and management of a patient experiencing a mild allergic or severe anaphylactic reaction. Another medication the AEMT may use in the arsenal for managing these patients is diphenhydramine. Although no real data exist regarding the use of diphenhydramine specifically, it is commonly used with oxygen and intravenous fluids for mild allergic reactions, whereas in severe allergic reactions diphenhydramine falls lower in the treatment regimen. Finally, it sees some use as an antiemetic and mild sedative. This is a drug, though, that the AEMT will have ample opportunity to consider using.

Respiratory distress is a very common complaint seen in prehospital medicine. Its prevalence cannot be estimated because of the diverse range of etiologies in which it occurs. However, it is known that 22 million individuals have asthma, more than 9 million have chronic bronchitis, and 2 million have emphysema. All these patients will likely experience dyspnea at some point, and many of them will receive the drug ipratropium for ongoing maintenance as well as for acute management. Because some EMS systems carry this medication for COPD patients, the AEMT should be familiar with this as well.

Thiamine is vitamin B_1, which is normally acquired in the diet. However, the AEMT may encounter certain patients (patients with alcoholism, prolonged diarrhea, and malnutrition) who are thiamine deficient. Thiamine deficiency has a relatively low incidence rate, but when it does occur it often causes significant pathophysiologic changes to the neurologic and cardiovascular systems of the body, especially in the presence of dextrose. Hence, the presence of this medication in the drug inventory of the AEMT

is needed to help counter this occasional, but important, syndrome in some patients.

Perhaps one of the most common symptoms that accompany many types of illnesses and injuries is the complaint of nausea and/or vomiting. It may be the initial reason for EMS being summoned, or may simply be part of the associated patient complaints. Its presence, though, is important for the AEMT to detect and manage in order to help keep the patient comfortable and possibly prevent the occurrence of vomiting, which is stressful to the patient and potentially detrimental to certain concurrent conditions.

Because nausea and vomiting are symptoms and not a distinct disease process, it is difficult to get an incidence or prevalence rate. However, any EMS provider can tell you after only days on the job that nausea and/or vomiting are common with the vast majority of patients treated and transported. A newer drug called ondansetron is gaining more widespread use in EMS for treatment of nausea and vomiting and may be administered by the AEMT with proper medical control.

PATHOPHYSIOLOGY

As discussed in the previous topics addressing cellular metabolism and pathophysiology, all disturbances of the body—resulting from trauma, illnesses, or otherwise—occur because of some disturbance that affects normal cellular activity. For example, the patient who is hypoxic because of a chest injury does not have the available oxygen in the bloodstream to maintain normal metabolism and energy production. The body quickly slips into anaerobic metabolism and a detrimental cascade of events, resulting in acid production and cellular death, ensues. With this death, critical masses of tissues and organs begin to fail, eventually resulting in system dysfunction and patient death. Thus, while the AEMT assesses for findings of dyspnea, the underlying hypoxia has already started to alter cellular function, which in turn creates the signs and symptoms that the AEMT recognizes.

As such, the administration of appropriate drugs in these (and other) situations is performed to *alter* cellular activity, not to make a cell do something it cannot normally do. A drug alters cellular activity by manipulating the target cell's receptor sites. This manipulation then alters intracellular activity.

There are basically two categories of cellular receptor sites—agonists and antagonists—that influence intracellular activity. Agonist receptor sites (and, hence, agonist drugs) are those that stimulate the receptor sites on the cells to cause an effect, whereas antagonists receptor sites (and drugs) inhibit certain cellular functions. This alteration of cellular activity in turn affects the action of the tissues and organ systems it is part of, culminating in the desired clinical effect.

Although Table 57-1 does not describe a pathologic process per se, it does illustrate how the medications used by the EMT can have an affect on the pathophysiology of a disease process and help move the body back toward homeostasis. For a more thorough discussion of these drugs, the AEMT can also refer to a pharmacologic text.

ASSESSMENT FINDINGS

To a large extent, many of the medical emergencies discussed in this chapter are also represented throughout the rest of this text in their own respective topics. As such,

TABLE 57-1	Drugs Used by the AEMT		
Generic Name	Common Trade Name(s)	Mechanism of Action	Indications and Administration
Activated charcoal	SuperChar, InstaChar, Actidose, Liqui-Char, Charcoaid	Activated charcoal is a fine black powder that is used in the emergency care of some patients who swallowed poisons. The charcoal is designed to adsorb or bind the poison to the charcoal. Once this occurs, the poison will be carried by the charcoal through the digestive tract and then eliminated in the bowel movement. This eliminates or largely diminishes the toxic effect the poison may have had on the body.	Activated charcoal should be used, on orders from medical direction, for a patient who has ingested poison by mouth. It is most effective when administered within 1 hour after the ingestion of the poison. The common dose of for activated charcoal is 1 gram/kg of body weight. It is commonly packaged premixed with water in a plastic bottle containing 12.5 grams.
Atropine sulfate	Atropine	Atropine is known to be a *parasympatholytic* (parasympathetic antagonist) drug. Atropine exerts its action by blocking muscarinic acetylcholine receptors in the autonomic nervous system, thereby inhibiting the effect of the neurotransmitter acetylcholine. This effect is bodywide, including influencing cholinergic receptors in the heart rate, bronchiole tone, GI smooth muscle, exocrine glands, and others.	The AEMT would likely give this drug to patients who sustained a cholinergic overdose (excessive para-sympathetic tone). Because atropine blocks this parasympathetic tone, it is the agent of choice. The dose for organophosphate poisoning is 2–3 mg IVP and should be given until sufficient abatement of the cholinergic influence has been removed. When used in pediatrics, the dose is 0.01–0.03 mg/kg IVP. The drug is commonly supplied in a syringe of 1 mg/10 mL.
Benzodiazepines • Diazepam • Lorazepam • Midazolam	Diazepam: • Valium Lorazepam: • Ativan Midazolam: • Versed	A classification of medications that share several similar actions on the central nervous system. The drug acts on the CNS by increasing the activity of GABA neurotransmitters (GABA agonist) which, in turn, causes a depressant effect on the CNS by inhibiting nerve transmission. This depressant effect is manifested by hypnotic, sedative, and amnestic properties. In addition, it causes calming, skeletal muscle relaxation and sleep with higher doses. Finally, the change in neurotransmitter activity can stop the spread of seizures, or in some instances, prevent their occurrence.	Multiple indications exist, including sedation due to general anxiety, as adjunct to endotracheal intubation, for ongoing sedation for patients who are vent dependent, and to suppress acute seizure activity. *Diazepam:* The adult patient commonly receives 2–10 mg slow IVP as an initial dose, which may repeat every 1–2 hours as needed. Pediatric patients should receive 0.5–2.0 mg slow IVP as needed. Supplied in 5 mg and 10 mg vials. *Midazolam:* The adult dose of midazolam is commonly 1.0–2.5 mg slow IVP over 1–2 minutes. The pediatric dose is 0.05–0.2 mg/kg slow IVP over 2–3 minutes. The drug is supplied as 2 mg, 5 mg, and 10 mg vials for parenteral injection. *Lorazepam:* The adult dosage is 0.5–2.0 mg slow IVP (average single dose is 2–4 mg), every 1–2 hours as needed in the acute situation. Pediatric patients should receive 0.03–0.05 mg/kg slow IVP up to 4 mg. Supplied as 2 mg vials.

Generic Name	Common Trade Name(s)	Mechanism of Action	Indications and Administration
Diphenhydramine	Benadryl	This drug is a first-generation anti-histamine used mainly to treat allergies. As an antihistamine, it blocks the effects of histamine on receptor sites (histamine antagonist) that cause the inflammatory reaction seen in allergic reactions. The drug also has a powerful hypnotic effect, and for this reason is often used as a nonprescription sleep aid and a mild anxiolytic. The drug also acts as an antiemetic.	Although it has many indications, the AEMT would use this drug primarily when a patient is displaying signs of a mild allergic reaction (hives, itching, watery eyes, mild wheezing). In a severe reaction, it could be given after the patient's airway and hemodynamics are stabilized. The adult dose is 25–50 mg slow IVP. Pediatric patients usually receive 12.5–25 mg slow IVP. Supplied as 50 mg/mL vials.
Ipratropium bromide	Atrovent Apovent Aerovent	Parasympathetic (cholinergic) blocking agent (parasympathetic antagonist), chemically related to atropine, that blocks the action of the parasympathetic neurotransmitter acetylcholine. This block causes a decrease in intracellular cyclic-GMP that promotes smooth muscle relaxation. Because it is inhaled, the effects occur primarily to bronchial smooth muscle, where it promotes better airflow for the dyspneic patient. It is *not* a fast-acting agent.	Used to promote bronchodilation in patients with COPD and acute bronchospasm not resolved by albuterol aerosol. Also used as a maintenance therapy for long-standing COPD disorders. The adult dosage of the drug is 500 mcg (unit dose vial) every 4–6 hours. If using an MDI, administer 2 inhalations every 4 hours. For inhalation purposes, the drug comes prepared in an 18 mcg/inhalation MDI. For nebulization, use a 0.02% solution. Pediatric dose (3–12 years) is 125–250 mcg nebulized, or 1–2 inhalations from an MDI.
Thiamine hydrochloride (vitamin B_1)	Thiamine	Thiamine (vitamin B_1) helps the body cells convert carbohydrates into energy. It is also essential for the functioning of the heart, muscles, and nervous system. A deficiency of thiamine can cause weakness, fatigue, psychosis, and nerve damage. Thiamine deficiency can lead to multiple medical conditions, including beriberi, and in severe cases brain damage can occur (Korsakoff syndrome or Wernicke disease). EMS typically sees thiamine deficiency in malnourished and alcoholic patients.	Thiamine is effective for the treatment of thiamine deficiency, dry beriberi (major symptoms related to the nervous system), or wet beriberi (major symptoms related to the cardiovascular system). Thiamine should also be used where rapid restoration of thiamine is necessary, as in Wernicke encephal-opathy, or when giving IV dextrose to individuals with marginal thiamine status to avoid precipitation of heart failure. The IV dose is 100 mg of the drug, which is supplied as a 100 mg/2 mL vial.
Ondansetron	Zofran	Ondansetron is a selective $5\text{-}HT_3$ receptor antagonist. Serotonin receptors of the $5\text{-}HT_3$ type are present on both peripheral vagal nerve terminals and in the central chemoreceptor trigger zone. By antagonizing the receptor sites, chemicals triggering nausea and vomiting are inhibited. This can prevent or manage these processes.	This medication is indicated for patients experiencing nausea and/or vomiting from disease processes, traumatic injuries, or medication administration. The adult dose is 4 mg of drug IV or IM. Pediatric dose is 0.1 mg/kg if the child weighs less than 40 kg. Supplied as 4 mg in a 2-mL vial (2 mg/mL).

the AEMT can refer to those sections for a more enhanced discussion on the patho-physiology, assessment findings, additional drug therapy, and treatment guidelines. However, for purposes of completeness, Table 57-2 provides an overview of common assessment findings for each of the medical emergencies the EMT may encounter that may result in the administration of a drug mentioned in this topic.

Note that no drug can be given to the patient by the AEMT without proper authorization by off-line or on-line medical control. For all prescribed medications, ensure that the patient's "six rights" (right person, drug, dose, time, route, and documentation) exist first.

TABLE 57-2   Assessment Findings and Drugs for Medical Emergencies

Medical Emergency	History Findings	Assessment Findings	Drug Name and Adult Dose
Ingested poisoning	Known or suspected ingestion of caustic substance. Possible psychiatric history or history of attempted suicide.	Visible burns to mouth, lips, and pharynx; abdominal pain; nausea and vomiting; diarrhea; possible change in mental status and changes in vital signs.	For certain types of ingested poisons, activated charcoal may be administered at 1 g/kg orally. Drug may need to be mixed in cold water.
Organophosphate poisoning	Organophosphates are substances commonly found in certain pesticides, which cause profound parasympathetic stimulation. Absorption of an organophosphate through the skin may result in a severe systemic reaction, leading to death. Other exposure could be from WMD deployment.	The effects of organophosphate poisoning are recalled using the mnemonic SLUDGE (salivation, lacrimation, urination, defecation, GI distress, emesis). In addition, bronchospasm, blurred vision, and profound bradycardia may result.	Atropine sulfate, 2–3 mg every 3–5 minutes IVP until heart rate improves and heavy oral secretions subside.
Seizure activity	The patient will likely have a history of epilepsy if seizures are recurrent per patient or family. Patient may also have medical history of diabetes, drug abuse, or a recent history of head trauma or strokes.	A generalized seizure is characterized by tonic–clonic activity to the flexor and extensor muscles of the body. The effects of a generalized seizure usually include the inability to breathe adequately, airway occlusion, skeletal trauma, and possible brain injury.	*Diazepam:* 2–10 mg slow IVP as an initial dose, which may repeat every 1–2 hours as needed. *Lorazepam:* 0.5–2.0 mg slow IVP every 1–2 hours as needed in the acute situation. Because of the longer-lasting effect of lorazepam, it is preferred over diazepam.
Mild allergic reaction	A patient with an allergic reaction will likely have a known exposure that initiates it. The patient may also have an EpiPen prescribed for a severe allergic reaction.	Mild allergic reactions are characterized by skin hives, redness, blotching, itching, and warm skin. The patient may have minor swelling to facial structures, runny eyes/nose, and mild wheezing.	Diphenhydramine 25–50 mg slow IVP.
Respiratory distress (COPD)	Asthma, emphysema, chronic bronchitis, subjective respiratory distress. Patient may also have home nebulized medications or MDI medications he takes regularly.	Tripod positioning, nasal flaring, diminishing pulse oximetry, abnormal breath sounds (crackles, wheezing, ronchi, or diminished), retractions, tachypnea, vital sign changes.	Remember oxygen! *Ipratropium:* 500 mcg every 4–6 hours. For nebulization use a 0.02% solution. If using an MDI, administer 2 inhalations every 4 hours. MDI delivers 18 mcg/inhalation.
Malnutrition/ thiamine deficiency	Although starvation is not as prevalent in the United States as in some other nations, the patient may have malnutrition if homeless. The patient may also have histories of persistent vomiting, GI disorders inhibiting normal absorption, breastfeeding mothers who have a poor diet, or alcoholism.	Because of the malnutrition, the patient may be physically emaciated. If thiamine deficiency has progressed to nervous system damage, the patient may display signs and symptoms of Wernicke-Korsakoff syndrome, including paralysis of the eyes, dementia, hypothermia, the inability to sort fiction from reality, and eventual coma.	Thiamine—the IV push dose is 100 mg of the drug.
Nausea and vomiting	The exact history is very nebulous, as almost any illness, traumatic injury, or medication use can cause nausea or vomiting.	Generally, the patient may have feelings of malaise. Sometimes the patient is guarding the abdominal area because of the pain, or may be in the fetal position. Evidence of active vomiting is obvious.	Ondansetron: 4–8 mg IV push or IM.

EMERGENCY MEDICAL CARE

Regardless of the specific etiology causing the medical emergency, salient assessment steps and interventions must always be performed for the patient, especially when drug therapy is warranted. Time is always of the essence for an unstable patient, so interventions that the AEMT employs must be completed efficiently and expediently. Remember also to repeat your assessment and assess the effectiveness of interventions that you are using to ensure that they are appropriate and working as best possible.

> No drug can be given to the patient by the AEMT without proper authorization by off-line or on-line medical control.

Finally, the AEMT may use other medications prior to the ones mentioned in this topic or described here. Always follow medical direction and ensure that the "six rights" are intact prior to any medication therapy.

1. **Ensure an open airway.** Use common airway techniques to guarantee this.

2. **Provide oxygen.** If the patient is breathing adequately, consider a nonrebreather mask (NRB) at 15 lpm. If the patient is breathing inadequately, provide PPV at 10 to 12/min with high-flow supplemental oxygen. Use pulse oximetry.

3. **Position the patient as appropriate.** If the patient has an altered mental status, a lateral recumbent position will help maintain the airway should the patient regurgitate.

4. **For patients with nausea or vomiting, administer 4 mg ondansetron** IVP or IM.

5. **For organophosphate overdose patients, administer atropine** 2 to 3 mg IVP every 3 to 5 minutes until the desired effect of heart rate and oral secretions are obtained.

6. **For patients with mild anaphylaxis, administer 25 to 50 mg IV push diphenhydramine** if local protocol allows.

7. **For patients who recently ingested poison, administer 1 g/kg activated charcoal** if the patient is able to swallow and local protocol allows.

8. **For dyspneic patients with a chronic pulmonary disease, consider ipratropium** according to route of administration (MDI or nebulization) if the patient is breathing adequately and local protocol allows. Also keep the patient in a semi- or high Fowler position to help ease breathing.

9. **For patients experiencing a generalized seizure, consider either lorazepam** at 0.5 to 2.0 mg IVP or diazepam at 2 to 10 mg IV push. Although many EMS systems carry it, diazepam is no longer considered the first choice for seizure control. If you have the choice between lorazepam and diazepam, use lorazepam.

10. **For malnourished, alcoholic with altered mental status, or unresponsive patients who look malnourished, consider thiamine hydrochloride** 100 mg IV push if local protocol allows.

11. **Arrange for ALS backup or intercept.** ALS providers can administer additional medications to help with the complications common to many of these patients.

12. **Ensure rapid transport to the emergency department.** Notify the receiving ED as early as possible. If the patient becomes pulseless and apneic (no pulse, no respirations), immediately apply the automated external defibrillator.

Administration of medications to patients is a very serious responsibility for the AEMT. As much as a medication may help alleviate a patient's condition, it may also be harmful or fatal should the medication be used inappropriately or given to the wrong patient or for the wrong condition. Before administering any medication, be sure you fully understand how the medication works, how the medication is administered, the appropriate dose, contraindications to the medications, and potential side effects.

Always operate within your local medical directives (whether off-line or on-line); if a situation arises in which the AEMT is not sure whether a medication should be administered or not, always consult medical direction at the receiving facility for additional guidance. Finally, following the administration of any medication, complete a reassessment of the patient to determine if any changes exist in their clinical status that may necessitate a change in your treatment goals.

TRANSITIONING ● ● ● ● ● ● ●

REVIEW ITEMS

1. If a drug causes a stimulatory effect on the body, thereby increasing its normal metabolic cellular activity, what type of effect is being provided to the receptor sites in the cellular wall?
   - a. agonist
   - b. antagonist
   - c. simulatory
   - d. depressant

2. If a drug causes the blood vessels of the body to constrict, thereby raising blood pressure, this would be known as what drug characteristic?
   - a. indications
   - b. side effect
   - c. contraindications
   - d. mechanism of action

3. A patient for whom you are caring needs activated charcoal administered. The patient weighs 240 pounds. What would be his total dose of medication?

    a. 87 grams   b. 109 grams

    c. 120 grams   d. 240 grams

4. A patient with emphysema presents to EMS extremely dyspneic. The patient has an altered mental status, minimal breath sounds in the bases of the lungs bilaterally, and the pulse oximeter is dropping. What drug would be most warranted in this situation?

    a. MDI   b. oxygen

    c. EpiPen   d. mechanical ventilation

5. Ondansetron is a medication that when administered, should have what effect in the body?

    a. increase the heart rate

    b. reduce feelings of nausea

    c. drop the systolic blood pressure

    d. increase the likelihood of vomiting

APPLIED PATHOPHYSIOLOGY

You are caring for an elderly female patient with respiratory distress. The patient has a history of emphysema. Currently she is speaking in full sentences with a respiratory rate of 26/minute, the pulse oximeter reads 94 percent on room air, bilateral breath sounds are present but diminished, and the blood pressure is 149/86 mmHg.

1. Given this presentation, list one drug and its corresponding dose mentioned in this chapter that may be appropriate for this patient.

2. Beyond oxygen, what other medications (and their respective dose) could be administered to a patient with epilepsy who is experiencing a grand-mal seizure?

CLINICAL DECISION MAKING

You encounter a 59-year-old male patient sitting on the front porch of his residence. As approach the patient, you see that he is struggling very hard to breathe. On the ground beside him is a yard rake and a can of aerosolized hornet/bee killer. After determining that the scene is safe, you approach the patient. He is sitting upright in a tripod position and appears to be in mild respiratory distress.

1. Based on the scene size-up characteristics, list the possible conditions you suspect the patient is experiencing.

The primary assessment reveals that the patient is anxious. His airway is clear, and he can speak in full sentences. The patient has a respiratory rate of 28/minute with normal chest rise and fall. The peripheral pulses are present, and his heart rate is 116 beats per minute. The skin is warm and flushed, and you note reddened hives on the body. The SpO_2 reading is 96 percent on room air.

2. What is the underlying pathology of this patient?

3. What immediate emergency care should you provide based on the initial assessment?

During the secondary assessment, inspection of the mouth reveals the mucous membranes to be slightly swollen; breath sounds are present with slight expiratory wheezing. The abdomen is unremarkable, pelvis is stable, and there are no deformities or evidence of trauma to the

extremities. The extremities are warm, flushed, and diaphoretic. The peripheral pulses are palpable.

The patient states that he is allergic to certain bee stings, for which he carries an EpiPen. "In fact," he states, "I shot myself with my EpiPen right after I got stung!" His medical history also includes mild asthma, for which he takes albuterol as needed. His last oral intake was 3 hours ago and consisted of a fast-food hamburger and fries. The blood pressure is 128/62 mmHg, heart rate is 118 beats per minute, and respirations are 26 per minute.

4. What conditions have your ruled out in your differential field diagnosis? Why?

5. Based on your differential diagnosis, what are the next steps in emergency care? Why?

6. Based on the history, what type of reaction is this patient experiencing?

7. For the pathophysiologic changes listed here, name the drug and its corresponding dose that would best correct the underlying disturbance:

    a. SpO_2 84%

    b. Bilateral wheezing

ECG MONITORING AND CARDIAC DYSRHYTHMIAS

TRANSITION *highlights*

- **Overview of basic information obtained by an electro-cardiograph tracing:**
  - Heart rate.
  - Rhythm regularity and irregularity.
  - Intervals for impulse conduction.
  - Conduction pathways that are irregular.

- **Description of specialized types of myocardial cells:**
  - Working cells.
  - Pacemaker cells.
  - Conduction cells.

- **Placing electrodes for 3- and 4-lead monitoring.**

- **Description and meaning of the ECG wave:**
  - P wave.
  - QRS complex.
  - T wave.
  - PRI interval.

- **Components to analyzing the ECG rhythm:**
  - Rate.
  - Regularity.
  - QRS width.
  - P waves.
  - P–R interval.

- **Review of common ECG dysrhythmias.**

- **Need for acquisition of a 12-lead ECG.**

- **Placing electrodes for a 12-lead ECG.**

- **Location of limb electrodes.**

- **Location of precordial electrodes.**

- **Methods to obtain a reliable 12-lead ECG tracing.**

INTRODUCTION

When treating a patient with an apparent cardiac problem, it is important to determine whether a mechanical or electrical dysfunction exists, as these are often the culprit for what is wrong with the patient. Much of what you need to know about the heart's activity cannot be determined through a traditional AEMT physical assessment of vital signs (BP, HR, skin characteristics), however. For example, if an electrical disturbance to the heart is causing it to beat too fast, cardiac output drops, as does the patient's blood pressure. In addition, conduction disturbances can also change the heart's ability to contract properly—and without being able to see the electrical disturbance, treatment is limited. An electrocardiogram (ECG), however, can reveal the presence of an abnormal rhythm or conduction disturbance, and when the ECG is coupled with the physical assessment, a clearer picture of the patient's problem is possible. Often, this information is critical to treatment decisions made for the patient.

Interpreting ECGs does not come without risks, however—improper rhythm identification will almost certainly lead to improper management. The ability to read and interpret an ECG is an essential skill in the management of patients with cardiovascular disturbances—but you must also be certain of your impression if you want the maximum effects from your care.

To assess the electrical activity of the heart, you need to know how to interpret the ECG. It is worth emphasizing early that the ECG provides information only about the electrical activity of the heart, not about the mechanical function (Table 58-1). To this end, it is possible for the ECG to look perfectly normal in the absence of any mechanical contraction. Always remember the popular phrase: "Treat the patient, not the monitor."

Electrophysiology (or the physiology of how the heart works on electricity) is often presented as complex, abstract, and frustrating. Many beginning students become so intimidated by the physiology that they never learn to interpret ECGs. The intent of this topic is to limit the amount of technical information to what you will need to identify the basic, life-threatening cardiac rhythms commonly seen in prehospital care. Once you have mastered basic rhythm recognition, we encourage you to tackle electrophysiology, which will increase your understanding of

TABLE 58-1	Information Obtainable from an ECG Strip	
Heart rate	Yes	
Rhythm regularity and irregularity	Yes	
Intervals for impulse conduction	Yes	
Conduction pathways that are irregular	Yes	
Pumping action of the heart		No
Blood pressure (systolic/diastolic)		No
Flow of blood through the heart		No
Flow of blood to the tissues of the body		No

cardiology. Electrophysiology, you will learn, becomes less overwhelming once you have a grasp of the basics.

The heart is a unique organ. It is made up of muscle tissue that has the property of automaticity. *Automaticity* is the ability of the heart, or any of its individual muscle cells, to contract on its own—without any nervous system control. In fact, if you quickly remove the heart from the body, place it in a saline bath, and provide it with oxygen and glucose, the heart will continue to beat for quite some time. If you cut it into tiny pieces and separate them, each chunk of heart muscle will beat separately! This is an amazing physiologic phenomenon and makes the heart dramatically different from any other organ in the body.

To contract, a myocardial cell must be depolarized. Depolarization is a process where a shift in the electrical properties of the cell occurs from the movement of electrically charged particles across the cell's membrane. When the electrical properties of the cell change, the cell is capable of contracting. Some areas of the heart have evolved to perform special functions, which are the result of three specialized types of myocardial cells: working cells, pacemaker cells, and conduction cells.

Working Cells

The physical contraction of the heart is caused by the myocardial working cells. These muscle cells are bundled into an interconnecting weave of muscle fibers. Contraction, or shortening, of these fibers causes a rapid decrease in the internal size of the atria and ventricles, which in turn ejects the blood from the chambers.

The actual contraction of the heart occurs when electrical depolarization is coupled with physical contraction. It is important to remember that the physical contraction—not the electrical activity—generates blood flow. However, the physical contraction requires organized electrical activity to occur. The organized electrical activity starts by the regular depolarization of pacemaker cells.

Pacemaker Cells

Pacemaker cells are specialized cardiac tissue that depolarizes regularly by controlling the flow of charged particles into and out of the cell. Pacemaker cells control the heart's rate and rhythm. Through influence from the autonomic (sympathetic and parasympathetic) nervous systems, the rate of the depolarization can be altered.

The primary pacemaker of the healthy heart is the sinoatrial (SA) node, a bundle of cardiac tissue that is located on the inner wall of the heart near the junction of the right atrium and the vena cava. Without nervous control, the SA node will normally depolarize 60 to 100 times per minute. If the body demands changes in cardiac output, the autonomic nervous system can increase (as a sympathetic action) or decrease (as a parasympathetic action) the rate at which the SA node emits impulses.

If the SA node fails to emit an impulse, some backup functions will ensure that the heart will continue to beat. If the SA node fails, the atrioventricular (AV) node at the junction of the atria and ventricles will take over as a pacemaker and will depolarize at a rate of 40 to 60 times per minute. If both the SA and AV nodes fail, the Purkinje fibers of the ventricles will depolarize at a rate of less than 40 times per minute.

Conduction Cells

The impulse from the pacemakers travels through the heart in several ways. It is the responsibility of the conduction cells to carry the electrical impulse throughout the heart in an organized fashion. To do so, internodal pathways connect the SA node to the AV node. In normal conduction, the SA node impulse must reach the AV node, as this is the only electrical connection between the atria and the ventricles of the heart; therefore, any stimulation for the ventricles to contract that

> **The ECG provides information only about the electrical activity of the heart, not about the mechanical function.**

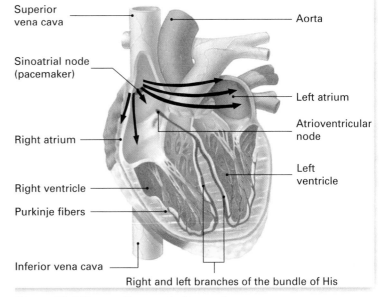

Superior vena cava
Aorta
Sinoatrial node (pacemaker)
Left atrium
Atrioventricular node
Right atrium
Left ventricle
Right ventricle
Purkinje fibers
Inferior vena cava
Right and left branches of the bundle of His

Figure 58-1 The cardiac conduction system.

originates above the ventricles must pass through the AV node. Below the AV node, the impulse for contraction travels through the bundle of His, the bundle branches, and the Purkinje fibers. These latter conduction pathways allow the ventricles to contract as a unit, propelling blood from the ventricles.

The overall cardiac conduction pathway in the normal heart (▶ Figure 58-1), therefore, is

> SA node → internodal pathways → AV node → bundle of His → right and left bundle branches → Purkinje fibers

TABLE 58-2   Electrode Locations on the Body

Three-Lead Monitoring System	Four-Lead Monitoring System
1. Just inferior to right clavicle on right anterior thorax	1. Just inferior to right clavicle on right anterior thorax
2. Just inferior to the left clavicle on the left anterior thorax	2. Just inferior to the left clavicle on the left anterior thorax
3. Approximately 5th ICS, midaxillary line of the left thorax	3. Approximately 5th ICS, midaxillary line of the left thorax
	4. Approximately 5th ICS, midaxillary line of the right thorax

THE ELECTROCARDIOGRAM

The body is a giant conductor of the electrical impulse transmission that occurs within the heart. These events can be detected by two electrodes—one positive and one negative—placed on the skin. Typically, the signal is amplified and then displayed on an oscilloscope or printed on graph paper. Theoretically, electrodes can be placed anywhere on the body, but this causes subtle differences in the relative size of each wave. For convenience and standardization, you should remember some conventional electrode placements.

▶ Figure 58-2 shows typical ECG monitoring leads using three-lead and four-lead placement configurations, and Table 58-2 describes where to place the electrodes on the body. If the AEMT wants to view a different lead on the monitor, he needs only to activate a switch on the ECG monitor panel, and the machine will change the lead polarity to the new view. This saves the EMS provider from rearranging the actual electrodes and wires on the patient.

Because it is the most common monitoring lead, all the rules and rhythm strips in this chapter are presented in Lead II. For Lead II (the standard monitoring lead), the positive cable (red) attaches to the electrode placed on the patient's lower left chest. The negative cable (white) attaches to the electrode placed inferior to the right clavicle. Finally, the black cable attaches to the electrode placed inferior to the left clavicle. If you are using a four-lead monitor, the remaining cable (green) would be attached to an electrode placed on the lower right chest (see Figure 58-2).

The electrical events of the heart rhythm produce waves that are labeled alphabetically, P through T. You should become familiar with these components of the normal ECG, as shown in ▶ Figure 58-3 and discussed in Table 58-3.

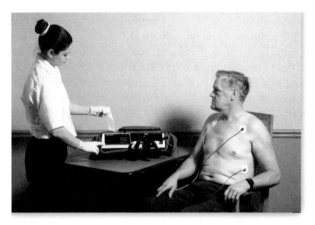

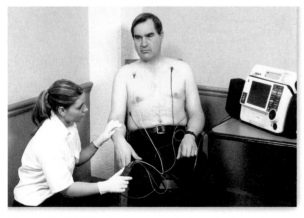

Figure 58-2 ECG placements: (a) three-lead configuration and (b) four-lead configuration. (© *Carl Leet*)

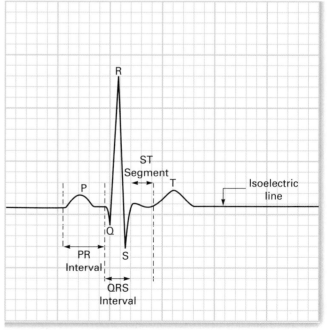

Figure 58-3 The electrocardiogram (ECG).

TABLE 58-3	ECG Waveform Names and Descriptions
ECG Wave	**Wave Description/Meaning**
P wave	This wave represents atrial contraction. In Lead II it should be upright.
QRS complex	This complex of waves represents ventricular contraction. It should be no wider than 3 mm, or 0.12 sec.
T wave	This wave represents ventricular repolarization. It should be upright in Lead II.
PRI interval	The distance from the beginning of the P wave to the beginning of the QRS should be 3–5 mm (0.12–0.20 sec)
ST segment	This is the distance from the end of the QRS to the beginning of the T wave. It should be isoelectric.
R–R interval	The distance between the tops of two consecutive QRS complexes should be regular and can help compute the heart rate.

the paper exits the machine at a constant speed, the horizontal boxes represent time: each large box represents 0.20 seconds, and each small box represents 0.04 seconds. The vertical boxes represent the magnitude of the electrical impulse in millivolts: two large boxes represent 1 mV. It is important to remember the time increments for each box, as they will be used extensively in ECG interpretation.

ANALYZING THE ECG

Now that you know how to identify each wave of the ECG, analyzing the cardiac rhythm simply becomes a matter of looking at a number of parameters and

Each wave discussed represents the summation of the depolarization or repolarization of a mass of heart tissue. As a review: Atrial depolarization, which is associated with mechanical contraction of the atria, produces the P wave. Ventricular depolarization, which correlates with mechanical contraction of the ventricles, produces the QRS complex, and ventricular repolarization produces the T wave. Atrial repolarization is buried in the QRS complex and is clinically irrelevant (▶ Figure 58-4).

Occasionally, there are variations in how the waves look from person to person. But all the waves discussed earlier should be present for a normal rhythm to be considered present. When they are not, alterations are the way you will be able to recognize that dysrhythmias are present. If you keep the aforementioned information in mind, dysrhythmia recognition becomes much easier.

MONITORING SYSTEMS

Many different cardiac monitors are on the market. They have numerous features, with various configurations of switches and buttons, but basically all cardiac monitors are the same. They generally consist of a screen (or oscilloscope) and usually have a printer that will print a hard copy of the patient's cardiac rhythm. Cardiac monitors print the ECG on a strip of graph paper (▶ Figure 58-5). Because

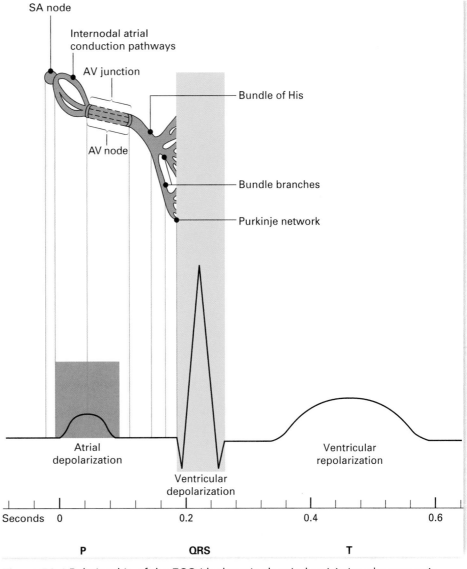

Figure 58-4 Relationship of the ECG (the heart's electrical activity) to the anatomic sequence of the heart's mechanical actions.

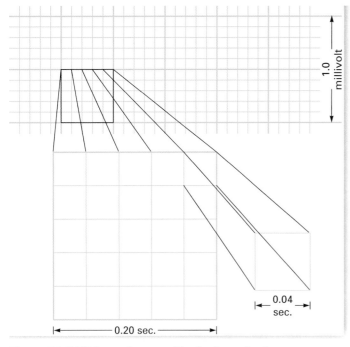

Figure 58-5 ECG graph paper. The horizontal axis represents elapsed time in seconds. The vertical axis represents the magnitude of the electrical impulse in millivolts.

TABLE 58-4	Five Parameters of ECG Assessment
Rate	• What is the rate? (Normally 60–100 per minute)
Regularity	• Is the rhythm regular? (Normally a variance of less than 0.04 seconds)
QRS complex	• Do all the QRS complexes look alike? (Normally yes) • What is the width of the QRS complex? (Normally less than 0.12 seconds)
P waves	• Is there a P wave before every QRS complex? (Normally yes) • Is there a QRS complex after every P wave? (Normally yes) • Are the P waves upright and rounded? (Normally yes)
P–R interval	• What is the P–R interval? (Normally less than 0.20 seconds) • Is the P–R interval constant? (Normally yes)

Assess the heart rate by looking at the number of QRS complexes in a given period of time.

- Rate
- Regularity
- QRS width
- P waves
- P–R interval

applying a couple of rules. We will use the "red flag" method of ECG interpretation. This method looks at five parameters in each ECG; by understanding what they mean, you will easily be able to interpret the ECG. The five parameters (Table 58-4) are:

Rate

As mentioned earlier, the SA node normally depolarizes 60 to 100 times a minute. This represents the normal range of heart rate. Any rate that is faster than 100 beats per minute is called *tachycardia*, and any rate slower than 60 beats per minute is *bradycardia*. We assess the rate by looking at the number of QRS complexes in a given period of time.

Two ways exist to determine the heart rate by looking at the ECG. The easiest way is to count the number of QRS complexes that occur in 6 seconds and multiply by 10. For convenience, ECG paper is often marked in 3- or 6-second increments. This method is best used to count irregular rhythms.

The second way to determine the heart rate is to look for a QRS complex that falls on one of the heavy lines on the strip (this is known as the R–R method). You then count how many large boxes are between this and the next QRS complex. Then divide that number into 300—because 300 large boxes represent 60 seconds, or 1 minute. Therefore, if the next QRS fell exactly three heavy lines away, the rate would be 100 beats per minute (300 ÷ 3 = 100). Usually, you are not lucky enough to have the subsequent QRS fall directly on a heavy line, so this technique is often used just to estimate the heart rate. Study ▶ Figure 58-6; can you see why the rate is estimated to be 70 on this strip?

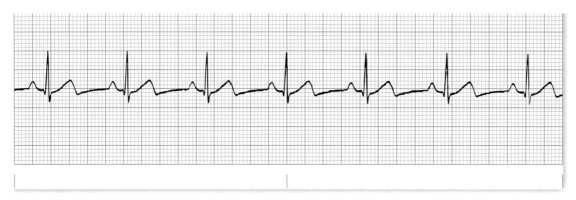

Figure 58-6 ECG strip with a heart rate of about 70 bpm.

Regularity

The next variable to analyze is the regularity of the rhythm. The normal heart rhythm is highly regular. A variance of more than 0.04 seconds, or one small box, between the complexes is considered abnormal. This is best analyzed using calipers. Simply measure the distance between two QRS complexes (R–R interval) and then check the distances between the next two complexes to determine whether they are within 0.04 seconds of each other.

QRS Complex

After evaluating the rate and the regularity of the rhythm, next analyze the QRS complexes. Remember that the QRS complex represents ventricular depolarization. Specifically, you are examining the QRS complexes to see whether they have the same morphology (look the same) and whether they are the same width. If all the QRS complexes look alike, they are all following the same conduction pathways below the AV node and are termed *monomorphic.*

The width of the QRS complex has special significance. If the QRS complex is narrow, defined as less than 0.12 seconds (three small boxes), the wave of depolarization is assumed to have followed the normal conduction pathways below the AV node. In other words, the beat did *not* originate in the ventricles.

If the QRS complex is wider, this generally means an abnormality is present. If the QRS complex is greater than 0.12 seconds (three small boxes), there are commonly three causes:

- The impulse may have originated in the ventricles, outside the normal conduction pathway.
- The impulse may have originated above the ventricles but circumvented the normal conduction pathway through the AV node. This is one form of *aberrant conduction.* Because it then enters the ventricle in a different area, the complex becomes wider.
- The impulse may have originated above the ventricles and traveled through the AV node but experienced a delay in one side of the ventricular conduction system (the bundle branches). This is called a *bundle branch block.* Bundle branch blocks are another type of aberrant conduction.

P Waves

Remember that the P wave represents atrial depolarization. There are three questions to ask about the P waves:

- Is there a P wave before every QRS complex? (Yes when normal.)
- Is there a QRS complex after every P wave? (Yes when normal.)
- Are the P waves upright and rounded? (Yes when normal.)

P–R Interval

The normal delay of conduction that occurs at the AV node is less than 0.20 seconds (one big box or five small boxes). You need to know two things about the P–R interval to correctly interpret the ECG:

- Is the P–R interval less than 0.20 seconds? (Yes when normal.)
- Is the P–R interval constant? (Yes when normal.)

BASIC ECG INTERPRETATION

Now that you know the five parameters for analyzing any ECG (rate, regularity, QRS complex, P waves, and P–R interval), interpreting and understanding cardiac rhythms simply becomes a matter of answering each question and applying a few rules. We call this the "red flag" method, because by knowing which of the five variables falls out of the normal range (raises a red flag), you can interpret the rhythm.

A word of caution: After you have analyzed many ECGs, you will have a tendency to cut to the chase and attempt to interpret the rhythm without going through each step of analysis. Although this will often result in a correct interpretation, you will sometimes miss important findings. We suggest that you use this sequential method of ECG analysis until you have gained considerable experience in ECG interpretation. Table 58-5 lists the red flags for several of the most common dysrhythmias.

Clinical Application

Generally speaking, the approach to managing the patient with a cardiac rhythm disturbance is rather straightforward. Prehospitally, the ALS provider rarely attempts to correct atrial disturbances. Rather, the goal is to manage the ventricular response to the atrial activity.

For example, if the patient is displaying a tachydysrhythmia as a result of a rapid atrial flutter, the paramedic will likely employ measures to slow the ventricular response to the massive number of atrial impulses assaulting the AV node. This may be done pharmacologically with medications that create a temporary block in the AV node slowing the impulses reaching the ventricles (thus slowing down the pulse rate), or it can be done with synchronous cardioversion (an electrical shock) from the defibrillator.

Likewise, if the patient is bradycardic because of sinus bradycardia or some type of heart block, the paramedic can administer medications that will increase the SA node discharge rate, which should in turn promote a faster ventricular rate, or the paramedic may employ transcutaneous pacing, which is using electricity to stimulate the heart to contract faster and thus improve cardiac output and blood pressure.

The goal is to maintain normal electrical activity within the heart to enable sequential and normal depolarization of muscle tissue so that blood flow may occur. Any disturbance to the electrical activity can have a negative impact on myocardial contraction; thus, the EMS provider must rapidly identify and correct underlying ECG disturbances.

The recognition of dysrhythmias is an important aspect in any ALS system and a necessary component of the patient assessment for any cardiac patient. Many clinicians become intimidated by the electrophysiology of the heart and fail to learn a systematic method of evaluating ECGs. By using the red flag method and applying a few rules and an understanding of the etiology of dysrhythmias, dysrhythmia recognition becomes much easier.

A brief word of caution: For clarity, we considered only one dysrhythmia at a time in Table 58-5. In real life, patients can exhibit multiple dysrhythmias at the same time. It is not uncommon, for example, to have a patient in sinus bradycardia with a first-degree heart block. For now, though, when you are first learning ECGs, it is much easier to consider "textbook" ECG strips one at a time to illustrate the concepts of dysrhythmia interpretation. With time and practice, you will become

TABLE 58-5	Common ECG Dysrhythmias	
Rhythm Name	ECG Example	Defining Characteristics (Red Flag)
Normal sinus rhythm	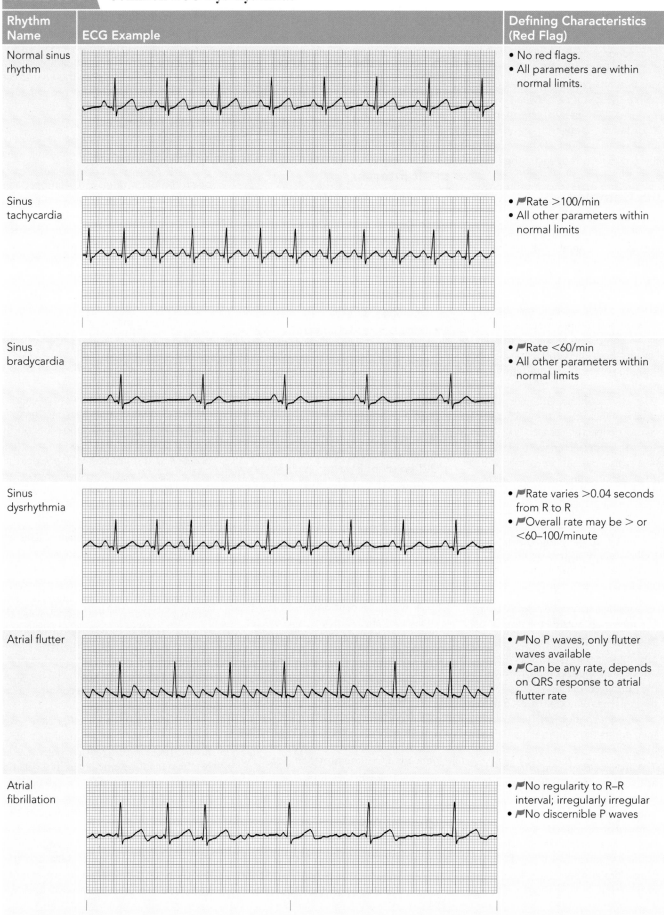	• No red flags. • All parameters are within normal limits.
Sinus tachycardia		• ⚑Rate >100/min • All other parameters within normal limits
Sinus bradycardia		• ⚑Rate <60/min • All other parameters within normal limits
Sinus dysrhythmia		• ⚑Rate varies >0.04 seconds from R to R • ⚑Overall rate may be > or <60–100/minute
Atrial flutter		• ⚑No P waves, only flutter waves available • ⚑Can be any rate, depends on QRS response to atrial flutter rate
Atrial fibrillation		• ⚑No regularity to R–R interval; irregularly irregular • ⚑No discernible P waves

Rhythm Name	ECG Example	Defining Characteristics (Red Flag)
Supraventricular tachycardia	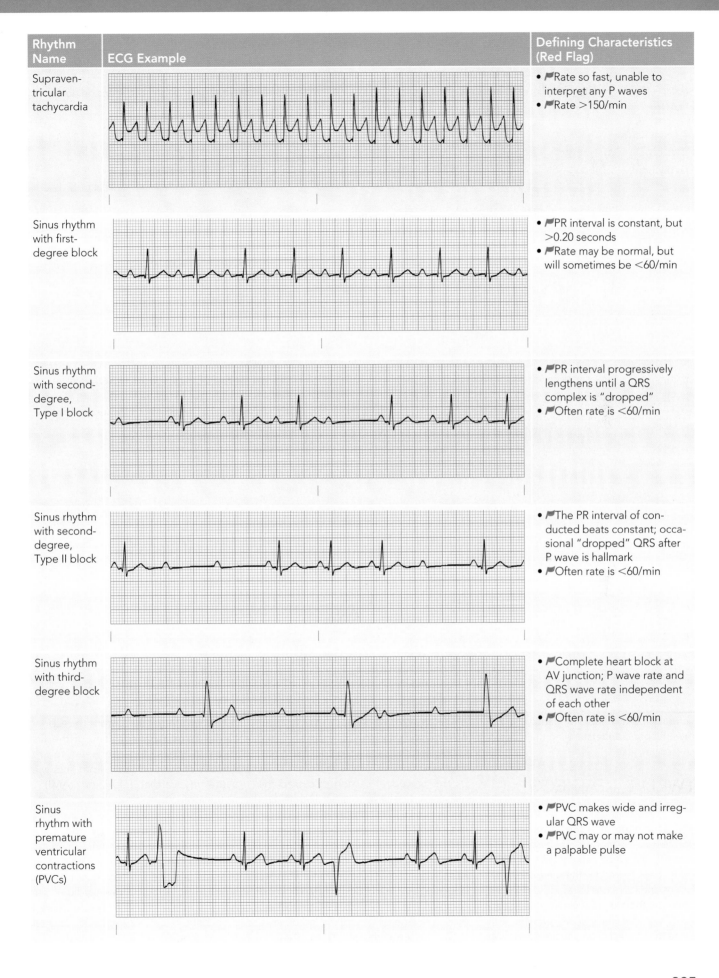	• 🚩Rate so fast, unable to interpret any P waves • 🚩Rate >150/min
Sinus rhythm with first-degree block		• 🚩PR interval is constant, but >0.20 seconds • 🚩Rate may be normal, but will sometimes be <60/min
Sinus rhythm with second-degree, Type I block		• 🚩PR interval progressively lengthens until a QRS complex is "dropped" • 🚩Often rate is <60/min
Sinus rhythm with second-degree, Type II block		• 🚩The PR interval of conducted beats constant; occasional "dropped" QRS after P wave is hallmark • 🚩Often rate is <60/min
Sinus rhythm with third-degree block		• 🚩Complete heart block at AV junction; P wave rate and QRS wave rate independent of each other • 🚩Often rate is <60/min
Sinus rhythm with premature ventricular contractions (PVCs)		• 🚩PVC makes wide and irregular QRS wave • 🚩PVC may or may not make a palpable pulse

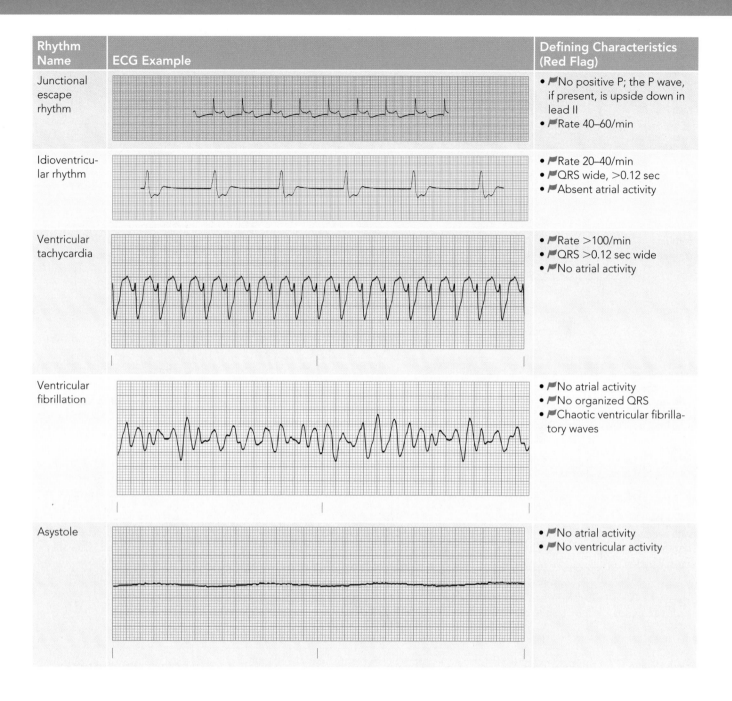

Rhythm Name	ECG Example	Defining Characteristics (Red Flag)
Junctional escape rhythm		• 🚩No positive P; the P wave, if present, is upside down in lead II • 🚩Rate 40–60/min
Idioventricular rhythm		• 🚩Rate 20–40/min • 🚩QRS wide, >0.12 sec • 🚩Absent atrial activity
Ventricular tachycardia		• 🚩Rate >100/min • 🚩QRS >0.12 sec wide • 🚩No atrial activity
Ventricular fibrillation		• 🚩No atrial activity • 🚩No organized QRS • 🚩Chaotic ventricular fibrillatory waves
Asystole		• 🚩No atrial activity • 🚩No ventricular activity

naturally more capable at identifying dysrhythmias and understanding their clinical consequences.

TWELVE-LEAD ECG ACQUISITION

The treatment of acute coronary syndromes has changed dramatically in the past 10 years. Whereas prehospital care providers have teamed with emergency physicians and surgeons to rapidly deliver the patient with traumatic injuries to the operating suite for many years, patients with acute myocardial infarction are now being treated using a similar approach. Because of the progressive destruction of myocardial muscle during an infarction, the expression that should guide the emergency provider is "time is muscle."

The preceding section discussed the recognition of basic cardiac rhythms and dysrhythmias. This section focuses on the use of the 12-lead electrocardiogram as an adjunct in the management of patients in the prehospital setting, and how the AEMT can assist the paramedic with obtaining a 12-lead ECG rapidly. The most common use of 12-lead ECG is to help recognize emerging cardiac syndromes.

To this end, the ability to obtain a 12-lead ECG is essential to activating the emergency care system to respond to the cardiac patient. One of the first steps in identifying the need for re-establishing blood flow in patients with acute myocardial infarction (AMI) is obtaining a diagnostic-quality ECG. By recognizing characteristic changes on the electrocardiogram by the paramedic indicative of ischemia or infarction, EMS can then set in motion a series of steps designed to help restore blood flow to the affected myocardium. The AEMT's role in this is to help acquire a diagnostic-quality 12-lead ECG, as often the paramedic will be busy with other patient care tasks.

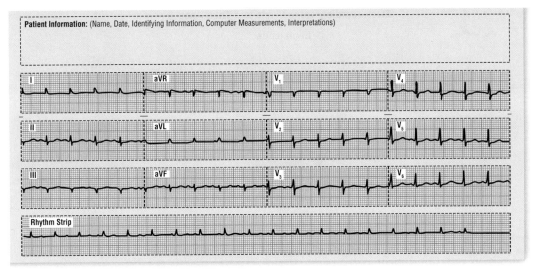

I   aVR   V₁   V₄

II   aVL   V₂   V₅

III   aVF   V₃   V₆

Rhythm Strip

Figure 58-7 Normal 12-lead ECG printout.

Twelve-Lead Configuration

If the AEMT works in an EMS system with 12-lead capability, he will be able to review multiple 12-lead tracings. In doing so, the AEMT must be familiar with the basic format of the 12-lead printout. Unlike a three- or four-lead tracing, as discussed previously, in which the paper printout is of only one lead tracing, the AEMT will notice 12 different tracings of the same cardiac activity on the 12-lead printout.

The first thing to note is that there commonly are four lines of ECG tracings. The first three lines are further subdivided into four smaller boxes, each representing 2.5 seconds of time, and each with a different "view" of the heart. Although most 12-lead machine printouts will label each smaller box, some will not, and the AEMT will need to have memorized the standard configuration for each lead tracing. The bottom tracing on the printout is a continuous tracing of (most commonly) lead II. Review the illustrated 12-lead printout (▶ Figure 58-7), and become familiar with each lead location.

Twelve-Lead ECG—Lead Placement

As mentioned earlier, the electrocardiogram is a representation of electrical events that are occurring within the heart as viewed by a variety of leads, sometimes referred to as "camera views" placed on the surface of the body. These cameras provide different views of the same electrical events that occur during the cardiac cycle. To do so, the AEMT will apply an electrode to various locations of the body, each of these electrodes will serve as the "camera" once the appropriate monitor cable is applied (most monitoring cables are labeled, so attach the correct wire to its corresponding electrode).

The first four electrodes that are attached to the body will be placed on the patient's limbs (Table 58-6). Three of these electrodes will be used by the 12-lead ECG machine to determine the *bipolar limb leads* known as leads I, II, and III (top of ▶ Figure 58-8). Three of these leads are also used by the 12-lead machine to determine the *augmented limb leads* that will view the electrical currents traveling from the center of the heart to the right arm (aVR), left arm (aVL), and left foot (aVF; bottom of Figure 58-8). As you can see from the figure, leads II, III, and aVF provide information about the inferior portions of the heart. Leads I and aVL are considered the lateral leads.

The six remaining views are obtained by examining the heart along the horizontal plane. These leads are referred to as the *precordial leads,* and the positive electrode for each lead proceeds from the right side of the chest (V₁) to the left chest (V₆) (▶ Figure 58-9). V₁ and V₂ provide information about the interventricular septum, V₃ and V₄ view primarily the anterior wall of the left ventricle, and V₅ and V₆ demonstrate the lateral wall of the left ventricle. Table 58-7 reviews the proper location for electrode placement on the chest for the precordial leads.

Thus, the 12-lead electrocardiogram records the electrical activity of the heart from the perspective of each of the limb leads (3), the augmented limb leads (3), and precordial leads (6; ▶ Figure 58-10):

When reviewing for ischemic changes on a 12-lead (basically elevated ST segment of greater than 1 mm in two anatomically contiguous leads), having an understanding of the correlation between ECG lead locations and the wall of the left ventricle viewed is a must (Table 58-8).

In most situations, the AEMT will not need to acquire a 12-lead ECG until after it has been determined that the patient has no immediate life-threatening conditions or fatal dysrhythmias as viewed with a three-lead ECG. In prehospital care, the 12-lead is most helpful in identifying patients who may be experiencing an acute coronary syndrome. In addition, it may also help your paramedic partner in distinguishing between possible types of similar dysrhythmias.

Hints for Obtaining a Reliable Tracing

Whereas a good quality 12-lead ECG is essential for determining whether myocardial ischemia or infarction is present, an unreliable tracing with excessive artifact is of no use and is essentially a waste of time. Because everything done in prehospital care is measured against the time it takes to complete it, taking an extra few moments to ensure a good-quality tracing the first time is extremely important. Generally, poor tracings occur

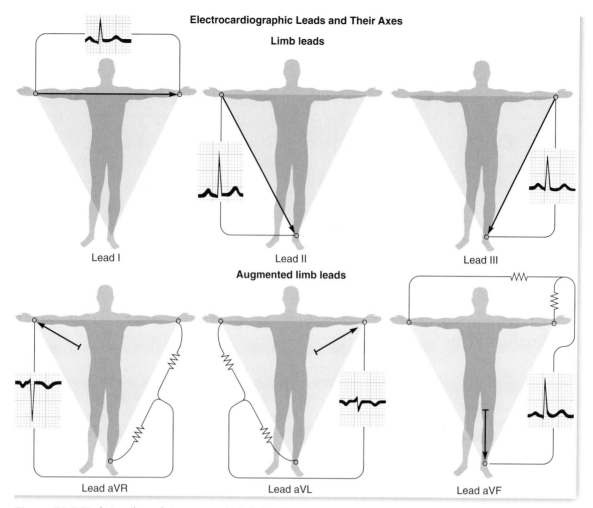

Electrocardiographic Leads and Their Axes

Limb leads

Lead I

Lead II

Lead III

Augmented limb leads

Lead aVR

Lead aVL

Lead aVF

Figure 58-8 Limb Leads and Augmented Limb Leads.

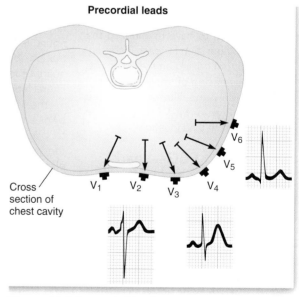

Precordial leads

Cross section of chest cavity

V_1 V_2 V_3 V_4 V_5 V_6

Figure 58-9 Precordial leads.

TABLE 58-6	Electrode Locations for Limb Leads
Electrode Name	**Anatomic Location**
Augmented voltage right (aVR)	Anterior surface of right arm, just proximal to wrist
Augmented voltage left (aVL)	Anterior surface of left arm, just proximal to wrist
Augmented voltage foot (aVF)	Medial surface of left leg, just proximal to ankle
Ground electrode	Medial surface of right leg, just proximal to ankle

TABLE 58-7	Locations for Precordial Leads
Electrode Name	Anatomic Location
V_1	4th ICS, right sternal boarder
V_2	4th ICS, left sternal border
V_3	Midway between V_2 and V_4
V_4	Left thorax, 5th ICS, midclavicular line
V_5	Left thorax, lateral to V_4, anterior axillary line
V_6	Left thorax, lateral to V_4 and V_5, midaxillary line

TABLE 58-8	Correlation of Infarction Sites and Leads
Site	Leads
Septal wall	V1 and V2
Anterior wall	V3 and V4
Lateral wall	Lead I, aVL, V5, and V6
Inferior wall	Lead II, Lead III, aVF

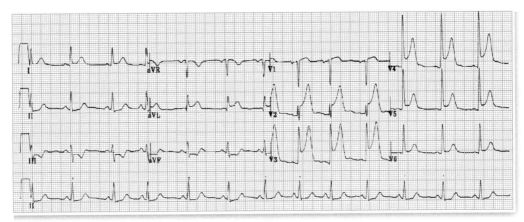

Figure 58-10 Anterolateral myocardial infarction.

as a result of bad adhesion of the electrode to the skin. The AEMT should use the following guidelines to help ensure that the first tracing obtained is the best tracing:

1. Wipe away any moisture or fluid from the skin.
2. Remove (shave or clip) excessive hair from the skin.
3. Keep the patient from moving (shaking, tremors, gripping the rails of the cot, etc.).
4. Do not allow the cables to be excessively taut or too loose and dangling.

5. Vehicle movement may distort tracing; stop the vehicle if necessary.
6. Electrical interference may occur; remove or shut down electrical equipment.
7. Ensure that aVR is negatively deflected (very rarely will it be positive).
8. Ensure that one complete cardiac cycle is captured for each of the 12 leads.

For many patients, the 12-lead ECG is a valuable adjunct to your physical examination and history taking skills. It can provide important information about the possibility of an acute coronary event that

may require rapid reperfusion. Being able to identify these patients and initiating the complex series of events that will lead to fibrinolysis or angioplasty is the hallmark of a well-coordinated and excellent EMS system. The AEMT can assist in this process by applying the electrodes, attaching the cables, and printing out the 12-lead ECG for the paramedic to review.

> **Generally, poor tracings occur as a result of bad adhesion of the electrode to the skin.**

TRANSITIONING

REVIEW ITEMS

1. If the patient has some type of cardiac disturbance that resulted in the atria no longer depolarizing appropriately, which ECG waveform would likely look abnormal?
   - a. P wave
   - b. QRS complex
   - c. T wave
   - d. ST segment

2. Each small box on the ECG paper represents how much time?
   - a. 0.40 second
   - b. 0.20 second
   - c. 0.08 second
   - d. 0.04 second

3. When using a three-lead ECG machine, the red wire (+) is attached to which electrode?
   a. right lateral lower chest
   b. left lateral lower chest
   c. inferior to the left clavicle
   d. inferior to the right clavicle

4. Your patient is has an ECG rhythm in which the only abnormality (red flag) is that the PR interval is too long. What is the most likely interpretation for this rhythm?
   a. sinus bradycardia
   b. first-degree heart block

c. second-degree heart block, Type I
d. second-degree heart block, Type II

5. When interpreting an ECG rhythm clinically, which one of the following variables cannot be determined?
   a. what the heart rate is
   b. if there is a block at the AV node
   c. whether the patient has a pulse
   d. what type of conduction disturbance is present

APPLIED PATHOPHYSIOLOGY

You and your paramedic partner have been called to a home of an elderly woman with chest pain and nausea. On arrival, your partner starts to perform an assessment while you place the patient on the pulse oximeter and give oxygen via nonrebreather mask. During the assessment, your paramedic partner turns to you and says, "Hey, why don't you hook up the monitor to see what is going on."

1. Given the patient's presentation thus far, would you set up for 3-lead monitoring or 12-lead monitoring?

2. If the patient displayed a rhythm that produced a heart rate over 120 beats per minute, what are at least three different dysrhythmias it may be?

CLINICAL DECISION MAKING

You encounter a 59 year-old male patient sitting on a park bench of a local hiking trail. As you approach the patient, you see that he is struggling very hard to breathe. After determining that the scene is safe, you approach the patient, who is sitting upright in a tripod position and is using accessory muscles to breathe. He says to you, in labored breaths, "Please help … I … I … can't breathe."

1. Based on the scene size-up characteristics, list the possible conditions you suspect the patient is experiencing.

The primary assessment reveals that the patient is anxious. His airway is clear, and he can speak only in broken sentences. The patient has a respiratory rate of 28/minute with diminished rise and fall. The peripheral pulses are present, and his heart rate is 126 beats per minute and slightly irregular. The SpO$_2$ reading is 93 percent without oxygen.

2. What immediate emergency care should you provide based on the primary assessment?

3. When applying the cardiac monitor, would it be wiser to obtain a 3-lead tracing or a 12-lead tracing initially? Explain your answer.

During the secondary assessment, breath sounds are present with inspiratory crackles and slight expiratory wheezing. The abdomen is unremarkable, the pelvis is stable, and there are no deformities or evidence of trauma to the extremities. The extremities are cool and diaphoretic. The peripheral pulses are palpable. The patient's medical history includes CHF and diabetes, for which he takes furosemide (Lasix), potassium, and regular insulin shots. He replies with a "no" when you ask him whether he has any allergies or any other complaints. His last oral intake was 4 hours ago and consisted of fruit at breakfast. The blood pressure is 138/72 mmHg, heart rate is still tachycardic, and his respirations are 28 per minute.

4. As you complete your differential diagnosis, from which two cardiac syndromes do you think this patient could be suffering?

5. The following is his three-lead ECG tracing. What is your interpretation?

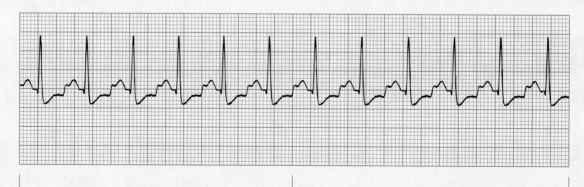

During your movement of the patient to the ambulance, he suddenly becomes lethargic. You glance at the monitor, which only you can see from your carrying vantage point, and see the following rhythm.

6. What rhythm would you tell your partner the patient just went into? ■

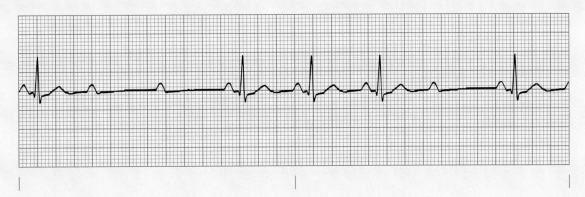

While in the ambulance, you and your partner continue high-flow oxygen, you start an IV of normal saline, and your paramedic partner sets up for transcutaneous pacing. You then witness the next ECG prior to the start of pacing.

7. What is it? ■

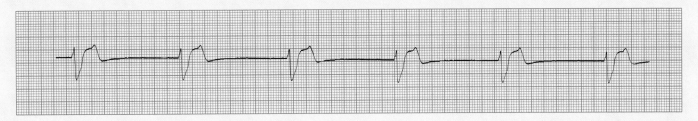

Despite the treatment rendered, the patient continues to deteriorate and goes into cardiac arrest.

8. Of the following rhythms, which one is most likely to not produce a palpable pulse? Why?

a.

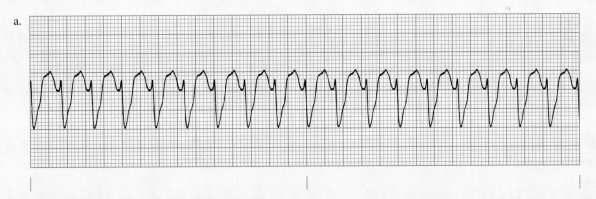

b.

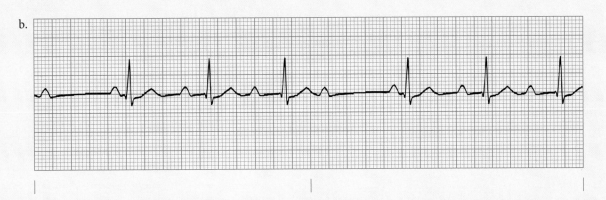

c.

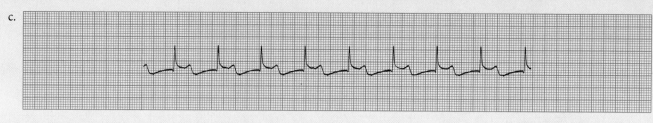

d.

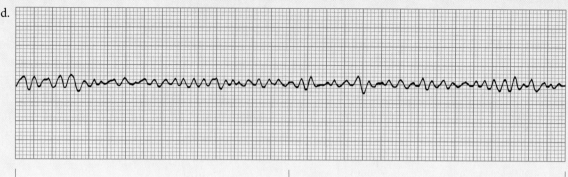

INDEX

Note: Page numbers followed by *f* represent figures and page numbers followed by *t* represent tables.

A

Abandonment, 18
Abbreviations (medical)
  accepted terms, 30–31
  "do not use" list, 31
Abdominal aneurysm, 179
Abdominal aortic aneurysm, 127
Abdominal cavity, 262
Abdominal distention, 292
Abdominal emergencies
  abdominal aortic aneurysm, 127
  abdominal pain, 125–126, *126f*
  appendicitis, 127
  assessment findings, 128
  cholecystitis, 127
  emergency medical care, 128–129
  epidemiology, 125
  esophageal varices, 127
  gastroenteritis, 127
  gastrointestinal bleeding, 126–127
  hernia, 127
  intestinal obstruction, 127
  pancreatitis, 127
  pathophysiology, 125–128
  peritonitis, 127
  ulcers, 127, *127f*
  vomiting/diarrhea/constipation, 127–128
Abdominal injuries, 265, 266
Abdominal organs, 125, *126f*
Abdominal pain, 125–126, *126f*
  acute, position for patient, *265f*
Abdominal quadrants
  contents of, *263f*, *264t*
Abdominal trauma, 263
  abdominal pain, 265
  assessment findings, 263–265
  compression injury, 263
  direct force injury, 263
  emergency medical care
    airway and breathing, 265
    circulation, 266
    treatment concerns, 266–267
  epidemiology, 262
  pathophysiology, 262
    blood vessels, 262
    hollow organs, 262
    solid organs, 262
  pediatric considerations, 265
  penetrating vs. blunt trauma, 264–265
    shearing/deceleration injury, 263
  wound
    dressing, *266f*
    open abdominal, *266f*
Abruptio placentae, 310. *See also* Placental abruption
Absence seizure, 120
Abuse
  as special reporting situation, 20
Accessory muscles, 37, *37t*
Access to emergency care, 19
Activated charcoal, 186–187, *187f*, 372
Acute anaphylaxis, *72t*
Acute coronary syndrome (ACS)
  angina pectoris, 165–166, *166f*
  assessment findings, 167–168
  emergency medical care, 168–169
  epidemiology, 164
  myocardial infarction, 165, 166–167, *167f*
  pathophysiology, 164–165
Acute myocardial infarction (AMI), 386
Acute renal failure (ARF), 218
Acute respiratory distress syndrome (ARDS), 200
Adenosine triphosphate (ATP), 25, 232
ADHD. *See* Attention deficit hyperactivity disorders (ADHD)
Adjustable-banded gastroplasty (ABG), 347
Adolescents, 59, *59f*
Adulthood
  assessment tips, 60
  early, 59
  late, 59–60
  middle, 59
Adult-oriented physical exam, 324
Advanced life support (ALS), 5
AED. *See* Automated external defibrillator (AED)
AEMT, additional pharmacology, 371–376
  assessment findings, 373–375
  drugs uses, *373t–374t*
  emergency medical care, 376
  epidemiology, 372
  medical emergencies
    assessment findings and drugs, *375t*
  nausea and vomiting, 372
  pathophysiology, 372–373
AEMT, advanced skills, 358–369
  administration
    preparation of medications, 366–369
  capnogram, *360f*
  capnometry, 359
  clinical applications, 360–363

AEMT, advanced skills (*continued*)
  colorimetric end-tidal CO$_2$ detector, *359f*
  CO$_2$ waveform, *361t*
  end-tidal carbon dioxide (ETCO$_2$), 359
  factors, 359
  glass ampules, *367f*
  glass medication vials, *367f*
  heparin lock/saline lock
    establishment of, 366
  heparin/saline lock, *366f*
  in-line capnography sensor, *360f*
  intubated patient, with CO$_2$ detection, *360f*
  IO needle
    insertion sites, *365f*
    procedure, 365
  IV piggyback medication, *368f,* 369
  IV therapy, 358
  nonconstituted drug vial, 368, *368f*
  prefilled syringes, *368f*
  proximal tibia, 364
  waveform capnography, use of, 360
  waveform changes, *362f–363f*
Aerobic metabolism, 25, *25f,* 239
Afterload, 50–51
Age-related etiology, of altered mental status, *106t*
Aging respiratory system, 330
Agitated delirium, 161
Agoraphobia, 159
Airway
  obstruction, 36, *36f*
  patency of, 36–37
Airway, breathing, circulation (ABC), 288
Airway and respiratory dysfunction
  airway, 79
  assessment findings, 76–79
  continuous positive airway pressure, 80–81, *80f*
  emergency medical care, 79–81
  epidemiology, 75
  lower airway dysfunction, 76
  pathophysiology, 75–76
  positive pressure ventilation, 80
  respiratory distress, 77, 79, *79f*
  respiratory failure, 77, 79–80
  upper airway dysfunction, 75–76, *76f*
Airway and ventilation (CAB), 234
Airway occlusion, 349
Airway resistance, 36, *37f*
Airway resistance disorders, 190–195
  assessment findings, 192–194
  bronchioles, pathophysiologic changes in, *191f*
  emergency medical care, 194–195
  epidemiology, 190–191
  lung/gas exchange disorders, 198–205
  nebulizer oxygen supply, *195f*
  pathophysiology
    acute bronchitis, 192
    asthma, 191–192
    chronic bronchitis, 192
  respiratory airway disorders findings
    for, *194t*

small-volume nebulizer, medication, *194f–195f*
  types of, 190
Alcohol, 184, 185, 186
Alcohol-based hand cleaners, 8
Alert, voice, pain, unresponsive (AVPU), 276
Allergic reactions. *See* Immunologic
    emergencies
ALS. *See* advanced life support (ALS)
Altered mental status
  age-related etiology of, *106t*
  assessment findings, 108–110
  emergency care, 110
  epidemiology, 106
  Glasgow Coma Scale, *109t*
  lesions as cause of, *108t*
  pathophysiology, 107–108
Alveolar/capillary gas exchange, 45–46
Alveoli, 39
Alzheimer disease, 160
Ambient air, composition of, 35–36, *36t*
American Heart Association, 177
Anabolism, 25
Anaerobic metabolism, 25–26, *25f*
Anaphylactic, 245
Anaphylactic reactions, 131–132
  common causes of, *132t*
  common signs and symptoms of, *135t*
Anaphylactoid reaction, 132
  common causes of, *132t*
Anaphylaxis, 76, 131, *133f*
Anemia, 213
Angina pectoris, 165–166, *166f*
  stable, 166
  unstable, 166
  variant, 166
Anorexia nervosa, 160
Anterior cord syndrome, 283
Anterior spinal artery supplies, 281
Antiepileptic drug therapy, 122, *122t*
Anxiety, 312
Anxiety disorders, 159
Aortic aneurysm (thoracic and abdominal),
    178–179, *179t*
Aortic dissection, 179, *179t*
Apgar scoring system, 324
Apnea monitors, 341
Appendicitis, 127
Arterial emboli, 306
Arteriosclerosis, 164
Arteriovenous malformation (AVM), 114
Arthritic spurs, 296
Asherman chest, 257
Asperger syndrome, 160
Assault, 18
Assessment
  as ongoing process, 86–87, *86f*
  as public health function, 62
Asthma, 191–192
Asystole, 232
Atherosclerosis, 164–165, *165f*

Atonic seizure, 121
ATP. *See* Adenosine triphosphate (ATP)
Atrial depolarization, 381
Atrial natriuretic hormone (ANH), 332
Atrioventricular (AV) node, 379
Attention deficit hyperactivity disorders (ADHD), 160
Autism spectrum disorders, 160
Automated external defibrillator (AED), 168, 232
Autonomic nervous system, 50, 51
AVM. *See* Arteriovenous malformation (AVM)

B

Bag-valve-mask (BVM), 344, 360
    ventilation, 317
Bariatric emergencies, 346
    assessment findings, 348–350
    bariatric devices, *348f*
    emergency care, 350
    epidemiology, 346–347
    excess weight, effects of, *347t*
    obese patient, assessment and care of, *348f*
    obesity, 346
        BMI for, 346
    pathophysiology, 347–348
        bariatric patients, complications, 348
        malabsorption surgical procedures, 347–348
        restrictive surgical procedures, 347
Bariatric surgery, 347
Baroreceptors, 53–54
Benzodiazepines (BZDs), 372
Bi-level positive airway pressure (BiPAP), 341
Binge eating disorder, 160
BiPAP. *See* Bi-level positive airway pressure (BiPAP)
Bipolar disorder, 159
Birth defects, 315
Biventricular failure, 173
Bleeding control, 248–251, 249
    assessment findings, 249
    emergency medical care
        bleeding control priority, 249
        bleeding control progression, 249–250
        direct pressure, 249
        dressings, 250
        hemostatic agents, 250
        intravenous fluid replacement, 251
        tourniquets, 250–251
    epidemiology, 248
    hemostatic agents
        Celox™, *250f*
    pathophysiology
        exsanguinating hemorrhage, 248–249
Blood
    composition, 48
    distribution, 49, *49t*
    hydrostatic pressure, 49, *49f*
Blood cells, 212
Blood pressure, 53–54, 296
    baroreceptors, 53–54
    chemoreceptors, 54

diastolic, 51, 52, 53
systolic, 51, 52, 53
Blunt abdominal, 287
Blunt trauma, 254, 264, *264f,* 265
BNP. *See* Brain-type natriuretic peptide (BNP)
Boyle law, 37, 305
Brain, 107–108, *107f–108f. See also* Altered mental status
Brainstem, 107
Brain-type natriuretic peptide (BNP), 172
Breathing, 199. *See also* Ventilation
    medical patient assessment, 101
    trauma patients' assessment, 91, 93
Bronchioles, 37
    pathophysiologic changes in, *191f*
Bronchiolitis, 191, 192, 193
Bronchitis, acute, 192
Bronchoconstriction, 134, 191
Brown-Séquard syndrome, 283
Bulimia nervosa, 160
Burn shock, 297
BVM. *See* Bag-valve-mask (BVM)

C

CAD. *See* Coronary artery disease (CAD)
Calling for help, 10
Cannabis products, 185, 186
Carbon dioxide transport, 45, *45f*
Cardiac arrest, 231–235, 232
    assessment findings, 233
    AutoPulse™ Model, *235f*
    close-up view, *235f*
    emergency medical care, 233–235
    epidemiology, 231–232
    high-concentration oxygen, ventilation, *234f*
    pathophysiology, 232–233
    patient's carotid pulse, *234f*
    survival rates, 234
Cardiac cell hypoxia. *See* Myocardial ischemia
Cardiac dysrhythmias
    anterolateral myocardial infarction, *389f*
    cardiac conduction system, *379f*
    conduction cells, 379–380
    electrocardiogram (ECG), 378–392,
        380–381, *380f*
        analyzing, 381–382
        information, *379t*
    electrode locations, *380t*
    infarction sites and leads
        correlation of, *389t*
    limb leads, *388f*
        electrode locations for, *388t*
    monitoring systems, 381
    pacemaker cells, 379
    precordial leads, *388f*
        locations for, *389t*
    working cells, 379
Cardiac function
    heart rate, 50
    microcirculation, 52–53, *53f*

Cardiac function (*continued*)
  stroke volume, 50–51
  systemic vascular resistance, 51–52
Cardiac output, 49–50
Cardiogenic pulmonary edema, 200
Cardiomyopathy, 326
Cardiothoracic pump, 234, 244
Cardiovascular disease (CVD), 231, 294
Cardiovascular dysfunction, cause of, 350
Cardiovascular emergencies
  aortic aneurysm, 178–179, *179t*
  aortic dissection, 179, *179t*
  assessment findings, 179–180
  congestive heart failure, 171–175
  emergency medical care, 180–181
  hypertensive and vascular, 177–181
Cardiovascular system
  body ages, 330
  calcium, 329
  medical terms for, *32t*
Case series/case reports, 4
Catabolism, 25
CDC. *See* Centers for Disease Control and Prevention (CDC)
Cellular metabolism
  aerobic, 25, *25f*
  anabolism and catabolism, 25
  anaerobic, 25–26, *25f*
  cellular respiration, 25
  clinical application of, 26–27
  described, 24
  of glucose, 148–149, *149f*
  sodium/potassium pump, 26, *26f*
  treatment of shock, 27
Cellular respiration, 25
Centers for Disease Control and Prevention (CDC), 139, 206, 354
Central chemoreceptors, 41–42
Central cord syndrome, 283
Cerebellum, 107
Cerebrospinal fluid (CSF), 273, 295, 331
Cerebrum, 107
Charcoal, 186–187, *187f*
Charles law, 306
Chemoreceptors, 54, 331
  central, 41–42
  peripheral, 42
Chest injuries, 257
  differential field diagnosis of, *259t*
Chest pain. *See also* Acute coronary syndrome (ACS); Angina pectoris
  aspirin and nitroglycerin for, 68
  differential diagnosis and, 85, *86f*
Chest trauma, 199
  assessment, 254–255
  emergency medical care
    flail chest, 257–258
    hemothorax, 258
    open pneumothorax/communicating pneumothorax, 256–257

pericardial tamponade, acute, 258–259
    tension pneumothorax, 255–256
  epidemiology, 253
  injury, mechanism of, 253–254
  pathophysiology, 254
CHF. *See* Congestive heart failure (CHF)
Children, communicating with, 15
Chlamydia trachomatis, 223
Cholecystitis, 127
Chronic obstructive pulmonary disease (COPD), 192, 201, 294
  disorders, 328
Chronic renal failure (CRF), 218
Circulatory system, 306
Citric acid cycle, 25
Clonic seizure, 121
Clostridium difficile (C-Dif), 8, 142
COBRA. *See* Consolidated Omnibus Budget Reconciliation Act (COBRA)
Cohort/concurrent control/case-control studies, 4
Colloid oncotic pressure. *See* Plasma oncotic pressure
Combining forms (medical terminology), 29–30, *32t–33t*
Communication
  challenges, 15
  facilitating techniques, *14t*
  guidelines for initial patient contact, 14
  nonverbal, 14, *14f, 14t*
  patient interview, 14–15
  process of, 13–14
  transcultural considerations, 15
Complex partial seizure, 120
Compliance, 37
Concealment, 10, *11f*
Confidentiality, patients' right to, 19
Congestive heart failure (CHF), 294
  assessment findings, 173
  clinical findings/pathophysiologic etiology of, *174f*
  emergency medical care, 173–175
  epidemiology, 171
  jugular vein distention, 172, *173f*
  left-sided failure, 172
  pathophysiology, 171–173
  right-sided failure, 172
  signs and symptoms of, *174f*
Congestive ventricular failure. *See* left ventricular failure
Consolidated Omnibus Budget Reconciliation Act (COBRA), 19
Constipation, 127–128
Contact and cover, 10
Contact officer, police work, 10
Contagious diseases. *See* Infectious disease
Continuous positive airway pressure, 80–81, *80f*
  in congestive heart failure, 173–174
Continuous positive airway pressure (CPAP), 341, 349
Control groups, 3
Coronary artery disease (CAD), 165
Coronary syndromes, acute
  treatment of, 386
Cover, 10, *10f*
Cover officer, police work, 10

Crackles, 202
Crime scene, as special reporting situation, 20
Critical thinking
    assessment as ongoing process, 86–87, *86f*
    careful/strategic/dynamic care plans, 87
    contradictions and challenges, 87
    defined, 83–84
    differential diagnostic process, 85–86, *85t*
    EMT as clinician, 84
    primary assessment, 84–85, *85f*
    technician *versus* clinician, 84
    treating life threats first, 84–85
Crossover sensations, 185
Crush injuries, 270, 271
    assess circulation, *271f*
    assessment findings
        compartment syndrome, 270–271
    direct force, *269f*
    emergency medical care, 271
        preventing, 271
        treating compartment syndrome, 271
    epidemiology, 269–270
        direct force, 270
        entrapment/weight-based compression, 270
        internal compression, 270
    pathophysiology
        compartment syndrome, 270
Cushing reflex, 275
Cystic fibrosis (CF), 199, 201, 203

D

Dalton law, 305
Dead space, 39
Decompression sickness, 305
Decontamination equipment, 8–9
Deep venous thromboembolism (DVT),
    200, 348
Defamation, 18
Deliriants. *See* Inhalants
Deoxyhemoglobin, 45
Depressants (narcotics/sedatives),
    184–185, 186
Diabetes mellitus
    pathophysiology, 148–149
    types of, 147–148
Diabetic ketoacidosis (DKA), 152,
    153–154
    assessment findings, 153–154
    electrolyte disturbance, 153
    metabolic acidosis, 153
    osmotic diuresis, 153
    pathophysiology of, 153
Diagnostic and Statistical Manual of Mental Disorders, Fourth
    Edition, 159
Dialysis, 343
Diarrhea, 127–128
Diffuse axonal injury (DAI), 274
    concussion, 274
Disabilities, communicating with patients having, 15

Diseases of concern (safety issues), 9, *9t*
Disposable equipment and supplies, 9
Disseminated intravascular coagulation (DIC), 240
Dissociative disorders, 159–160
Diuresis, 153
Divers alert network (DAN), 305
Diving-related injuries
    assessment findings
        circulatory system, 306
        complicated diving injuries, 306
        decompression sickness, 306–307
        nervous system, 306
        respiratory system, 306
    emergency medical care, 307
        appropriate transport, 307
    epidemiology, 305
    pathophysiology
        arterial emboli, 306
        Boyle law, 305
        Charles law, 306
        Dalton law, 305–306
        dysbarism, 305
        Henry law, 306
DNR. *See* Do not resuscitate (DNR)
Dog bites, as special reporting situation, 21
Do not resuscitate (DNR), 20
Dorsal respiratory group (DRG), 43
Dressings, 250
DRG. *See* Dorsal respiratory group (DRG)
Dumping syndrome, 350
Duty to act, 19
Dysbarism, 305
Dyspnea
    causes of, *331f*
Dysthymic disorder, 159

E

Early adulthood, 59
Ears, medical terms for, *32t*
Eating disorder, 160
Ectopic pregnancy, 310
Elastin, 38
Electrocardiogram (ECG) monitoring
    analyzing, 381–383
        P–R interval, 383
        P wave, 383
        QRS complex, 383
        rate, 382
        regularity, 383
    assessment parameters, *382t*
    basic interpretation, 383–386
        clinical application, 383–386
        hints for, 387–389
        twelve-lead configuration, 387
    cardiac dysrhythmias, 378–392
    dysrhythmias, *384f–386f*
    graph paper, *382f*
    with heart rate, *382f*
    monitoring systems, 381

Electrocardiogram (ECG) monitoring (*continued*)
normal 12-lead printout, *387f*
placements, *380f*
relationship of, *381f*
waveform names and descriptions, *381t*
Electrolyte disturbance, 153
Electromechanical dissociation (EMD), 290
Electrophysiology, 378
Embolic stroke, 113
Emergency Medical Services for Children (EMSC)
program, 326
Emergency Medical Treatment and Active Labor Act
(EMTALA), 19
Emphysema, 199
EMT
parent's response, 323
EMTALA. *See* Emergency Medical Treatment and Active
Labor Act (EMTALA)
Endocrine emergencies
diabetes mellitus, 147–150
hyperglycemic disorders,
152–155
hypoglycemia, 149–150
Endocrine systems, medical terms for, *32t*
Epidural hematoma, 274, 275
Epiglottis, 36
Epinephrine, 137
Epistaxis, 228
Esophageal varices, 127
Ethical behavior, 19
Exhalation, accessory muscles of, 37, *37t*
Eye injuries, 228
lens placement, *228f*
Morgan Lens, *228f*
Eyes, ears, nose, and throat emergency,
226–229
assessment, 227–228
emergency care, 228
epidemiology, 226
epistaxis, 228–229
eye injuries, 228
pathophysiology, 226–227
Eyes, medical terms for, *32t*
EZ-IO device
with needles, *364f*

F

Face protection, 8
Facial fractures
types of, 227
Factitious disorders, 159
False imprisonment, 18
Febrile seizure, 120
Feeding tubes, 343
Female reproductive system, 221
Flail chest, 257, *257f*
Floppy baby, 317
Flu and pandemic flu, 142–143

G

Gastroenteritis, 127
Gastrointestinal bleeding, 125, 126–127
signs and symptoms of, 127
Gastrointestinal system, medical terms for, *32t*
Gastrointestinal (GI) tract, 203
Gender identity disorders, 160
Generalized anxiety disorder, 159
Generalized tonic–clonic seizure, 121–122, *121f*
Geriatric patient, 296
aging effects, *329t, 330f*
assessment findings, 332
clinical findings, *333t–334t*
clues, *334t*
dyspnea, causes of, *331t*
emergency medical care, 332–336
epidemiology, 328
geriatric patient, assessment of, *335t*
medications, *329f*
pathophysiology, 328–332
cardiovascular system, 329–330
endocrine system, 332
gastrointestinal system, 331–332
integumentary system, 332
musculoskeletal system, 332
nervous system, 331
renal system, 332
respiratory system, 330–331
Geriatric patients, 294
altered mental status, *106t*
cardiac events, special considerations in, *169t*
communicating with, 15
trauma, manifestations of, *297t*
Geriatric population, 297
Geriatric trauma patient
management of, 298
Glasgow Coma Scale (GCS), *109t*, 273, 288
Glottic opening, 36
Glucagon, 148
Glucose, cell metabolism of, 148–149, *149f*
Glycogen, 319
Glycolysis, 25, 26
Good Samaritan laws, 19
Gunshot wounds, 301
Gynecologic emergencies, 221
assessment, 224–225
emergency medical care, 225
epidemiology, 221
pathophysiology
pelvic inflammatory disease (PID), 223
pregnancy, 223–224
sexual assault, 224
vaginal bleeding, 221–222
vaginal bleeding, traumatic, 222–223

H

Hallucinogens, 185, 186
Hand washing, 142, *142f*

Head injuries, 273
  assessment of, 276
Head trauma, 295
Head/traumatic brain injury (TBI), 273
  assessment findings, 276–277
  for deformities, depressions, lacerations/impaled
      objects, 277f
  emergency medical care, 277–278
  epidemiology, 273
  epidural hematoma, 274f
  Glasgow Coma Scale, 277t
  pathophysiology
    diffuse axonal injury (DAI), 274
    epidural hematoma, 274–275
    intracerebral hemorrhage, 274
    subdural hematoma, 275–276
  posturing, 276f
  subdural hematoma, 275f
  vital signs, changes, 278t
Health care proxy (medical power of attorney), 20
Health Insurance Portability and Accountability Act
      (HIPAA), 19
Heart rates, 50, 319
Heart's electrical activity, 381. See also Electrocardiogram
      (ECG) monitoring
Hematology
  assessment findings, 214
  blood disorders, 212–215
  emergency medical care, 214–245
  epidemiology, 212
  oxygen is transported, 213f
  pathophysiology, 212
    platelet diseases/clotting disorders, 214
    red blood cell diseases, 213–214
    white blood cell diseases, 214
Hemoglobin, 45
Hemorrhage, 248, 249
  controlled/uncontrolled, 245
Hemorrhagic stroke, 113–114
Hemostatic agents, 250
Hemothorax, 258, 258f
Henry law, 306
Hepatitis, 139–140
Hernia, 127
High-visibility ANSI-approved vests, 9, 9f
Highway scenes, safety of, 9–10, 9f
HIPAA. See Health Insurance Portability and Accountability
      Act (HIPAA)
Histamine, 133
Hives (urticaria), 134f
H1N1 influenza, 143
Hollow organs, abdominal cavity,
      125, 126f
Hostile patients, 15
Hydrostatic pressure, 49, 49f
Hypercapnic drive, 42
Hypercarbic drive, 42
Hyperglycemic disorders
  diabetic ketoacidosis, 152, 153–154
  emergency medical care, 155

epidemiology, 152
hyperglycemic hyperosmolar nonketotic syndrome, 152,
      154–155
signs and symptoms of, 155t
Hyperglycemic hyperosmolar nonketotic syndrome (HHNS)
  assessment findings, 154–155
  emergency medical care, 155
  pathophysiology of, 154
Hypertension, 180
  chronic, 178
  primary, 178
  secondary, 178
Hypertensive emergencies, 178
Hyperventilation
  dangers of, 290
Hypoglycemia, 149–150
  assessment findings, 149
  emergency medical care, 149–150
  signs and symptoms of, 150t
Hypoperfusion, 113, 239
Hypotension, 276
Hypotonia, 317
Hypoxia, 282, 289
Hypoxic drive, 42–43

I

ICH. See intracerebral hemorrhage (ICH)
Immune system, medical terms for, 32t
Immunologic emergencies
  anaphylactic reactions, 131–132, 132t
  anaphylactoid reaction, 132, 132t
  assessment findings, 134, 136
  bronchoconstriction and, 134
  decreased vascular smooth muscle tone, 133
  emergency care, 136–137
  epinephrine, 137
  increased bronchial smooth muscle tone, 134
  increased capillary permeability, 133
  increased mucus secretion in the tracheobronchial tract, 134
Immunology, 372
Implied consent, 20
Impulse control disorders, 160
Incident command system (ICS), 353
Increased capillary permeability, 133
Infants, 316
  assessment tips, 58
  developmental milestones for, 57t
  developmental stage, 56–58
  feeding for, 319
  respiratory systems of, 325
Infectious disease
  EMS and public health, 143–144, 144t
  exposure, as special reporting situation, 21
  flu and pandemic flu, 142–143
  hepatitis, 139–140
  HIV/AIDS, 140–141
  measles and mumps, 143
  pertussis, 143
  tuberculosis (TB), 141–142

Inflammation, 126
Influenza A H1N1, 143
Informed consent, 19
Inhalants, 185, 186
Inhalation, accessory muscles of, 37, *37t*
Institute of Medicine (IOM), 62
Insulin, 148
Insulin shock. *See* Hypoglycemia
Integumentary system, medical terms for, *32t*
Intentional torts, 18
Interview, patient, 14–15
Intestinal obstruction, 127
Intracerebral hemorrhage (ICH), 114, 274
Intracranial pressure (ICP), 275, 343
Intraosseous (IO) cannulation, 363
Intraventricular shunts, 343
IOM. *See* Institute of Medicine (IOM)
Irritant receptors, 43
Ischemia, 126
Ischemic stroke, 111–113, *112f*
    classification by supplying vessel, 113
    pathophysiology of thrombus formation in, 113
IV fluid replacement, 251

J

J-receptors, 43. *See also* Lung receptors

K

Kidney disease, 217. *See also* Renal disorders
Kidney failure, 218
Kidneys
    fluid and electrolyte balance, 332
Kidney stones, *218f*
Krebs cycle, 25
Kussmaul respirations, 154, *154f*

L

Language barriers, 15
Laryngospasm, 37
Larynx, 37
Late adulthood, 59–60
LDL. *See* low-density lipoproteins (LDL)
Left-sided failure congestive heart failure, 172
Left ventricular failure, 51
Legal issues
    legal terms, 18–19
    patients' rights, 19–20
    special reporting situations, 20–21
Leukocytes. *See* Blood cells
Life span development
    adolescents, 59, *59f*
    early adulthood, 59
    infants, 56–58, *57t*
    late adulthood, 59–60, *60f*
    middle adulthood, 59
    school-age children, 58–59, *59f*

stages, *56t*
    toddlers and preschoolers, 58, *58t*
Lifting, 11, *11f*
Lithotripsy, 218
Liver, 332
Living wills, 20
Low-density lipoproteins (LDL), 165
Lower airway dysfunction, 76
Lung collapse, 201
Lung compliance, 198
    changes, 199
    treatment for, 203
Lung receptors, 43

M

Major depressive disorder, 159
Malingering, 159
Measles, 143
Medical direction, 19
Medical patient, assessment of
    airway, 101
    body system approach to common medical complaints, 103, *103t*
    breathing, 101
    circulation, 101–102
    history, 102–103, *102f*
    primary assessment, 101–102, *101f*
    priority determination, 102
    reassessment, 104, *104f*
    scene size-up, 100–101
    secondary assessment, 102–103, *102f*
    vital signs, 103–104
Medical power of attorney (POA), 20
Medical terminology
    accepted terms/abbreviations, 30–31
    common combining forms, *32t–33t*
    common prefixes, *31t*
    common suffixes, *31t*
    "do not use" list of abbreviations, 31
    origins, 29
    reading/defining terms, 30
    structure, 29–30
Medulla oblongata, 107
Meta-analysis, 4–5
Metabolic acidosis, 153
Metarterioles, 52
Metered-dose inhaler (MDI), 209
Methicillin-resistant *Staphylococcus aureus* (MRSA), 141–142
Midbrain, 107
Middle adulthood, 59
Minute ventilation (minute volume), 38–39
Miscarriage, 312
Mood disorders, 159
Morbidity and Mortality Weekly Report, 63
Motor vehicle collision (MVC), 295, *295f*
Motor vehicle trauma, 288
MRSA. *See* Methicillin-resistant *Staphylococcus aureus* (MRSA)
Multidrug-resistant organisms, 141

Multiple-casualty incident (MCI), 353
   branch units
      communications, 355
      follow-through, 355
      staging, 355
      transport, 355
      treatment, 355
      triage, 354–355
   components of
      communications and information management, 353
      preparedness, 353
      resource management, 353
   incident commander, *354f*
   incident command system (ICS), 353–354
   management of, 353–355
   psychological stress, 355
   treatment
      order of priority, *355f*
Mumps, 143
Munchausen syndrome by proxy, 159
Musculoskeletal system
   medical terms for, *32t*
Mycobacterium tuberculosis, 141
Myocardial contractility, 50
Myocardial infarction (MI), 165, 166–167, *167f,*
      238, 294
Myocardial ischemia, 165, 167
Myoclonic seizure, 121

N

Narrow pulse pressure, 52
Nasopharynx, 36
National Association of Emergency Medical Technicians, 19
National Health Interview Survey, 198
National Incident Management System (NIMS), 353
National Survey on Drug Use and Health (NSDUH), 183
National Trauma Triage Protocol, 92
Neck injuries, 227, 295, *295f*
Neglect
   as special reporting situation, 20
Negligence, 18, 19
Neisseria gonorrhoeae, 223
Neonatology, 315–320
   ABCs, 317–319
   assessment, 316–320
   chest compressions, *318f*
   death, causes of
      by age group, *316f*
   don't ever forget glucose! (DEFG), 319
   emergency care, 316–320
   epidemiology, 315–316
   hypothermia (H), 319
   infection (I), 319–320
   positive pressure ventilation, *317f*
   safely transport, 320
   terminology, 316
Nervous system, 306
Neurologic assessment, 285
Neurologic disorder, 331

Neurologic function, 282
Neurologic system, 331
Neurology/psychology, medical terms for, *32t*
Neuromuscular diseases, 340
Newton, Isaac, 263
Noncardiogenic pulmonary edema, 200
Noncoital reproductive tract injuries, 223
Nonfatal injuries, 288
Nonverbal communication, 14, *14f, 14t*
Nosebleed, *229f*
NSDUH. *See* National Survey on Drug Use and
      Health (NSDUH)

O

Obesity, 340, 346
   body mass index (BMI) of, 346
   weight control, 347
Obsessive-compulsive disorder, 159
Obstetrics, 309
   abortion, types of, *312t*
   abruptio placentae, *310f*
   antepartum complications
      signs and symptoms, *313t*
   assessment, 312–313
   ectopic pregnancy, *311f*
   emergency care, 313
   epidemiology, 309
   pathophysiology
      abruptio placentae, 310
      ectopic pregnancy, 310–311
      placenta previa, 309–310
      preeclampsia/eclampsia, 311–312
      spontaneous abortion, 312
   placenta previa, *310f*
Organ donation, 20
Oropharynx, 36
Osmosis, 153
Osmotic diuresis, 153
Osteoporosis, 296
OTC. *See* over-the-counter (OTC) medications
Over-the-counter (OTC) medications, 183
Overweight, 346
Oxidation, 25
Oxygen transport, 45, *45f*
   in blood, 213
Oxyhemoglobin, 45

P

Pacemaker cells, 379
Pain. *See also* Chest pain
   abdominal, 125–126, *126f*
   parietal, 126
   referred, 126
   visceral, 125
Pancreatitis, 127
Pandemic influenza, 143
Panic disorder, 159

Parietal pain, 126. *See also* Abdominal pain
Partial seizure, 120
"Patient dumping," 19
Patient interview, 14–15
Patient's diastolic pressure, 302
Patients' rights
    access to emergency care, 19
    advance directives, 20
    consent, 19–20
    organ donation, 20
    privacy and confidentiality, 19
    refusing care, 20
Patient's speech patterns, 344
Pediatric assessment triangle (PAT), 324
Pediatric injuries, 288
Pediatric pedestrians, 290
Pediatrics, 322–326
    anxiety, 322
    approaching the child, 322–323
    case study, 325–326
        circulation, 326
        pediatric champion, 326
        pump failure, 326
        treatment guidelines, 326
    parents and caretakers, 323–324
    pediatric assessment triangle
        appearance, 324–325
        breathing, 325
    pediatric patient, assessment of, 324–325
Pelvic inflammatory disease (PID), 223
Penicillin allergy, *134f*
Perfusion, 35
    disturbances, 44
Perialveolar capillary membranes, 296
Pericardial tamponade, *258f*
Peripheral chemoreceptors, 42
Peripheral vascular resistance (PVR), 258
Peritonitis, 127
Personality disorders, 160
Pertussis, 143, 206, 207
    complications of, 207
    treatment of, 209
Pharmacology (prehospital), 67–73
    assessment findings, 69
    drugs for medical emergencies, *71t–72t*
    emergency medical care, 69–73
    epidemiology, 68–69
    medications commonly used by EMTs,
        70t, 71f–72f
    pathophysiology, 69
    preventing medication errors, 68
Pharynx, 36
Placental abruption, 310
Placenta previa, 309
    risk factors, 309
Plasma oncotic pressure, 49, *49f*
Platelet diseases/clotting disorders, 214
    disseminated intravascular coagulation (DIC), 214
    hemophilia, 214
    myeloma, 214

    thrombocytopenia, 214
    thrombocytosis, 214
    von Willebrand disease, 214
Platelets, 213
Pleural space, 37–38, *38f*
Pneumonia, 206, 207, 209
Pneumothorax, 258
    open, *256f*
    tension, *255f*
Pons, 107
Positive end-expiratory pressure (PEEP), 255
    use of, 318
Positive pressure ventilation (PPV), 80, 234,
        298, 350
Posttraumatic stress disorder, 159
Preeclampsia, 311
Prefix, 30, *31t*
Pregnancy, 223, 312, 313
    anatomy of, *302f*
    born, prematurely, 315
    complication of, 310
Pregnant women
    falls and physical abuse, 301
Preload, 50
Prenatal
    fetal/*in utero* period, 316
Preschoolers, 58, *58t*
Primary hypertension, 178
Prinzmetal angina. *See* Variant angina
Privacy, patients' right to, 19
Prospective *versus* retrospective studies, 3
Proteinuria, 312
Psychiatric disorders
    Alzheimer disease, 160
    anxiety disorders, 159
    attention deficit hyperactivity disorders (ADHD), 160
    autism spectrum disorders, 160
    dissociative disorders, 159–160
    eating disorder, 160
    emergency medical care, 161–162
    epidemiology, 158
    factitious disorders, 159
    impulse control disorders, 160
    pathophysiology, 158–160
    personality disorders, 160
    psychosis, 159
    restraint and patient safety, 161
    schizophrenia, 159
    sexual and gender identity disorders, 160
    somatoform disorders, 159
    substance-related disorders, 160
    suicide, 160
Psychosis, 159
Public health
    achievements of, 63–64
    core functions/essential services, *63t*
    EMS interface with, 64–65, *64f*
    versus individual patient care, 62
    laws/regulations/guidelines, 64
Public Health in America, 62

Pulmonary air embolism
  signs of, 307
Pulmonary blood flow
  lack of, 290
Pulmonary complications, 201
Pulmonary diseases
  chronic, 192
Pulmonary dysfunction, 331
Pulmonary edema, 198
  acute, 199
Pulmonary embolism, 198, 202
Pulseless electrical activity (PEA), 290
Pulselessness
  determination of, 233
Pulse pressure, 52
Purkinje fibers, 380
Pyruvic acid, 25

R

Rales. *See* Crackles
Randomization, 3
Randomized controlled trials (RCT), 3–4
Red blood cell diseases, 213–214
  anemia, 213–214
    types of, 213
  polycythemia, 214
  thalassemia, 214
Referred pain, 126. *See also* Abdominal pain
Renal disorders, 217
  assessment findings, 218–219
  emergency medical care, 219
  epidemiology, 217
  kidney stones, *218f*
  pathophysiology, 217
    dialysis, 218
    hemodialysis, 218
    kidney stones, 218
    peritoneal dialysis, 218
    renal conditions, 217–218
    renal (kidney) failure, 218
Renal emergency, *217f*
Reproductive system, medical terms for, *32t–33t*
Research, EMS, 1–5
  basics of, 2–5
  case series/case reports, 4
  cohort/concurrent control/case-control studies, 4
  control groups, 3
  meta-analysis, 4–5
  prospective *versus* retrospective, 3
  randomization, 3
  randomized controlled trials (RCT), 3–4
  study group similarity, 3
  systematic review, 3
Respiratory distress, 77, 79, *79f*, 372
Respiratory emergencies
  airway resistance disorders, 190–195, *See also* Airway resistance
    disorders
  airway restriction
    mucus plugs and inflammation cause, *192f*

infectious disorders, 206–210
  assessment findings, 208–209
  emergency medical care, 209–210
  epidemiology, 206–207
  pathophysiology, 207–208
  pertussis, 207, 209
  pneumonia, 207
  pneumonia, emergency medical care for, 209
  pneumonia, signs/symptoms of, 208–209
  viral respiratory infection, 209
  viral respiratory infections, 207–208
  VRI cases, 209–210
lung/gas exchange disorders
  assessment findings, 202–203
  cystic fibrosis (CF), 201
  differential assessment findings, *203t*
  differential assessment findings for, *203t*
  emergency medical care, 203–204
  emphysema, 199
  emphysema, pathophysiologic changes, *199f*
  epidemiology, 198–199
  pathophysiology, 199–201
  pneumothorax, *201f*
  pulmonary artery, blocking blood flow, *201f*
  pulmonary edema, 199–200, *200f*
  pulmonary embolism, 200
  spontaneous pneumothorax, 201
Respiratory failure, 77, 79–80. *See also* Airway and
    respiratory dysfunction
Respiratory resistance disorder, 193
  crackles, 193
  rhonchi, 193
  wheezing, 193
Respiratory rhythm, 208
Respiratory syncytial virus (RSV), 191, 208
Respiratory system, 306
  of infant, 325
  medical terms for, *33t*
Resuscitation, 231–235
Retreat, 10
Retrospective *versus* prospective studies, 3
Reversible ischemic neurologic deficit (RIND), 113
Rib fractures, pain, 257
Right-sided failure congestive heart failure, 172
RIND. *See* Reversible ischemic neurologic deficit (RIND)
Ringer's lactate, 228

S

SAH. *See* subarachnoid hemorrhage (SAH)
Scene size-up, 9–11
Schizo-affective disorder, 159
Schizophrenia, 159
School-age children, 58–59, *59f*
Scope of practice, 18
Secondary hypertension, 178
Seizures
  absence seizure, 120
  antiepileptic drug therapy, 122, *122t*
  assessment findings, 122–123, *123t*

Seizures (*continued*)
  atonic seizure, 121
  clonic seizure, 121
  complex partial seizure, 120
  emergency care, 123–124
  epidemiology, 119
  febrile seizure, 120
  generalized tonic–clonic seizure, 121–122, *121f*
  myoclonic seizure, 121
  pathophysiology, 119–120
  phases, 120–122
  simple partial seizure, 120
  status epilepticus, 122
  tonic seizures, 121
  types of, 120–122
Sexual assault, 224
Sexual disorders, 160
Sexually transmitted disease (STD), 223
Shock, 238–245
  assessment findings, 241–242
  body organs, effects of, *240t*
  characteristics of, *244t*
  defined, 26
  emergency medical care, 242
    airway considerations, 243
    breathing considerations, 243–244
    cardiogenic etiology, 245
    circulatory considerations, 244–245
    hemorrhage, 245
    intravenous therapy, 245
    spinal immobilization considerations, 242–243
    vasodilation etiology, 245
    volume loss etiology, 245
  epidemiology, 238–239
  etiologies of, *243t*
    pump failure, *243f*
    vasodilation, *244f*
  hypoperfusion, compensatory mechanisms in, 240, *240t*
  pathophysiology, 239–240
    etiologies of, 241
    stages of, 239–241
  progressive stage of, 239
  severity of, 241, *241f*
  treatment of, 27
  types of, 242
Sickle cell disease, 213
Simple partial seizure, 120
Sinoatrial (SA) node, 50
Skeletal injuries, 292
Social phobia, 159
Sodium/potassium pump, 26, *26f*
Soft tissue injuries
  surface of, *271f*
Solid organs, abdominal cavity, 125, *126f*
Somatoform disorders, 159
Sovereign immunity, 19
Special challenges
  assessment and management, 343–344
  EMT, ventilation, *344f*
  epidemiology, 338–339

excess weight, effects of, *341t*
  mental retardation, causes of, *340t*
  pathophysiology
    child abuse, 339
    disabilities, 340–341
    mental illnesses, 339
    physical abuse, *339f*
    sexual abuse, 339
    technology assistance/dependency, 341–343
  peripherally inserted central catheter (PICC), *342f*
  tracheostomy tube, *352f*
Spinal cord, 280
  anatomy, 280–282
  cross sections of, 283
Spinal cord injury (SCI), 280, 291
  anatomy, 280–282
  assessment findings, 284–285
  cross section of, *282f, 283f*
  differential assessment findings, *284t*
  emergency medical care, 285
  incomplete spinal cord injury syndrome, *283t*
  level of loss of sensation, *285t*
  ligaments and intervertebral disks, *284f*
  motor assessment, *284t*
  pathophysiology
    anterior cord syndrome, 283
    Brown-Séquard syndrome, 283
    central cord syndrome, 283
    complete, 282
    incomplete, 282–283
    spinal shock, 283–284
  spinal nerves, illustration of, *281f*
Spinal cord injury without radiologic abnormality (SCIWORA), 291
Spinal shock, 282, 283
Spinothalamic nerve tracts, 282
Spontaneous abortion, 312
Stable angina, 166
Stab wounds, 301
Standard of care, 18
Standard Precautions, 7–8, *7f*
Stanton, Bonita, 15
Status asthmaticus, 192
Status epilepticus, 122
Statute of limitations, 19
ST-elevation myocardial infarction (STEMI), 180
STEMI. *See* ST-elevation myocardial infarction (STEMI)
Stimulants, 184, 186
Stretch receptors, 43
Stroke
  assessment of, 114–116
  assessment scales, 116–117, *116t*
  embolic stroke, 113
  emergency medical care, 117
  epidemiology, 111
  hemorrhagic stroke, 113–114
  hypoperfusion, 113
  ischemic stroke, 111–113, *112f*
  neurologic dysfunction and damage in, 114
  pathophysiology, 111

reversible ischemic neurologic deficit (RIND), 113
   signs and symptoms of, 114–116, *115f*
   thrombotic stroke, 112
   transient ischemic attack (TIA), 113
Stroke patient, *270f*
Stroke volume, 50–51
Study group similarity, 3
Subarachnoid hemorrhage (SAH), 114, 275
Subdural hematoma, 275
Substance-related disorders, 160
Sudden cardiac arrest (SCA), 232
Suffix, 30, *31t*
Suicide, 160
Supine position, 243
Supraventricular tachycardia (SVT), 326
Surrogate decision maker, 20
Systematic review, 3
Systemic vascular resistance (SVR), 319
   blood pressure, 319
Systolic blood pressure, 276

T

Tension pneumothorax, 256
Thermoregulation, 291
Thiamine, 372
Thoracic trauma, 287
Throat injuries, 227
Thrombotic stroke, 112
TIA. *See* Transient ischemic attack (TIA)
Tidal volume, 38–39
Toddlers, 58, *58t*
Tonic seizures, 121
Tourniquets, 250
   bleeding control, 251
   placement of, 251
Toxicology (street drugs)
   alcohol, 185
   assessment findings, 185–186
   cannabis products, 185
   commonly abused drugs, *184t*
   depressants (narcotics/sedatives), 184–185
   emergency medical care, 186–188
   epidemiology, 183–184
   hallucinogens, 185
   inhalants, 185
   pathophysiology, 184–185
   stimulants, 184
Toxidrome, 184
Trachea, 37, 317
Tracheostomy, 341
Transient ischemic attack (TIA), 113
Transport
   of incapacitated or patients against their will, 21
   legal issues, 20
   lifting and moving, 11, *11f*
Trauma, in special populations
   pediatrics, 287–292
      abdomen and pelvis, 292
      airway, oxygenation, and ventilation, 289

      anatomic, 288–289
      assessment, 288–292
      breathing, 289–290
      chest, 291
      circulation, 290
      emergency care, 288–292
      epidemiology, 288
      head, neck, and spine, 290–291
      multiorgan system trauma, 291–292
      physiologic differences, 288–289
      scoring systems, 288
      skeletal injuries, 292
   pregnancy, complications of
      abruptio placentae, 302
      anatomy/physiology, 302
      assessment findings, 303
      cardiopulmonary arrest, 303
      emergency medical care, 303
      epidemiology, 301
      hemorrhage/shock, 303
      pelvic fractures, 303
      penetrating trauma, 303
      preterm labor, 302
      spontaneous abortion, 302
      uterine contractions, 302
      uterine rupture, 303
Trauma patients, assessment of
   airway, 91
   breathing, 91, 93
   circulation, 93
   general impression, 91
   history, 93
   interventions and transport, *96f*
   National Trauma Triage Protocol, 92
   primary assessment, 91, 93, *93f*
   priority determination, 93
   reassessment, 98, *98f*
   scene size-up, 90–91
   secondary assessment, 93–98,
      94f–96f, 97t
   vital signs, 93, *95f*, 96, 97–98, *97t*
Traumatic brain injury (TBI), 273
Traumatized patients, 340
Triage, illness
   dead/fatally injured, 354
   mental status, 355
   perfusion status, 355
   respiratory status, 354–355
   serious but not life-threatening, 354
   treatable life-threatening, 354
   treatment
      order of priority, *355f*
   walking wounded, 354
Triage systems, 288
Tuberculosis (TB), 141–142
   methicillin-resistant *Staphylococcus aureus* (MRSA),
      141–142
   multidrug-resistant organisms, 141
Type 1 diabetes mellitus, 147
Type 2 diabetes mellitus, 147–148

U

Ulcers, 127, *127f*
Unmotivated patients, 15
Unstable angina, 166
Upper airway dysfunction, 75–76, *76f*
Upper respiratory infection (URI), 191
Urinary catheters, 344
Urinary system, medical terms for, *33t*
Urticaria (hives), *134f*
U.S. Public Health Service (USPHS), 62
USPHS. *See* U.S. Public Health Service (USPHS)
Uterine bleeding, 221
Uterus, 302
    blood, flow of, 309
    fetus, growing, 302

V

Vaginal bleeding, 221, 303, 310
Vaginal lacerations, 222
Vancomycin-resistant enterococci (VRE), 142
Variant angina, 166
Vascular access devices (VADs), 342
Vascular structures, abdominal cavity, 125
Vascular system, systemic vascular resistance, 51–52
Vasodilation, 51
Vena cava
    compression of, 255
Venous system, 49
Ventilation
    accessory muscles, 37, *37t*
    alveolar, 39
    alveolar/capillary gas exchange, 45–46
    carbon dioxide transport, 45, *45f*
    cell/capillary gas exchange, 46
    chemoreceptors, 41–42
    factors affecting, 37–39
    mechanics, 37–39
    oxygen transport, 45, *45f*
    pressure imbalances, 43–44
    regulation, 41–43
    specialized respiratory centers, 43
    ventilation/perfusion (V/Q) ratio, 43–44
Ventilators, 342
Ventral respiratory group (VRG), 43
Violence, 10
Viral infection, 325
Viral respiratory tract infections (VRIs), 207, 208
Visceral pain, 125. *See also* Abdominal pain
Vital signs
    medical patient assessment, 103–104
    normal, 60, *60t*
    trauma patients' assessment, 93, *95f*, 96, 97–98, *97t*
Vomiting, 127–128
VRE. *See* Vancomycin-resistant enterococci (VRE)
VRG. *See* ventral respiratory group (VRG)

W

Weapons of mass destruction (WMD)-type exposures, 372
White blood cell diseases, 214
    leukemia, 214
    leukocytosis, 214
    leukopenia/neutropenia, 214
    lymphoma, 214
WHO. *See* World Health Organization (WHO)
Whooping cough. *See* Pertussis
Winslow, C. E. A., 62
Workforce safety and wellness
    diseases of concern, 9, *9t*
    exposure prevention, 8–9
    highway scenes, 9–10, *9f*
    lifting and moving, 11, *11f*
    protection from disease (Standard Precautions), 7–8
    reacting to danger, 10–11
    scene size-up, 9–11
    violence, 10
World Health Organization (WHO), 139
Wounds
    gunshot and stab, 301